The Neuroscience
of Clinical Psychiatry

The Pathophysiology of Behavior
and Mental Illness

The Neuroscience of Clinical Psychiatry

The Pathophysiology of Behavior and Mental Illness

Third Edition

Edmund S. Higgins, MD
Clinical Associate Professor of Psychiatry and Family Medicine
Medical University of South Carolina
Charleston, South Carolina

Mark S. George, MD
Distinguished Professor of Psychiatry, Radiology, and Neurosciences
Layton McCurdy Endowed Chair
Director, Brain Stimulation Laboratory (BSL)
Editor-in-Chief, *Brain Stimulation*
Medical University of South Carolina
Charleston, South Carolina

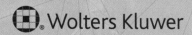 Wolters Kluwer

Philadelphia · Baltimore · New York · London
Buenos Aires · Hong Kong · Sydney · Tokyo

Acquisitions Editor: Chris Teja
Editorial Coordinator: Emily Buccieri
Strategic Marketing Manager: Rachel Mante Leung
Production Project Manager: Linda Van Pelt
Design Coordinator: Elaine Kasmer
Manufacturing Coordinator: Beth Welsh

Prepress Vendor: TNQ Books and Journals
Third edition
Copyright © 2019 Wolters Kluwer.

9   8   7   6   5   4

Printed in China

Library of Congress Cataloging-in-Publication Data

Names: Higgins, Edmund S., author. | George, Mark S. (Mark Stork), 1958-author.
Title: The neuroscience of clinical psychiatry : the pathophysiology of behavior and mental illness / Edmund S. Higgins, Mark S. George.
Description: Third edition. | Philadelphia : Wolters Kluwer, [2019] | Includes bibliographical references and index.
Identifiers: LCCN 2017058724 | ISBN 9781496372000 (alk. paper)
Subjects: | MESH: Mental Disorders–physiopathology | Nervous System–physiopathology | Neuropsychology–methods
Classification: LCC RC483 | NLM WM 140 | DDC 616.89–dc23 LC record available at https://lccn.loc.gov/2017058724

To my two sons, who assisted with
the artwork on Tuesday mornings at local
coffee shops while waiting for school to start.

—ESH

To my many mentors—four formally
designated in research fellowships, numerous
others who've just helped and taught along
the way—and the students and patients who have
taught me so much as well. May we all be lifelong
students!!

—MSG

Preface

Neuroscience is the basic science of psychiatry. Neuroscience describes the brain mechanisms that

- gather information from the external and internal world,
- analyze the information, and
- execute the best response.

Psychiatric disorders are the result of problems with these mechanisms.

The increased accessibility to the workings of the brain in the past 30 years has resulted in an explosion of information about neuroscience. Different lines of research such as brain imaging and animal studies along with more traditional postmortem analysis, study of medication effects, and genetic studies have transformed the way we conceptualize normal and abnormal behavior.

Bits and pieces of the neuroscience literature have filtered up to the practicing clinician, but a comprehensive understanding of the field is almost inaccessible to all but the most dedicated self-educators. The jargon is foreign and difficult to navigate. The standard textbooks are thick with contributions from multiple authors and almost impossible to read cover to cover. The relevance to the practice of psychiatry can sometimes be hard to appreciate.

We hope this book will provide a way for residents and practicing clinicians to gain a thorough appreciation for the mechanisms within the brain that are stimulating (or failing to stimulate) their patients. We also hope that the reader will have more accurate answers for the patient who asks, "What's causing my problem?" Likewise, we hope the reader will be better prepared for the increasingly difficult neuroscience questions that appear on board certification tests.

If we've learned anything from our studies on the brain, it is that LEARNING IS WORK! The brain increases its metabolism when conducting academic assignments. The process of focusing one's attention, understanding the concepts, and storing the new information requires energy. There is no passive learning.

Consequently, when learning is interesting and relevant it requires less energy. We have made every effort to make this material appealing and easy to consume. Pictures, drawings, and graphs have been liberally incorporated to allow the reader to learn the concepts quickly and efficiently. Every effort has been made to keep the material short and concise, but not too simple. Finally, we think information that is relevant to the reader is easier to retain, so we have tried to keep bringing the focus back to the practice of psychiatry.

We intend our book to be for three populations. First, it is for those in training: psychiatrists, psychologists, counselors, and allied physicians. Second, it is for psychiatric residents seeking to review the topics in preparation for their board examinations. And last, it is for the practicing clinician who was trained before the revolution in neuroscience and who would like to become more up-to-date and familiar with the field.

We hope that the reader will have a thorough—soup to nuts—understanding of the important topics in neuroscience and will henceforth be able to read and comprehend the future research in this field.

Edmund S. Higgins, MD
Mark S. George, MD

Acknowledgments

The authors wish to thank the following people for their assistance with this manuscript: Sherri A. Brown for her assistance with the artwork; Pamela J. Wright-Etter, MD, and Robert J. Malcolm Jr, MD, who reviewed individual chapters; and Laura G. Hancock, DO, and L. William Mulbry, MD, residents who reviewed the entire book. We also wish to thank all those readers who pointed out the typos in the first edition.

Figures 3.5–3.7 and 22.2 and the dolphin in Chapter 15, Sleep, were drawn by Fess Higgins.

For the third edition we would like to thank Eric Brueckner, DO, and Edward M. Kantor, MD, for facilitating a review of the book by the MUSC fourth year residents—and all the helpful feedback they offered.

About the Authors

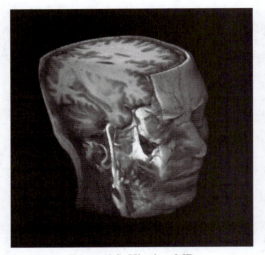

Edmund S. Higgins, MD

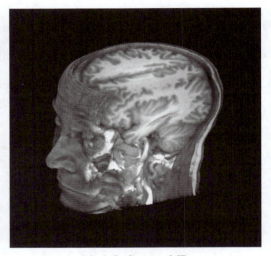

Mark S. George, MD

Edmund S. Higgins, MD, is a Clinical Associate Professor of Psychiatry and Family Medicine at the Medical University of South Carolina (MUSC). He received his medical degree from Case Western Reserve University School of Medicine. He completed residencies in family practice and psychiatry at MUSC. He is currently providing psychiatric care for South Carolina Department of Corrections and has a tiny private psychiatric practice. He lives on Sullivan's Island, SC.

Mark S. George, MD, is a Distinguished Professor of Psychiatry, Radiology, and Neuroscience as well as Director of the Brain Stimulation Division, Psychiatry at the Medical University of South Carolina (MUSC), Charleston. He also holds the Layton McCurdy Endowed Chair in Psychiatry and was the original director of the Center for Advanced Imaging Research at MUSC. He received his medical degree and completed dual residencies at MUSC in both neurology and psychiatry and is board certified in both areas. After a fellowship in London and 4 years at the National Institute of Mental Health, he returned to Charleston where he has conducted pioneering work with functional imaging of the brain, transcranial magnetic stimulation and vagus nerve stimulation, and other forms of brain stimulation. He is on several editorial review boards, has published over 500 scientific articles or book chapters, and has written or edited 6 books. He has been the editor-in-chief of *Brain Stimulation* for the past decade since it began, a journal published by Elsevier. He also resides on Sullivan's Island, SC.

Contents

SECTION I **The Neuroscience Model**

1 Introduction   2

2 Neuroanatomy   15

3 Cells and Circuits   29

4 Neurotransmitters   41

5 Receptors and Signaling the Nucleus   53

6 Genetics and Epigenetics   64

SECTION II **Modulators**

7 Hormones and the Brain   79

8 Plasticity and Adult Development   92

9 Immunity and Inflammation   108

10 The Electrical Brain   122

SECTION III **Behaviors**

11 Pain   133

12 Pleasure   148

13 Appetite   164

14 Anger and Aggression   177

15 Sleep   191

16 Sex and the Brain   207

17 Social Attachment   222

18 Memory   237

19 Intelligence   249

20 Attention   261

SECTION IV **Disorders**

21 Depression   274

22 Anxiety   288

23 Schizophrenia   302

24 Alzheimer's Disease   316

Bibliography   328
Answers to End-of-Chapter Questions   346
Index   348

The Neuroscience Model

CHAPTER 1

Introduction

OVERVIEW

The brain has not always been of great interest to humankind. Most ancient cultures did not consider the brain to be an important organ. Both the Bible and Talmud fail to mention diseases related to the central nervous system (CNS). Egyptians carefully embalmed the liver and the heart but had no use for the brain; they actually scooped it out and threw it away. (If there really is an Egyptian afterlife—those poor pharaohs are spending eternity without a brain.) Now we are in the *Neurocentric Age* and view the brain as the most complex organ in the universe. George H. W. Bush, the former President of the United States dedicated an entire decade to the study of the brain. You don't see the gastrointestinal tract get that kind of attention. We've come a long way.

This book is intended to bring you an up-to-date review of how the brain does all the amazing things we now recognize it is capable of doing. The best way to read this book is from cover to cover, which should give you a thorough, but easily digestible, understanding of the mechanisms of normal behavior and mental illness. Before we get started, we want to review a few basic principles or themes that run through this book.

Heredity

It has long been recognized that mental illness travels in families. In 1651 in *The Anatomy of Melancholy*, Robert Burton succinctly summarized this concept at least for alcoholism when he wrote: "One drunkard begets another." Fast forward to the 20th century and in-depth family studies provide similar, although less colorful, findings. For example, with schizophrenia, if one family member has the illness, the likelihood that a relative will also develop the disease increases the more closely they are related. The determining variable appears to be the percentage of shared DNA (Figure 1.1).

The domestication of animals provides another example of the genetic control of behavior. Charles Darwin, without any knowledge of genes, believed the temperament of domestic animals was inherited. Dmitry Belyaev, a Russian geneticist, validated this with his famous farm-fox experiment in Siberia.

Belyaev domesticated wild foxes simply by selecting and breeding the tamest animals. He started with 130 wild foxes and used a simple test of tameness. Humans approached the caged foxes, and those that were most tolerant were mated. The process was repeated with the offspring, each time mating the tamest animals from the litter. Within 20 years the foxes were domesticated. Within 40 years, the offspring of wild foxes were literally house pets. Of interest, the brains of the domesticated foxes produced less corticosteroids (the stress hormones) and higher levels of serotonin than did the wild foxes.

It is a bit unsettling to accept that our personalities, seemingly molded by the events of our lives, are actually hardwired from our genes. Eccentric, stingy, gregarious, thin-skinned, etc., are more a product of our genes than our environment. But what role does the environment play in the development of our personalities?

Bouchard and others have tried to tease out *nature* and *nurture* by looking at personality characteristics in monozygotic (identical) and dizygotic (fraternal) twins—reared together and reared apart. Using personality tests to assess the five major personality traits, they found more correlations for monozygotic twins compared with dizygotic twins regardless of whether they were raised together or apart (Table 1.1). In other words, the monozygotic twins reared apart shared more personality

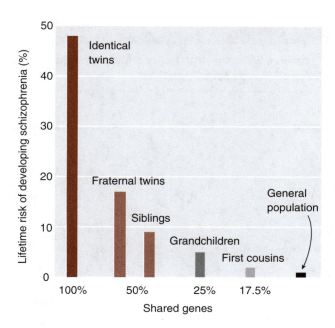

FIGURE 1.1 As the shared genetic profile with someone having schizophrenia increases, the risk of developing schizophrenia also increases. (Data from Gottesman II. *Schizophrenia Genesis*. New York: W.H. Freeman; 1991.)

characteristics than did the dizygotic twins reared in the same household. Bouchard concluded that personality traits are strongly influenced by inheritance and only modestly affected by environment. (The lay press unfortunately summarized this research as "Parents Don't Matter.")

Figure 1.2 shows a remarkable example of identical twins separated at birth (5 days old) and raised in different households—one in Brooklyn, the other in New Jersey. They did not meet again until they were 31 years old. Both are firefighters, bachelors, with mustaches and metal frame glasses. Not only do they have the same mannerisms, but they also laugh at the same jokes and enjoy the same hobbies. Yet, they were exposed to entirely different environmental influences throughout their lives. Our individuality—who we are, how we socialize, what we like, even our religious beliefs—are likely influenced more by the brain we are born with than by the experiences we have along the way.

A word of caution: even though there is about a 50% concurrence between monozygotic twins for personality traits and schizophrenia, the other 50% are out of sync—*yet they share the same DNA*. This is also true for bipolar disorder, alcoholism, and panic disorder. About half the monozygotic twins have the same illnesses, whereas the other half do not.

Clearly, our brains are more programmed by our genes than we previously believed, but that does not explain everything. Experiences during our lives impact our personality, particularly trauma, and especially when the trauma occurs early in life. The challenge for us is to unravel the brain mechanisms that are predetermined by genetics and understand how they can change in response to the environment.

The Brain Is Dynamic

In 1894, Santiago Ramón y Cajal, maybe the first neuroscientist, stated in a lecture to the Royal Society of London, "the ability of neurons to grow in an adult and their power to create new connections can explain learning." This is often cited as the origin of the synaptic theory of memory. Hebb, a Canadian psychologist, wrote in 1949 a phrase that is loosely paraphrased as *neurons that fire together, wire together*. These men surmised that the brain must change in some way for details to be remembered, but their tools were not sophisticated enough to identify the mechanisms.

Proving that the adult brain can change in response to experience (plasticity) has been the most exciting discovery in neuroscience. Although many individuals have been involved in this research, no single individual has done more than *Eric Kandel*. Kandel was able to prove what Ramón y Cajal could only speculate about—that learning changes the cells of the brain and even the chemical composition of those cells. Kandel worked with the simple sea snail *Aplysia* because

TABLE 1.1

The Correlations for Five Personality Traits in Monozygotic Twins and Dizygotic Twins Reared Apart and Together[a]

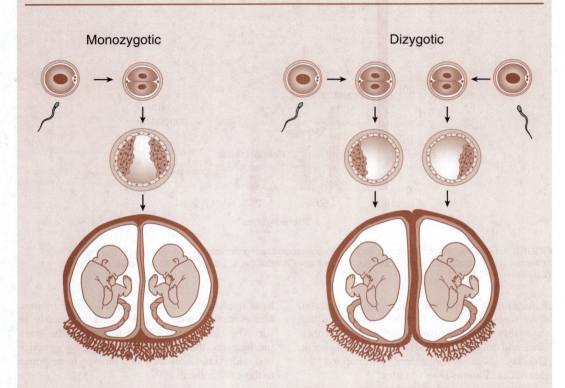

Monozygotic Raised Apart	Monozygotic Raised Together	Personality Trait	Dizygotic Raised Apart	Dizygotic Raised Together
0.41	0.54	Extraversion	0.0	0.19
0.49	0.48	Neuroticism	0.44	0.19
0.54	0.54	Conscientiousness	0.07	0.29
0.24	0.39	Agreeableness	0.09	0.11
0.57	0.43	Openness	0.09	0.11
0.45	**0.48**	**Mean**	**0.17**	**0.18**

[a]The mean correlations are surprisingly similar to the lifetime risk of developing schizophrenia for identical (monozygotic) and fraternal (dizygotic) twins shown in Figure 1.1.

it can remember and has only about 20,000 neurons in its entire CNS (compared with 100 billion in humans). Kandel taught the snail a few simple tasks—habituation (gradually ignoring an innocuous stimulus) and sensitization (remembering an aversive stimulus) (Figure 1.3).

For *Aplysia*, the gill with its siphon is a sensitive and important organ—one that quickly withdraws with any sign of danger. Habituation is induced by sequentially touching the siphon with a soft brush. With repetition, the snail learns to ignore the gentle stimuli. Sensitization, on the other hand, is elicited with an electrical shock to the tail coupled with the soft brush of the siphon. This is something not to forget. Indeed, after many sessions the gill is still retracted with great vigor. After training *Aplysia* to habituate or react (forget or remember), Kandel and his colleagues dissected and analyzed the

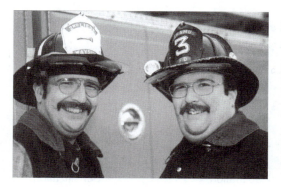

FIGURE 1.2 Gerald Levy *(left)* and Mark Newman *(right)* are identical twins who were separated at birth, yet have made many of the same choices in life. (With permission from The Image Works, Woodstock, New York.)

changes in the sensory neurons. With habituation the neurons regressed (*don't need them*), whereas with sensitization the number and size of the synaptic terminals grew (Figure 1.4). Kandel wrote, "we could see for the first time that the number of synapses in the brain is not fixed – it changes with learning!" And there may be nothing more important in a brain than learning and memory.

Making the Diagnosis

Another theme in this book is the difficulty making an accurate diagnosis. We are not big fans of the *Diagnostic and Statistical Manual* now in its fifth edition (*DSM-5*) or the *International Classification of Diseases* now in its tenth revision (*ICD-10*). Both of these classification systems are based on symptoms, not actual neurophysiology. It is all self-reported. Therefore patients who are stoic are likely to underreport symptoms, and hysterical patients are... well, all over the place. The former may not receive a diagnosis, and the latter receives too many. Neither gets a diagnosis that accurately reflects what occurs in the brain.

Further complicating the symptom-based categorization is that the brain only has a few ways to show distress: psychosis, depression, anxiety, autistic behavior, etc. However, there are probably hundreds of different causes for any of these symptoms. Figure 1.5 shows a metaphor for this concept. Just as all the aquifers and streams in the Midwest ultimately coalesce into the mighty Mississippi River, all enduring psychosis (for example) will be called schizophrenia, even though many different genes and negative experiences are responsible. With symptom-based categorization, we cannot differentiate one form

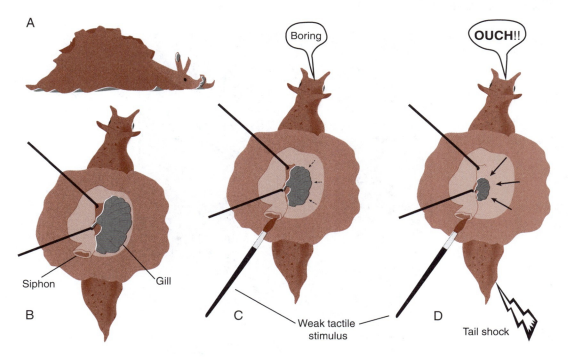

FIGURE 1.3 *Aplysia's* gill-withdrawal reflex. **A:** Aplasia slugging along. **B:** Resting state with gill exposed. **C:** Gill withdrawal to mild stimulus to the siphon. Habituation to this stimulus will develop with repeated exposure. **D:** A strong gill-withdrawal reflex persists when a strong stimulus is applied to the tail. (Adapted from Kandel ER. *In Search of Memory: The Emergence of a New Science of the Mind*. New York: W. W. Norton & Company; 2006.)

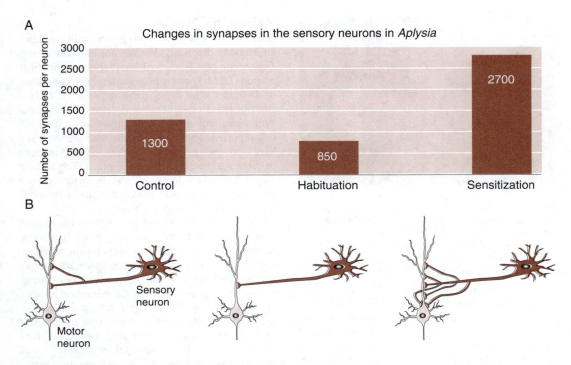

FIGURE 1.4 A: The number of synapses from the average sensory neuron to the motor neuron changes with learning. **B:** A schematic representation of morphologic changes in the connections between sensory and motor neurons. (Adapted from Kandel ER. *In Search of Memory: The Emergence of a New Science of the Mind.* New York: W.W. Norton & Company; 2006.)

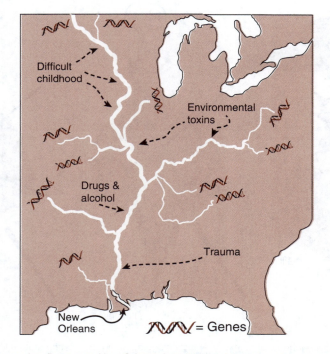

FIGURE 1.5 All the water that flows past New Orleans is called the Mississippi River, even though it comes from many different locations. Psychiatric disorders develop from heterogeneous pathophysiology, but, within a diagnostic class, all presentations are given the same name.

of schizophrenia from another. The biology may be different, but the symptoms are the same. The main point is this: there are no laboratory tests, X-rays, brain scans, or genetic profiles that can assist in separating the different forms of mental illness—with the possible exception of Alzheimer's disease.

We believe psychiatric diagnosis is about where pneumonia was in the mid-19th century. At that time, pneumonia was described by several symptoms: cough, sputum production, fever, etc. It was not until the recognition of the germ theory that the different causes of pneumonia were accurately identified. Andrew Solomon, in his book *Far From the Tree*, provides a similar change in nomenclature that has occurred for some forms of autism.

> Autism is a catchall category for an unexplained constellation of symptoms. Whenever a subtype of autism with a specific mechanism is discovered, it ceases to be called autism and is assigned its own diagnostic name. Rett syndrome produces autistic symptoms; so, often, do phenylketonuria (PKU), tuberous sclerosis, neurofibromatosis, cortical dysplasia-focal epilepsy, Timothy syndrome, fragile X syndrome, and Joubert syndrome. People with these diagnoses are usually described as having "autistic-type behaviors," but not autism per se.

This is an excellent description of how our diagnostic terms (such as autism, schizophrenia, depression, etc.) are typically reserved for that which we cannot explain. Once we find the mechanism, we give it a medical name. Ostensibly, all psychiatric disorders will have a medical name in the future. We simply haven't discovered them yet.

Tom Insel, the former director of the NIMH, would like to see our field move toward diagnostic criteria that incorporate biomarkers: genetics, neuroimaging, and metabolic findings, along with signs and symptoms. The NIMH has launched the Research Domain Criteria (RDoC) to classify mental disorders with more biomedical precision. Insel would like to see mental health evaluations identifying and intervening before the problems develop into a full disorder, similar to the way we treat hyperlipidemia and hypertension to prevent heart disease. Unfortunately, with our current knowledge, the neurobiologic markers are not precise enough... yet.

The Spectrums of Brain Functions

We believe psychiatric disorders occur along spectrums rather than in discrete categories. Recent findings with *prosopagnosia* provide a good example of a spectrum. Prosopagnosia, "face blindness," is a neurologic disorder in which patients, who are otherwise intellectually intact, are unable to recognize human faces—even their own face. It can be quite problematic, for example, when a mother picks up the wrong child at school. We all have this to some degree, but patients with the disorder are significantly further along the impairment scale.

Prosopagnosia was described in the 19th century. What is new is the other end of the spectrum, what Russell and his colleagues call "super-recognizers: people with extraordinary face recognition ability" in their 2009 paper. Apparently, Scotland Yard employs super-recognizers to review video footage of crimes and identify the culprit. Russell et al. stated, "these 'super-recognizers' are about as good at face recognition and perception as developmental prosopagnosics are bad."

Facial recognition is a good example of a brain function that occurs along a spectrum from "severely impaired" to "exceptional," with most of us residing in the middle. We believe psychiatric disorders reside along similar spectrums, which are best understood as thoughts/feelings/behaviors controlled by the brain, with most of us having average capacity and some individuals functioning at either extreme.

Localizing of Function

Before the 1860s the brain was seen as a single multipurpose organ, much the way we currently view the liver or pancreas. The French physician *Paul Broca* with his famous case in 1861 confirmed for the first time that certain functions were localized to specific regions of the brain (Figure 1.6). Broca's

Central sulcus

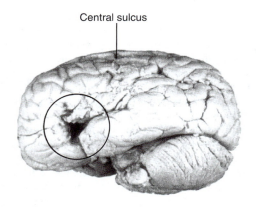

FIGURE 1.6 The preserved brain of the patient who helped Broca convince physicians that some functions—in this case the ability to speak—were localized in the cerebrum. (Adapted from Bear MF, Connors BW, Paradiso MA, eds. *Neuroscience: Exploring the Brain*. 4th ed. Baltimore: Lippincott Williams & Wilkins; 2015.)

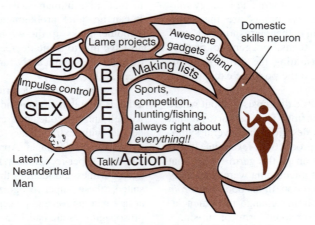

Activating the Beer neurons tends to excite the latent
Neanderthal Man as well as the Ego & SEX neurons
but inhibits the Impulse Control sulcus.

FIGURE 1.7 Localization of function in the male brain. Intuitively correct, but not supported by research.

patient developed a sudden loss of articulate speech. All he could say was one syllable: "tan." His utterances could convey great emotional tone (he retained oral dexterity, and he could hear and comprehend), but one syllable was all he could express. After his death, an autopsy revealed a lesion of his left frontal lobe—what is now called *Broca's aphasia*. The fact that almost all similar cases were on the left hemisphere and that similar right hemispheric lesions did not affect speech also led Broca to identify left/right dominance for some functions.

The belief that one function or emotion resides in a specific area in the brain appeals to our desire for uncomplicated organization. Figure 1.7 shows the sort of characterization of the male brain that we would like to believe is possible. It is rarely this simple, particularly with behavior. When we do find discrete regions of the brain, which appear to control one function, it is usually what we would consider in the realm of neurology: motor, sensory, sleep, speech, etc. Typically, behaviors (and consequently mental illness) are a confluence of networks communicating back and forth between different regions of the brain. It can be confusing and convoluted. This is why it has been so difficult to determine where behaviors arise in the brain and to identify what goes wrong in mental illness. Consequently, we need to be cautious when reading new studies that purport to have localized a specific behavior to a discrete region of the brain.

MODERN RESEARCH: HOW WE STUDY THE BRAIN

Dissection

We do not biopsy psychiatric brains. Probably the only time live brains are touched in psychiatric patients occurs in those rare occasions when a patient undergoes neurosurgery for a separate disorder. In all other instances, as with Broca, we have to wait for the patient to die to examine the brain tissue..., and Broca had it easy. Examining one brain from a psychiatric patient has been of little value in understanding the pathology of psychiatric disorders. Because psychiatric symptoms likely reside in diffuse networks, finding and identifying the pathology has been difficult, so researchers need to compare many diseased and "normal" brains. This approach has spawned the creation of brain banks.

Brain banks (not FDIC insured) are laboratories that collect and store brains from patients with known disorders. The largest consortium in the United States is the NIH NeuroBioBank, which includes six centers (Harvard, Mt Sinai, the Universities of Maryland, Pittsburgh, and Miami, and UCLA) and has about 12,000 brains in storage. They collect brains from patients who had bipolar disorder, schizophrenia, borderline personality disorder, and autism (to name a few). Studies typically involve only a small amount of tissue so that one brain can be used in many different studies. Dr Michelle Freund of NIH recently stated that 10,000 samples of tissue were analyzed in various studies in the past 2 years. The new trend in brain banks is to gather clinical information premortem to compare and contrast with postmortem findings. This particularly applies to studies of Alzheimer's disease. Of interest, the brain banks are always in need of normal brains. Give them a call if you think you have one.

The brain has the consistency of gelatin. To see nerve cells, it is necessary to fix the brain before cutting thin slices. One of the advantages of central administration of the NIH brain banks is the ability to establish uniform criteria for preparing and storing the brains. This enables analysis of brains from different centers in the same study.

Brain cells are not easily identified in an unstained brain. In 1873 an Italian physician, *Camillo Golgi*, discovered a selective silver stain that allowed researchers to visualize the individual nerve cells in what would otherwise be a uniform blob of color. Termed the Golgi stain, and still used today, researchers can see sharp black images of individual nerve cells and identify specific parts such as the cell body and the dendritic branches (Figure 1.8). The morphology of the neuron (meaning the shape and structure) is a topic that comes up time and again in this book. We discuss alterations in neuron morphology as an indication that something is different in the brains of those

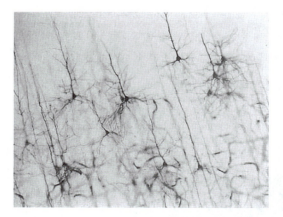

FIGURE 1.8 Pyramidal nerve cells after incubation with Golgi's silver stain. Only about 1% of the neurons absorb the stain, which allows for the identification of individual cells in what would otherwise be a very crowded slice. (Adapted from Bear MF, Connors BW, Paradiso MA, eds. *Neuroscience: Exploring the Brain*. 4th ed. Baltimore: Lippincott Williams & Wilkins; 2015.)

with certain disorders: mental retardation, substance abuse, schizophrenia, etc.

Imaging

Noninvasive analysis of the CNS has transformed the way we study behavior and mental disorders. Early attempts to image the brain were unhelpful, painful, and even dangerous. An ordinary X-ray provides little information because the brain is soft and is not radiopaque. Back in the day, searching for displacement of calcified structures (indirect evidence of a mass) was about the best they could hope for. Pneumoencephalography, in which cerebrospinal fluid is removed and replaced with air to enhance visualization of the CNS, is an example of the painful and dangerous extremes that were foisted on patients in earlier times.

The development of noninvasive imaging techniques (Table 1.2) has led to a small revolution in neuroscience. Although the functional studies (positron emission tomography [PET], single photon emission computed tomography [SPECT], and functional magnetic resonance imaging [fMRI]) remain largely limited to research, the noninvasive structural analyses (computed tomography [CT] and magnetic resonance imaging [MRI]) have transformed the practice of neurology. Diffusion tensor imaging (DTI), a technique using MRI scans to measure the movement of water in tissue, creates images of white matter tracts.

A word of caution regarding brain imaging studies and psychiatric disorders: throughout this book, we mention numerous studies examining brain volume or brain function for various psychiatric disorders. However, Ioannidis reviewed brain volume studies and found that the reported number of positive studies far exceeded what would be expected based on the power estimates of the studies. He believes the studies that do *not* find a significant difference between control subjects and patients are seldom published.

More recently, Daniel Weinberger, one of the original leaders in psychiatric brain imaging, wrote an editorial urging caution before uncritically accepting reports purporting to find "the elusive psychiatric 'lesion.'" Weinberger noted that common variables more likely found in patients than controls (smoking, substance abuse, excessive weight, stress, medication use, and head motion, to name a few) can confound the results and give the illusion of a neurobiologic finding. Ioannidis and Weinberger remind us that, in spite of the significant statistics and impressive images provided in journals, the studies may be more artifact than actual differences.

TABLE 1.2

A Brief History of Imaging Methods Used to Analyze the Central Nervous System

Date	Initials	Name	Method	Specifics
1918	X-ray	Pneumoencephalography	Replacing cerebrospinal fluid with air	Painful and dangerous
1927	X-ray	Cerebral angiography	Injecting contrast into circulation	Visualizes the cerebral vasculature
1970s	CT	Computed tomography	Ionizing radiation	Changed the way we practiced medicine
	PET	Positron emission tomography	Decay of positron-emitting radionuclides	Measures activity of brain by analyzing blood flow
	SPECT	Single photon emission computed tomography	Single photon emission	More widely available than PET, but lower resolution
1980s	MRI	Magnetic resonance imaging	Magnetic changes induced in molecules	No radiation, noninvasive, high resolution
	fMRI	Functional magnetic resonance imaging	Measures changes in blood oxygen used by the brain	Allows noninvasive exploration of brain function
1990s	DTI	Diffusion tensor imaging	Assesses direction of movement of water in tissue	Allows visualization of white matter tracts

POINT OF INTEREST

The figure shows a method of using imaging studies frequently found in the literature. That is, one functional study is subtracted from another and the result is superimposed on a structural image. In this case the subject is performing a finger opposition task with his right fingers while in a SPECT scanner (A). The white arrow shows the activation of the left motor cortex. (B) A SPECT scan in the controlled state (not moving) is also produced. (C) The control image is subtracted from the task image. (D) The results are superimposed on an MRI of the same location, and drawings of the human homunculus along the motor cortex are added for further understanding.

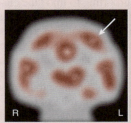
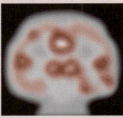
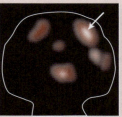
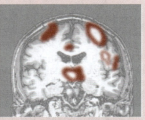

(A) Finger opposition task

(B) Control

(C) Task minus control

(D) Superimposed on MRI

Nonhuman Animal Studies

Nonhuman animal studies provide another approach to understanding the marvels of the brain. The nonhuman animal brain is accessible in ways that are beyond the ethics of human research. Although they might have paws and whiskers, non-human brains have much in common with those of humans. The protein-coding regions of the mouse and human genomes are 85% identical. Nature is conservative, and many of the molecular and cellular mechanisms that underlie behavior are preserved from one species to the next. However, animals do not possess a similarly developed human cerebral cortex, nor can we ever be sure they actually have the psychiatric symptoms being studied. In spite of these limitations, tweaking animal brains has been invaluable in enhancing our understanding of the functions of the brain. Ablation studies—removing part of the brain and observing how the animal behaves—are the crudest animal studies. Electrical stimulation provides more precision and has been the bedrock of neuroscience research. However, the more modern approaches have focused on the genes.

Markers of Gene Activation

Two words of advice we would give to any student interested in neuroscience: *gene expression*. The DNA that gets turned on (or alternatively turned off) is referred to as "gene expression," and this process controls the growth and activity of the brain. Understanding which genes are responsible is the key to understanding the brain and behavior. Researchers can now measure mRNA or proteins that result from gene expression. Cyclic adenosine monophosphate responsive element–binding protein (CREB) and proteins in the Fos family are two transcription factors that are frequently used as markers of gene expression. Identifying CREB or c-Fos in a postmortem brain slice helps pinpoint the areas in the brain that were active in the animal during the experimental manipulation.

Knockout Mice

Animals (typically mice) can be engineered so that specific genes are turned off—rendered mute. Animals with silenced genes are called *knockout mice*. They are raised (if possible) and observed for changes in behavior compared with control mice—often called "wild" mice. Knockout mice have been used to understand obesity, substance abuse, and anxiety. Although these studies represent a valuable research tool, one has to be cautious about generalizing from the results. The downstream effects of silencing the gene during development can never be fully appreciated.

Transgenic Mice

Transgenic mice are genetically engineered creatures. DNA from one organism is introduced into the DNA of a mouse egg, which is then fertilized. The adult mouse incorporates the foreign DNA into its genome. For example, DNA from jellyfish encoding for fluorescent proteins has been inserted into the mouse genome. Brain slices from these mice "light up" when viewed under fluorescent microscopes. Likewise, the ability to insert disease-causing DNA into mice and then observe the damage it causes to the brain has revolutionized neurology.

Viral-Mediated Gene Transfer

Viruses can be used as a vehicle to insert a section of DNA into the brain of living animals at specific locations. When the DNA is incorporated into the host DNA, new genes are expressed with possible alterations in behavior. For example, a virus was used to implant the DNA for the vasopressin receptor in the ventral pallidum of promiscuous voles. Responding voles were transformed into monogamous, family-oriented, card-carrying social conservatives (specifics in Chapter 17, Attachment).

Lighting Up the Brain

Despite all these wonderful techniques to investigate the brain, we still do not have a good grasp of what is actually going on. That is, how activity in cells and networks gives rise to memories, thoughts, and feelings. Furthermore, we only vaguely grasp the failures that produce psychiatric disorders. *Optogenetics* is a new technique that gives more precision in understanding the effects of distinct neural circuits and behavior in animals.

Optogenetics describes the combination of optics and genetics to make neurons respond to light. Figure 1.9 provides the basics of this method. It starts with green algae, which possess receptors that, when exposed to light, open and allow ions to pass. When the DNA for these receptors is inserted into DNA in neurons in rodents, light will open the receptor allowing ions to pass and "fire" the neuron. Then, conveniently, shining a light on the neurons can activate the specific network and allow researchers to observe changes in behavior when those neurons are turned "on" and "off." This technique has been used to elucidate neural circuits in animal models of anxiety, depression, schizophrenia, addiction, and social dysfunction.

Following the DNA

The rapid growth of genetic knowledge requires its own chapter, but there are two techniques for analyzing the brain that are worth mentioning now.

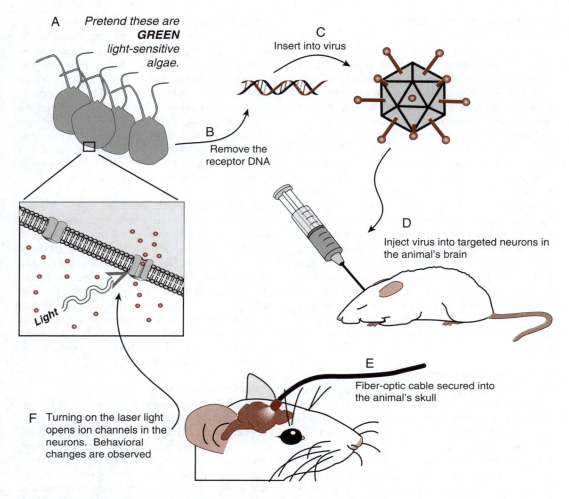

FIGURE 1.9 The DNA from light-sensitive algae, when inserted into the DNA of a rodent, enables the neuron to fire in the presence of a laser light—a process that is called optogenetics.

Microarrays

DNA microarrays (also called gene chips) enable researchers to compare the mRNA (and therefore gene activity) found in tissue samples with DNA of known identity. The microarray is a chip no bigger than a postage stamp with thousands of different DNA molecules, multiplied, segregated, and attached in separate tiny locations (Figure 1.10).

The mRNA from the tissue being studied is transcribed to DNA, labeled with fluorescent markers, and dropped onto the microarray chip. The single-stranded DNA from the tissue sample will bind with similar single-stranded DNA on the microarray. The chip is then read in a scanner that calculates the amount of binding between the tissue DNA and the chip DNA in each discrete spot, giving an estimate of that specific gene activity in the tissue. As an example, this procedure was done with small samples from the prefrontal cortex of schizophrenic and control postmortem brain. The schizophrenic brains showed reduced expression of myelination-related genes, suggesting a disruption in the myelin as part of the pathogenesis of schizophrenia (see Chapter 23, Schizophrenia).

Growing Brain Cells: Induced Pluripotent Stem Cells

In 2006, Shinya Yamanaka found a way to turn fully differentiated adult cells back into pluripotent stem cells. This means, cells already formed into tissuelike skin or fibroblasts, after some manipulation, act like embryonic stem cells and can develop into any type of cell in the body—without all the ethical questions provoked by using human embryos. Called *induced pluripotent stem cells*, the trick is to fool the cell into removing the "breaks"

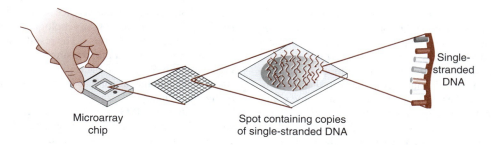

Single-stranded DNA

Microarray chip

Spot containing copies of single-stranded DNA

FIGURE 1.10 The microarray chip contains multiple copies of many different genes so that a broad spectrum of gene activity can be analyzed quickly in a scanner. (Adapted from Friend SH, Stoughton RB. The magic of microarrays. *Sci Am*. 2002;286:44–53.)

that constrain cellular differentiation. With considerable trial and error, Yamanaka, who went on to win a Nobel Prize in 2012, discovered that, by introducing into the cell four genes for transcription factors, he could turn back the cellular "clock" (Figure 1.11).

Fred Gage's laboratory (the Salk Institute for Biological Studies) unitized this procedure to study neurons from bipolar patients—without having to biopsy the brains. They reprogrammed fibroblasts and grew hippocampal dentate gyrus–like neurons from bipolar patients who were "lithium responders" and compared them with bipolar patients who were nonresponders to lithium and normal controls. They found hyperexcitability in the neurons from bipolar patients, which was

reversed by lithium, but only in those patients who responded to lithium. It is unclear if this specific finding will have enduring significance, but what it represents (disease in a dish, as some have called it) is an extraordinary way to study the physiology of neurons from patients with mental illness.

The Controlled Trial

It is discouraging that the brain is so resistant to change. It is more discouraging to read about eccentric clinicians, parents, teachers, and other meddlers expounding the effectiveness of unproven interventions to reduce symptoms or improve behavior. Sugar and hyperactivity were "known" to have a cause-and-effect relationship that has failed to materialize in controlled trials.

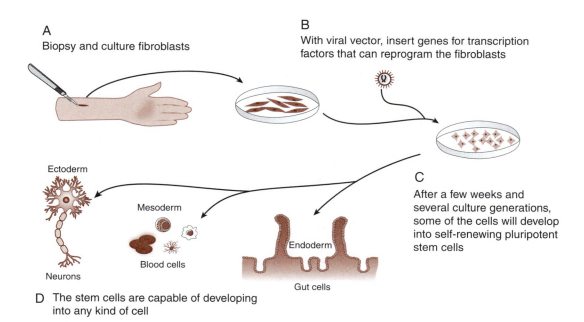

A
Biopsy and culture fibroblasts

B
With viral vector, insert genes for transcription factors that can reprogram the fibroblasts

C
After a few weeks and several culture generations, some of the cells will develop into self-renewing pluripotent stem cells

Ectoderm

Mesoderm

Endoderm

Neurons

Blood cells

Gut cells

D   The stem cells are capable of developing into any kind of cell

FIGURE 1.11 The creation of pluripotent stem cells from fibroblasts enables researchers to grow "minibrains" and may enable the development of better models of neuropsychiatric disorders.

It is important to prove that our efforts to heal are actually helping. Unfortunately, there are many instances of treatments that proved to be ineffective and too many that are even harmful. Perhaps the greatest research tool in health care has been the randomized controlled clinical trial. With controlled studies we can determine with some confidence how effective interventions might be, which then gives us some insight into the workings of the brain. But replication of studies is the hallmark of effective treatment.

Sexy, innovative studies are like catnip to journal editors and NPR news. However, a recent study in *Science* suggests that we need to do more to "verify whether we know what we think we know."

The authors of the Open Science Collaboration attempted to replicate 100 psychological studies from three prominent journals. The results the second time around were embarrassingly disappointing. Although 97% of the original studies were statistically significant, only 36% were so in the replication. Ouch!

We (ESH & MSG) are guilty of hearing the siren call of new, innovative studies and falling in love with the results. In this third edition we have made considerable efforts to substantiate previous findings and throw overboard the ones that have not stood the test of time.

CHAPTER 2

Neuroanatomy

CEREBRAL CORTEX

There are many large textbooks with extensive writings and illustrations providing all the known specifics about the anatomy of the nervous system. If you are looking for that sort of detail, then you are reading the wrong book. We—on the other hand—have tried to limit our discussion of neuro-anatomy to those structures frequently identified in the scientific articles that are relevant to the clinician treating mental illness. First, we feel compelled to review a bit about the developing brain. You can best understand how brain anatomy is organized by remembering how it formed itself in the first place.

Development

The fertilized egg quickly divides and differentiates into an embryo with three cell lines: the ectoderm, mesoderm, and endoderm (see Figure 1.11 as example). A portion of the ectoderm folds and forms the neural tube, which becomes the rudimentary nervous system. The most anterior cells of the nervous system spend the ensuing weeks proliferating, migrating, and developing into the different regions of the brain.

The process of differentiating is almost unbelievable. How one undeveloped cell decides it should be a neuron while a similar one becomes an astrocyte is simply amazing. The evidence suggests that chemical signals between cells turn the DNA on and off, which then controls the destiny, but orchestrating all this is almost beyond comprehension.

The migration of cells to their appropriate location in the brain is another remarkable aspect of the developing brain. Neuroblasts (undeveloped neural cells) multiply in an area called the ventricular zone. Then they shinny up radial cells (specialized glial cells), which form a kind of scaffolding to build the cerebral cortex (Figure 2.1). As the neuroblasts reach the surface of the brain, they differentiate into the various mature neurons and astrocytes that make up the gray matter.

Other neuroblasts migrate tangentially from the bottom of the ventricles. These neuroblasts typically develop into the inhibitory interneurons. They start in a different location and must come up and around before they intermingle with the other neuroblasts climbing the radial cells. It boggles the mind that all these cells find their correct location and make the right connections while we can barely find what we are looking for in Walmart.

A residual portion of the ventricular zone remains in the adult brain and allows limited neurogenesis to continue beyond the fetal stage—more on this topic in Chapter 8, Plasticity and Adult Development.

DISORDER

MENTAL RETARDATION

The migration of neurons to their specific location is a critical and venerable period of brain development. Fetal alcohol syndrome may in part be a result of aberrant migration due to the toxic effects of ethanol. Radiation is another insult that deters the traveling neuron. Studies of pregnant Japanese women, who were in proximity to the epicenter when the atomic bombs were dropped, found that 80% of the children who developed severe mental retardation were exposed to the radiation between 8 and 16 weeks after conception—the time of peak migration.

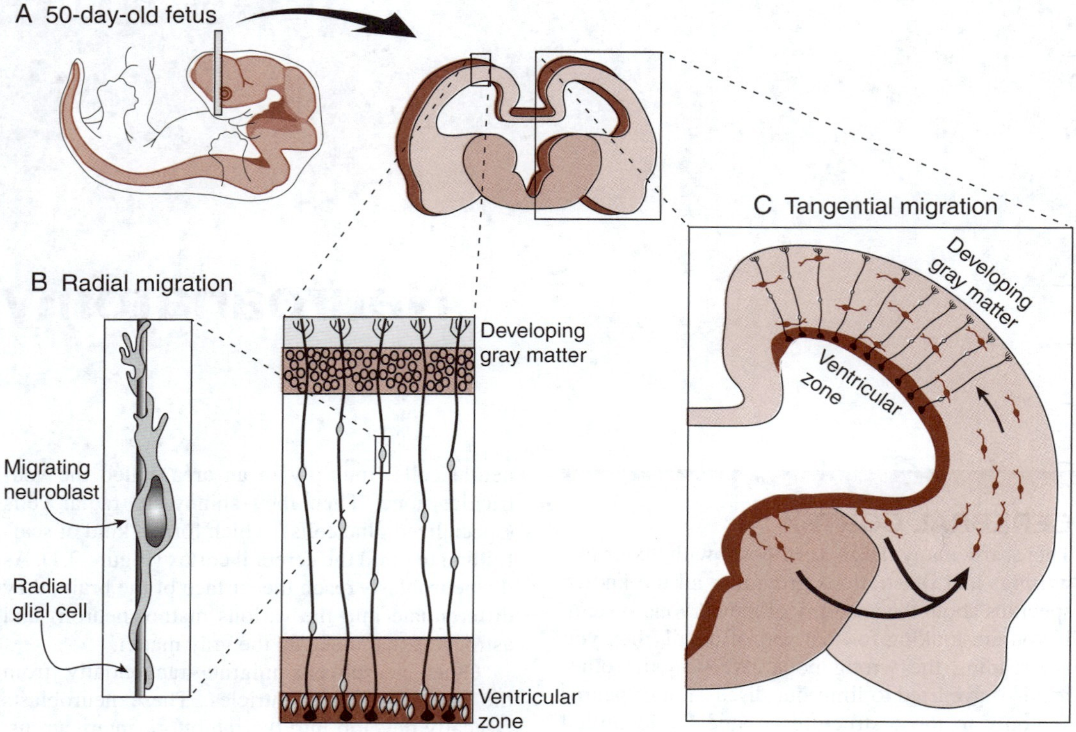

FIGURE 2.1 A: Cross section of the brain of a 50-day-old fetus. **B:** Neuroblasts climb up the radial glial cells to the developing gray matter. **C:** Inhibitory neurons develop from neuroblasts that migrate tangentially from lower regions of the brain.

The migrating and differentiating neuroblasts slowly form into the six layers of the cerebral cortex. Figure 2.2 shows how the process proceeds. The inner layers are formed first: layer IV, then layer V, and so on. This means that cells destined for the outer layers must climb past the other neurons before locating their place in the brain.

The cerebral cortex is made up of white matter and gray matter (Figure 2.3). The gray matter is where the nerve cells and synapses reside. This is where the action occurs psychologically—where we think and feel—where depression, schizophrenia, and dementia likely develop. The white matter is primarily myelinated axons transporting impulses between the gray matter and lower brain structures. The white matter makes up the circuits that connect the regions of the brain.

When we say a "neuron," we are usually thinking of the large pyramidal neurons with their triangular-shaped cell bodies. They make up approximately 75% of the cortical neurons. They have a single apical dendrite pointed toward the pial surface and a number of basilar dendrite branches projecting horizontally. The axons project

(and send impulses) to other cortical regions or the deeper structures of the subcortex.

The pyramidal neurons receive signals from the other brain regions as well as from the local interneurons. The afferent signals from other regions are typically excitatory signals that encourage the neuron to generate its own impulse. The interneurons are typically γ-aminobutyric acid neurons, which inhibit the pyramidal neuron and reduce the likelihood that it will fire.

Brodmann's Areas

In the early part of the 20th century, many neuroanatomists were struggling to divide the neocortex into structurally distinct regions. Korbinian Brodmann, a German neurologist, was working in a psychiatric clinic where he was influenced by Alois Alzheimer to pursue a career in neuroscience basic research. After extensive analysis of the human and monkey neocortex, he published in 1909 his classic work *Comparative Localization Studies in the Brain Cortex, Its Fundamentals Represented on the Basis of Its Cellular Architecture*. He had divided the

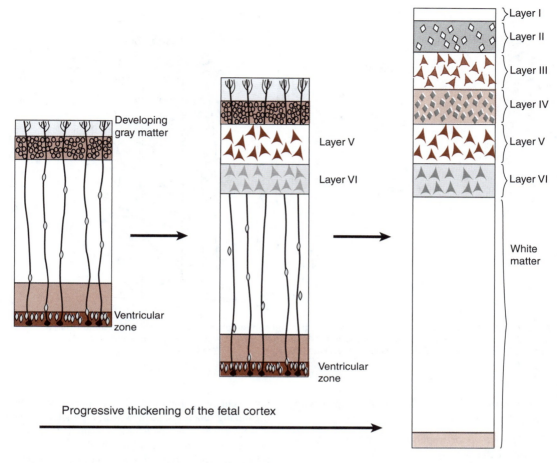

FIGURE 2.2 The six layers of the cerebral cortex develop in reverse order as the neuroblasts migrate up from the ventricular zone. (Adapted from Bear MF, Connors BW, Paradiso MA, eds. *Neuroscience: Exploring the Brain*. 4th ed. Baltimore: Lippincott Williams & Wilkins; 2015.)

neocortex into 52 regions based on the size, number, and density of the cells, as well as the local connections and long tract projections to and from the subcortical regions (Figure 2.4). Brodmann's scheme is still widely used and often mentioned in the scientific literature to locate the area in question.

Prefrontal Cortex

Who doesn't love the prefrontal cortex (PFC)? It is one of the anatomic structures that distinguishes humans from other mammals. Technically, the PFC is the part of the cortex in front of the motor cortex. Brodmann calculated that the PFC as a percentage of the total cortex is 3.5% in the cat, 7% in the dog, 8.5% in the lemur, 11.5% in the macaque, 17% in the chimpanzee, and 29% in humans. Dysfunction in the

PFC is implicated as a possible source of pathology in many psychiatric disorders—depression, schizophrenia, anxiety, and attention deficit hyperactivity disorder (ADHD), as well as disorders of anger and violence.

There are four regions of the PFC that are frequently mentioned in the scientific literature (Figure 2.5): lateral, orbital, and medial PFC as well as the cingulate gyrus. Modifying terms are often added to more precisely define the area of interest; for example, *dorso*lateral, *ventro*medial, and *anterior* cingulate are particularly popular. The ever-expanding jargon of the scientific writers is one of the great challenges of understanding neuroscience.

Neurologists, assessing and following patients with injuries (e.g., Phineas Gage—Figure 14.4),

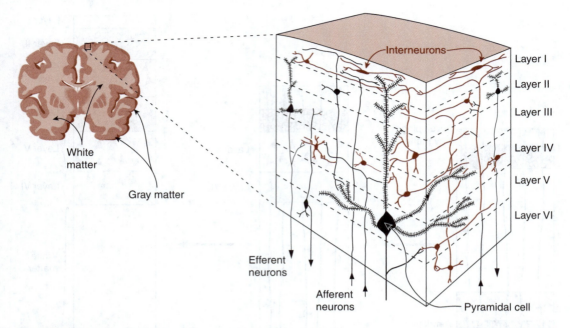

FIGURE 2.3 The six layers of the neocortex, from the pial surface above layer I to the white matter below layer VI. (From Snell RS. *Clinical Neuroanatomy: An Illustrated Review with Questions and Explanations*. 3rd ed. Philadelphia: Lippincott Williams & Wilkins; 2001.)

have identified three syndromes associated with frontal lobe damage.

Disinhibited—poor impulse control and inappropriate behavior
Disorganized—memory deficits and poor planning
Apathetic—unmotivated and paucity of spontaneous behavior

Next time you are sitting in front of a patient with old scars across his or her forehead or a history of traumatic brain injury, ask about these syndromes. Typically, patients are more aware of the disinhibition and disorganization but less cognizant of the apathy.

A lot goes on in the frontal lobes, including language and motor functions. But it is the executive functions (attention, working memory, planning, and inhibitory control) along with the emotional and social functions that are of most interest to us. As we discussed in the previous chapter, it is difficult to resist the urge to match functions with regions of the PFC. Joaquin Fuster, who recently finished the fifth edition of his book *The Prefrontal Cortex*, has written that the functions of the PFC are "interrelated and widely distributed." Here is his best attempt to assign functions to regions: "At most… the lateral prefrontal cortex is predominantly, but

not exclusively, involved in time integration and organizing functions, such as working memory. On the other hand, the medical and ventral prefrontal cortices are predominantly involved in such emotional and social functions as control of impulse, mood and empathy. However, any attempt to localize any such function, exclusively and specifically, in one prefrontal area or another is implausible." So we must not give in to the desire to put functions in boxes in the brain.

Insula Cortex

The insula is a part of the PFC that is hidden within folds of the lateral cortex and temporal lobes, which is not readily visible if you hold a brain in your hand like a neuropathologist Hamlet. We mention the insula in this edition because of a fascinating recent study out of Stanford University. The researchers collected over 15,000 MRI brain scans—roughly half of them patients and half of them controls. The scans were all from studies that had compared cases with matched controls. The difference in this study was that the patient group lumped together subjects with schizophrenia, bipolar disorder, major depression, substance abuse disorder, obsessive–compulsive disorder (OCD), and several anxiety disorders.

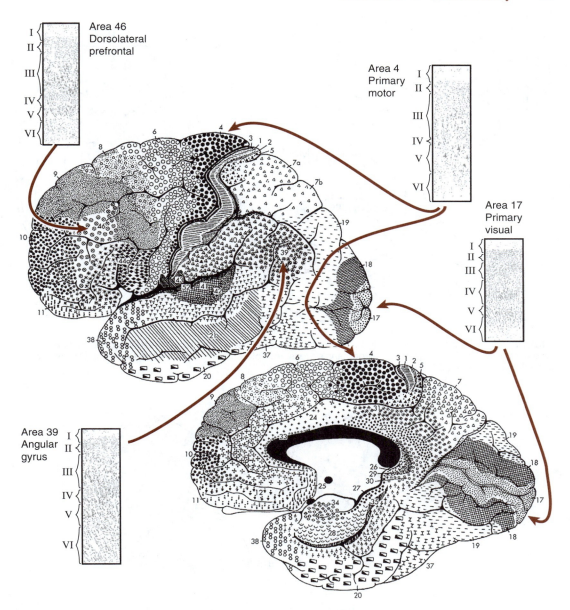

FIGURE 2.4 The human cerebral cortex as delineated by Brodmann in his 1909 publication. The different regions are defined by the composition of the gray matter. Four examples are shown.

Remarkably, the authors found that the mentally ill patients had more common deficits than differences. Specifically, they found gray matter loss in the insula and anterior cingulate (see Figure 2.6). What this means is that patients with an array of different symptoms and different diagnoses have a similar gray matter loss not found in the healthy controls. The authors called this a "shared neural substrate" and proposed that it is a common

pathway that appears to involve executive function—a frequent finding of major mental illness.

Hippocampus

The hippocampus and the amygdala are the essential structures of what is commonly called the *limbic lobe*—although there is no specific lobe. The hippocampus is a folded structure incorporated within the temporal lobe—dorsal to other

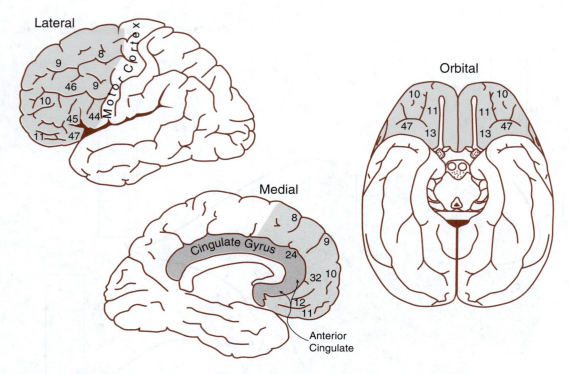

FIGURE 2.5 The important regions of the prefrontal cortex frequently mentioned in studies of normal behavior and mental illness. The numbers are Brodmann's areas. (Adapted from Fuster JM. *The Prefrontal Cortex*. 5th ed. Philadelphia: Elsevier; 2015.)

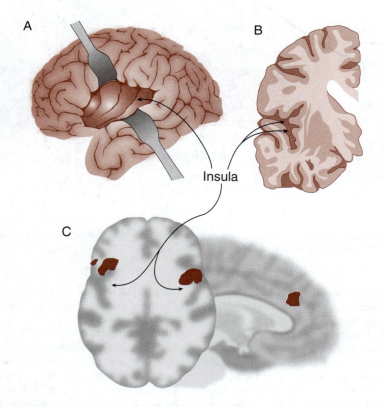

FIGURE 2.6 Lateral **(A)** and coronal **(B)** view of insula. Shared patterns of decreased gray matter (in *brown*) in the anterior insula and dorsal anterior cingulate **(C)**. (**C:** Data from Goodkind M, Eickhoff SB, Oathes DJ. Identification of a common neurobiological substrate for mental illness. *JAMA Psych.* 2015;72[4]:305–315.)

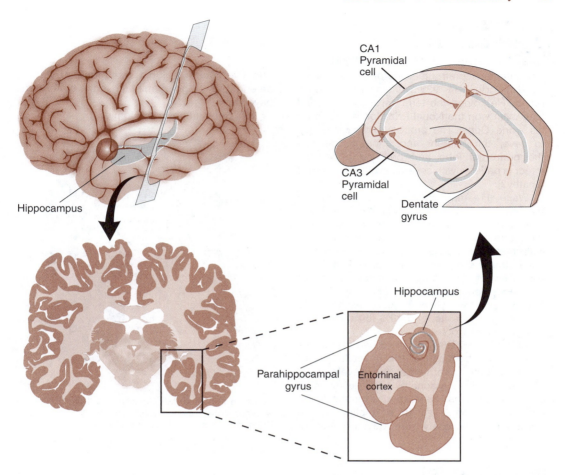

FIGURE 2.7 Different views of the hippocampus. (Adapted from Bear MF, Connors BW, Paradiso MA, eds. *Neuroscience: Exploring the Brain*. 4th ed. Baltimore: Lippincott Williams & Wilkins; 2015; and Kandel ER, Schwartz JH, Jessell TM, eds. *Principles of Neural Science*. 4th ed. New York: McGraw-Hill; 2000.)

important cortical structures of the rhinal sulcus (or primitive smell brain). The hippocampus is made up of two thin sets of neurons that look like facing "C"s—the dentate gyrus and the Ammon's horn. Ammon's horn has four regions, of which only CA3 and CA1 are shown in Figure 2.7.

The hippocampus plays an essential role in the development of memories (see Chapter 18, Memory) and is one of the few locations in the brain where neurogenesis persists in adults (see Chapter 8, Plasticity and Adult Development). Additionally, the volume of the hippocampus is decreased in various psychiatric disorders (e.g., posttraumatic stress disorder, Alzheimer's disease, and major depression), suggesting that this region may play a role in the pathogenesis of these disorders.

Amygdala

The amygdala lies within the temporal lobe just anterior to the hippocampus (Figure 2.8). Using the anatomy and connections, the amygdala can be divided into three regions: the medial group, the central group, and the basolateral group. The basolateral group, which is particularly large in humans, receives input from all the major sensory systems. The central nucleus sends output to the hypothalamus and brain stem regions. Therefore, the amygdala links sensory input from cortical regions with hypothalamic and brain stem effectors. The amygdala is active when people are anxious and/or angry, which will be discussed further in subsequent chapters. Likewise, when the organ is removed, these emotions are impaired.

TREATMENT

PREFRONTAL LOBOTOMY

The infamous prefrontal lobotomy was developed in Portugal in 1935 by the neurologist Egas Moniz. He coined the term *psychosurgery* and later even won the Nobel Prize for Medicine for his work. Oops! The procedure was intended to sever the afferent and efferent fibers of the prefrontal lobe and produce a calming effect in patients with severe psychiatric disease (apathy?).

Walter Freeman popularized and simplified the procedure in the United States. He developed a minimally invasive technique, shown in the figure, called the *transorbital lobotomy*. An instrument resembling an ice pick was inserted under the eyelid through the orbital roof and blindly swept left and right. It is hard to believe what Freeman reported in 1950—that of 711 lobotomies, 45% yielded good results, 33% produced fair results, and 19% left the patient unimproved or worse.

Although initially received with enthusiasm, in part because of the unavailability of other effective treatments, the development of unacceptable personality changes (such as unresponsiveness, decreased attention span, disinhibition, etc.) led to a decline in the procedure. Ultimately, the development of effective pharmacologic treatments brought an end to the biggest mistake in the history of psychiatry.

Transorbital frontal lobotomy.

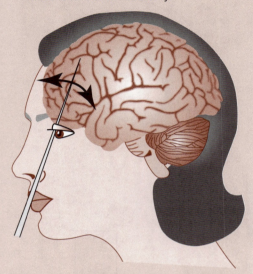

(Adapted from Bear MF, Connors BW, Paradiso MA, eds. *Neuroscience: Exploring the Brain*. 4th ed. Baltimore: Lippincott Williams & Wilkins; 2015.)

DISORDER

LIMBIC LOBE

The limbic lobe concept is a term that occasionally appears in psychiatric literature, but not one that we will use. It was originally introduced in 1878 by Broca, who noted that the cingulate gyrus, hippocampus, and their connecting bridges formed a circle on the medial side of the hemispheres. He called the structure *le grand lobe limbique*. Paul MacLean in the mid-1950s popularized the concept by linking the structure to emotional functions. Historically, this was a big step in associating emotions with neuroanatomy and had a large impact on biologic psychiatry.

Exactly what constitutes the limbic system has never been well defined nor is it clear that the structures involved (amygdala, hippocampus, and cingulate gyrus) have unique connections that process emotions. The problem originates from the attempt to impose emotional functions onto a number of closely related structures, rather than trying to find which structures are responsible for particular emotions. We prefer to identify the neuroanatomy involved with a specific emotion instead of using the more ambiguous limbic system concept.

Hypothalamus

If there is a tiny person that sits inside our head, watching the "control panel" from our body and making decisions about internal settings, he or she is sitting at the hypothalamus. This small cluster of nuclei makes up less than 1% of the brain mass yet has powerful effects on the body's homeostasis. The hypothalamus controls basic functions such as eating, drinking, sleeping, and temperature regulation, to name a few. A small lesion in the hypothalamus has devastating effects on the body's basic functions. The suprachiasmatic nucleus is an

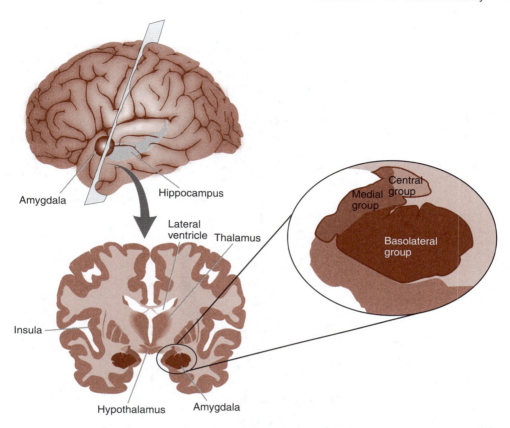

FIGURE 2.8 The location and groups (often called *nuclei*) of the amygdala. (Adapted from Bear MF, Connors BW, Paradiso MA, eds. *Neuroscience: Exploring the Brain*. 4th ed. Baltimore: Lippincott Williams & Wilkins; 2015.)

example of a small cluster of cells within the hypothalamus that has a profound impact on sleep–wake cycles (see Figure 15.8).

The hypothalamus sits in a commanding position within the central nervous system (CNS), between the cortex and brain stem (Figure 2.9). It receives input from four sources: the higher cortex, the brain stem, internal chemoreceptors, and hormonal feedback. The cortex relays filtered cognitive and emotional information about the external environment. The sensory neurons in the body send signals about the internal milieu up through the brain stem. The hypothalamus has its own chemoreceptors that measure glucose, osmolarity, temperature, and so on in the blood. Finally, the hypothalamus receives feedback from the steroid hormones and neuropeptides.

The hypothalamus lies on either side of the third ventricle and is divided into three zones. The lateral zone controls arousal and motivated behavior. The medial zone is more involved with homeostasis and reproduction. The periventricular zone is of most interest to us. It includes the suprachiasmatic nucleus, the cells that control the autonomic nervous system (ANS) and the neurosecretory neurons that extend into the pituitary (see Chapter 7, Hormones and the Brain).

AUTONOMIC NERVOUS SYSTEM

The two branches of ANS can be thought of as the brain's conduit to the vital organs of the body (Figure 2.10). One branch is the sympathetic division, which originates in the posterolateral region of the periventricular zone of the hypothalamus. The other branch is the parasympathetic division, which originates in the anterior cells of the same zone in the hypothalamus. The sympathetic and parasympathetic divisions appear to operate in parallel but with opposite effects, using different neurotransmitters.

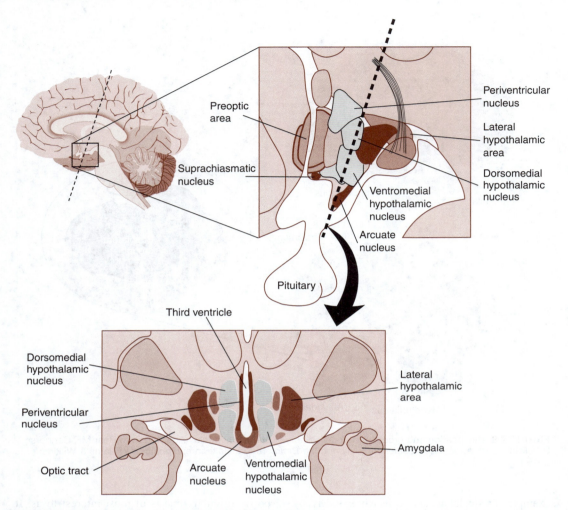

FIGURE 2.9 The hypothalamus lies on either side of the third ventricle in close proximity to the pituitary gland. The hypothalamus can be subdivided into multiple nuclei, many of which are not shown. (Adapted from Kandel ER, Schwartz JH, Jessell TM, eds. *Principles of Neural Science*. 4th ed. New York: McGraw-Hill; 2000.)

The sympathetic division, in a simplified sense, controls the fight–flight response and plays a prominent role in the physical symptoms of anxiety, for example, racing heart. These neurons send out axons from the thoracic and lumbar regions to preganglionic neurons, which primarily reside in the sympathetic chain on either side of the spinal cord. The postganglionic sympathetic neurons innervate the smooth muscles of the vital organs as well as the walls of blood vessels. The preganglionic neurons are cholinergic, whereas the postganglionic neurons use norepinephrine. The postganglionic norepinephrine receptors likely explain why β-blockers can be used to quell the physical symptoms of anxiety.

The parasympathetic neurons mediate functions that the body performs in times of calm, for example, digesting food. These neurons emerge from the brain stem and sacral region of the spinal cord. The axons travel longer distances and innervate ganglia typically located at the end organ. Unlike the sympathetic neurons, the parasympathetic neurons are exclusively cholinergic.

For the psychiatrist, the ANS occasionally complicates the treatment of mental disorders—particularly when using the tricyclic antidepressants. Side effects such as dry mouth, tachycardia, and constipation can be seen as an imbalance between the sympathetic and parasympathetic divisions. These symptoms are not so much the result of sympathetic stimulation as they are the result of parasympathetic blockade. The likely culprit is blockade of the muscarinic receptor in the cholinergic neurons of the parasympathetic division.

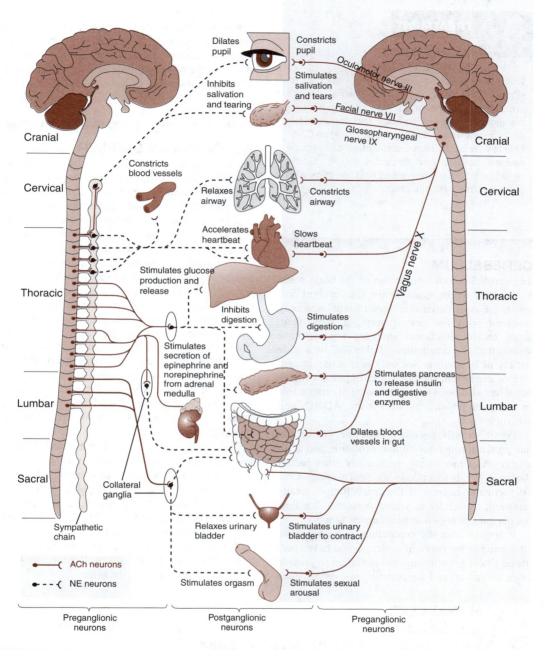

Sympathetic division

Parasympathetic division

Dilates pupil

Constricts pupil

Inhibits salivation and tearing

Stimulates salivation and tears

Oculomotor nerve III

Facial nerve VII

Glossopharyngeal nerve IX

Cranial

Cranial

Cervical

Constricts blood vessels

Relaxes airway

Constricts airway

Cervical

Accelerates heartbeat

Slows heartbeat

Stimulates glucose production and release

Thoracic

Inhibits digestion

Stimulates digestion

Thoracic

Vagus nerve X

Stimulates secretion of epinephrine and norepinephrine from adrenal medulla

Stimulates pancreas to release insulin and digestive enzymes

Lumbar

Lumbar

Dilates blood vessels in gut

Sacral

Collateral ganglia

Sacral

Sympathetic chain

Relaxes urinary bladder

Stimulates urinary bladder to contract

•—(ACh neurons

•- - -(NE neurons

Stimulates orgasm

Stimulates sexual arousal

Preganglionic neurons

Postganglionic neurons

Preganglionic neurons

FIGURE 2.10 The two divisions of the autonomic nervous system and the end organs they innervate. (Adapted from Bear MF, Connors BW, Paradiso MA, eds. *Neuroscience: Exploring the Brain*. 4th ed. Baltimore: Lippincott Williams & Wilkins; 2015.)

DISORDER

CARDIAC AUTONOMIC ACTIVITY

A 2016 prospective study of 1 million Swedish recruits found that heart rate at the age of 18 years was associated with psychiatric disorders as they became adults. Men with resting heart rates above 82 beats per minute (compared to 62 bpm) were at increased risk for OCD, schizophrenia, and anxiety disorder. In contrast, men with lower resting heart rates were more likely to exhibit substance use disorders and violent behavior. Similar associations were observed with blood pressure.

VAGUS NERVE STIMULATION

The ANS actually is a two-way street. That is, signals originating from the internal organs proceed up to the brain. Remarkably 80% of the signals traveling through the vagus nerve are afferent—from the organs toward the CNS. This is why vagus nerve stimulation can reduce seizure activity and improve mood. Some smart people have remarked that we think with our body, not just our brain.

CEREBELLUM

The cerebellum sits on the top of the brain stem, at the back of the skull, below the cerebral cortex. Once considered the "lesser brain" and only involved with the coordination of movement, more recent functional imaging studies have shown that the cerebellum "lights up" in a wide variety of behaviors. Not only is it active in sensation, cognition, memory, and impulse control, but it has also been suggested to be playing a role in the pathophysiology of autism, ADHD, and schizophrenia.

Fossil records document that the cerebellum has grown throughout human evolution and actually contains more neurons than any other part of the brain. Yet its function is not clearly understood. Of particular interest, if the cerebellum is totally removed, especially in young persons, with time the person can regain almost normal function.

It appears that the cerebellum is a supportive structure for the cerebral cortex. Some have speculated that it grew throughout evolution to provide extra computational support for an overburdened cortex. This reasoning proposes that the cerebellum is not responsible for any one particular task but rather functions as an auxiliary structure for the entire cerebral cortex—not just motor coordination. In the future we anticipate increased reports of the important role of the cerebellum in mental illness.

BLOOD–BRAIN BARRIER

The brain needs to be bathed in a pristine extracellular environment. If the brain is exposed to the fluctuations in hormones, amino acids, or ions as occurs in the rest of the body, unexpected neuronal activity could result. The brain uses the *blood–brain barrier* (BBB) to live in a more muted environment buffered from the hysterical fluctuations of the body.

Historically, it was thought that the barrier was produced by the astrocytes that hold the capillaries with their foot processes. Later it became clear that it is the *tight junctions* between the endothelial cells of the capillaries that prevent many substances from leaking into the CNS (Figure 2.11). There are a few areas of the brain that have gaps in the BBB. The pituitary gland and some parts of the hypothalamus are two examples of these BBB gap regions. This is appropriate because these areas need to receive unfiltered feedback regarding the status of the endocrine system by way of the circulating blood.

The BBB is not an impenetrable wall because the brain needs constant supplies to perform its functions. Lipid-soluble substances can readily diffuse through the lipophilic cell walls. Conversely, water-soluble substances are deflected by the endothelial cell wall. Yet the brain needs some water-soluble substances, such as glucose, and indeed there are active transport mechanisms within the endothelial cell wall to bring these essential substances into the brain.

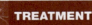

BREACHING THE BLOOD–BRAIN BARRIER

Approximately 98% of small molecules and nearly all the large molecules do not cross the BBB. Overcoming this obstacle is of utmost importance if new therapeutic agents are to reach their target. Several options are being explored—some more reasonable than others.

(1) Implants—medications impregnated in biodegradable wafers placed in the brain. (2) Administering high-frequency ultrasound or transcranial magnetic stimulation to disrupt the BBB and increase penetration of the drug into the brain. (3) Intranasal delivery. (4) Trojan horse—attach the medication to a molecule that binds with a transcytosis receptor. The medication then sneaks into the brain by endocytosis. (5) If all else fails, direct injection into the brain—always a favorite.

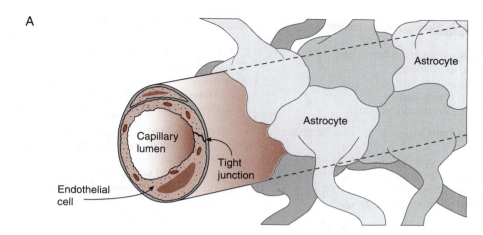

A

Astrocyte

Astrocyte

Capillary
lumen

Tight
junction

Endothelial
cell

B

Capillary lumen

Brain tissue

Passive exclusion:
Water soluble
e.g., dopamine

Active removal
(P-glycoprotein)
e.g., glycine

Passive diffusion:
Lipid soluble
e.g., O_2, ethanol

Active transport
e.g., glucose

Transcytosis
(receptor-mediated)
e.g., insulin, transferrin

FIGURE 2.11 A: The tight junctions formed by the brain endothelial cells along with the astrocytes make up the blood–brain barrier. **B:** Transport mechanisms facilitate or impede the movement of substances between the brain and blood stream. (**A:** Adapted from Goldstein GW, Betz AL. The blood-brain barrier. *Sci Am.* 1986;255[3]:74–83. Figure adapted from original by Patricia J. Wynne.)

The endothelial cells also actively transport offensive substances out of the brain's extracellular environment. The P-glycoprotein is such a transporter. Found in the gut as well as the brain, this protein actively removes a wide variety of drugs and deposits them in the capillary lumen. For example, the newer antihistamines are excluded from the CNS by this protein so they can work their magic on allergens in the body but not sedate the brain. Some psychiatrists speculate that a very active P-glycoprotein transporter contributes to treatment resistance by diminishing the cerebral concentration of medications; for example, olanzapine and risperidone are substrates for P-glycoprotein.

QUESTIONS

1. Brodmann's areas are differentiated by the
   a. Cortical morphology.
   b. Cellular architecture.
   c. Afferent connections.
   d. Predominant neurotransmitter.

2. The orbitofrontal aspect of the PFC describes the area
   a. Above the corpus callosum.
   b. Posterior to the amygdala.
   c. At the base of the PFC.
   d. Anterior to the cingulate gyrus.

3. Lesions of the medical (also ventromedial) PFC are associated with
   a. Paucity of spontaneous behavior—apathetic.
   b. Disorganized cognitive function.
   c. Concrete thinking.
   d. Poor impulse control.

4. All of the following are true about the hippocampus except that it
   a. Is smaller in some psychiatric disorders.
   b. Is involved with memory.
   c. Is disrupted by frontal lobotomy.
   d. Contains undifferentiated stem cells.

5. The "command center" of the brain is the
   a. Hippocampus.
   b. Amygdala.
   c. Autonomic nervous system.
   d. Hypothalamus.

6. All of the following are true about the sympathetic nervous system except that it
   a. Stimulates digestion.
   b. Is associated with anxiety.
   c. Stimulates secretions from the adrenal medulla.
   d. Relaxes the airways.

7. The cerebellum
   a. Solely functions to support movement.
   b. Has been implicated with autism.
   c. Is similar to the motor cortex.
   d. Is relatively small in humans.

8. The BBB can be crossed by all of the following except
   a. Lipid-soluble molecules.
   b. Active transport across the cell wall.
   c. Breaches in the tight junctions.
   d. Most medications.

See Answers section at the end of this book.

CHAPTER 3

Cells and Circuits

THE NEURONAL CELL

The human brain is the most complex organ known to exist in the universe. Its weight is just 3% of the body, but it consumes 17% of the body's energy. The workhorse of the brain is the neuron. It is estimated that we have 100 billion neurons with 100 trillion connections. When we think of a neuron, we are typically thinking of a pyramidal neuron in the cerebral cortex. These neurons have a diamond-shaped cell body and usually reside in layers III or V of the gray matter (Figure 3.1).

Let's start with a brief review of cell biology. The cell body of the neuron is full of the usual assortment of organelles, although not in the same proportions as seen in nonneural cells. Structures such as the *endoplasmic reticulum* (ER) and *mitochondria* are found more frequently in neurons than in other brain cells, presumably because of the increased need for protein synthesis and energy production. The instructions for the functioning of the cell are contained in the DNA, which resides in the nucleus. The instructions are read when the DNA is *transcribed* into messenger ribonucleic acid (mRNA), which is *translated* into proteins in the cytoplasm (Figure 3.2). As mentioned in Chapter 1, Introduction, this process is often called *gene expression*—two of our favorite words.

The *ribosome* is the organelle in which mRNA is translated into proteins (Figure 3.3). The ribosomes are usually attached to the rough ER but can also be floating freely in the cytoplasm. The proteins, once they are refined, are used by the cell for structural (e.g., receptors), functional (e.g., enzymes), or communication (e.g., neuropeptides) purposes, to name a few.

The *Golgi apparatus*, which looks like ER without the ribosomes, is where much of the "post-translation" refinement, sorting, and storage of proteins occurs. This structure enables proteins to be appropriately transported to distant sites within the cell.

The *mitochondria* are the remarkably abundant energy generators of the neuron. The brain requires considerable energy, even at rest, just to maintain an electrical gradient poised to respond at a moment's notice. The mitochondria convert adenosine diphosphate (ADP) into adenosine triphosphate (ATP), and it is ATP that the cell uses to perform its functions.

POINT OF INTEREST

One of our former patients, a very bright man with bipolar disorder and diabetes, could lower his blood glucose level (when it was high) by solving calculus equations—a good example of the propensity of the brain to be an energy hog (and the effort needed to master calculus).

The *dendrites* are the part of the neuron that sprout off the cell body and look like tree branches. They are often called the *ears* of the neuron for they receive input from other neurons and relay the signal to the cell body. Most dendrites have "little knobs" along their stalks that are called *dendritic spines*. Each spine is the postsynaptic receptor for an incoming signal from another neuron (Figure 3.4).

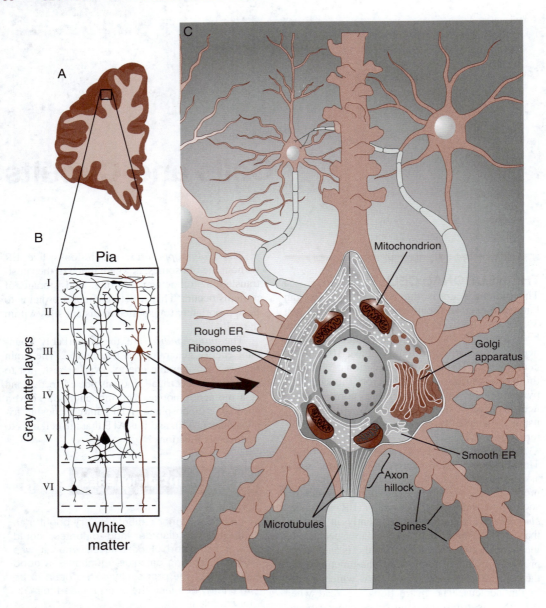

FIGURE 3.1 A: Cross section of the right prefrontal cortex (PFC). **B:** The six layers of neurons in the gray matter of the PFC. **C:** A stereotypical pyramidal neuron found in layer III of the cerebral cortex. ER, endoplasmic reticulum. (Adapted from Bear MF, Connors BW, Paradiso MA, eds. *Neuroscience: Exploring the Brain*. 4th ed. Baltimore: Lippincott Williams & Wilkins; 2015.)

The morphology (structure and density) of the dendritic spines has been a source of considerable interest since Ramón y Cajal first identified them over one hundred years ago. Spines can change in shape, volume, and number with remarkable speed and frequency. This plasticity is one of the great discoveries of modern neuroscience. We mention spines throughout this book as their morphology changes in a number of conditions, including substance abuse, mental retardation, schizophrenia, and learning (see Point of Interest).

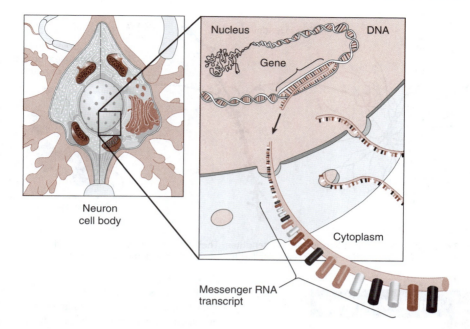

FIGURE 3.2 Messenger ribonucleic acid (mRNA) carries the genetic instructions from the nucleus to the cytoplasm where translation into proteins occurs. (Adapted from Bear MF, Connors BW, Paradiso MA, eds. *Neuroscience: Exploring the Brain*. 4th ed. Baltimore: Lippincott Williams & Wilkins; 2015.)

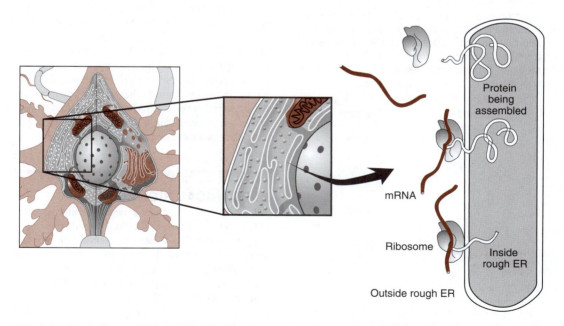

FIGURE 3.3 Messenger ribonucleic acid (mRNA) binds to a ribosome, initiating protein synthesis. Proteins synthesized on the rough endoplasmic reticulum (ER) as shown are eventually inserted into the membrane. Proteins synthesized on free ribosomes (not shown) are utilized in the cytosol. (Adapted from Bear MF, Connors BW, Paradiso MA, eds. *Neuroscience: Exploring the Brain*. 4th ed. Baltimore: Lippincott Williams & Wilkins; 2015.)

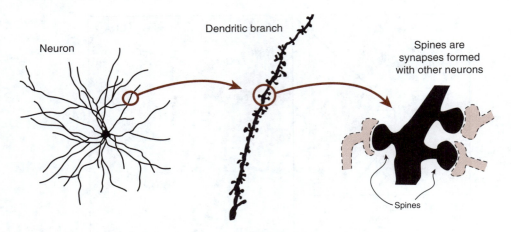

Neuron

Dendritic branch

Spines are synapses formed with other neurons

Spines

FIGURE 3.4 Spines are the "little knobs" on the dendrites. They are on the receiving side of the electrochemical signal from other neurons—also called the postsynaptic membrane.

POINT OF INTEREST

Enhanced branching and spine formation have been found consistently in rats raised in enriched environments when compared with rats raised in standard wire cages. The neurons in the following figure are from rats raised in different environments. Note the increased branching (also called *arborization*) of the neuron from the rat raised in the enriched environment. Abundant dendritic branching with multiple connections seems to be a microscopic sign of a healthy active brain.

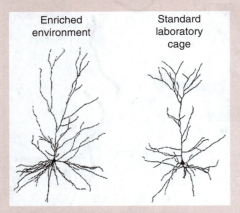

Enriched environment

Standard laboratory cage

(Reprinted from Kolb B, Forgie M, Gibb R, et al. Age, experience and the changing brain. *Neurosci Biobehav Rev*. 1998;22[2]:143–159. Copyright 1998 with permission from Elsevier.)

The *axon* is perhaps the most unique structure of the neuron. Starting at the *axon hillock* and running anywhere from a few micrometers to the entire length of the spinal cord, the axon can transmit a signal quickly without degradation to other neurons or end organs. For this reason the axon is often conceptualized as the telephone wire of the brain. Because the axon is devoid of ribosomes and incapable of protein synthesis, a process called *axoplasmic transport* enables the neuron to send material down the microtubules to the distal ends of the cell.

The terminal end of the axon forms the synapse (Figure 3.5). This is where one neuron talks to another—if the dendrites are the ears, the synapse is the voice. Here the electrical signal streaming down the axon is converted into a chemical signal, so the impulse can pass from one cell to another. The neurotransmitters that form the basis of the chemical signal are stored in vesicles. When released, they diffuse across the synaptic cleft to receptors on the postsynaptic dendrite (more on this later in the chapter).

ELECTRICAL SIGNALING

All living cells maintain a negative internal electronic charge relative to the fluid outside the cell—roughly—60 mV in a neuron. Nerve cells use the depolarization (rapid change in the electrical charge) to communicate with other nerves or end organs. There are two basic steps in this process. The neuron first receives signals through the dendrites—what are called *postsynaptic potentials*. Second, the cell sums the incoming impulses, and if they are high enough, then it sends an impulse down the axon—an *action potential*.

Postsynaptic Potentials

A single pyramidal cell will receive input from 1 to 100,000 neurons through the postsynaptic

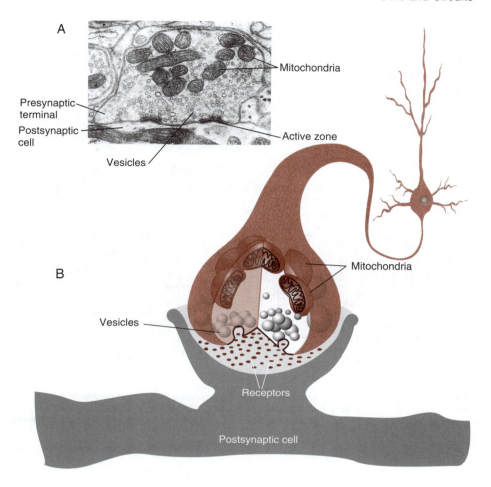

FIGURE 3.5 A synapse seen with an electron microscope **(A)** and in a schematic drawing **(B)**. Note the high concentration of vesicles filled with neurotransmitter and mitochondria to power the rapid processing. (Adapted from Bear MF, Connors BW, Paradiso MA, eds. *Neuroscience: Exploring the Brain*. 4th ed. Baltimore: Lippincott Williams & Wilkins; 2015.)

synapses (spines) on the dendrites and cell body. When the neurotransmitters bind with the receptor at the postsynaptic synapse, ions flow into the neuron and change the electrical potential, making it more positive or more negative—or what is called depolarization and hyperpolarization.

This proceeds in two ways:

Depolarize (excitatory) with an influx of positive ions such as Na+.
Hyperpolarize (inhibitory) with an influx of negative ions such as Cl−.

These are appropriately called *excitatory postsynaptic potentials* (*EPSPs*) and *inhibitory postsynaptic potentials* (*IPSPs*) (Figures 3.6 and 3.7). The EPSP and IPSP are, respectively, the accelerator and brake for the brain. An EPSP is more likely to generate an action potential; an IPSP inhibits the generation of an action potential. The goal for a healthy brain is to maintain the correct balance—if there is too much excitation, one can have a seizure; if there is too much inhibition, the brain is sluggish, even comatose. Actually, most of us want our brains to be excited during the day and inhibited at night—something our residual paleolithic brains are not always wired to accommodate.

The Action Potential

The decision to fire an action potential is made at the axon hillock. Moment to moment, the sum of all the incoming EPSPs and IPSPs at the axon hillock determines whether the neuron sends an impulse down the axon. If the potential has depolarized to the threshold, then an action potential is generated. Figure 3.8 shows how the neuron requires enough depolarization (excitation) but not too much hyperpolarization (inhibition) to generate an action potential.

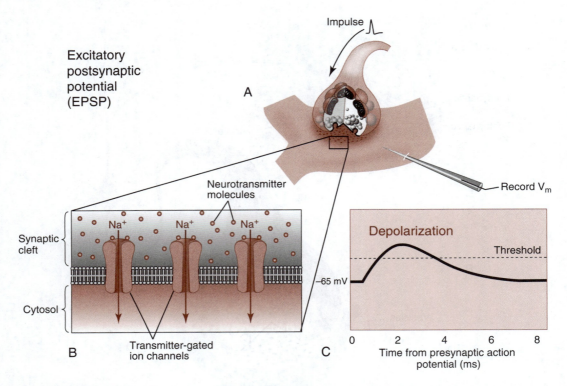

FIGURE 3.6 Neurotransmission from an *excitatory* neuron **(A)** promotes the entry of *positively* charged sodium ions into the dendrite **(B)**. The resulting depolarization generates an EPSP **(C)**. (Adapted from Bear MF, Connors BW, Paradiso MA, eds. *Neuroscience: Exploring the Brain*. 4th ed. Baltimore: Lippincott Williams & Wilkins; 2015.)

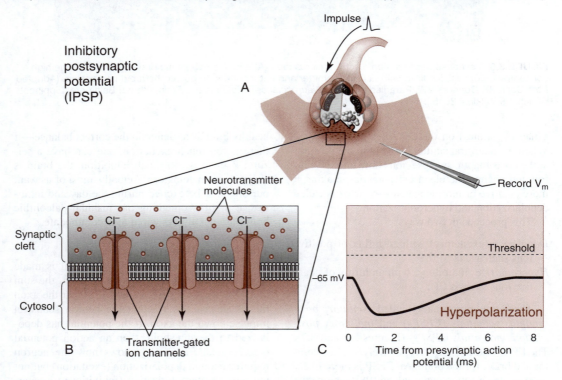

FIGURE 3.7 Neurotransmission from an *inhibitory* neuron **(A)** promotes the entry of *negatively* charged chloride ions into the dendrite **(B)**. The resulting hyperpolarization generates an IPSP **(C)**. (Adapted from Bear MF, Connors BW, Paradiso MA, eds. *Neuroscience: Exploring the Brain*. 4th ed. Baltimore: Lippincott Williams & Wilkins; 2015.)

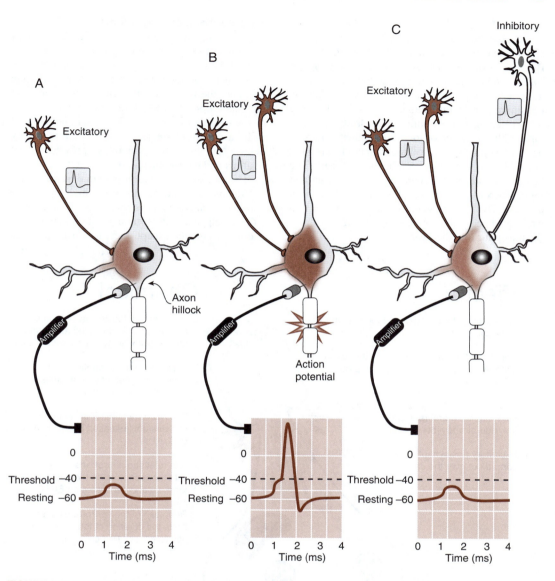

FIGURE 3.8 A signal from one excitatory neuron **(A)** increases the excitatory postsynaptic potential (EPSP) but is not sufficient to reach the threshold. Two excitatory impulses reaching the neuron at the same time **(B)** generate an EPSP that reaches the threshold at the axon hillock, and an action potential is fired. However, with inhibitory input from a third neuron **(C)**, the membrane potential again fails to reach the threshold.

TREATMENT

CALM DOWN

We often treat patients who have too much cerebral activity. Anxiety, attention deficit hyperactivity disorder, insomnia, and mania are four conditions in which the brain is going too fast. Such patients have too much excitation and not enough inhibition. It is encouraging that more research is being directed toward treatments that increase inhibitory potentials (e.g., γ-aminobutyric acid). The challenge is to selectively inhibit the annoying trait without slowing down the whole brain: calmer but not dumber.

Once the threshold (−40 mV) has been reached at the axon hillock, the neuron "pulls the trigger" and shoots an action potential down the axon. Because of the unique design of the *voltage-gated sodium channels*, the action potential maintains its integrity as it proceeds along the axon—there is no diminution in the signal. This occurs because the voltage-gated sodium channels facilitate a rapid influx of positive ions. Like other ion channels, the voltage-gated sodium channel is a protein embedded in the lipid member of the cell. The "gated" nature of the channel allows a large and rapid influx of the ions once the threshold has been crossed. The voltage-gated channel is like a trap waiting to be sprung. When the switch is tripped, the ions pour into the axon.

Electrochemical Signaling

Otto Loewi demonstrated in 1921 that the communication within the nervous system is *both* electrical and chemical. Figure 3.9 shows a representation of the arrival of the action potential at the synaptic terminal, the release of the neurotransmitters, and the generation of an EPSP or IPSP in the dendrite of the neighboring neuron. This example happens to be a dopamine neuron, which is an excitatory neuron, but the same principles apply to all the neurons and neurotransmitters.

The arrival of the action potential at the terminal depolarizes the membrane, which opens the *voltage-gated calcium channels*. The voltage-gated calcium channels are similar to the voltage-gated sodium channels except they are permeable to

Electro

1. The action potential arrives at the presynaptic terminal.

2. Depolarization causes voltage-gated calcium channels to open and results in a large influx of Ca^{2+}.

3. Exocytosis: Ca^{2+} causes the vesicles to fuse with the membrane and release the neurotransmitter.

4. Excitatory postsynaptic potentials (EPSPs) spread out over the dendrite.

Chemical

A. Precursor molecules and enzymes are transported down the axon from the cell body along the microtubules.

B. Enzymes in the synaptic terminal convert the precursor molecules into active neurotransmitter.

C. The neurotransmitter is stored in the vesicles until released by the influx of Ca^{2+}.

D. The released neurotransmitter binds with the receptors on the postsynaptic terminal and generates an EPSP.

E. Reuptake of the neurotransmitter limits the duration of the signal and allows the cell to recycle the neurotransmitter.

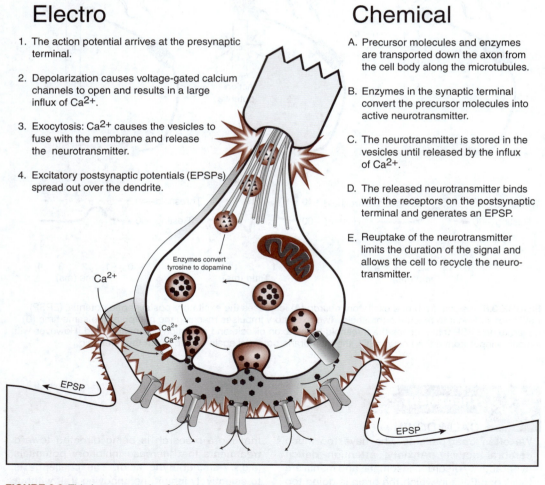

Enzymes convert tyrosine to dopamine

Ca^{2+}

Ca^{2+}
Ca^{2+}

EPSP

EPSP

FIGURE 3.9 This is an example of the electrochemical signaling from a dopamine neuron. If this were an inhibitory neuron, γ-aminobutyric acid or glycine for example, the postsynaptic potential would be an inhibitory postsynaptic potential and not an excitatory postsynaptic potential. (Adapted from Rosenzweig MR, Watson NV. *Biological Psychology*. 7th ed. Sunderland, MA: Sinauer; 2013, by permission of Oxford University Press, USA.)

Ca^{2+}. Consequently, there is a large and rapid influx of Ca^{2+}, which is required for *exocytosis* and the release of the neurotransmitter.

NONNEURONAL CELLS

The glial cells that make up the rest of the cells in the central nervous system (CNS) actually outnumber the neurons by 9:1. Traditionally seen as supportive cells with no role in communication, recent research has shown that glial cells modulate the synaptic activity. There are three kinds of glial cells: astrocyte, oligodendrocyte, and microglia. The microglia are similar to macrophages found in the peripheral tissue. They respond to injury with a dramatic increase in their numbers and remove cellular debris from the damaged area. (For more information on the microglia, refer Chapter 9, Immunity and Inflammation.)

The oligodendrocyte is considered the CNS equivalent of the Schwann cell in the peripheral nervous system (Figures 3.10 and 23.10). They are the cells that wrap myelin around the axons of the neurons, and by acting as an electrical insulator, they greatly increase the speed of the transmission of the action potential. This process of myelinization is not complete at birth and proceeds rapidly in the first years of life, which has a dramatic effect on behavior. In children, this process results in improved motor skills as they mature. Complete myelinization of the prefrontal cortex (PFC) is delayed until the second and even third decade of life. Hence why we worry about our teens—the bodies of adults without the brakes of matured frontal lobes.

Demyelinating disorders such as multiple sclerosis and Guillain–Barré have devastating effects on patients. Clearly, a neuron without its myelin is not as effective. Regarding mental illness, recent research suggests that some failure in myelination may play a role in schizophrenia.

The astrocyte is the star-shaped cell that fills the spaces between the neurons (Figure 3.11). We have already seen that the astrocyte plays a role in maintaining the blood–brain barrier, but other functions include regulating the chemistry of the extracellular fluid, providing structural support, and bringing nutrients to the neurons. Even more interesting is the role the astrocyte plays in modulating the electrical activity at the synapse. Research has shown that astrocytes encircle the synapse and have receptors that respond to the neurotransmitters released by the neuron. The astrocyte may in turn release its own neurotransmitter, which enhances the transmission of the signal. This may facilitate learning and memory. Additionally, there is evidence that the presence of astrocytes or their proteins increases the number of synapses a neuron

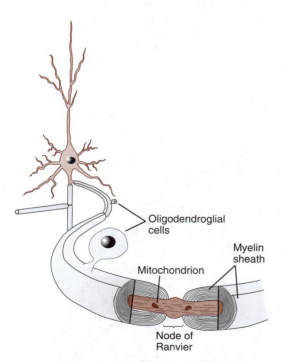

FIGURE 3.10 Oligodendroglial cells wrap a myelin sheath around the axon, providing electrical insulation. This can improve the speed of the transmission of an action potential up to 15 times. (Adapted from Bear MF, Connors BW, Paradiso MA, eds. *Neuroscience: Exploring the Brain*. 4th ed. Baltimore: Lippincott Williams & Wilkins; 2015.)

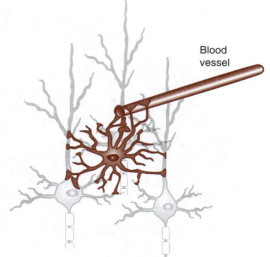

FIGURE 3.11 The astrocyte not only supports the neurons and blood vessels but also has some role in modulating the transmission of information.

will form. The lowly glial cells are more involved in the communication within the brain than previously thought.

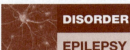

DISORDER

EPILEPSY

Increasing evidence is pointing to the astrocyte as playing an instigating role in epilepsy—a problem historically assigned to dysfunctional neurons. Analysis of specimens after surgical resection for epilepsy often shows prominent gliosis. Glutamate released from astrocytes can trigger experimental models of seizures. Finally, several effective antiepileptic drugs (such as valproate, gabapentin, and phenytoin) potently reduce astrocytic Ca^{2+} signaling—an event believed to precede seizure activity. If aberrant astrocytes are the nidus for seizures, then new treatments might be developed that can calm the astrocytes without dulling the neurons.

CIRCUITS

The capacity to communicate quickly over long distances (relative to the size of a cell) is the most unique feature of the nerve cell. Sending a signal, receiving feedback, and adjusting further responses are the essence of communication—cellular or social. The white matter tracts—bundles of axons just underneath the gray matter—connect the nerve cells with other regions of the cortex, subcortical nuclei, and end organs such as muscles and glands (Figure 3.12).

A new imaging technique, called diffusion tensor imaging (DTI), has been developed to assess the quality of the white matter tracts. Using an magnetic resonance imaging scanner, the technique involves following the movement of water (diffusion) in the brain. In most tissue the water molecules move in every direction. In the white matter tracts, the water molecules tend to move along the length of the axons. Thus, with some Herculean number crunching by the MRI computer, images can be produced showing remarkable detail of the white matter tracts (Figure 3.13). Although still a research tool, DTI is being used to identify white matter abnormalities in patients with psychiatric disorders.

The networks that coordinate a behavior are called circuits. A simple example of a circuit is evident in substance abuse. The addict is reminded of getting high and feels a compulsion to use but does not have enough control to abstain and does extraordinary things to get the drug. The interplay of regions involving memories, urges, and control (or absence of control) fails in the substance abuser.

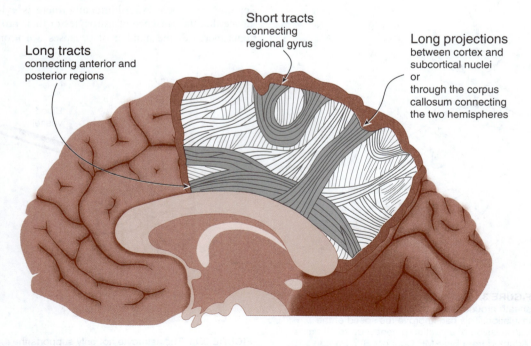

Short tracts
connecting
regional gyrus

Long tracts
connecting anterior and
posterior regions

Long projections
between cortex and
subcortical nuclei
or
through the corpus
callosum connecting
the two hemispheres

FIGURE 3.12 Beneath the gray matter are white matter tracts that allow communication between widely separated regions of the brain or between the brain and end organs. (Adapted from Rosenzweig MR, Watson NV. *Biological Psychology.* 7th ed. Sunderland, MA: Sinauer; 2013, by permission of Oxford University Press, USA.)

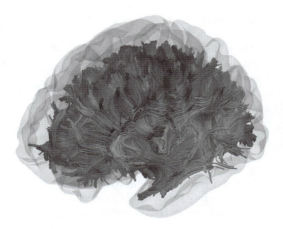

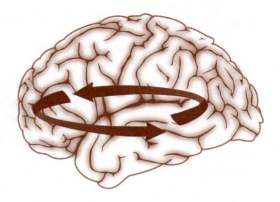

FIGURE 3.14 Dysfunctional circuits may explain behavioral and cognitive symptoms in psychiatric disorders.

FIGURE 3.13 Visualization of white matter tracts in the brain using diffusion tensor imaging technology. (Courtesy of G. Russel Glenn, Medical University of South Carolina, 2016.)

It is the coordination of the circuit—not one particular location in the brain—that goes awry in the substance abuser.

The elusive nature of the biologic causes of mental disorders has been the bane of psychiatry. Although Broca could pinpoint the damaged region to explain his aphasic patients, conspicuous lesions corresponding to psychiatric conditions have not been possible to locate. Increasing evidence suggests that problems in brain circuits may explain variants in behavior. Perhaps this is because it is not one specific region that is at fault but rather the dysfunction of the communication. However, this is difficult to measure.

Figure 3.14 shows a schematic representation of a hypothetical circuit between the PFC, temporal cortex, and subcortical regions. Imaging studies suggest that dysfunction of emotional circuits may explain some psychiatric disorders—particularly depression, anxiety, and substance abuse. One common example involves the PFC. Insufficient activity from the PFC allows the expression of impulses from lower regions of the brain—a problem we will address when we discuss anger, attention, and anxiety.

QUESTIONS

1. The pyramidal cells in the gray matter reside predominantly in which layers?
   a. I and III.
   b. II and IV.
   c. III and V.
   d. IV and VI.

2. Protein synthesis requires all of the following except
   a. Rough ER.
   b. Gene expression.
   c. Transcription and translation.
   d. Messenger RNA.

3. Enhanced arborization of the dendrites is found with
   a. Mental retardation.
   b. Stimulating environments.
   c. Usual laboratory environments.
   d. Schizophrenia.

4. An IPSP
   a. Results from the influx of sodium ions.
   b. Depolarizes the cell.
   c. Can induce seizures.
   d. Hyperpolarizes the cell.

5. The neuron generates an action potential based on the postsynaptic potential at the
   a. Axon hillock.
   b. Synapse.
   c. Nucleus.
   d. Node of Ranvier.

6. Exocytosis of the neurotransmitters at the synapse requires opening of the
   a. Voltage-gated sodium channels.
   b. Voltage-gated calcium channels.
   c. Excitatory postsynaptic channels.
   d. Inhibitory postsynaptic channels.

7. The cell responsible for myelin in the CNS is
   a. Astrocyte.
   b. Microglia.
   c. Schwann cell.
   d. Oligodendrocyte.

8. Modulates electrochemical activity at the synapse:
   a. Astrocyte.
   b. Microglia.
   c. Schwann cell.
   d. Oligodendrocyte.

See Answers section at the end of this book.

CHAPTER 4

Neurotransmitters

A "neurotransmitter" is technically defined by meeting three criteria:

1. The substance must be stored in the presynaptic neuron.
2. It must be released with depolarization of the presynaptic neuron induced by the influx of Ca^{2+}.
3. The substance must bind with a specific receptor on the postsynaptic neuron.

Neurotransmitters differ from hormones by their close physical proximity of the release to the receptor—although this turns out to be less straightforward than one might imagine.

The classic neurotransmitters—the ones we frequently discuss—are small molecules designed for economy of use. For neurotransmitters, the body needs a substrate that can be

produced quickly, with ease, and be recycled—much like the daily newspaper. Figure 4.1 shows some representative neurotransmitters compared with a neuropeptide substance P. The common neurotransmitters such as γ-aminobutyric acid (GABA) and norepinephrine (NE) are small and constructed with elements that are easy for the body to find. This facilitates the rapid creation and release of the signals that are the essential features of neural communication.

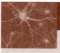

POINT OF INTEREST

The body—in all its wisdom—has developed only a small number of neurotransmitters. Rather than having a billion separate molecules, each transmitting a specific message, the body has a limited number of neurotransmitters that mean different things in different places. Much like the alphabets where 26 letters can create innumerable words, the body uses only a few hundred neurotransmitters to coordinate the most complex organ in the universe.

POINT OF INTEREST

It is not uncommon in our practices for patients to announce at the initial evaluation, "Doc, I have a chemical imbalance," as though it is some sort of *Diagnostic and Statistical Manual of Mental Disorders* (DSM) diagnosis. It is not likely that a "chemical imbalance" is the source of mental illness, but most assuredly the manipulation of these chemicals remains the bread and butter of psychiatry. They are the *chemical* part of the "electrochemical" communication and the focus of this chapter.

An extensive review of all known neurotransmitters is beyond the scope of this book. We will focus on the relevant molecules in the following three basic categories:

1. The classic neurotransmitters
2. Neuropeptides
3. Unconventional neurotransmitters

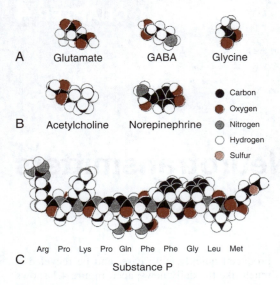

FIGURE 4.1 A sample of neurotransmitters showing the relative size of the amino acids **(A)**, two of the amines **(B)**, and a neuropeptide **(C)**. GABA, γ-aminobutyric acid. (Adapted from Bear MF, Connors BW, Paradiso MA, eds. *Neuroscience: Exploring the Brain*. 4th ed. Baltimore: Lippincott Williams & Wilkins; 2015.)

CLASSIC NEUROTRANSMITTERS

Amino Acids
Glutamate

This is the major workhorse of the brain, with glutamate neurons making up more than half of the *excitatory* neurons. Without glutamate, the brain does not get started or keep running. Glutamate and

another excitatory transmitter *aspartate* are nonessential amino acids that do not cross the blood–brain barrier—otherwise our diet could alter our neural activity. Consequently, glutamate must be synthesized in the brain from glucose and other precursors. Glial cells assist in the reuptake, degradation, and resupply of glutamate for neurons.

DISORDERS

Glutamate neurons seemed to be involved with all the important brain activities—memory formation, motor skills, plasticity, mental illness, etc. They are everywhere! If the brain does it, most likely glutamate was there. However, too much glutamate, as occurs with a stroke, is toxic to the nerve cells. Not only is the cell deprived of oxygen but also the glutamate that is released from the dying cell results in further damage. Efforts are under way to find an agent that will block the toxic effects of glutamate (excitotoxicity inhibitors) during ischemic events to limit the secondary neuronal damage.

γ-Aminobutyric Acid and Glycine

GABA is the major inhibitory transmitter in the brain and is used by approximately 25% of the cortical neurons. Glycine is the other, but less common, inhibitory amino acid. GABA puts the brakes on the brain: not enough GABA, one can have seizures. The GABA neurons are primarily the interneurons in the gray matter. They provide local constraint over too much cortical circuitry. Figure 3.7 shows an example of a

POINT OF INTEREST

Of the classic neurotransmitters, the monoamines are the ones we typically talk about. Hanging around psychiatrists, one might imagine that the brain is predominately made up of dopamine (DA), serotonin, and NE. Amazingly, these agents are in the minority in the brain. The largest number of neurons and the ones that do the heavy lifting in the brain come from the amino acid group, of which glutamate and GABA are the most prominent. The pie chart gives a very rough estimate of the relative proportion of several important neurotransmitters. The neuropeptides (discussed later) would only be a line on this chart.

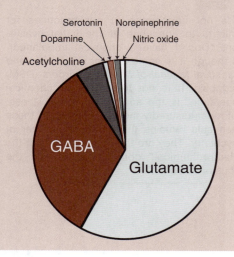

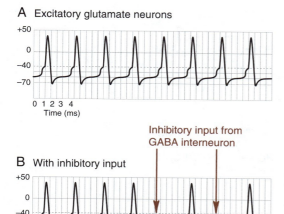

A Excitatory glutamate neurons

B With inhibitory input

Inhibitory input from
GABA interneuron

FIGURE 4.2 Effects of inhibitory input. **A:** Without GABA inhibition (or any other inhibition), the neuron fires regularly. **B:** With input from a GABA interneuron (in *brown*), some action potentials are inhibited. GABA, γ-aminobutyric acid.

GABA neuron hyperpolarizing the receiving neuron, so that it is less likely to fire an action potential.

Similarly, Figure 4.2 shows how input from a GABA interneuron quiets an overactive glutamate neuron. One can see how increasing GABAergic activity can be an effective treatment for epilepsy. More recently, increasing GABAergic activity has been used to treat insomnia, pain, and anxiety and to assist in the management of mania—all situations where too much central nervous system (CNS) activity is a component of the disorder.

Monoamines

The monoamines modulate the activity of the excitatory and inhibitory neurons. Although small in total number compared with glutamate or GABA, the monoamine neurons project widely throughout the brain. They have the capacity to "fine-tune" and coordinate the response of the major neurons.

There are two principal classes of monoamines: *catecholamines* (DA, NE, and epinephrine) and *indoleamines* (serotonin and melatonin). After being released, monoamines are degraded or reprocessed by the neuron. (Clinicians often refer to this as the reuptake pump, but neuroscientists call this the *transporter*, e.g., the DA transporter.) The class of enzymes in the terminal that degrades the neurotransmitters is the monoamine oxidases (MAOs). MAO inhibitors cause an increase in monoamines (e.g., DA, NE, and serotonin), by limiting the degradation process, with well-known benefits for depression and anxiety.

Unfortunately, some food products and medications enhance the release of NE. When the MAOs are inhibited, an excessive amount of NE is released. This can result in dangerous elevations in blood pressure, which has resulted in stroke and even death in some cases.

Catecholamines

The catecholamines begin as the essential amino acid tyrosine (Figure 4.3), which must be introduced in the diet. L-DOPA is the molecule made famous in the Oliver Sacks story *Awakenings* and remains the gold standard treatment for Parkinson's disease. The structures of DA, NE, and epinephrine are remarkably similar yet have different functions in the brain.

Dopamine

The DA neurons constitute only about half a million of the cells in the brain—a tiny percentage out of the 100 billion total cells (Figure 4.4). Three nuclei contain the cell bodies that project the three primary branches of the DA network. The *substantia nigra* located in the ventral midbrain has primary projections to the caudate and putamen (collectively called the *striatum*). This pathway is called the *nigrostriatal system* or *mesostriatal system*. As part of the basal ganglia, this pathway is integral to voluntary movement. Parkinson's disease is the result of a loss of DA neurons in the substantia nigra. The extrapyramidal side effects due to antipsychotic medications can induce parkinsonian symptoms by blockade of these neurons.

The cells of the *ventral tegmental area*, also in the ventral midbrain, project to the nucleus accumbens, prefrontal cortex, amygdala, and hippocampus. These innervations, called the *mesolimbocortical DA system*, are particularly dense in primates. Some writers subdivide these branches into the *mesolimbic* (nucleus accumbens, amygdala, and hippocampus) and *mesocortical* (prefrontal cortex), which seems artificial, as they originate from the same cell bodies.

DISORDERS

The branches to the nucleus accumbens are involved with reward and substance abuse. The branches to the prefrontal cortex are involved with attention and cognition and seem to be impaired in patients with attention deficit hyperactivity disorder (ADHD). Some speculate that problems with the mesolimbic system cause the positive symptoms of schizophrenia, whereas negative symptoms are caused by impairment in the mesocortical system.

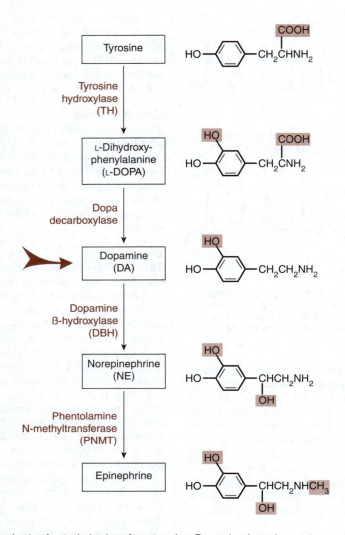

FIGURE 4.3 The synthesis of catecholamines from tyrosine. Dopamine *(arrow)* cannot cross the blood–brain barrier, although some L-DOPA can sneak through. By giving patients dopa decarboxylase inhibitors, such as carbidopa, along with L-DOPA, the half-life of L-DOPA is extended and more crosses into the brain. Furthermore, carbidopa does not cross the blood–brain barrier, so L-DOPA can be converted into dopamine in the brain, and the Parkinson's patient moves with greater ease.

The short tracts in the *arcuate nucleus* of the hypothalamus—called the *tuberoinfundibular DA system*—release DA into the portal veins of the pituitary gland. The synthesis and release of prolactin in the anterior pituitary is inhibited by DA. Any interruption between the DA and the prolactin-producing cells will lead to hyperprolactinemia. Hence, antipsychotic medications that block the DA receptor can cause an increase in prolactin, although it appears to be less with the newer antipsychotic agents for unclear reasons.

Norepinephrine

NE is *noradrenaline* in the United Kingdom, and hence neurons that produce NE are called noradrenergic neurons. These neurons contain an additional enzyme in their terminal buds, which converts DA to NE. Approximately 50% of the NE neurons have their cell bodies located in the locus coeruleus—small nuclei, one on each side of the brain stem. In total there are only about 24,000 neurons in both nuclei. The remainder of the NE neurons is found in loose clusters in the medullary reticular formation (Figure 4.5).

Dopaminergic
neurons

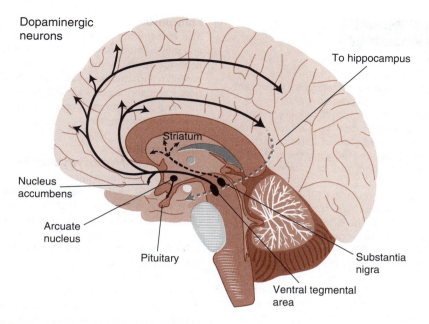

FIGURE 4.4 The three major pathways of the dopaminergic system. The substantia nigra forms the nigrostriatal pathways to the caudate and putamen. The ventral tegmental area projects to the nucleus accumbens and cortex. The arcuate nucleus of the hypothalamus projects to the tuberoinfundibular area of the hypothalamus.

The noradrenergic neurons project to virtually every area of the brain and spinal cord. Although small in number, they are essential for survival of the organism. For example, knockout mice that are deficient in NE cannot survive. The NE neurons play an important role in alertness. The firing of the locus coeruleus increases along a spectrum from drowsy to alert, with the lowest found when we sleep and the highest when we are hypervigilant. Clearly, the noradrenergic neurons are important in handling danger. In a threatening situation, the locus coeruleus is active as are the sympathetic neurons of the autonomic nervous system (ANS) where the peripheral noradrenergic neurons are found.

Noradrenergic
neurons

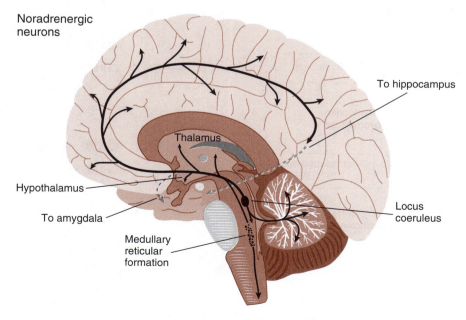

FIGURE 4.5 The noradrenergic system. With projections to almost every area of the brain and spinal cord, the norepinephrine system plays an important role in alertness and anxiety.

TREATMENT

Inappropriate noradrenergic activity, both centrally and peripherally, plays an important role in anxiety and depression. Not only is a rapid heart rate a symptom of anxiety but also a high resting heart rate after a motor vehicle accident is a predictor of later posttraumatic stress disorder. Reducing the activity of these neurons is one goal of pharmacologic treatment.

Vagus nerve stimulation (VNS) is a treatment for medication-resistant depression. Incoming signals to the brain from the vagus nerve give the locus coeruleus information about the state of the internal organs. In a hypervigilant condition such as chronic anxiety, the information from the vagus nerve increases the activity of the locus coeruleus and the NE neurons. VNS may work by regulating the locus coeruleus and the NE system.

NE is cleared from the synaptic cleft by a reuptake transporter that is also capable of taking up DA—most likely due to the structural similarity of these two transmitters (Figure 4.4). This may explain why atomoxetine, an NE reuptake inhibitor, results in an increase in DA (as well as NE) in the prefrontal cortex, even though it does not inhibit the DA reuptake pump.

Epinephrine

The *epinephrine* (or adrenaline) neurons are few and play a minor role in the CNS. Most of the epinephrine in the body is produced in the adrenal medulla and excreted with sympathetic stimulation. Epinephrine plays a much greater role outside the brain as a hormone, compared with its role as a CNS neurotransmitter.

Indoleamines
Serotonin (5-Hydroxytryptamine)

No other neurotransmitter is more closely associated with modern neuropsychopharmacology than serotonin. Also called *5-hydroxytryptamine* (*5-HT*), serotonin is found in many parts of the body outside the CNS, such as platelets and mast cells. Only about 1% to 2% of the body's serotonin is located in the brain.

Serotonin is synthesized from tryptophan, another essential amino acid that cannot be synthesized in the body (Figure 4.6). Unlike the catecholamines, levels of serotonin in the brain can be significantly lowered with insufficient dietary tryptophan (grains, meats, and dairy products are good sources of tryptophan). In the pineal gland, there are two additional enzymes that convert serotonin to *melatonin*, the other indoleamine.

The location of the cell bodies and distribution of the serotonin neurons are similar to those of the catecholamines (Figure 4.7). The cell bodies are relatively few in number (approximately 200,000) and reside in the raphe nuclei in the brain stem. As with NE, the serotonin neurons project to virtually all areas of the brain.

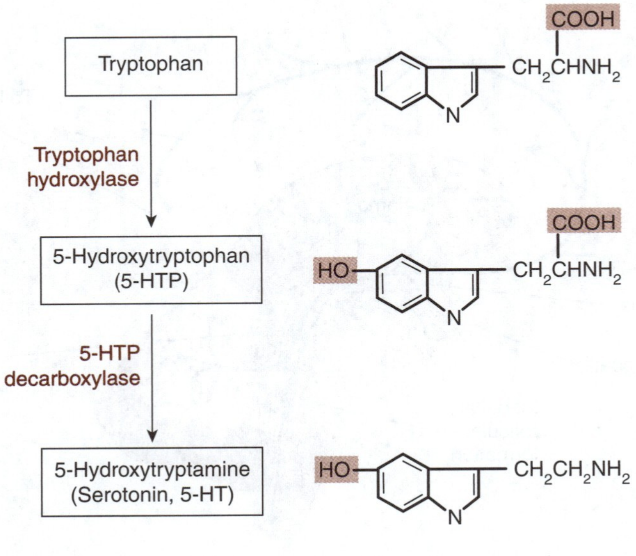

FIGURE 4.6 Serotonin synthesis.

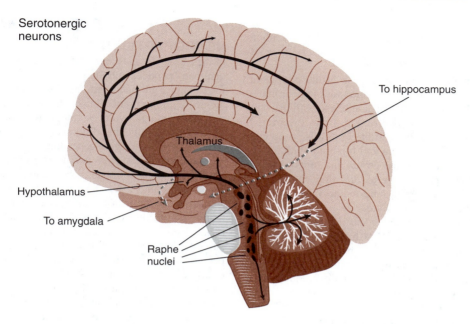

Serotonergic neurons

To hippocampus

Thalamus

Hypothalamus

To amygdala

Raphe nuclei

FIGURE 4.7 The serotonergic system. The cluster of raphe nuclei along the brain stem has projections to most of the brain and spinal cord. These neurons play an important role in mood and anxiety and in the sleep–wake cycle.

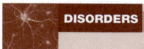

DISORDERS

Serotonin, as with the catecholamines, is removed from the synaptic cleft by the reuptake of the transmitter with the serotonin transporter. It is the blockade of this process that is believed to result in the therapeutic effect of the commonly prescribed antidepressants. Although increasing the availability of serotonin in the synaptic cleft has proven therapeutic value for the treatment of depression, it remains unclear if insufficient serotonin is part of the cause of the disorder.

Histamine

Histamine is not just for itching anymore. Although histamine is released from mast cells as part of an allergic reaction in the peripheral tissue, in the brain it is involved in arousal and attention. Most of the cell bodies start in the tuberomammillary nucleus of the posterior hypothalamus, with sparse but widespread projections to all regions of the brain and spinal cord. The histamine neurons are quiet when mammals are sleeping. As prescribers, we are often struggling with unintended sedation due to blocking of the histamine transmission (antihistamines), for example, tricyclic antidepressants (TCAs), clozapine, or olanzapine.

Alternatively, when the histamine neurons are active, mammals are physically and cognitively alert. Modafinil indirectly activates the histamine neurons and has been used successfully as a treatment for narcolepsy, excessive sleepiness, and ADHD. Histamine-3 receptor antagonists are research medications that also have potential to brighten the brain. Current interests include possible benefits for Alzheimer's disease, ADHD, and drug abuse.

Orexin/Hypocretin

In 1998, two laboratories, almost simultaneously, discovered the same neurotransmitter. One group called them orexins, and the other group named them hypocretin. The scientific community cannot agree on one name. It's so annoying! The orexin/hypocretin (O/H) neurons are remarkably similar to the histamine neurons (which makes things confusing). The cell bodies reside in the hypothalamus and have projections throughout the brain and spinal cord. Furthermore, the O/H neurons modulate sleep and wakefulness, except in the opposite direction of the histamines. Recently, orexin receptor antagonists have been developed and FDA-approved for the treatment of insomnia.

Acetylcholine

In the 1920s, acetylcholine (ACh) was the first molecule to be identified as a neurotransmitter. ACh is the only small molecule transmitter that is not an amino acid or directly derived from one. ACh is actually not a monoamine but is often grouped with these neurotransmitters because of similar size and distribution.

ACh plays a prominent role in the peripheral ANS and is the neurotransmitter at the neuromuscular junction. Its relative ease of accessibility outside the cranium is one reason it was discovered first. The ACh neurons in the CNS arise from cell bodies in the brain stem and forebrain with prominent projections to the cortex and hippocampus. These later projections to the hippocampus are involved with learning and memory and are disrupted in Alzheimer's disease.

ACh is also synthesized in interneurons in the CNS. In the striatum, the ACh neurons balance the dopaminergic input from the substantia nigra to coordinate extrapyramidal motor control. Disruption of this balance with DA-blocking antipsychotic agents can result in extrapyramidal side effects. We often give anticholinergic agents to restore the ACh/DA balance and restore normal movement.

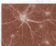

CONCERN

The cholinergic system plays an important but poorly understood role in cognition. Anticholinergic medications (such as Benadryl, TCAs, etc.) have been linked to cognitive decline. Recently, a group at Indiana University conducted a longitudinal study of elderly adults with normal cognition. They found that those taking anticholinergic medications had poorer memory, increased brain atrophy, and worse performance on cognitive tests.

POINT OF INTEREST

Henry Dale, who shared the 1936 Nobel Prize with Otto Loewi, started the convention of identifying neurons by the neurotransmitter they release, for example, "adrenergic" and "cholinergic." This was based on Dale's belief that a neuron can synthesize just one neurotransmitter. We now know neurons can release different transmitters with opposing functions, for example, the excitatory ACh and inhibitory glycine have been found in the same neuron. Furthermore, small molecule neurotransmitters, such as those discussed in the preceding text, often inhabit the same neuron with neuropeptides—referred to as *colocalization*.

NEUROPEPTIDES

In the late 1960s and early 1970s, it was established that many peptides initially discovered in the body, for example, gut and heart, are also produced and are active in the brain. This is another example of the parsimonious evolution of neurotransmitters: The same transmitter has different functions in various organs or brain region depending on its location.

These peptides such as adrenocorticotropic hormone, luteinizing hormone, somatostatin, and vasopressin (to name a few favorites) have important endocrine functions in the body, such as the regulation of reproduction, growth, water intake, salt metabolism, temperature control, and so on. In the past 40 years, it has been established that these same peptides are synthesized in nerve cells and have effects on behaviors such as learning, attachment, mood, and anxiety. This has generated tremendous interest in further analysis of the effects of these neuroactive peptides on behavior. Table 4.1 gives examples of neuropeptides from the five classes.

The neuropeptides are small chains of amino acids (Figure 4.1) and are considerably larger than the classic neurotransmitters. Additionally, the formation, release, and inactivation of the neuropeptides differ from those of the monoamines. Figure 4.8 shows the life of a neuropeptide in relation to a classic neurotransmitter. Peptides must be transcribed from mRNA on the ribosomes of the endoplasmic reticulum. Initially the peptide is a large *propeptide* precursor, which is cleaved into an active neuropeptide as it is moved from the Golgi apparatus into large dense core vesicles that are stored at the terminal bud of the neuron. Unlike the monoamines, neuropeptides are not recycled by the neuron but rather are broken down by degradative enzymes (*peptidases*) on the receptor membrane.

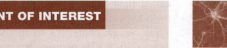

POINT OF INTEREST

In some cases the neuropeptides travel relatively long distances from their release to a receptor. This begs the question: Are they transmitters or hormones? Further complicating our understanding of the role of neuropeptides, it has been shown that they do not always evoke an action potential. They sometimes play a gentle role—often called *modulation*—in facilitating or enhancing the effects elicited by the classic neurotransmitters, and they are often stored in the same neuron as 5-HT, NE, or DA. It appears that neuropeptides act as transmitters, hormones, or modulators depending on the tissue, synapse, and frequency of stimulation.

TABLE 4.1

The Five Classes of Neuropeptides and Some Examples

Peptide Class	Example
Gut–brain peptides	Substance P
	Cholecystokinin
	Galanin
Pituitary peptides	Adrenocorticotropic hormone
	Luteinizing hormone
	Oxytocin
	Vasopressin
Hypothalamic releasing peptides	Corticotropin-releasing factor
	Gonadotropin-releasing hormone
	Thyrotropin-releasing hormone
	Somatostatin
Opioid peptides	β-Endorphin
	Enkephalins
Other peptides	Angiotensin
	Bradykinin

UNCONVENTIONAL NEUROTRANSMITTERS

It would be foolish to think that we have discovered all the neurotransmitters—or even all the transmitter classes. For example, two unconventional neurotransmitters (nitric oxide [NO] and the endocannabinoids) are being studied that are expanding our understanding of how the brain communicates and what constitutes being a neurotransmitter.

Gases

Most commonly associated with erectile dysfunction, *NO* is a gas that is formed in glutamate neurons when arginine is converted into citrulline and NO. NO has the ability to diffuse (without obstruction) out of the originating cell, through the extracellular medium and into any neighboring cell that it meets. NO converts guanosine triphosphate (GTP) into cyclic guanosine monophosphate (cGMP) that acts as a second messenger. Cells containing the NO synthase (the enzyme that creates NO)

TREATMENT

Since the serendipitous discovery in the 1950s that patients treated for tuberculosis with an agent that inhibited MAO showed improvement in mood, there has been an explosion in the manipulation of monoamines as treatment for depression and anxiety: TCAs, selective serotonin reuptake inhibitors, and so on. Although this has resulted in incalculable relief for millions of patients, the newer medications are in many ways just refinements of the original concept. They all increase the monoamines in the synaptic cleft. The neuropeptides offer the possibility of a unique mechanism for the treatment of psychiatric disorders.

Several pharmaceutical companies are investigating neuropeptide systems as novel therapeutic targets for depression, anxiety, and pain. Unfortunately, none have come to the market, and some have been withdrawn from investigation. The problem may be that the desired effects are only mild and are not robust enough to justify seeking full FDA approval. This may reflect the modulating role that neuropeptides have in the CNS. Additionally, the blood has circulating peptidases that degrade neuropeptides, which compromises oral or IV administration.

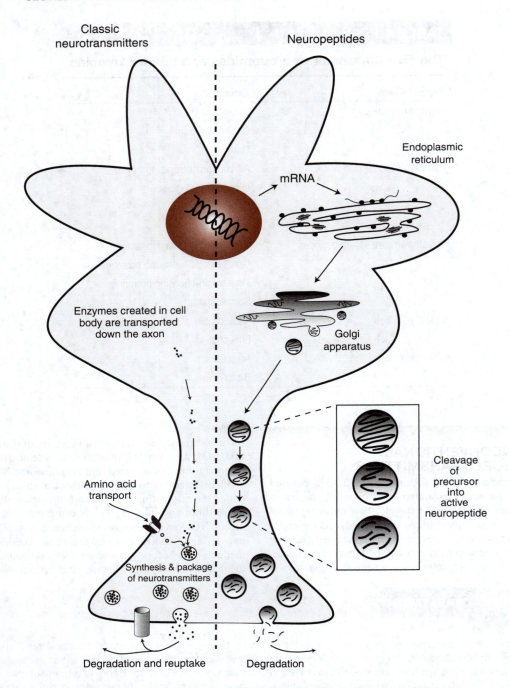

FIGURE 4.8 Comparison of classic neurotransmitters and neuropeptides.

constitute only approximately 1% of neuronal cells in the brain but reach out so extensively that nearly every cell in the brain may encounter NO. It is hard to imagine this gas as a neurotransmitter in the traditional sense if for no other reason than it cannot be stored in vesicles to await for the appropriate signal to be released. But NO does send a message to the neighboring cells that signals an increase in

activity—almost like turning on the porch lights to show our neighbors we're home.

Endocannabinoids

The journey from recognizing an effect of a substance on behavior to identifying the endogenous substrate and receptor is a common and fascinating story. Reserpine and the monoamines, as well as morphine and the enkephalins, are two well-known examples of this process. Marijuana and the endocannabinoids are the latest in this history of searching for the mechanisms to explain an effect. The main active compound of marijuana is Δ^9-tetrahydrocannabinol, which binds to the cannabinoid receptor and induces euphoria, calming, distorted cognition, and "munchies." Following the discovery of the receptor, there was an active search for the naturally occurring neurotransmitter that activates the receptor. Subsequently, the endogenous cannabinoids, called *endocannabinoids*, were identified.

 DISORDERS

The question remains: What effect does NO have on behavior and mental disorders? Little is known about this, but NO may be involved with aggression and sexual behavior, as well as migraine headaches. Knockout mice, bred without NO synthase, are extraordinarily aggressive and sexual, although their behavior is mediated by testosterone and absent in females. These findings suggest that NO may restrain aggressive and sexual behavior. It is worth noting that the medications for erectile dysfunction have not been associated with any adverse effects on mental function. This may be due to the inability of these medications in their current form to cross the blood–brain barrier.

The cannabinoid receptor (CB_1) is widely expressed throughout the brain on presynaptic terminals. The endocannabinoids are retrograde messengers residing in the postsynaptic neuron. When released, they diffuse back across the synaptic space. When coupled with a CB_1 receptor, the endocannabinoids inhibit the release of the presynaptic neurotransmitter. This simple description explains the calming effect of marijuana—it reduces neural activity.

There is considerable interest in the therapeutic effects of pharmacologic manipulation of various components of the endocannabinoid signaling pathways. The issue of medical marijuana highlights the potential benefits of activating the CB_1 receptor for pain, nausea, and glaucoma. But this is also not without potential CNS problems, e.g., psychosis and depression. Likewise, blocking the CB_1 receptor offers an alternative array of potential benefits. For a short time, CB_1 receptor blockers (antagonists) were available in Europe to treat obesity and smoking cessation but were eventually removed because of psychiatric complications. Medications that enhance or reduce the endocannabinoids will likely continue to be developed, as these neurotransmitters have such potential.

QUESTIONS

1. Which is an indoleamine?
   a. Dopamine.
   b. Norepinephrine.
   c. Melatonin.
   d. Aspartate.

2. Which pathway is believed to result in the negative symptoms of schizophrenia?
   a. Nigrostriatal.
   b. Mesocortical.
   c. Mesolimbic.
   d. Tuberoinfundibular.

3. Which pathway mediates prolactin?
   a. Nigrostriatal.
   b. Mesocortical.
   c. Mesolimbic.
   d. Tuberoinfundibular.

4. The cell bodies of the NE neurons are located in the locus coeruleus and the
   a. Medullary reticular formation.
   b. Raphe nuclei.
   c. Arcuate nucleus.
   d. Tuberomammillary nucleus.

5. Most of the cell bodies for histamine neurons reside in the
   a. Medullary reticular formation.
   b. Raphe nuclei.
   c. Arcuate nucleus.
   d. Tuberomammillary nucleus.

6. Which statement is not true regarding NO?
   a. It is quickly degraded.
   b. It converts GTP into cGMP.
   c. It is stored in dense core vesicles.
   d. It is formed from arginine.

7. All of the following are neuropeptides except
   a. Cannabinoid peptides.
   b. Pituitary peptides.
   c. Opioid peptides.
   d. Hypothalamic releasing peptides.

8. The most common neurotransmitter in the brain is
   a. Serotonin.
   b. Dopamine.
   c. γ-Aminobutyric acid.
   d. Glutamate.

See Answers section at the end of this book.

CHAPTER 5

Receptors and Signaling the Nucleus

INTRODUCTION

In this chapter we continue our discussion about events at the cellular level and explore what happens at receptors, after neurotransmitters make contact.

Electrochemical communication continues at the receptor on the postsynaptic membrane. Without a receptor, the neurotransmitter is like a tree falling in the woods with no one to hear it. The binding of the neurotransmitter with the receptor initiates a series of events that change the postsynaptic cell in some way. Receptors are protein units embedded in the lipid layer of the cell membrane. There are two basic types of receptors activated by neurotransmitters (more on this below), and the response generated depends on what type of receptor is engaged.

Agonists and Antagonists

Most neuropsychiatric medications work their magic by enhancing or limiting the effects of the neurotransmitter at the receptor. Figure 5.1 shows a schematic representation of a receptor, a neurotransmitter, and the opposing effects of contrasting medications. Pharmacologists and neuroscientists use the terms *ligand*, *agonist*, and *antagonists*, but in this book we will also use the more self-explanatory terms such as *transmitter*, *drug/medication*, *stimulate*, and *block*.

FAST RECEPTORS: CHEMICAL

There are two basic types of receptors for neurotransmitters. The one we usually think of is shown in Figure 5.1—an ion channel (also called *transmitter-gated ion channel*). A neurotransmitter or medication stimulates the opening of the pore inside the receptor, and ions rapidly flow into the cell. Receptors that allow the entry of positive ions

such as Na^+ or Ca^{2+} result in an excitatory postsynaptic potential (EPSP). Acetylcholine (ACh) and glutamate result in such activation and are considered excitatory.

Receptors permeable to negative ions, such as Cl^-, will result in inhibitory postsynaptic potentials. γ-Aminobutyric acid (GABA) and glycine, both considered inhibitory, cause this kind of activation. The essential point regarding these transmitter-gated ion channels is that they are FAST. These receptors are magnificent little machines that rapidly allow the entry of large currents with great precision. The ions pour into the cell, and the signal from the proceeding neuron, whether excitatory or inhibitory, is quickly propagated along the membrane of the target cell. As we reviewed in Chapter 3, Cells and Circuits, an action potential is only generated if enough EPSPs bring the resting potential of the postsynaptic cell above the threshold at the axon hillock.

Amino Acid Receptors

The amino acid receptors mediate most of the fast transmitter-gated channels in the brain, the two prominent ones being glutamate and GABA.

POINT OF INTEREST

The receptors, unlike the transmitter, come in a variety of styles—a relationship that is much like feet and shoes. You only have two feet but many shoes. Serotonin is one example: there are 14 different receptor subtypes for this one neurotransmitter. Some receptors are categorized as different classes, whereas others are just different subtypes within a class. It is not entirely clear why some differences constitute a new class and others just warrant a new subtype. Most likely a committee decided.

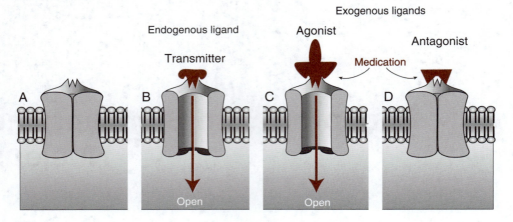

FIGURE 5.1 An unbound receptor in closed state **(A)**. A natural ligand (neurotransmitter) stimulates the receptor, which then opens to allow entry of ions **(B)**. Medication *simulates* the action of the natural ligand, and the receptor opens **(C)**. An antagonist *blocks* the action of the ligand, so the receptor cannot be opened **(D)**.

Glutamate

There are three prominent glutamate receptors: *N-methyl-D-aspartate(NMDA),α-amino-3-hydroxy-5-methyl-4-isoxazole propionate (AMPA)*, and *kainate*, each with several subtypes. They are named after the artificial agonist that selectively activates them. For example, NMDA activates the NMDA receptor, but not the AMPA, or kainate receptors. NMDA and AMPA constitute the bulk of fast excitatory synaptic transmission in the brain. The role of kainate is not clearly understood.

NMDA and AMPA receptors, which often coexist on the same postsynaptic receptor, both allow the rapid entry of Na^+ into the cell (and the simultaneous exit of K^+) that generates the depolarization of the postsynaptic cell. NMDA receptors are unique in that they also allow the entry of Ca^{2+} that can act as a second messenger inside the cell. This can have a profound impact on the cell resulting in lasting changes, as will be shown at the end of this chapter when we discuss long-term memory.

The NMDA receptor is further unique in that it requires both the glutamate transmitter and a change in the voltage to open before it will allow the entry of Na^+ and Ca^{2+}. This property is due to the presence of Mg^{2+} ions, which clog the NMDA receptor at resting voltage. Figure 5.2 shows how the AMPA receptor works in conjunction with the NMDA receptor to depolarize the cell and bring Ca^{2+} into the cell. This property has a significant impact on the capacity of the neurons to change.

The glutamate receptor is increasingly being explored as a novel target for psychiatric conditions. Studies have shown that a single IV infusion of ketamine (an NMDA antagonist) can rapidly and temporarily reduce depression. In Chapter 18, Memory, we discuss the potential benefits of D-cycloserine, a partial NMDA agonist, in reducing fear when given in conjunction with exposure therapy. Additionally, the pharmaceutical industry is funding research efforts to explore development of glutamatergic antipsychotic medications.

γ-Aminobutyric Acid

GABA and *glycine* are the primary inhibitory neurons in the brain; inhibition is a process that must be tightly regulated. Too much inhibition causes the brain to dumb down—even lose consciousness. Not enough inhibition and the electrical activity can get out of control—evoke a seizure. GABA is the most common inhibitory receptor.

The GABA receptor is made up of five protein subunits, which vary for different subclasses of the receptor. The GABA$_A$ receptor (Figure 5.3) is the focus of much pharmacologic interest. There are several other sites on the GABA$_A$ receptor where chemicals can modulate its function. For example, *barbiturates* and *benzodiazepines* have their own distinct sites on the GABA receptor. These medications by themselves do not open the GABA channel, but they enhance the strength or frequency of the opening. Benzodiazepines plus GABA result in more Cl$^-$ entering the cell and a greater inhibitory effect.

Ethanol is another popular drug that enhances the function of the GABA receptor. Long-term use

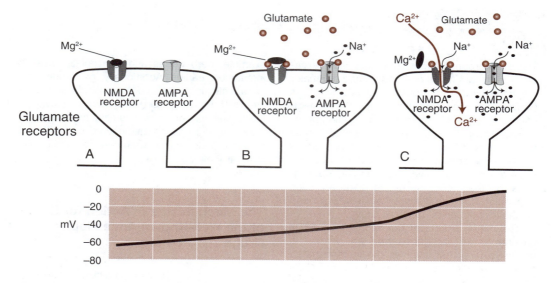

FIGURE 5.2 A: A postsynaptic glutamate terminal with both receptors closed. **B:** The presence of glutamate transmitters opens the AMPA receptor but not the NMDA receptor. **C:** When the voltage in the postsynaptic neuron gets above −35 mV, the magnesium ion blocking the receptor falls off, and Na⁺ and Ca²⁺ ions pour into the cell. AMPA, α-amino-3-hydroxy-5-methyl-4-isoxazole propionate; NMDA, N-methyl-D-aspartate.

of ethanol decreases the expression of the GABA receptor, which may explain the tolerance that develops with alcoholism. Whether the receptor alterations contribute to the propensity for seizures when the alcohol is withdrawn remains unclear.

The steroid hormones also modulate GABA receptors (sometimes called *neurosteroids* when they have effects on neurons) (see Figure 7.1). This may explain the psychiatric symptoms that develop at times when the sex hormones are reduced, for

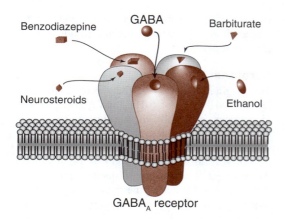

FIGURE 5.3 The GABA receptor showing other drugs that can modify and enhance the inhibitory effect of these receptors. GABA, γ-aminobutyric acid.

example, premenstrual syndrome, menopause, and chemical castration for men. Additionally, researchers have found that some steroid hormone levels drop in patients during a panic attack. Others have shown that medications such as olanzapine and fluoxetine—known to decrease anxiety—increase steroid hormone levels.

SLOW RECEPTORS: METABOLIC

Starting in the 1950s, researchers teased out the details of a second type of receptor—one that activates a cascade of biochemical events in the cytosol of the receptor cell, which ultimately modifies the function of target proteins or the DNA. This type of receptor, called a *G protein–coupled receptor*, is perhaps even more relevant to the effect of psychiatric medications than the transmitter-gated ion channel. G protein is the short form for guanosine triphosphate–binding protein. Although there are many types of G protein–coupled receptors, the basic style involves three steps:

1. A neurotransmitter binds to the receptor.
2. The receptor activates the G protein, which moves along the intracellular membrane.
3. The G protein activates the "effector" protein.

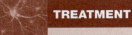

ANTIEPILEPTIC DRUGS

The background about inhibitory and excitatory receptors helps one understand the major mechanisms of action of the antiepileptic drugs (AEDs). The goal of treatment with these medications is to modify the aberrant bursting properties, synchronization, and spread of abnormal firing without affecting ordinary electrical activity. These effects, although intended to control seizure disorders, have wide-ranging applications to other neuropsychiatric disorders such as bipolar affective disorder, anxiety, pain, and alcohol dependence, to name a few.

The major effects of the well-known AEDs fall into three categories and are shown in the table. The first involves the voltage-gated sodium channel discussed in Chapter 3, Cells and Circuits. Remember that these are the pores that allow rapid entry of sodium into the cell to propagate the action potential along the axon. Modulation of these channels is believed to account for some of the effectiveness of several AEDs. The second category involves the voltage-gated calcium channels, which are located on the terminals of the neuron and instigate the release of neurotransmitters into the synaptic cleft. Blockade of these channels decreases the neurotransmitter release and ultimately decreases excitability.

The final mechanism of action involves the GABA receptor and increasing inhibition, for example, barbiturates and benzodiazepines as mentioned earlier. Additionally, valproate and gabapentin increase GABA synthesis and turnover with the net effect of increased activity of these inhibitory neurons. It is easy to understand the rationale for trying medications with different mechanisms of action when one medication fails to control the disorder.

The Mechanisms of Action for Some of the Well-Known Antiepileptic Drugs

	Sodium Channels $\geq$	Calcium Channels $\geq$	GABA System
Phenytoin	X	—	—
Carbamazepine	X	—	—
Lamotrigine	X	X	—
Valproate	X	X	↑ turnover
Gabapentin	—	X	↑ turnover
Phenobarbital	—	X	X
Benzodiazepines	—	—	X

GABA, γ-aminobutyric acid.

The activated "effector" protein can have a variety of functions, including just opening traditional ion channels (not shown). However, the more interesting effector proteins are enzymes that trigger a process called a *secondary messenger cascade* (Figure 5.4). The neurotransmitter activates the G protein, which slides along the membrane and stimulates the effector protein. The activated effector protein then converts adenosine triphosphate into cyclic adenosine monophosphate (cAMP): the secondary messenger, which will diffuse away into the cytosol where it can change the neuronal operations. With the exception of serotonin type 3 receptor (5-hydroxytryptamine$_3$ [5-HT$_3$]), all the monoamine receptors belong to the G protein–coupled family—which means that most psychiatric medications deliver their punch through secondary messengers.

Serotonin Receptors

The original discovery of the serotonin receptor led to two subtypes: 5-HT$_1$ and 5-HT$_2$. Further discoveries, especially the application of molecular cloning techniques, have resulted in multiple subdivisions of these two receptors and the addition of several more for a total of 14. Although the prospect of activating or blocking the various receptors for further refinement of psychopharmacologic treatment is an enticing possibility, the clinical results with a few exceptions have been limited.

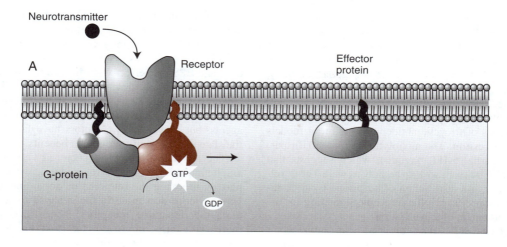

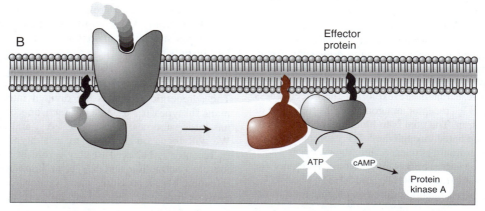

FIGURE 5.4 The initiation of the secondary messenger cascade starts with a neurotransmitter binding with G protein receptor **(A)** and ends with the conversion of ATP into cAMP **(B)**. ATP, adenosine triphosphate; cAMP, cyclic adenosine monophosphate; GDP, guanosine diphosphate; GTP, guanosine triphosphate.

POINT OF INTEREST

Autoreceptors reside on the cell body or terminal of the *presynaptic neuron*. They sense the presence of the neurotransmitter and provide negative feedback to the neuron. That is, if too much of the neurotransmitter is present, these receptors activate a secondary messenger and turn off further release of the neurotransmitter—and in some cases reduce synthesis of the neurotransmitter. The figure shows an example of this type of receptor using the 5-HT$_{1A}$ (anxiety-related) and 5-HT$_{1D}$ (migraine-related) receptors. Similar autoreceptors are known for other transmitters such as dopamine and norepinephrine. Blocking these specific receptors may provide unique ways to alleviate specific symptoms.

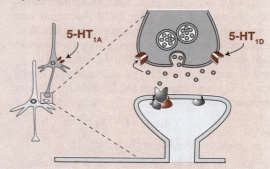

The 5-HT$_1$ receptors make up the largest subtype with 5-HT$_{1A}$, 5-HT$_{1B}$, 5-HT$_{1D}$, 5-HT$_{1E}$, and 5-HT$_{1F}$. 5-HT$_{1A}$ has received the most interest and seems to play a prominent role in depression and anxiety. It is an autoreceptor on the cell body, which curtails the release of serotonin when stimulated. How this would improve mood is unclear, but blocking this receptor has decreased the effectiveness of tricyclic antidepressants in rat models of depression. The anxiolytic buspirone (Buspar) is a partial 5-HT$_{1A}$ agonist, which suggests that 5-HT$_{1A}$ has some role in anxiety as well. The development and distribution of buspirone is an example of specific serotonin receptor targeting for the development of a medication.

The 5-HT$_{1D}$ receptor is also an autoreceptor but is located on the nerve terminal at the synapse. Here it appears to function to sense the serotonin in the synaptic cleft and turn off release of more serotonin when stimulated. The 5-HT$_{1D}$ receptor is stimulated by the antimigraine drug sumatriptan (Imitrex) although the importance of this effect in the overall efficacy of the medication is unclear. Some researchers are exploring the effectiveness of a 5-HT$_{1D}$ receptor antagonist for the treatment of depression. The goal is to block the negative feedback mediated through the 5-HT$_{1D}$ receptor, so that more serotonin is released into the synapse.

Some other important serotonin receptors for the psychiatrist are 5-HT$_{2A}$ and 5-HT$_{2C}$. The 5-HT$_{2A}$ receptor has been identified as playing an important role in the "atypicalness" of the second-generation antipsychotic agents (such as clozapine, risperidone, olanzapine, etc.). These newer agents have a greater capacity to block 5-HT$_{2A}$ receptors than do the traditional agents such as haloperidol, which may explain the observed decrease in the extrapyramidal symptom (EPS).

Dopamine Receptors

The dopamine receptors are involved in a wide range of functions, including locomotion, cognition, psychosis, and even neuroendocrine secretion. It became clear after 1979 that there was more than one dopamine receptor: D$_1$ and D$_2$. More recently with molecular cloning they have identified three more receptors: D$_3$, D$_4$, and D$_5$. The D$_3$ and D$_4$ receptors are "D$_2$-like," and the D$_5$ receptor is "D$_1$-like." However, the D$_1$ and D$_2$ receptors remain the most important.

$$\text{``D}_1\text{-like''} = \text{D}_1 \text{ and } \text{D}_5$$

$$\text{``D}_2\text{-like''} = \text{D}_2, \text{D}_3, \text{ and } \text{D}_4$$

The D$_1$ and D$_2$ receptors have been distinguished by their differing affinity for binding with traditional antipsychotic agents such as haloperidol: The D$_2$ receptor has high affinity, whereas the D$_1$ receptor has low affinity. Increased D$_2$ receptor antagonism correlates with the therapeutic efficacy and EPS side effect with the traditional antipsychotics. There is great interest in the "D$_2$-like" receptors (D$_3$ and D$_4$) as possible alternative sites for therapeutic potentiation with antipsychotic agents, but as yet these receptors have failed to translate into clinically significant benefits.

The psychostimulants (such as cocaine, amphetamine, and methylphenidate) work in part by blocking the reuptake of dopamine and leaving more dopamine in the synapse to stimulate the dopamine receptors. The effects are increased energy, improved cognition, and even psychosis. The effects on reward and cognition seem to be more prominently mediated by the D$_1$ receptor. Augmenting D$_1$ and D$_2$ receptors (agonists) is the mainstay of treatment for Parkinson's disease.

Adrenergic Receptors

The adrenergic receptors are divided into three main subtypes α_1, α_2, and β. Each one of these has three subtypes: α_{1a}, α_{1b}, α_{1d}, α_{2a}, and so on. We will focus on the three main subtypes. The α_1 receptor is believed to play a role in smooth muscle contraction and has been implicated in effecting blood pressure, nasal congestion, and prostate function. Although widely expressed in the central nervous system (CNS), the central role of the α_1 receptor remains to be determined. Locomotor activation and arousal have been suggested by some studies. Stimulation of the α_1 receptor may synergistically increase the activity of the serotonin neurons in the raphe nucleus, although stimulation of the α_2 receptor may have just the opposite effect.

The α_2 receptor subtypes in the CNS inhibit the firing of the norepinephrine neurons through autoreceptors. This mechanism of action is believed to mediate the sedative and hypotensive effects of the α_2 receptor agonist clonidine. Additionally, stimulation of the α_2 receptors decreases sympathetic activity, which may explain the therapeutic utility of clonidine for suppressing the heightened sympathetic state for patients in opiate withdrawal.

The β receptor subtypes are more famous for their part in slowing cardiac rhythm and lowering blood pressure. The functions of the β receptors in the CNS, although widely distributed, are not well understood. It is not uncommon to use a β blocker, for example, propranolol, for treating performance anxiety or antipsychotic-induced akathisia.

Whether these benefits come from a central or peripheral blockage of the β receptor, or both, is not known.

Histamine Receptors

There are four histamine receptors, although H_4 is predominately present in the periphery and only recently discovered. The H_1 receptor is the target for the classic antihistamines, which highlights its role in sedation and arousal. Of great interest to psychiatrists is the role of H_1 in weight gain. Recent analysis has shown that the potential to gain weight with antipsychotic agents correlates with the antagonism for the H_1 receptor. For example, clozapine and olanzapine have the most affinity for the H_1 receptor and the most weight gain, whereas aripiprazolde and ziprasidone have the least.

The H_2 receptor is more traditionally associated with the gut. Blockade of the H_2 receptor has been a widely used treatment for peptic ulcer disease. The H_3 receptor functions as an inhibitory receptor on the histamine neurons as well as other nonhistamine nerve terminals. The role of this receptor is not clearly understood but may be involved in appetite, arousal, and cognition.

Cholinergic Receptors

It was with the cholinergic receptor that scientists first realized that one neurotransmitter (ACh) could have different receptors. The initial subtypes were identified and named after the drug that distinguished its effect. For example, nicotine will stimulate cholinergic receptors in skeletal muscle but not in the heart. Conversely, muscarine will stimulate the heart but has no effect on skeletal muscle. Therefore, the two receptors can be identified by the actions of different drugs, and the receptors were named after those drugs: nicotinic and muscarinic. Unfortunately, it has been hard to find a drug with unique action on each receptor subtype, so we are stuck with designations such as 1A, 2B, and so on.

Many more subtypes of the nicotinic and muscarinic receptors have been identified since the early days of receptor delineation, but the significance of these various subtypes for the psychiatrist remains obscure. Clearly, ACh is important in cognition and memory as noted by the benefits of inhibiting acetylcholinesterase as a treatment for Alzheimer's disease. Likewise, the blockage of the muscarinic receptor by tricyclic antidepressants and antipsychotic medications results in troublesome dry mouth, constipation, and urinary hesitancy (which we generically call the anticholinergic side effects). However, the importance of one receptor subtype over another has not been shown.

DISORDERS

Myasthenia gravis is an autoimmune disease in which the body produces antibodies to the nicotinic ACh receptor. Patients complain of weakness and fatigue in the voluntary muscles resulting from the interruption of the chemical signal at the neuromuscular junction. Muscarinic receptors in the heart and CNS are unaffected.

ACh, unlike the monoamines, is cleared from the synaptic cleft by an enzyme, acetylcholinesterase. One treatment for myasthenia gravis is with the acetylcholinesterase inhibitors, such as edrophonium (Tensilon), that prolong the life of the released ACh.

SIGNALING THE NUCLEUS

After the neurotransmitter has stimulated the G protein to slide across the membrane and activate an enzyme (which is the case with most of the catecholamines), a cascade of events with secondary messengers transpires to modify neuronal function. Neurons use many different secondary messengers as signals within the cytosol—two of which we have discussed: Ca^{2+} and cAMP. The secondary messengers regulate neuronal function by activating enzymes that will add a phosphate group (*phosphorylation*) to other proteins in the cell. The *protein kinases*, of which there are wide varieties, are the enzymes that add a phosphate group to other proteins. Protein kinase A and calcium/calmodulin protein kinase are two examples of this sort of enzyme. Once proteins are phosphorylated, they are "turned on" and can execute a broad range of cellular functions such as regulating enzyme activity or ion channels.

Additionally, the protein kinases can induce our two favorite words—*gene expression*. The protein kinases can "turn on" the DNA and start the synthesis of messenger ribonucleic acid. This process takes longer but can have large and relatively stable effects on the cell, for example, upregulation of receptors or the production of growth factor proteins. Figure 5.5 shows an example of how two different types of receptors—a G protein–coupled receptor and a transmitter-gated ion channel—can activate a secondary messenger that will stimulate the production of new proteins.

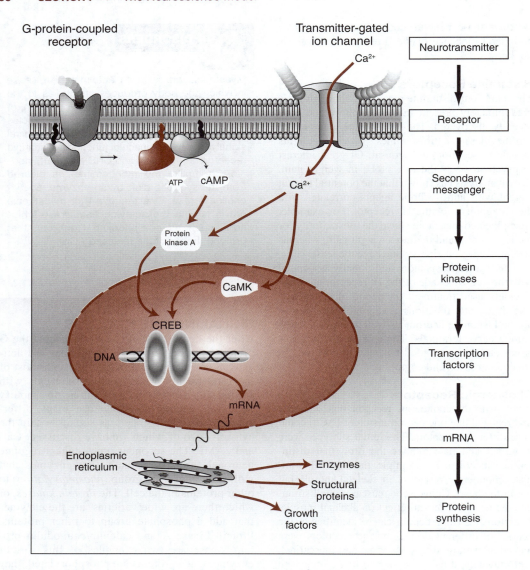

FIGURE 5.5 Signaling the nucleus. The neurotransmitters stimulate a cascade of events that ultimately leads to activation of the DNA (gene expression) and the synthesis of proteins that can modify the function of the cell. ATP, adenosine triphosphate; CaMK, calcium/calmodulin protein kinase; cAMP, cyclic adenosine monophosphate; CREB, cyclic adenosine monophosphate response element–binding protein; mRNA, messenger ribonucleic acid.

LONG-TERM POTENTIATION: A SUMMARY EXAMPLE

Understanding long-term potentiation (LTP) is a way to apply what has been discussed in the past few chapters to a topic of great relevance to neuroscience: learning and memory. LTP is a laboratory example of learning that was discovered accidentally. As we have seen, applying a single stimulus to a neuron generates an excitatory impulse (EPSP) in the cell. Applying high-frequency stimuli—hundreds of impulses within a second—generates a higher EPSP in the cell. What was found accidentally was that once a neuron has been exposed to high-frequency stimulation, something changes, and now a single stimulus will generate a high EPSP. This sort of change has been shown to last for several months if not longer. Figure 5.6 shows these three steps.

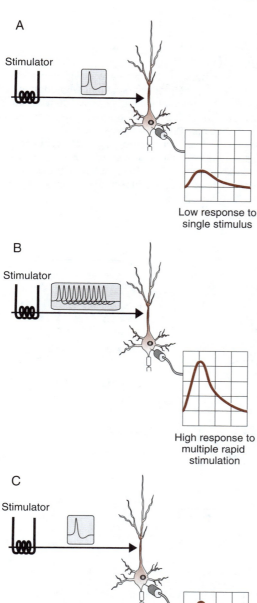

A

Stimulator

Low response to
single stimulus

B

Stimulator

High response to
multiple rapid
stimulation

C

Stimulator

High response to
single stimulation

FIGURE 5.6 Long-term potentiation. In **(A)** the neuron receives a single stimulus that generates a small impulse in the cell body. In **(B)** a high-frequency stimulus generates a big response in the cell body. This process changes something in the cell, and following this high-frequency testing, the original single stimulus **(C)** generates a big response in the cell body.

LTP sounds like one of those topics that neuroscientists discuss ad nauseam but which has little relevance to practicing clinicians. *Oh contraire!* LTP is a demonstration—although artificial—that neurons can incorporate lasting changes, an essential step to developing memories and skills. And what is life without memories? Unfortunately, some memories are haunting. LTP is an example, at the cellular level, of what may happen for people who experience overwhelming trauma and develop posttraumatic stress disorder.

The changes brought about with LTP can be analyzed at the molecular level. Researchers have shown that both glutamate receptors (NMDA and AMPA) must be operational for the process to work. Likewise, others have shown that calcium (a secondary messenger) and the kinases are required for LTP. Of even greater interest is the demonstration that protein synthesis (gene expression!) is an essential part of the development of LTP. All the processes shown in Figure 5.5 are involved in LTP.

What happens inside the cell with the induction of LTP? Clearly, there is some strengthening of the connection between the two cells that are communicating when LTP occurs. Figure 5.7 depicts the events that transpire when the presynaptic cell is hyperstimulated, the postsynaptic cell signals its nucleus, and the connection between the two cells is enhanced by the insertion of more glutamate receptors. Additional evidence has shown that a retrograde signal such as nitric oxide diffuses back across the synaptic cleft and induces the presynaptic neuron to release more transmitters. The combined result is increased sensitivity and responsiveness at the synapse: more transmitters and more receptors resulting in a stronger signal.

Amazingly, the structural changes to the synapse can actually be seen under the right experimental circumstances. Engert and Bonhoeffer filled neurons from the hippocampus with fluorescent dye and then induced LTP. They captured the development of new spines on the postsynaptic dendrite as shown in Figure 5.8. This research is consistent with other data that suggest that the development of spines is possibly the structural manifestation of learning and memory.

LTP demonstrates that electrical, molecular, and structural changes are involved in the process of storing information. It is a small leap to conclude that highly charged events in our lives—the emotional equivalent of high-frequency stimulation—leave enduring changes to neuronal connections in a manner similar to LTP.

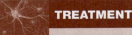

TREATMENT

TRANSCRANIAL MAGNETIC STIMULATION

LTP has not been established in humans for obvious ethical reasons. Repetitive transcranial magnetic stimulation offers a possible noninvasive method of stimulating conscious human subjects that can mimic the effects of LTP. The prospect of inducing long-lasting changes to the human cortex through non-invasive stimulation offers the hope of a new kind of treatment applicable to a wide range of mental disorders.

Preliminary studies have demonstrated changes in motor skills consistent with changes seen with LTP when subjects receive continuous stimulation at the motor cortex. The changes lasted up to 60 minutes beyond the period of stimulation. Although the utility of a change lasting only 60 minutes is of little clinical value, the opportunity to alter the function of the cortex without breaching the blood–brain barrier is an exciting possibility.

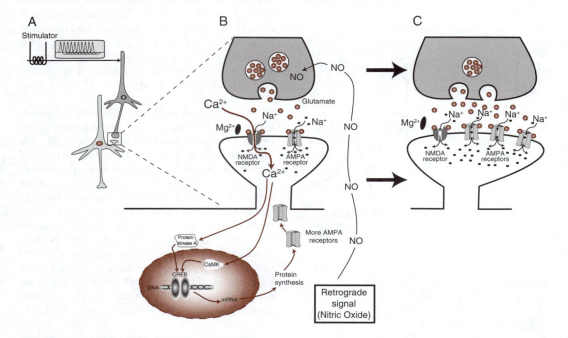

FIGURE 5.7 Long-term potentiation inducing a change at the synapse. **A:** Hyperstimulation of the presynaptic neuron. **B:** The NMDA and AMPA receptors open, allowing the entry of the secondary messenger, calcium, which signals the nucleus to synthesize more receptors. **C:** The new AMPA receptors are inserted into the membrane, which has the effect of increasing the cell's responsiveness to future stimulation. AMPA, α-amino-3-hydroxy-5-methyl-4-isoxazole propionate; NMDA, N-methyl-ᴅ-aspartate; NO, nitric oxide.

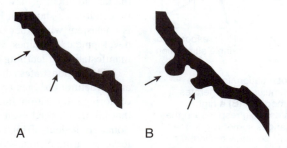

FIGURE 5.8 With the induction of long-term potentiation (LTP) in neurons from the hippocampus, new spines developed on the dendrite within an hour as shown by the *arrows*: **(A)** spines before LTP and **(B)** spines one hour after LTP. (Adapted with permission from Macmillan Publishers Ltd. Engert F, Bonhoeffer T. Dendritic spine changes associated with hippocampal long-term synaptic plasticity. *Nature*. 1999;399[6731]:66–70. Copyright 1999.)

QUESTIONS

1. Which equation is correct?
   a. *Antagonist = stimulate.*
   b. *Agonist = block.*
   c. *Agonist = transmitter.*
   d. *Antagonist = endogenous ligand.*

2. Which is not a glutamate receptor?
   a. NMDA.
   b. cAMP.
   c. AMPA.
   d. Kainate.

3. The strength of the GABA inhibitory signal is enhanced by all of the following except
   a. Ethanol.
   b. Phenobarbital.
   c. Carbamazepine.
   d. Neurosteroids.

4. The AEDs exert their major effects through all of the following except
   a. Decreasing glutamate activity.
   b. Modulation of the voltage-gated sodium channels.
   c. Blockade of the voltage-gated calcium channels.
   d. Increasing GABA activity.

5. Which of the following is true?
   a. Mg^{2+} is a common secondary messenger.
   b. Most monoamine receptors are fast receptors.
   c. Fast receptors typically lead to gene expression.
   d. Autoreceptors give negative feedback to the neuron.

6. Gene expression stimulated by a neurotransmitter involves all of the following except
   a. Phosphorylation.
   b. Long-term potentiation.
   c. Protein kinases.
   d. G protein–coupled receptor.

7. All of the following about LTP are true except
   a. Enhanced EPSP.
   b. Increased receptors.
   c. Gene expression.
   d. Enhanced ligand binding.

8. Which describes LTP best?
   a. It was discovered by accident.
   b. Neuroscientists love to pontificate on this topic.
   c. It is an example of learning.
   d. All of the above.

See Answers section at the end of this book.

CHAPTER 6

Genetics and Epigenetics

Woody Guthrie, the depression era folk singer ("This Land Is Your Land"), developed Huntington's disease late in his 30s. The disease is an autosomal dominant neurodegenerative disorder, which often isn't expressed until middle age. Woody's son, Arlo Guthrie, who popularized the Vietnam era song about Alice's Restaurant, has not developed the disorder, as he did not inherit the deviant gene from his father. Huntington's disease is an example of simple Mendelian genetics—one dominant gene leads to the disorder. With other simple Mendelian disorders, such as cystic fibrosis or sickle cell disease, the affected individual must inherit two recessive genes—one from each parent. Single gene changes with large effects.

Unfortunately, the genetic patterns of the common psychiatric disorders are not this simple. As a matter of fact, they remain incomprehensibly complex. We have yet to find a gene or a set of genes that can explain any major psychiatric disorder. Analysis of the human genome has revealed that the genetic mechanisms are more complex than we had imagined. Furthermore, events from the environment (such as toxins, abuse, isolation, etc.) can alter gene expression by changing the molecules *around* the DNA. The genetics of mental illness largely remains a mystery, although we know a lot more about genetics overall than we used to.

HERITABILITY OF MENTAL ILLNESS

There is no question that psychiatric disorders are genetically linked. The twin and adoption studies (Figure 1.1 and Table 1.1) show that behavioral traits and mental illness run in families. The DNA that puts individuals at risk for mental disorders is passed from parent to child. Geneticists use the term *heritability*, which they define as the proportion of observed variance in a group of individuals that can be explained by genetic variance. What does that mean? Well, heritability (h^2) of a trait is the total proportion of the total variance that is genetic ($h^2 = V_G/V_P$). Clear as mud. A better way to understand heritability is shown in Table 6.1.

Kenneth Kendler created the scale in Table 6.1 to correlate heritability percentages with common traits. Language and religion have zero genetic influence. Asian babies raised by American families speak English without an accent and vice versa. At the other extreme of the scale is height. In the absence of malnutrition or a pituitary tumor, height is almost completely determined by the genes inherited from the parents. Monozygotic twins rarely differ in height by more than half an inch.

The heritability of psychiatric disorders is placed next to this scale for comparison. We cannot think of any psychiatric condition that does not have some genetic influence. Even traumatic brain injury, which should be the result of a random accident, is probably, in some people, linked to impulsive and risk-taking genes. The common psychiatric disorders have moderate heritability, whereas the serious mental disorders have strong genetic components. The take-home message is clear—mental disorders are influenced by genes—although some more than others. But which genes are causing the problems? First, a word about the human genome.

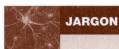

JARGON

The comedian Steve Martin said, "Those French... they have a different word for EVERYTHING!!!" At times it seems like geneticists are speaking French, only without the passion. For example, gene is the term to describe a unit of heredity—a portion of DNA that codes for proteins or RNA. An allele is one of the two or more forms of the DNA sequence for a gene. Such a gene is polymorphic. It gets worse. For example, the protein catechol-*O*-methyltransferase has a common polymorphism (Val158Met) at the chromosome 22q11.2. Ugh! We try to minimize the jargon and stick to simple terms. Sacré bleu!

HUMAN GENOME PROJECT

Genome is the term used to refer to the sum total of genetic information in a particular organism. The human genome is the entire DNA code contained in the chromosomes in each nucleated cell. The Human Genome Project was a large international scientific study focused on sequencing the nucleic acids (called base pairs) for the entire human genome. It was the Manhattan Project for biologists. They started in 1990 and completed the project in 2003. Important findings included the following:

- the human genome is made up of 3 billion base pairs,
- less than 2% of the DNA codes for proteins, and
- there are only approximately 23,000 protein-coding genes.

Although it is hard to find an example in which the Human Genome Project has advanced our medical treatment, it certainly has transformed our conceptualization of the storage of genetic information. The most shocking aspect is that we have so few protein-coding genes—just about 23,000. This is a bit unsettling especially when one considers that *Caenorhabditis elegans* (a flat worm ~1 mm in length) has about 20,000 protein-coding genes. The governor of South Carolina seems so much more intelligent than a flat worm, yet they have about the same number of protein-coding genes? How can this be? Clearly, there is more to complexity than the total number of protein-coding genes.

Protein-Coding Genes

For decades the central dogma of biology purported that DNA makes RNA, which in turn makes proteins. Here is the key point: it was presumed that proteins orchestrate all the important functions in a cell—regulatory, metabolic, structural, etc. So, how can the governor of South Carolina and a flat worm have roughly the same number of protein-coding genes? The answer seems to be hidden in the other 98% of the genome that is not coding for proteins. This portion of the genome, which has been called "junk DNA," was presumed to be useless, inert DNA that was only there to connect the important sections together. In fact the "junk DNA" is more active and more important than most people had imagined.

It's an RNA World

A new respect for the "junk DNA" developed after the mouse genome was sequenced and compared with the human genome. Mice and people share

---

TABLE 6.1

Benchmarks for a Scale of Heritability for General Traits and Psychiatric Disorders

Human Traits/Disease	Heritability	Heritability of Psychiatric Conditions
Language, religion	0%	—
Myocardial infarct, breast cancer	20%–40%	Anxiety, depression, and eating disorders
Cholesterol, blood pressure	40%–60%	Alcohol and drug dependence
Weight, intelligence	60%–80%	—
Height	80%–100%	Schizophrenia, bipolar disorder, autism, and attention deficit hyperactivity disorder

many of the same protein-coding genes—this was expected. However, much to everyone's amazement, the two species also share vast regions of "junk DNA." This was remarkable because the mouse and human lineage diverged over 75 million years ago. If large sections of "junk" DNA were preserved over that time, then they must be important for the function of the cell. Equally revealing, it appears that the complexity of an organism is related to non–protein-coding DNA. Figure 6.1 shows how the percent of non–protein-coding DNA increases with the complexity of the organism.

Further evidence of the importance of RNA comes from analysis of the transcriptional activity of the DNA. Even though less than 2% of the DNA codes for proteins, fully 85% of the genome is transcribed into RNA. The scientific literature has exploded with a dazzling array of various newly discovered non–protein-coding RNA molecules that differ from our old friend messenger RNA (mRNA) (see Figure 3.2). Molecules with names such as microRNA, long noncoding RNA, and small nucleolar RNA are examples of RNA that are transcribed throughout the genome. Even introns, the RNA spliced out of the protein-coding mRNA, seem to be functional.

A New Level of Gene Regulation

We believe that the cell would not expend energy transcribing the DNA into RNA if it was not beneficial. But what are all the non–protein-coding RNA molecules doing? Some of the functions that have been identified are as follows:

- maintaining DNA integrity
- transcriptional regulation
- posttranscriptional modification
- viral defense
- epigenetic modification

MicroRNA provides a good example of what the non–protein-coding RNA may be doing in the cell. MicroRNAs have the capacity to silence gene expression by blocking the mRNA. MicroRNAs have complementary nucleic acids that bind to the nucleic acids on the mRNA, effectively shutting down any translation of the mRNA into protein—like putting gum in a typewriter. Mechanisms such as this and others that are beyond the scope of this book enable non–protein-coding RNA to affect and influence gene expression.

This new view of the genome is relevant for mental illness because non–protein-coding RNA is highly expressed in the brain. Small changes in these RNA molecules can affect the expression of multiple genes and may underlie neurodevelopmental, neurodegenerative, and psychiatric disorders. Recent studies have shown that some microRNAs are downregulated, whereas others are upregulated in schizophrenia.

Percentage of genome that is non-protein coding

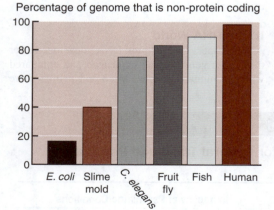

FIGURE 6.1 The percent of the genome that does not code for proteins increases as the complexity of the organism increases. This may explain one reason why the governor of South Carolina is more complex than a *C. elegans*. (Adapted from Taft RJ, et al. 2007. The relationship between non-protein-coding DNA and eukaryotic complexity. *BioEssays*. 29:288–299.)

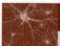 **AN RNA WORLD**

The origins of life in the primordial world remain a mystery. The development of a mechanism to pass along the instructions for building, maintaining, and replicating the cell was an essential step for sustaining any life form. It has been assumed that life started with DNA. Yet DNA requires proteins to build RNA, which in turn makes the required proteins. It is a chicken and egg dilemma. New thinking postulates that RNA was the original hereditary molecule. Lincoln and Joyce from the Scripps Research Institute recently created a self-replicating RNA, which can, by itself, reproduce indefinitely. Possibly, DNA developed later in evolution as a more stable form of storage, and proteins evolved as molecules more adapted to control the functions of the cell.

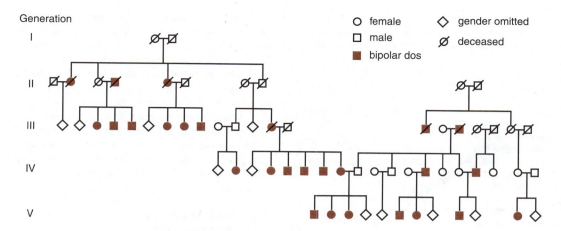

FIGURE 6.2 The high prevalence of bipolar disorder in this Amish family is shown in this pedigree. Linkage studies suggested a single gene located on chromosome 11. (Adapted from Law A, et al. Genetic linkage analysis of bipolar affective disorder in an Old Order Amish pedigree. *Hum Genet*. 1992;88:562–568, with permission of Springer.)

FINDING THE OFFENDING GENES

Our DNA is subjected to a constant cycle of damage and repair. Radiation, toxins, and the natural decay of molecules take a toll on the DNA. Most damage is irrelevant, as it is quickly repaired or results in cell death. Changes to the DNA that endure can have an effect on the cell that occurs along a spectrum from benign to pathogenic. Finding the changes that affect the behavior of the organism is the Holy Grail of psychiatric genetics.

It is easier to find the offending genes if the pathophysiology of a disease is known. For example, an abnormal type of hemoglobin is known to be the cause of sickle cell anemia, and the errant gene has been identified down to the single altered nucleotide. The pathophysiologies of psychiatric disorders, however, remain obscure. For many years the prevailing theories about psychiatric pathology developed from the effects of psychiatric medications—the monoamine hypothesis or dopamine hypothesis—what we call the "chemical imbalance" theories. However, analyses of genes that control for serotonin and dopamine or their receptors have failed to locate abnormalities that correlate with the frequency of the disorder. When such genes are identified, they are either too common in the unaffected population or fail to replicate in further studies.

Single Genes
Linkage Studies

Before the era of genome-wide studies, one used to see in the literature reports linking a specific gene or chromosomal region with a particular disease. This was done by analyzing families with an illness and searching for the genes. Figure 6.2 shows a pedigree for an Amish family with bipolar disorder. The heritability of the disorder is readily apparent. The location of the gene or genes causing the problem is much harder to locate.

Researchers used linkage studies to narrow down the location of the problematic gene. Linkage studies are based on the understanding that genes are located on the arms of chromosomes and that during meiosis some swapping of genes occurs between the arms. The closer the two genes are to each other on the chromosome arm, the more "linked" they are (less likely to swap). Consequently, using known locations for various genes, and the cooccurrence with the disorder, researchers can estimate where the gene might be. In this situation the gene was narrowed down to the tip of the short arm of chromosome 11. Unfortunately, as is the problem with most single gene studies, subsequent research failed to replicate the initial finding.

Few single gene linkage studies have yielded enduring results for mental illness. The apolipoprotein E gene is one exception. The E4 allele (there are three common alleles) is associated with late-onset Alzheimer's disease. People with two copies of the gene have 15 times the risk of

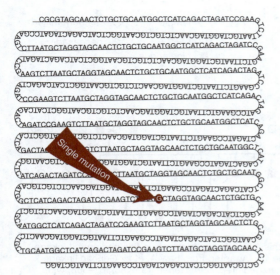

FIGURE 6.3 A hypothetical example of a single nucleotide polymorphism. In this single strand of DNA, a "C" has been replaced with a "G." This is roughly one nucleotide change in a strand of 1000 nucleotides, which is about the difference between any two humans.

developing the disease than do those without the E4 allele. People with any copies of the gene who sustain head trauma suffer more residual cognitive problems. Unfortunately, there are few other single gene linkage studies with such significant findings in our field. And with the ability to assess the entire genome, linkage studies have been left in the dust.

Many Small Changes
Single Nucleotide Polymorphism

If single problematic genes do not cause the common psychiatric disorders, then maybe the disorders arise from many minor changes—not one big bang but the cumulative effect of many small hits. Small changes in the DNA are one-letter variations called single nucleotide polymorphisms (SNPs—pronounced "snips") (Figure 6.3). Genome-wide studies have identified that humans have numerous SNPs that seem to have little effect on observable characteristics (phenotype) of the person. For example, James Watson (of Watson and Crick fame) had his genome sequenced. They discovered that he had 3.3 million SNPs. Of interest, 10,000 of the SNPs occurred in protein-coding genes, which could cause malfunctions in building an important protein—yet he still won a Nobel Prize and is alive in his 80s. On the other hand, Watson's eldest son, whom he openly discusses, is diagnosed with schizophrenia.

Many of the common SNPs cooccur with various diseases. However, the majority of people who have a particular SNP do not develop the disease—that is, a particular SNP by itself has low predictive value of developing the disease. But maybe common diseases are caused when enough of the common SNPs show up in the same unlucky person. Therefore the natural next step has been huge studies with large numbers of subjects attempting to correlate numerous SNPs with the disease states. Unfortunately, the studies thus far have been a big disappointment. The findings continue to have low predictive value.

Structural Variation
Copy Number Variation

It was not until 1956 that geneticists could identify and count the number of human chromosomes—called karyotyping. They were surprised to find 46 chromosomes instead of 48 as they had expected (the great apes have 48). Subsequently, curious clinicians looked at the chromosomes of children with inherited disorders. In 1959, Jérôme Lejeune, a French pediatrician and geneticist, karyotyped the chromosomes in children with Down syndrome—what was called mongolism at the time. Lejeune discovered that these children had an extra chromosome, which was later identified as chromosome 21 (Figure 6.4A).

The presence of the extra chromosome in Down syndrome, or in some cases just an extra part of the chromosome, has profound effects on the cognitive and physical development of the child. Although it is not clear what molecular problems result from the additional DNA, we know something goes awry. It may be that the extra DNA results in excessive gene expression, which overwhelms the precise mechanisms of normal development—like having too many cooks in the kitchen.

Henry Turner, an endocrinologist in Illinois, first reported in 1938 a syndrome in girls of short stature and undeveloped secondary sexual characteristics. It was not until 1959 that the syndrome, which has since taken his name, was recognized as resulting from the absence of an X chromosome. Affected women have 45 chromosomes—only one X. Down syndrome and Turner syndrome are examples of genetic abnormalities at the macro level—large additions or deletions in the total quantity of DNA. SNPs, on the other hand, are at the other end of the spectrum—single letter changes. There must be something between these two extremes (whole chromosome

A Large variation in chromosomal number

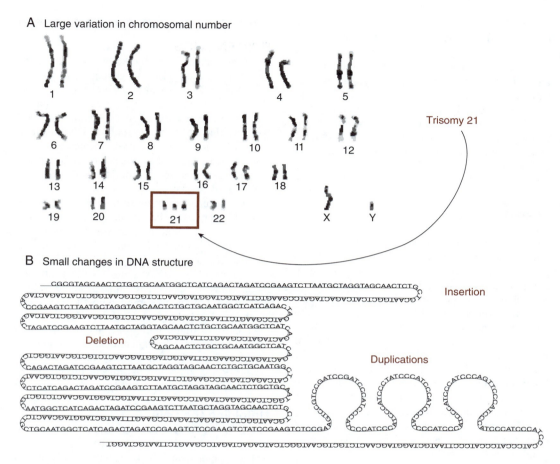

B Small changes in DNA structure

FIGURE 6.4 Structural variation—macro and micro. **A:** The karyotype of a male child with Down syndrome showing the addition of an extra chromosome. **B:** Copy number variations are smaller insertions, deletions, or duplications within the DNA strand.

additions/deletions and SNPs). They are called copy number variations (CNVs).

CNV is a term that describes more than a few base pair insertions, deletions, or duplications within the DNA molecule (Figure 6.4B). CNVs range in size from hundreds up to millions of base pairs of DNA. Remarkably, they are harder to detect than SNPs because it requires microarray technology, which is different than the method used to sequence the genome. Recently, attention has turned to the role CNVs may play in mental illness. Many laboratories are comparing CNVs in normal populations with CNVs in those with disorders. Studies suggest that CNVs play a role in schizophrenia, autism, and attention deficit hyperactivity disorder (ADHD). A recent study in ADHD highlights some of the problems. 410 children with ADHD were compared with 1156 healthy, matched controls. 14% of the ADHD children had large rare CNVs, whereas only 7% of the controls had similar genetic deficits. Although this is a significant difference, it is also discouraging because it shows that most children with ADHD do not have CNVs and many healthy controls do.

Younger Gametes

We have known for many years that older mothers have an increased risk for having children with Down syndrome. Turns out, older fathers have their own risks—older sperm is more damaged. A study in Iceland found that compared with 20-year-old men, 37-year old-men pass along twice as many mutations, whereas 70-year-old men pass on eight times as many. A different study in Sweden looked at mental illness and the age of the father, and replicated findings from previous studies. That is, children of older fathers have increased incidence of autism, psychosis, and bipolar disorder. In addition, using siblings and cousins as comparison, they found increased risk for ADHD, suicide attempts, substance abuse problems, and low educational attainment in children born to fathers who were 47 compared with fathers in their early 20s.

This is troubling information. Many people reading this book (including the authors) will have delayed starting a family in pursuit of education and a career. We do not have an easy solution to this vexing dilemma.

Shared Genes

We envision psychiatric disorders as discrete entities—different chapters in the book, if you will. We believe that anxiety, depression, schizophrenia, etc. are different disorders because they come from different problems in the brain, with divergent symptoms and illness progressions. But what seems like different categories may have more in common than we would imagine.

One of our training residents tells a story of meeting the family of a bipolar patient whom he was treating in the hospital. As the resident recalls, Mom suffered with depression and anxiety, Dad was finally clean and sober (but just barely), Uncle was in prison, the grandfather had been institutionalized for many years, and Junior was bouncing off the walls during the meeting. They all had a problem but not the same one.

A better understanding of the genetics of mental illness should help us understand the boundaries between syndromes (or the overlapping foundations). A recent genome-wide analysis of 33,000 patients with autism spectrum disorder, ADHD, bipolar disorder, major depression, and schizophrenia (compared to 27,000 healthy controls) identified a number of SNPs in common. In other words, what we think of as distinct disorders may have similar genetic origins.

Missing Heritability

In spite of the technological advances in analyzing the genome, the genetic causes of the common medical and psychiatric disorders remain elusive. At this time a good family history remains more clinically useful than expensive genetic sequencing. Where is the missing heritability? One answer is that the genetic mechanisms are more complicated than previously expected. Another answer may be that events from the environment can alter the gene expression, further complicating the picture.

EPIGENETICS

Every nucleated cell in the body contains a complete copy of the organism's genetic code. Cardiac cells, liver cells, and neurons, all contain the same DNA. Yet only a fraction of the genes in any particular cell are expressed. Most are literally switched "off" so that only the appropriate DNA is transcribed for any given cell line. During embryonic development, different cell lines emerge by turning on some genes (at the appropriate time) and turning off all the rest.

Understandably, transcription is under tight control in any cell. Having the correct "key" to a particular gene is one mechanism the cell uses to limit transcription. Each gene has a sequence of DNA called the promoter region that signals the starting point for RNA synthesis. Transcription factor proteins specific for that promoter, along with RNA polymerase, bind with the DNA and synthesize RNA (Figure 6.5). (Less is known about the control of transcription of non–protein-coding RNA.) Another mechanism to control gene expression is for a cell to limit access to the promoter region. Remarkably, events during the course of one's life can affect these mechanisms.

Unfolding the DNA

The DNA in each of our 46 chromosomes is one long strand of a double-helix fiber, which would measure approximately a meter if laid end to end. The cell must package these strands into the nucleus (Figure 6.6). This is accomplished by using dense proteins called histones—vacuum storage bags at the cellular level. The DNA, which is negatively charged, wraps around a series of positively charged histones. These "beads on a string" are then folded into a compact structure called chromatin. The chromatin is further coiled and folded to form the chromosome.

The histones do more than just packaging the DNA. They also regulate gene expression. DNA is inaccessible to regulatory signals when it is folded in its chromatin structure. Transcription factors cannot initiate gene expression when they cannot physically reach the promoter region of the DNA. Transcription of the gene requires the unfolding of the chromatin, the unwrapping of the histone, and the exposure of the promoter region.

Concealing the Gene

The attachment of other molecules to the DNA or histones can have a tremendous impact on gene

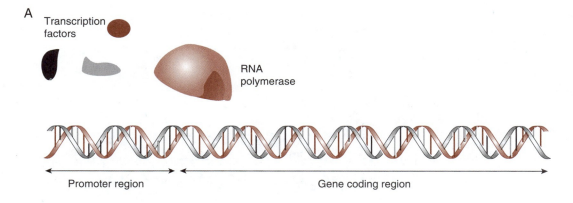

A

Transcription factors

RNA polymerase

Promoter region

Gene coding region

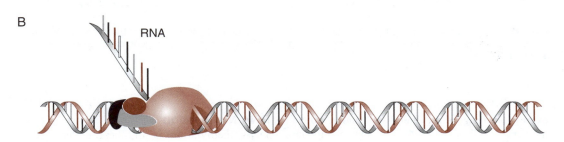

B

RNA

FIGURE 6.5 Transcription factors and RNA polymerase **(A)** must combine and lock onto the promoter region of the gene before the DNA can be transcribed into mRNA **(B)**.

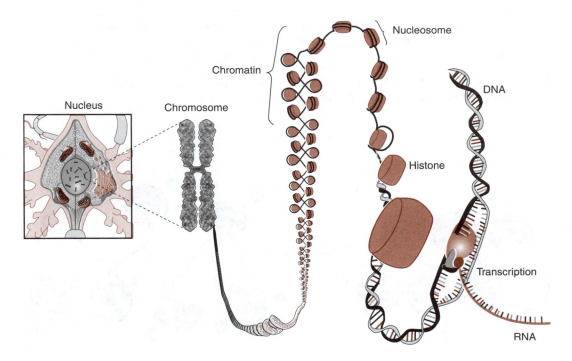

Nucleosome

Chromatin

DNA

Nucleus

Chromosome

Histone

Transcription

RNA

FIGURE 6.6 The DNA must be properly packaged to fit into the nucleus. For gene expression (transcription) to occur, the appropriate section must be unfolded and exposed.

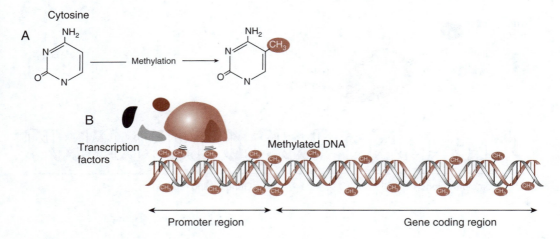

FIGURE 6.7 **A:** Addition of a methyl group to the cytosine nucleotide. **B:** Methylation of the promoter region of the gene prevents transcription factors from locking onto the DNA and prevents gene expression, which silences the gene.

expression. Epigenetics (literally meaning "above the genetics") has come to mean changes in gene expression that take place without a change in the sequence of A, T, C, and G nucleotides. In other words, the specific genetic code is not changed, but the accessory molecules hanging on the nucleotides and/or histones may conceal or expose the DNA which can alter gene expression. In particular the addition (or subsequent removal) of methyl or acetyl groups to the DNA or the histone proteins can alter access to the promoter region of the gene. Typically, methyl groups decrease gene expression, whereas acetyl groups increase gene expression.

DNA Methylation

DNA methylation is the best understood of the epigenetic alterations. DNA methylation involves the addition of a methyl group (CH_3) to one of the nucleotides—in this case, cytosine (Figure 6.7). The methyl group is only a problem when it is added to cytosines found in the promoter region of genes. DNA methylation of the cytosine nucleotide in the promoter region effectively silences that gene by preventing the transcription factors from binding with the DNA. If transcription cannot get started, gene expression does not occur.

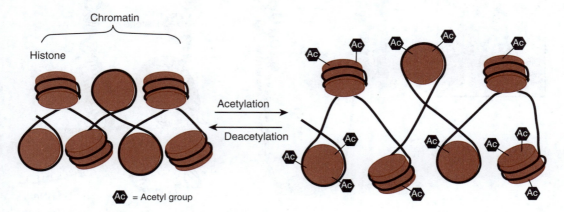

FIGURE 6.8 The addition of acetyl groups to the histones opens up the chromatin and allows greater access to the genes. The result is generally increased gene expression.

Chromatin Remodeling

Chromatin remodeling is another epigenetic mechanism regulating gene expression. The addition or deletion of various molecules to the histone proteins can affect the structure of the chromatin. The chromatin structure can be more tightly wrapped or more loosely exposed depending on which molecules are attached to the histone. Open chromatin structure allows greater access to the promoter region of a gene and enhances gene expression.

There are many molecules that can be attached to the histone, but the two most widely reported in behavioral studies are methyl and acetyl groups. The methyl groups tend to compress the chromatic structure and silence the gene. Acetylation, on the other hand, opens up the chromatin structure and allows the transcription factors greater access to the DNA and hence greater gene expression (Figure 6.8).

Environmental Events and Epigenetics

Now, this is where it gets really interesting! It turns out stimuli from the environment (such as toxins, radiation, trauma, etc.) can alter gene expression through epigenetic mechanisms. Physical or emotional events during one's life can literally alter gene expression through epigenetic mechanisms— without changing the genetic code. For example, smoking can increase the risk of cancer through epigenetic mechanisms. Smoking can turn off tumor suppressor genes. Without the tumor suppressor genes producing suppressor proteins, tumors can grow unimpeded. The individual's behavior has negative health effects through epigenetic mechanisms.

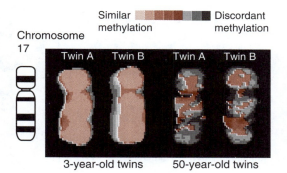

FIGURE 6.9 Color is used to show similar or discordant methylation patterns for each set of twins. The study suggests that epigenetic markers, similar when young, change over the course of one's life. (Adapted from Fraga MF, Ballestar E, Paz MF, et al. Epigenetic differences arise during the lifetime of monozygotic twins. *Proc Natl Acad Sci U S A*. 2005;102:10604–10609. Copyright [2005] National Academy of Sciences, U.S.A.)

Epigenetics may also explain why identical twins do not always develop the same diseases— an issue broached in Chapter 1, Introduction. Although genetically identical, the twins do not live identical lives and grow increasingly discordant for epigenetic markers as they age. Figure 6.9 shows chromosome 17 stained for methylation from two sets of twins—one 3 years old and the other 50 years old. The methylation pattern is practically identical in the young twins but much more out of sync in the older twins. The events of one's life are recorded on the epigenome.

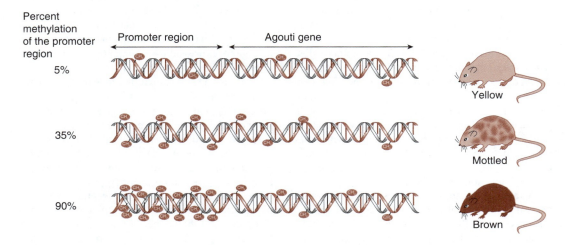

FIGURE 6.10 The Agouti gene causes the mouse to have a yellow coat and predisposes the mouse to obesity, diabetes, and cancer. With increased methylation of the promoter region of the gene, the gene is not expressed and the mouse is brown and healthy.

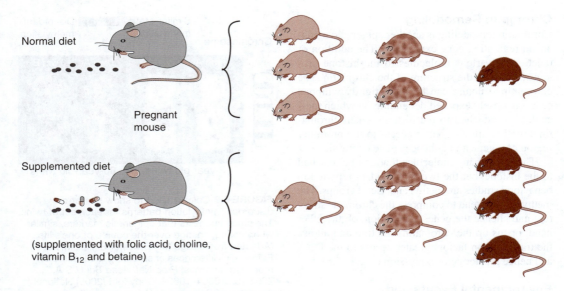

Normal diet

Pregnant
mouse

Supplemented diet

(supplemented with folic acid, choline,
vitamin B$_{12}$ and betaine)

FIGURE 6.11 Pregnant mice fed with a supplemental diet high in methyl groups will produce more pups with a silenced Agouti gene because of increased methylation of the gene.

Agouti Gene

The Agouti gene in mice is a wonderful example of how environmental factors—in this case the mother's diet—can affect health through epigenetic changes. The Agouti gene is a problem. It not only turns the mouse's hair yellow but also predisposes it to diabetes, obesity, and cancer. Fortunately, the Agouti gene can be turned off if the promoter region in front of the gene is methylated—transcription factors cannot attach to the gene, and it is silenced. This is good for the mouse. Figure 6.10 shows the results of study by Waterland and Jirtle analyzing the methylation of the Agouti gene and the coat of the mouse. More methylation results in a browner and healthier mouse.

What is more remarkable is that a mother's diet when she's pregnant can affect the methylation of the Agouti gene in her pups. Mother mice fed with a supplemental diet high in methyl groups (such as folic acid, vitamin B$_{12}$, choline, and betaine) will produce a greater percentage of brown, healthy pups (Figure 6.11). This study shows a clear connection between an environmental event (in this case diet) and subsequent epigenetic effects on physical appearance and health.

A fascinating study conducted in Sweden suggests that the diet of our *grandparents* has enduring epigenetic effects on our health. Researchers studied a small, isolated community in northern Sweden, which was subjected to periods of feast and famine in the 19th and early 20th centuries. People who enjoyed bountiful harvests during their preadolescent years had grandchildren who died younger. On the other hand, people who were underfed when they were between the ages of 8 and 12 years sired grandchildren who lived longer. In other words, the diet of our grandparents during their preadolescent years may have epigenetic effects that are passed on to future generations. If this is true, what will the current epidemic of obesity in children have on future generations?

Epigenetics is of particular relevance to understanding mental illness. We know that environmental events (such as trauma, relationships, drugs, poverty, etc.) play a large role in the development of mental disorders. Epigenetic mechanisms may explain the link between events in the environment and gene expression—a topic that appears frequently in the coming chapters.

Perhaps one reason it is so hard to find the genes of mental illness is that epigenetic factors obscure the real culprits. If the genome is the hardware of inheritance, then epigenetics describes the software. A problem with *both* the hardware (the actual genetic code) and software (the environment and how life events affect gene expression) would be especially difficult to identify.

A final thought about epigenetics. We give psychiatric medications as treatments for mental disorders, and they appear to modify behavior by turning genes off or on. For example, in adolescent rats, methylphenidate unregulated more than 700 genes, many of which are involved in synaptic plasticity. Ostensibly this all transpires through epigenetic mechanisms. The question is... Are these changes transient or do they endure even after the medication is discontinued?

We know that some of our medications cause long-term side effects, e.g., tardive dyskinesia from antipsychotics. It seems reasonable to assume that this results from permanent epigenetic changes although we do not know what causes tardive dyskinesia, so we do not know where to look. With addiction, we know something changes in the addict's brain with extended exposure to drugs, and we have a better sense of where to look. In animal models, Nestler has shown epigenetic changes including methylation and acetylation to the histones, DNA, and noncoding RNA in the reward systems after repeated exposure to drugs of abuse. It does not take too much of a leap to postulate that psychiatric medications could induce molecular changes with effects that last long after the medications are stopped.

Multifactorial

All mental disorders likely result from some problem with gene expression: too much or too little—either starting during embryonic development or beginning later in life. Yet finding the genes involved remains hidden at this point. The genome has proved to be more complex than we imagined. Disorders are likely caused by hundreds of additions, substitutions, or deletions, each having a small effect. Epigenetic effects compound the difficulty of finding the offending genes. Furthermore, what appears to be one illness such as anxiety or schizophrenia could be many different conditions that share a similar final common pathway. Clearly the predisposition to a major mental illness is to some degree inherited, but the sources of the errors are too numerous and mysterious to identify with our current technology. The search continues.

One final thought. Siddhartha Mukherjee wrote in his wonderful book *The Gene: An Intimate History*, "Every genetic 'illness' is a mismatch between an organism's genome and its environment." This is particularly true of many psychiatric disorders, e.g., the fifth grade boy, who might be at in his element running around rural Missouri like Tom Sawyer, gets medicated because he cannot sit still in class. Likewise, posttraumatic stress disorder and addictions do not develop unless vulnerable individuals are in the wrong setting. Sometimes the problem is not the biology of the patient in front of us but the environment in which the patient has landed.

TELOMERE

Telomeres are the molecular caps on the end of each strand of DNA. Like a knot at the end of a rope, they identify the terminal portion of the chromosome. This ensures that the enzymes that repair the DNA will not mistake the end for a break in the strand and attempt to connect it to some other free end—a process that normally preserves the DNA but under these circumstances scrambles the genetic code.

Telomeres shorten with every cell division. Telomere shortening is an inevitable and unfortunate consequence of aging. As the telomeres grow shorter, eventually the cells reach the limit of their replicative capacity and progress to senescence or death (apoptosis). Consequently, telomere length can be considered a rough measure of cell age (see the figure).

Patients with mental disorders have been found to have accelerated shortening of their telomeres. Patients with mood disorders, schizophrenia, Alzheimer's disease, and a history of childhood abuse have shorter telomeres when compared with healthy controls. Exercise appears to preserve telomere length.

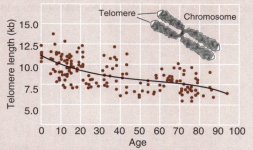

(Adapted from Calado RT, Young NS. Telomere diseases. *New Engl J Med*. 2009;361:2353–2365. Copyright © 2009 Massachusetts Medical Society. Reprinted with permission from Massachusetts Medical Society.)

Cancer is the result of cells that replicate continuously and without constraint. The telomeres, although small, are preserved. In many cancers an enzyme called telomerase is produced that adds nucleotides back onto the end of the DNA and preserves the telomeres—and the cell. Actually, every cell has the capacity to synthesize telomerase, but only a few do. Some people speculate that harnessing telomerase may be the fountain of youth.

THE NEUROSCIENCE MODEL

Up until this point in this book, we have been reviewing the basic parts of the brain. We started with the big organ and got increasingly small: from cortical structures, to cells, down to molecules. In this chapter we have gone to the deepest level, the DNA—where it all begins. If you view this sequence of chapters in the opposite order: genes to molecules to cells to networks to behaviors and then the effects of the behaviors on the DNA, this is what we call the neuroscience model (Figure 6.12). The most up-to-date model for understanding normal behavior and mental illness.

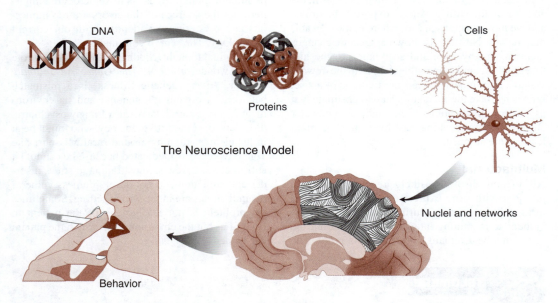

FIGURE 6.12 The neuroscience model. Although the term is not used, this is the prevailing model of understanding the physiology of normal behavior and mental illness.

QUESTIONS

1. Why does the governor of South Carolina have so few protein-coding genes?
   a. The governor believes protein-coding genes are another example of too much government control.
   b. The governor is closely related to *Caenorhabditis elegans*.
   c. The governor sold off the vast majority of protein-coding genes in an attempt to balance the State budget.
   d. Because much of the complexity of the human species is controlled by other parts of the DNA.

2. All of the following lead us to believe "junk DNA" is important except
   a. Non–protein-coding sections are highly expressed in the brain.
   b. RNA has more capacity to control functions in a cell than previously recognized.
   c. Defects in "junk DNA" have been identified in autism.
   d. Some microRNAs have been implicated in schizophrenia.

3. What has happened to the "chemical imbalance" theories of mental illness in the genomic era?
   a. Genome-wide studies fail to implicate genes that are associated with neurotransmitters or their receptors.
   b. Genes for the serotonin receptor have been identified in families with bipolar disorder in multiple linkage studies.
   c. The dopamine transporter gene on chromosome 11 is altered in most patients with childhood-onset schizophrenia.
   d. A significant number of patients with panic disorder are lacking the gene for the A section of the GABA receptor.

4. Understanding epigenetics helps us understand
   a. Why non–protein-coding sections are so highly expressed in the brain.
   b. How events in the environment can alter gene expression.
   c. The cognitive effects of trisomy 21.
   d. The increased potential for insertions, deletions, and duplications in the seriously mentally ill.

5. Which of the following is the most accurate?
   a. Methylation increases gene expression and acetylation increases it.
   b. Methylation increases gene expression and acetylation reduces it.
   c. Methylation reduces gene expression and acetylation increases it.
   d. Methylation reduces gene expression and acetylation reduces it.

6. All of the following is true of the Agouti gene in mice except
   a. Methylation of the promoter region produces more brown pups.
   b. What the pregnant mothers eat can have enduring effects on the DNA of the pups.
   c. Pups with less expression of the Agouti gene are healthier.
   d. A pregnant mother's diet high in polyunsaturated fats will silence the Agouti gene.

7. All of the following are true about telomeres except
   a. They identify the terminal end of a chromosome.
   b. They are altered by the diet of one's grandparents.
   c. They grow shorter with increasing replication.
   d. They are believed to correlate with some mental disorders.

See Answers section at the end of this book.

Modulators

CHAPTER 7

Hormones and the Brain

CHARACTERISTICS OF A HORMONE

In the preceding chapters we reviewed the electro-chemical connection between neurons. This is the predominant method of communication within the brain and the focus of much attention from psychiatrists. The next four chapters describe systems that modulate the electrochemical connections. We will start with hormones—molecular messengers sent through the bloodstream.

Neurons and neurotransmitters can be compared to telephone wires connecting one phone to another. Hormones are like TV signals that are broadcast across the skies and only recognized by appropriate receivers. With the advent of cell phones and cable TV, the distinction between direct and broadcast communication has blurred. This blurring has also occurred in the brain—traditional neurotransmitters sometimes function as hormones, and hormones sometimes function as neurotransmitters. For example, epinephrine can be a neurotransmitter but functions as a hormone when released from the adrenal medulla with a signal from the sympathetic division of the autonomic nervous system (ANS).

Although they can act in a similar manner, hormones differ from neurotransmitters in several key ways. Hormones tend to do the following:

1. Affect behavior and physiology in a gradual manner over days and weeks.
2. Receive reciprocal feedback.
3. Secrete in small pulsatile bursts.
4. Fluctuate with circadian rhythm.
5. Assorted effects on different organs.

The last point (no. 5) is of great interest to us and will be a large part of the focus of this chapter.

The γ-aminobutyric acid (GABA) receptor provides an example of a hormone modulating an electrochemical communication. Steroid hormones, as well as other molecules, influence the GABA receptor (see Figure 5.3). Figure 7.1 shows how a progesterone metabolite enhances the influx of Cl^- ions through the GABA receptor. This will reduce the potential of the postsynaptic neuron to fire, effectively calming the neuron. This may explain the emergence of psychiatric symptoms with sex hormone fluctuations.

The difference between hormones and neurotransmitters is further blurred by the existence of *neuroendocrine* cells (sometimes called *neurosecretory cells*). Neuroendocrine cells are hybrids of neurons and endocrine cells (Figure 7.2). They receive neural signals but secrete a hormone into the bloodstream. For example, the neuroendocrine cells of hypothalamus receive electrical impulses from the cerebral cortex and then signal the pituitary through the bloodstream.

Classification

There are three types of hormones, which can be grouped by their chemical structure: (1) protein, (2) amine, and (3) steroid (Table 7.1). Protein hormones, such as neuropeptides, are large molecules composed of strings of amino acids. Amine hormones are small molecules derived from amino acids. Steroid hormones are composed of four interlocking rings synthesized from dietary cholesterol. This last group, also called *neurosteroids*, is known to make GABA more inhibitory (Figure 7.1) and behaviorally have anxiolytic, anticonvulsant, and sedative effects. Changes in neurosteroids might explain the emergence of psychiatric symptoms often seen with fluctuations in hormones. There is

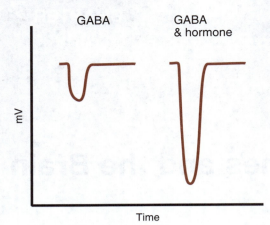

FIGURE 7.1 The Cl⁻ current is enhanced when a progesterone metabolite is added to γ–aminobutyric acid (GABA). Cl, chlorine. (Adapted from Rupprecht R, Holsboer F. Neuroactive steroids: mechanisms of action and neuropsychopharmacologic perspectives. *Trends Neurosci.* 1999;22[9]:410–460. Copyright 1999 with permission from Elsevier.)

Neurotransmitter

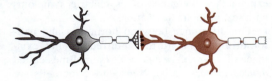

Endocrine

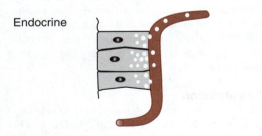

Neuroendocrine

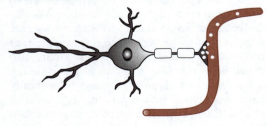

FIGURE 7.2 Chemical communication systems in humans.

TABLE 7.1
The Major Classes of Hormones

Protein Hormones
  Oxytocin
  Vasopressin
  Releasing Hormones
    Corticotropin-releasing hormone
    Thyrotropin-releasing hormone
    Gonadotropin-releasing hormone
    Growth hormone–releasing factor
  Tropic Hormones
    Adrenocorticotropic hormone
    Thyroid-stimulating hormone
    Luteinizing hormone
    Follicle-stimulating hormone
    Growth hormone
    Prolactin

Amine Hormones
  Epinephrine
  Norepinephrine
  Thyroid hormone
  Melatonin

Steroid Hormones (neurosteroids)
  Estrogens
  Progestins
  Androgens
  Glucocorticoids
  Mineralocorticoids

considerable interest in the neurosteroids as potential novel therapeutic agents for psychiatric disorders, although nothing, as yet, has proven effective and safe.

Effects on Target Cells

Hormones have two primary effects on target cells:

1. Promote differentiation and development.
2. Modulate the rate of function.

Hormones bind to specific receptors on or in the target cell in three ways. Most of the protein and amine hormones exert their effects by binding with receptors imbedded in the cell wall (as is the case with the classic neurotransmitters). The steroid hormones and thyroid hormones are lipophilic and can pass directly through the cell wall. They bind with receptors inside the cell. The steroid hormones bind with a receptor in the cytoplasm, which initiates protein synthesis when the complex couples with the DNA. The thyroid hormone

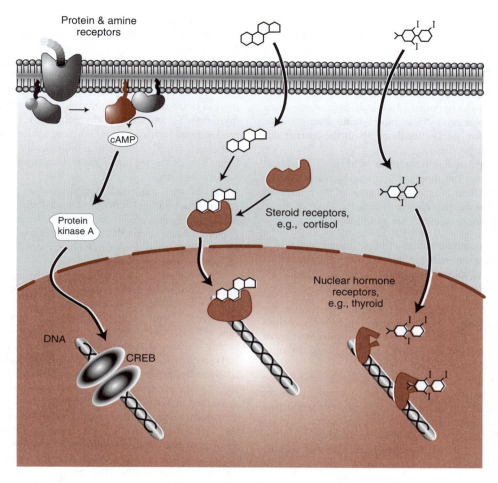

FIGURE 7.3 The three types of receptors used by different hormones. cAMP, cyclic adenosine monophosphate; CREB, cyclic adenosine monophosphate response element–binding protein.

receptor belongs to a family of nuclear hormone receptors. These receptors reside in the nucleus on the gene and suppress gene expression until activated by a thyroid hormone (specifically T_3). Figure 7.3 shows these three different receptors.

In all cases, the hormones change the function of the target cell by stimulating gene expression. This process is called a *genomic effect*. Some hormones affect neurons without stimulating the transcription of genes by modulating ion receptors: a *nongenomic effect*.

CENTRAL NERVOUS SYSTEM AND HORMONES

The primary endocrine glands in the brain are the hypothalamus and the pituitary gland. The hypothalamus appears to be the command center

that integrates information about the state of the brain and the body by way of neuronal projections and intrinsic chemosensitive neurons. The hypothalamus coordinates the actions of the pituitary gland to maintain homeostasis in response to changes in the body and environment. Some of the essential somatic functions controlled by the hypothalamus and pituitary gland are as follows:

1. Control of blood flow (e.g., drinking, blood osmolarity, and renal clearance)
2. Regulation of energy metabolism (e.g., feeding, metabolic rate, and temperature)
3. Regulation of reproductive activity
4. Coordination of response to threats
5. Modulating circadian rhythms

The remarkable number of functions governed by these relatively small glands is possible because of the diversity of neuronal projections sent to the hypothalamus from the brain and the spinal cord. Additionally, the hypothalamus and pituitary gland have a multitude of intrinsic chemosensitive neurons that respond to circulating levels of various hormones. The pituitary gland, as well as some areas of the hypothalamus, is an area of the brain not protected by the blood–brain barrier. This allows for quicker feedback about the current status of target organs.

Of particular interest to behavioral neuroscientists are the direct afferent projections that the hypothalamus receives from areas of the brain with well-known psychiatric functions. Four of these important projections are as follows:

1. Corticohypothalamic fibers: frontal cortex
2. Hippocampohypothalamic fibers: hippocampus
3. Amygdalohypothalamic fibers: amygdala
4. Thalamohypothalamic fibers: thalamus

These afferent fibers play a large role in the stimulation, or lack of stimulation, to the hypothalamus and the pituitary gland that results in many of the endocrine abnormalities found during different behavioral conditions.

Figure 7.4 shows the complex relationship between the cortex, hypothalamus, pituitary gland, and target organs for the neuroendocrine system. The figure illustrates the central location of the hypothalamus, the two sides of the pituitary, the variety of target organs affected, and the feedback mechanisms. Figure 7.5 shows most of the hormones associated with the anterior pituitary gland, particularly the releasing hormones excreted by the neuroendocrine cells of the hypothalamus, which stimulate the release of the tropic hormones.

Although most of the hormones affect the brain in one way or another, we will only focus on the two systems most relevant to mental illness: the hypothalamic–pituitary–thyroid (HPT) axis and the hypothalamic–pituitary–adrenal (HPA) axis.

THYROID: THE HYPOTHALAMIC–PITUITARY–THYROID AXIS

Thyroid hormones are involved in maintaining optimal metabolism in nearly every organ system and are integral to the temperature regulation of the body. The secretion of thyroid hormones is controlled by the HPT axis shown in Figure 7.6. The neuroendocrine cells in the hypothalamus secrete thyrotropin-releasing hormone (TRH) into the portal circulation of the pituitary. TRH binds with receptors on the thyrotroph cells of

the anterior pituitary and stimulates the release of thyroid-stimulating hormone (TSH). The hypothalamic neuroendocrine cells also synthesize and release somatostatin, which inhibits the release of TSH (as well as growth hormone).

TSH stimulates the synthesis and release of two thyroid hormones from the thyroid gland: triiodothyronine (T_3) and tetraiodothyronine (T_4). T_4 is the predominant form of thyroid hormones released by the gland, but T_3 is the more biologically potent form. T_4 is converted into T_3 by the target organs as well as the brain.

In humans, congenital hypothyroidism causes severe structural and functional neurologic abnormalities known as cretinism. This disorder is easily corrected but a disaster if missed. It is one of the few medical conditions routinely screened for in the newborn nursery.

The role of thyroid hormones in the maintenance of the mature brain is less understood. The brain maintains tight control over the level of thyroid hormone in the central nervous system (CNS), and thyroid nuclear receptors are highly expressed throughout the brain, particularly within the hippocampus. Clinical features of hypothyroidism and hyperthyroidism, including significant neuropsychiatric symptoms, are described in Table 7.2.

Additionally, clinical studies have shown that the T_3 hormone can augment other medications used to treat patients with treatment-resistant depression, as well as accelerate the response to antidepressants when initiating treatment for depression. However, meta-analysis of augmenting and accelerating studies found the trials to be small in number and not uniformly positive. The efficacy of liothyronine augmentation was compared with that of lithium augmentation as the third step for treatment-resistant depression in the STAR*D study. Both groups showed only modest remission rates (liothyronine 24.7% vs lithium 15.9%) and were not statistically significantly different.

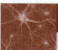

POINT OF INTEREST

Thyroid hormones are the only substance produced by the body that contains iodine. Without enough iodine, the thyroid gland swells (stimulated by excessive TSH), producing a goiter. The addition of small amounts of iodine to salt prevents the development of this diet-induced hypothyroidism.

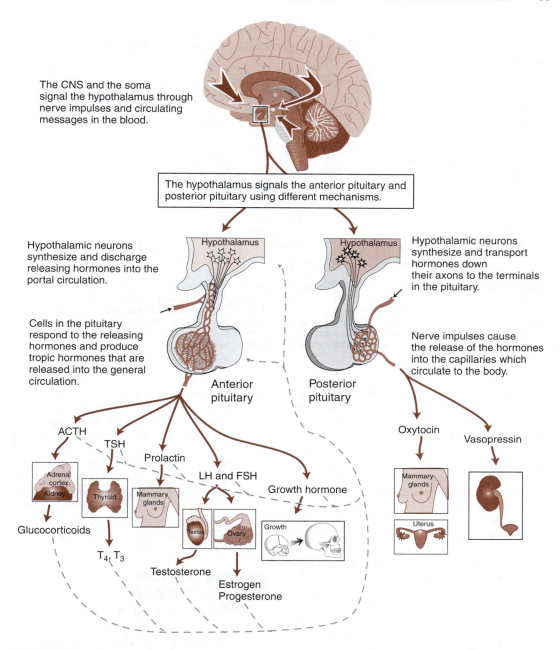

The CNS and the soma signal the hypothalamus through nerve impulses and circulating messages in the blood.

The hypothalamus signals the anterior pituitary and posterior pituitary using different mechanisms.

Hypothalamic neurons synthesize and discharge releasing hormones into the portal circulation.

Hypothalamus

Hypothalamus

Hypothalamic neurons synthesize and transport hormones down their axons to the terminals in the pituitary.

Cells in the pituitary respond to the releasing hormones and produce tropic hormones that are released into the general circulation.

Nerve impulses cause the release of the hormones into the capillaries which circulate to the body.

Anterior pituitary

Posterior pituitary

ACTH

TSH

Prolactin

LH and FSH

Growth hormone

Oxytocin

Vasopressin

Adrenal cortex
Kidney

Thyroid

Mammary glands

Testes   Ovary

Growth

Mammary glands

Uterus

Glucocorticoids

T_4, T_3

Testosterone

Estrogen
Progesterone

FIGURE 7.4 Information from the cerebral cortex and bloodstream converges on the hypothalamus, which instigates a cascade of actions and in turn responds to feedback from the target organs. ACTH, adrenocorticotropic hormone; CNS, central nervous system; FSH, follicle-stimulating hormone; LH, luteinizing hormone; TSH, thyroid-stimulating hormone; T_3, triiodothyronine; T_4, tetraiodothyronine.

Thyroid hormones are important for the function of the adult brain, but the underlying molecular mechanism by which the HPT axis influences neuropsychiatric conditions remains unclear. Many authors in psychiatry postulate that the cognitive and emotional symptoms associated with thyroid disorders are related to changes in serotonin, norepinephrine (NE), and dopamine. Indeed, studies on rats have found increased serotonergic transmission concomitant with decreased 5-hydroxytryptamine$_{1A}$ (5-HT$_{1A}$) sensitivity and increased 5-HT$_{2A}$ sensitivity with exogenous thyroid. With regard to NE, Gordan et al. have demonstrated anterograde transport of T_3 from the cell bodies in the locus

Releasing hormones	CRH	TRH	PRH	GnRH	GHRH	Hypothalamus
Tropic hormones	ACTH	TSH	Prolactin	LH and FHS	Growth Hormone	Anterior pituitary
Target organs	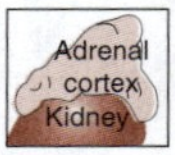 Adrenal cortex Kidney	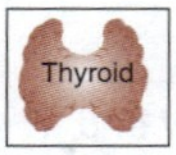 Thyroid	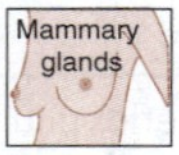 Mammary glands	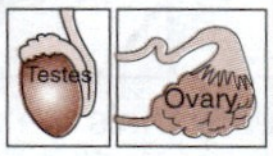 Testes Ovary	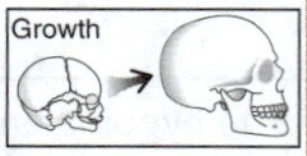 Growth	
Peripheral hormones	Gluco-corticoids	T_4, T_3		Testosterone Estrogen Progesterone		

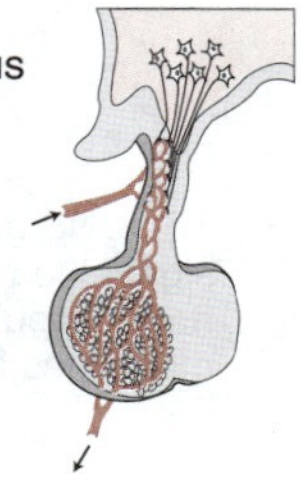

FIGURE 7.5 The anterior pituitary. Releasing hormones excreted by the hypothalamus stimulate the release of tropic hormones from the anterior pituitary. The tropic hormones then stimulate the target organ to change or release its own hormone. ACTH, adrenocorticotropic hormone; CRH, corticotropin-releasing hormone; FSH, follicle-stimulating hormone; GHRH, growth hormone–releasing hormone; GnRH, gonadotropin-releasing hormone; LH, luteinizing hormone; PRH, prolactin-releasing hormone; TRH, thyrotropin-releasing hormone; TSH, thyroid-stimulating hormone; T_3, triiodothyronine; T_4, tetraiodothyronine.

coeruleus to the nerve terminals in the hippocampus and cerebral cortex. They believe that T_3 functions as a cotransmitter along with NE. This suggests that sufficient T_3 is needed for proper NE activity.

An alternative explanation for the influence of thyroid hormones on the psychiatric status of the mature brain revolves around their role with nerve growth factors. Nerve growth factor genes are activated by T_3 during development, although growth factors, such as brain-derived neurotrophic factor (BDNF), are unaltered by thyroid hormone in the adult brain. Recently, Vaidya et al. established that 5-HT$_{1A}$ stimulation with chronic T_3 administration altered the production of BDNF in the hippocampus, although neither did so alone. They postulate a synergistic relationship between 5-HT$_{1A}$ receptors and thyroid hormones in the expression of BDNF (see Chapter 21, Depression, for more information on the role of BDNF in depression).

The most compelling explanation for the correlation between mood disorders and thyroid hormones appears to be related to the general effect that thyroid has on brain metabolism, much like the effect on peripheral metabolism. Positron emission tomography studies on patients with hypothyroidism show global reduction in brain activity and as much as a 23% reduction in cerebral blood flow in the patients compared with controls. In a remarkable study at the National Institutes of Mental Health, Marangell et al. examined TSH in medication-free patients with mood disorders, none of whom had overt thyroid disease. The study found an inverse relationship between TSH and global cerebral blood flow: TSH was up when cerebral blood flow was down. The areas with the greatest reduction in blood flow were the areas of the brain associated with depression: left dorsolateral prefrontal cortex (PFC) and medial PFC. One can postulate that the hypothalamus is responding to the reduced metabolism of the PFC (by way of the afferent fibers) as a result of the depression and reacts by stimulating the release of TSH. In essence, the HPT axis is seeking to correct the brain disorder.

DISORDER

MOOD DISORDERS

Although it is clear that thyroid disorders cause neuropsychiatric symptoms and that adding thyroid hormone can accelerate and augment the treatment of mood disorders, relatively few psychiatric patients have thyroid disease. Two analyses of clinical patients with depression found a 2% to 2.5% incidence of thyroid disease. The researchers concluded that routine screening for thyroid disease was not justified. Furthermore, although some patients with affective disorders can have mild laboratory changes, often referred to as *subclinical thyroid disease*, almost all anomalies resolve with effective treatment of the psychiatric disorder.

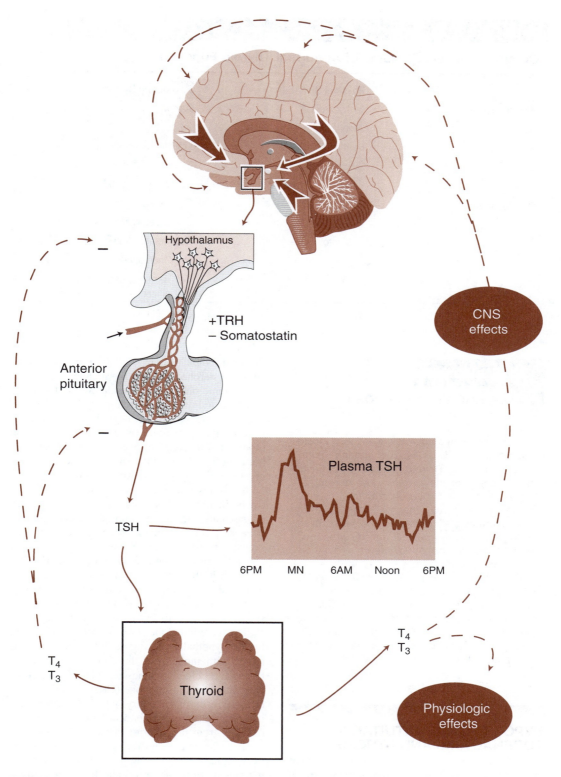

FIGURE 7.6 The hypothalamic–pituitary–thyroid axis showing the complex relationship between the brain and thyroid hormones. The important point is that tetraiodothyronine (T_4) and triiodothyronine (T_3) have direct effects on the brain as well as the body. CNS, central nervous system; TRH, thyrotropin-releasing hormone; TSH, thyroid-stimulating hormone.

TABLE 7.2

Common Clinical Features of Abnormal Thyroid Function

	Physical Symptoms	Psychiatric Symptoms
Hyperthyroidism	Tachycardia	Anxiety
	Weight loss	Irritability
	Heat intolerance	Trouble concentrating
	Sweating	Emotionally labile
		Psychomotor agitation
Hypothyroidism	Fatigue	Depressed mood
	Weight gain	Decreased libido
	Cold intolerance	Psychomotor retardation
	Dry skin	Poor memory
		Severe forms: delusions and hallucinations

DISORDER

ANOREXIA NERVOSA

Women with anorexia nervosa, when purging and undernourished, often have symptoms that resemble hypothyroidism (such as cold intolerance, bradycardia, low resting metabolic rate, etc.). Thyroid studies of patients in this condition have found low normal T_4, low T_3, and normal TSH. Additionally, reverse T_3, the metabolically inactive enantiomer of T_3, is increased. This thyroid profile is called *euthyroid sick syndrome*. It can be produced by starvation in normal volunteers and is corrected with weight gain.

This decrease in active T_3 thyroid profile seems like a physiologic adaptation to malnutrition, with the goal of preserving calories and limiting the expenditure of energy. Some patients with eating disorders will surreptitiously take exogenous thyroid to stimulate their metabolism and try to lose weight.

HYPOTHALAMIC–PITUITARY–ADRENAL AXIS AND STRESS

The HPA axis controls the synthesis and release of the corticosteroids. The corticosteroids are derived from dietary cholesterol in the adrenal cortex and include the mineralocorticoids, sex hormones, and glucocorticoids (Figure 7.7). The mineralocorticoid aldosterone assists in the maintenance of the proper ionic balance by stimulating the kidney to conserve sodium and excrete potassium. The sex hormones are secreted in negligible amounts, but have physiologic significance, and are covered in more detail in Chapter 16, Sex and the Brain. The hormone of greatest interest to the mental health community is the glucocorticoid cortisol.

Cortisol is of interest because it mobilizes energy (by promoting catabolic activity) and increases cardiovascular tone. At the same time, cortisol suppresses anabolic activity, such as reproduction, growth, digestion, and immunity. The release of cortisol varies throughout the day, with maximal secretion in the early morning hours to effectively prepare the brain and body for the rigors of the day. Cortisol also plays a large part in acute and chronic stress, which we will discuss subsequently.

The secretion of the adrenal cortex is controlled by the hypothalamus (Figure 7.8). The hypothalamus, with input from the cortex and feedback through the blood, synthesizes and releases corticotropin-releasing hormone (CRH) into the portal circulation of the pituitary, which in turn stimulates the release of adrenocorticotropic hormone (ACTH) from the anterior pituitary. The input to the hypothalamus from the cortex includes inhibitory signals from the hippocampus and activating signals from the amygdala. In other words, a healthy hippocampus turns down the HPA axis, whereas an active amygdala turns it up. This is

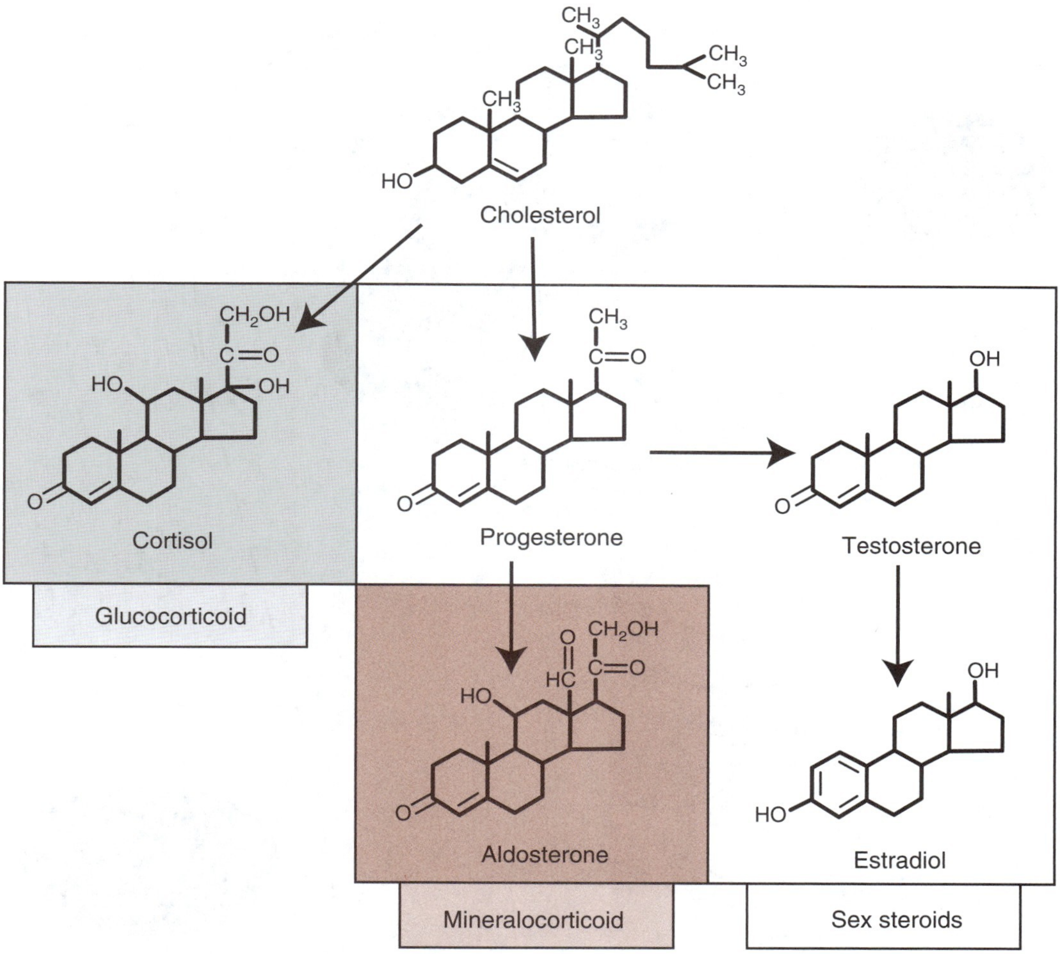

Cholesterol

Cortisol

Glucocorticoid

Progesterone

Testosterone

Aldosterone

Mineralocorticoid

Estradiol

Sex steroids

FIGURE 7.7 The corticosteroids are built from the sterol backbone of cholesterol by the addition or removal of side groups.

important in understanding the endocrine role in depression and anxiety.

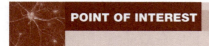

POINT OF INTEREST

CRH is an example of a hormone that has multiple functions. The primary role of CRH is the stimulation of ACTH, but CRH receptors can be found throughout the brain, not just on the anterior pituitary, suggesting other, as yet unknown, effects for this hormone.

ACTH is released into the systemic circulation from the anterior pituitary. ACTH starts as a large propeptide precursor that is cleaved into smaller segments, some of which (such as ACTH) are biologically active (see Figure 16.13). ACTH stimulates the release of cortisol from the adrenal cortex. This has a variety of physiologic effects, including changes in the CNS. The high incidence of psychiatric symptoms in patients with primary endocrine disorders, such as Cushing's disease and Addison's disease, is supportive evidence of the direct effects of cortisol on the brain.

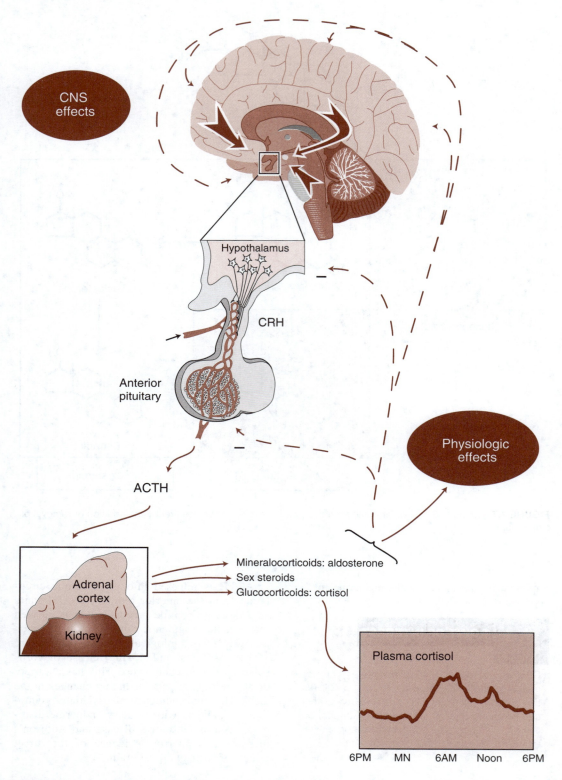

FIGURE 7.8 The hypothalamic–pituitary–adrenal axis. Note that adrenocorticotropic hormone (ACTH) releases an array of hormones with a diurnal variation. As with all hormones, there are direct effects on the cerebral cortex. CNS, central nervous system; CRH, corticotropin-releasing hormone.

DISORDER

ADDISON'S AND CUSHING'S DISEASES

Addison's disease, first described by Thomas Addison in 1855, results from a loss of cortisol and aldosterone secretion due to the near-total or total destruction of both the adrenal glands. Classic symptoms include anorexia, nausea, and hypotension, along with neuropsychiatric symptoms of apathy, fatigue, irritability, and cognitive impairment.

Cushing's disease is named after the neurosurgeon Harvey Cushing, who in 1932 linked adrenal hyperplasia and hypercortisolemia with a pituitary adenoma. The somatic effects of excessive cortisol include easy bruising, truncal obesity, muscle atrophy, osteoporosis, and impaired immune response. The psychiatric symptoms are similar to endogenous depression: irritability, depressed mood, insomnia, and trouble with memory/concentration. Patients can also experience euphoria and even hypomania, as well as psychosis. However, these symptoms are more common in patients taking glucocorticoid medications. With both Addison's and Cushing's diseases, most psychiatric symptoms remit with the resumption of normal endocrine status.

Stress

In his book, *Why Zebras Don't Get Ulcers*, Sapolsky uses a clever example to illustrate the difference between the acute physical stress that a zebra experiences when running from a lion and the chronic psychological stress that many people experience in modern industrial societies. The acute response is the biologic equivalent of mobilizing troops to handle a perceived threat. The sympathetic activation by the ANS and the liberation of cortisol bring the body and brain to an alert, fight or flight orientation. Cortisol has the effect of mobilizing energy, increasing cerebral glucose, and turning down the nonessential functions (i.e., erections, digestions, etc.). Ultimately, the brain becomes more focused and vigilant.

The body and brain pay a price for maintaining a heightened state of alertness when the stress persists, and the person cannot adapt. As seen with Addison's and Cushing's diseases, too little or too much cortisol is problematic. The benefits of cortisol can be graphed as an upside-down "U." Moderation is best.

Chronic stress is best defined as an adverse experience that induces heightened and sustained arousal over which one has little control. One of the effects of chronic stress is that the brain is unable to turn down the HPA axis, which exposes the brain and body to excess glucocorticoids. Although most of the data come from patients on glucocorticoid medications with Cushing's disease or from laboratory animal studies, the adverse consequences are believed to be similar to that of the harried stressed-out individual.

Pathologic consequences of heightened sympathetic activity and HPA activation are hypertension, formation of atherosclerotic plaque, diabetes, ulcers, and impaired immune function. In the brain, the most dramatic negative effect involves the hippocampus, a structure with ample glucocorticoid receptors (GRs) and afferent fibers to the hypothalamus. The hippocampus is well known for its role in memory, and excess glucocorticoids have indeed been shown to have the following effects:

1. Impair memory performance.
2. Disrupt long-term potentiation (LTP).
3. Induce atrophy of hippocampal dendrites.
4. Shrink the hippocampus.
5. Decrease neurogenesis (next chapter).

These cognitive changes do not develop without an active amygdala. The amygdala, well known for its role in anxiety, is stimulated by glucocorticoids, which in turn potentiates the hippocampus (see Figure 7.9). Chronic stress increases the dendritic arborization of neurons in the basolateral amygdala, which may be a reason people have trouble forgetting traumatic events.

Cushing's Disease

Excessive glucocorticoid levels, for any reason, have been shown to cause impairments in declarative memory as well as hippocampal atrophy. In a remarkable analysis of patients with Cushing's disease who underwent neurosurgical resection, Starkman et al. showed that decreasing urinary cortisol correlated with increase in the hippocampal volume. In a follow-up study, they showed that a greater improvement in memory (word list learning) was associated with greater increase in hippocampal volume.

Aging

There is evidence that glucocorticoids may contribute to age-related neuronal atrophy and cognitive decline. An essential aspect of a healthy, adaptive stress response is the ability to shut off the system when the threat has passed. Studies on rats have shown that the HPA axis is slower to turn off as the animal ages. With age, it is exposed to more continuous high levels of glucocorticoids.

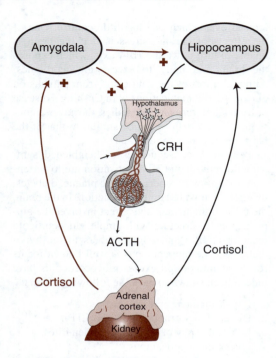

FIGURE 7.9 A schematic representation of the connections and feedback between the hypothalamic–pituitary–adrenal axis and the amygdala and hippocampus. ACTH, adrenocorticotropic hormone; CRH, corticotropin-releasing hormone.

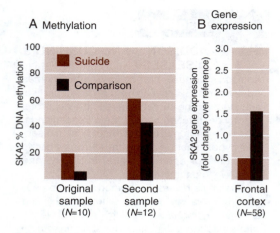

FIGURE 7.10 A: Two separate postmortem samples of suicide victims showing increased methylation of the SKA2 gene. **B:** Conversely, expression of the SKA2 gene is reduced in the suicide victims. (Adapted from Guivtivano J, Brown T, Newcomer A, et al. Identification and replication of a combined epigenetic and genetic biomarker predicting suicide and suicide behaviors. *Am J Psych.* 2014;171: 1287–1296. Reprinted with permission from the *American Journal of Psychiatry* [Copyright © 2014]. American Psychiatric Association. All Rights Reserved.)

In humans, the ability to turn off the HPA axis and the sympathetic nervous system in tranquil times is a variable trait. Some people are able to do this more effectively than others. Possibly this is a feature of being more resilient.

Lupien et al. followed up 51 healthy volunteers over 6 years and annually measured 24-hour plasma cortisol. They assessed memory and hippocampal volume in subgroups of those with high levels of cortisol and compared those findings with those of the groups with lower levels of cortisol. They found greater impairments in memory and a 14% reduction in the volume of the hippocampus in the group with high cortisol levels. This suggests that prolonged exposure to glucocorticoids either reduces the ability of neurons to resist insults or directly damages the neurons.

Depression and Anxiety

There is a long history of correlating alterations in the HPA axis with anxiety and depression. A few recent studies demonstrate the application of new research to this correlation. One research group in the Netherlands has analyzed GR number before military deployment and then assessed psychiatric symptoms on return from combat. They found

greater numbers of GR's, predeployment, in those individuals who developed depression and post-traumatic stress disorder (PTSD). For PTSD, they found that with an increase of every 1000 GRs, the risk for developing the disorder increased 7.5-fold. A different group at Emory University found that polymorphisms of the CRH receptor and a history of child abuse increased the risk of depression as an adult.

In 2014 a group from Johns Hopkins identified a gene with effects on the HPA axis that is a marker for suicidal behavior. The SKA2 gene produces a protein that appears to "chaperone" the GR from the cytoplasm into the nucleus (Figure 7.3). In a postmortem study of suicide completers the Hopkins researchers analyzed the gene from prefrontal neurons. In two independent samples, the SKA2 gene was more methylated in the suicide subjects (Figure 7.10A). And, as one would imagine, gene expression of the protein was reduced because of the methylation (Figure 7.10B). All this may blunt the suppression of cortisol in stressful situations.

These are just a few studies showing that dysregulation of the HPA axis can have detrimental effects on mood. The pharmaceutical industry has made a number of attempts to develop treatments for depression by manipulating the HPA axis. Unfortunately, nothing to date has been successful.

QUESTIONS

1. The primary mechanism by which the estrogen molecule stimulates the cell is
   a. Binding to a protein receptor imbedded in the cell wall.
   b. Activating a G protein–coupled receptor.
   c. Binding with a receptor in the cytoplasm.
   d. Coupling with a receptor in the nucleus.

2. Which of the following are true?
   a. Thyroid hormone can enhance the GABA current.
   b. Protein hormones bind a receptor on the DNA.
   c. Hormones are used for fast signals.
   d. Neuroendocrine cells excrete directly into the circulation.

3. Which of the following is correct?
   a. GnRH → LH → Estrogen.
   b. GHRH → LH → Testosterone.
   c. TRH → TSH → Prolactin.
   d. CRH → TSH → Cortisol.

4. Possible explanations for the role of thyroid hormone in mood disorders include all of the following except
   a. Changes in brain metabolism.
   b. Effects on growth hormones.
   c. Changes in GRs.
   d. Effects on 5-HT receptors.

5. Women in the acute phase of anorexia nervosa exhibit a thyroid profile called "euthyroid sick syndrome" that includes all of the following except
   a. Low T_3.
   b. Low reverse T_3.
   c. Low–normal T_4.
   d. Normal TSH.

6. The triad of hippocampal atrophy, hypercortisolemia, and cognitive impairment has been found with all the following except
   a. Cushing's disease.
   b. Addison's disease.
   c. Alzheimer's disease.
   d. Major depression.

7. All of the following go together except
   a. Amygdala atrophy.
   b. Hippocampal atrophy.
   c. Memory deficit.
   d. LTP disruption.

See Answers section at the end of this book.

CHAPTER 8

Plasticity and Adult Development

In a video produced in 1996 by Robert Sapolsky for the Teaching Company entitled *Biology and Human Behavior*, Dr Sapolsky stated,

"To the greater extent you've got all the neurons you're ever going to have to deal with by the time we're 4 or 5 years old and, unfortunately, all you do from there is lose them."

Until recently this belief—stated by Dr Sapolsky such a short time ago—was shared by almost all clinicians and neuroscientists. We are not criticizing Dr Sapolsky, whose outstanding contributions to the field were cited in the previous chapter. Rather, we wish to show that even astute Stanford professors once believed the brain was a static organ. The authors of this book were no more enlightened at that time.

Additionally, an abundance of new research has established that the brain is not the fixed structure we used to envision. Our brains have more plasticity (or ability to change) than we previously imagined. Although the rate of change is especially prominent early in life, altering the structure of the brain in response to environmental factors remains a feature across the entire life span.

The almost unbelievable prenatal development of the central nervous system (CNS) is a topic we briefly touched on in Chapter 2, Neuroanatomy. The fundamental miracle of the brain is that a single fertilized egg ultimately develops into 100 billion neurons with 100 trillion connections. In utero, this process is largely genetically driven. After birth, interactions with the environment play a greater role in determining the direction of development.

PHASES OF DEVELOPMENT

The cellular events can be divided into four phases:

1. *Neurogenesis*: The production, migration, and development of distinct new cell types—nerve or glial—from undifferentiated stem cells.
2. *Cell expansion*: The branching of axons and dendrites to make synaptic connections.
3. *Connection refinement*: The elimination of excessive branching and synaptic connections.
4. *Apoptosis*: Programmed neuronal cell death.

Neurogenesis

The cells of the intestinal epithelium are turned over every 2 weeks, whereas skin cells are replaced every 1 to 2 months. The adult brain is not nearly this prolific but is not barren either. In 1998, unequivocal newborn neurons were identified in the hippocampus of elderly subjects whose brains were examined shortly after death. We now know that undifferentiated neural stem cells remain in the CNS and continue to divide throughout life (Figure 8.1). Neural stem cells can develop into neural precursors that grow into neurons or support cells. However, they must migrate away from the stem cell's milieu before they can differentiate, and only about half the cells successfully move and transform.

Clear evidence for adult neurogenesis has been established in two areas of the brain: the subgranular zone (SGZ) in the dentate gyrus of the hippocampus and the subventricular zone (SVZ) of the lateral ventricles (Figures 8.2 and 8.3). Newborn cells are identified by tagging them with

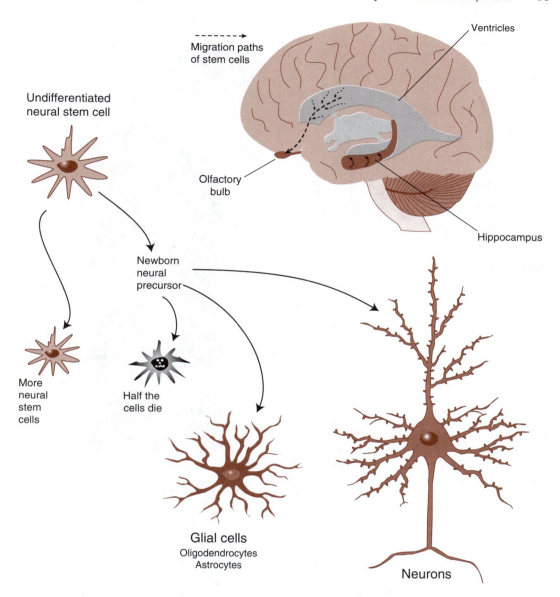

FIGURE 8.1 The process of neurogenesis starts with an undifferentiated neural stem cell that has the capacity to migrate and transform into functioning nerve cells. (Adapted from Gage FH. Brain, repair yourself. *Sci Am*. 2003;289[3]:46–53. Figure adapted from original by Alice Y. Chen.)

bromodeoxyuridine (BrdU), a thymidine analogue that can be incorporated into newly synthesized DNA. A fluorescent antibody specific for BrdU is then used to detect the incorporated molecule and thereby indicate recent DNA replication.

The use of creating new neurons in the human brain remains a mystery. The SGZ is part of the hippocampus, and neurogenesis may facilitate the stabilization of new memories. The cells born in the SVZ, on the other hand, primarily migrate

to the olfactory bulb. This might be helpful for a dog, but it is hard to imagine how this benefits humans.

In 1999, Gould et al. identified newborn nerve cells in the neocortex (prefrontal, temporal, and parietal) of adult monkeys. They established that neural stem cells migrated through the white matter and differentiated into neurons and extended axons (Figure 8.3). Unfortunately, the number of new cells is less than that found in the hippocampus or

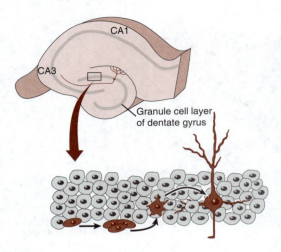

FIGURE 8.2 The granule cell layer just under the dentate gyrus (called the subgranular zone) is the most studied location of neurogenesis.

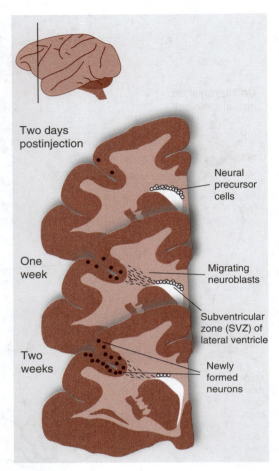

FIGURE 8.3 Adult macaque monkeys were injected with BrdU and sacrificed 2 hours, 1 week, and 2 weeks later. These sections from the prefrontal cortex show the development and migration of neural precursor cells from the subventricular zone, through the white matter to the neocortex. Additional tests established that some of the cells were newly formed neurons. (Adapted from Gould E, Reeves AJ, Graziano MS, et al. Neurogenesis in the neocortex of adult primates. *Science*. 1999;286[5439]:548–552. Reprinted with permission from AAAS.)

olfactory bulb and inadequate for significant CNS repair. Future neurologic treatments may come from finding methods (such as medications, exercise, magnetic stimulation, etc.) to invigorate the limited primate neurogenesis so as to replace damaged tissue.

A remarkable recent study seems to establish that adult neurogenesis does *not* generate new neurons capable of productive work in the gray matter. Swedish researchers used a vestige of the cold war to determine the age of neurons and nonneural brain cells in postmortem cortical biopsies.

For most of history, the amount of ^{14}C in the atmosphere and in living cells has remained constant. Aboveground nuclear bomb testing in the 50s and 60s resulted in an explosive increase in ^{14}C, which then steadily declined after the Test Ban Treaty in 1963. The amount of ^{14}C in a cell's DNA can be used to give the accurate date of the cell's birth when plotted on the known curve of ^{14}C available in the atmosphere over the past 50 years. The neuroscientists in Sweden used this technique to determine the age of brain cells in seven individuals who died unexpectedly.

The researchers were able to separate nuclei of neurons and nonneuronal cells from four regions of the cortex. Then the DNA was extracted, analyzed for ^{14}C, and plotted on the known levels of ^{14}C in the atmosphere. The results are shown in Figure 8.4. These results seem to establish that all the adult human neurons in the *neocortex* were created perinatally with none developing after birth. Nonneuronal brain cells continued to form and were born, on average, 5 years after the birth of the individual. The Swedish researchers did a

second study using autopsied brains from cancer patients who had received injections of BrdU months before death. They found neurons in SGZ of the dentate gyrus (where they are formed), but the only BrdU-labeled cells in the neocortex were nonneuronal (glial).

In summary, it appears that neurons are born in the SGZ and the SVZ throughout the life of humans, but after birth they are not inserted as functional neurons into the cerebral cortex—at least in healthy brains. So why is it that the brain continues to make new neurons until we die?

Rate of Neurogenesis

The rate of neurogenesis is modulated by various factors. It is known that enriched environments and exercise will increase neurogenesis (Figure 8.5). Additional research suggests that gonadal steroid hormones may also enhance new cell production. For example, testosterone will stimulate nerve cell production in songbirds (and possibly middle-aged men seeking to recapture the vigor of their youth). The point is that various factors may promote neurogenesis, which appears to be an indication of the health status of the brain.

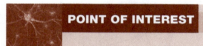

POINT OF INTEREST

The studies establishing an increase in neurogenesis with enriched environments for mice have also documented increased size of the dentate gyrus of the hippocampus. Additionally, the mice showed improved memory performance on hippocampal-dependent memory tasks (water maze). These findings validate the link between neurogenesis, neuronal growth, hippocampal size, and memory.

Stress, for example, has an inhibitory effect on neurogenesis. Extended maternal separation is a well-characterized model of early life stress for a rodent. As adults, such rodents will show protracted elevations of corticotropin-releasing factor, adrenocorticotropic hormone, and corticosterone (cortisol equivalent in a rat), as well as behavioral inhibition in response to stress. Work from Gould's laboratory has shown that rats exposed to prolonged maternal separation will have an enduring blunting of neurogenesis. When the corticosterone is experimentally lowered, the neurogenesis rebounds to normal levels—suggesting that hypersensitivity to corticosterone may be the mechanism of action that suppresses neurogenesis.

The relation between early stress, the hypothalamic–pituitary–adrenal (HPA) axis, and neurogenesis is particularly interesting because of the role of the hippocampus in modulating the HPA axis. We can conceptualize that a healthy hippocampus is necessary to put the brakes on an activated HPA axis after the stressful event dissipates. The above research suggests that early stress (e.g., an unavailable mother) leads to a smaller hippocampus because of insufficient neurogenesis, which results in an overactive HPA axis and all those secondary problems discussed in the previous chapter.

Stem Cells

One potential way to rebuild a damaged brain is to implant human embryonic stem cells that have been isolated from a very immature embryo (only 100 to 200 cells). So far it has been difficult to get these immature cells to differentiate into functioning neurons outside the olfactory bulb and hippocampus. The problem may be the absence of biochemical signals that normally prompt the developing stem cell to migrate and differentiate.

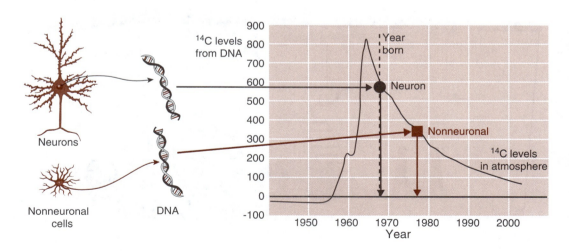

FIGURE 8.4 Postmortem analysis of ^{14}C levels in DNA from neurons and nonneuronal brain cells shows that the neurons were created at the time of this individual's birth. (Right side adapted from Bhardwaj RD, Curtis MA, Spalding KL, et al. Neocortical neurogenesis in humans is restricted to development. *Proc Natl Acad Sci U S A.* 2006;103[33]:12564–12568. Copyright [2006] National Academy of Sciences, U.S.A.)

Parkinson's disease involves the loss of dopamine (DA) neurons. Stem cells offer a potential source for cell replacement therapy. A group in Japan reported a successful treatment in monkeys with chemically induced Parkinson's disease. The important difference may have been a "cocktail" of several growth factors that coaxed the undifferentiated cells to develop into neurons and then into authentic DA neurons. These cells were injected into the bilateral putamen of the "Parkinsonian" monkeys. Figure 8.6 shows a diagram of the procedure and some results.

You would think if there were any illness that is amenable to stem cell transplantation it would be Parkinson's disease, but studies with humans have been disappointing. Almost two decades ago,

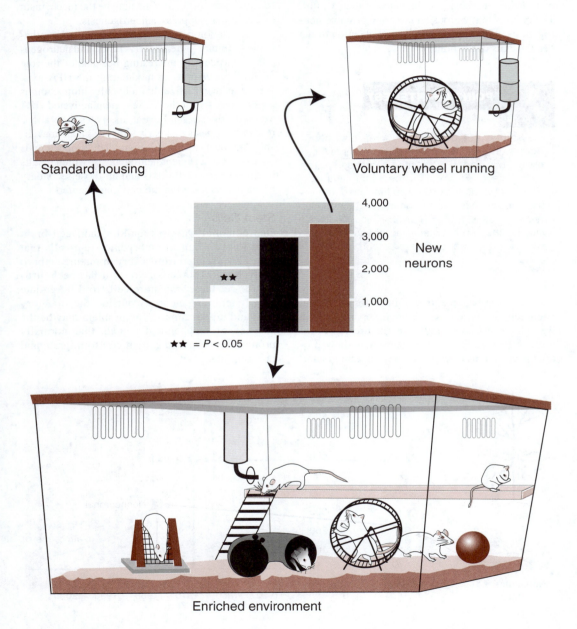

FIGURE 8.5 A study by Brown et al. showed that an enriched environment and physical exercise stimulated neurogenesis in the hippocampus but not in the olfactory bulb in mice. (Graph adapted from Brown J, Cooper-Kuhn CM, Kempermann G, et al. [2003.] Enriched environment and physical activity stimulate hippocampal but not olfactory bulb neurogenesis. *Eur J Neurosci*. 17[10]:2042–2046.)

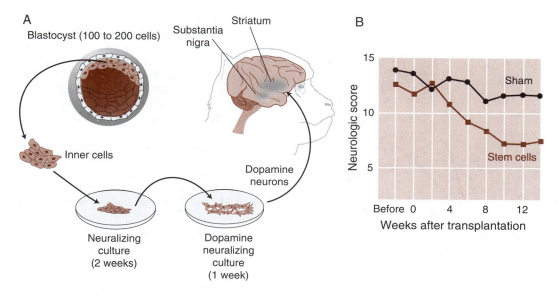

FIGURE 8.6 A: Harvesting embryonic stem cells, stimulating the development of dopamine neurons in several cultures, and injecting them into a monkey with chemically induced Parkinson's disease. **B:** Improved neurologic scores over 14 weeks. (Adapted from Takagi Y, Takahashi J, Saiki H, et al. Dopaminergic neurons generated from monkey embryonic stem cells function in a Parkinson primate model. *J Clin Invest.* 2005;115[1]:102–109.)

controlled studies with fetal tissue established that the treatment can work and, indeed, transplanted neurons remained alive and functional until death over a decade later in some patients. However, the treatment was not without problems and the studies were stopped.

More recently, studies have resumed with pluripotent stem cells, which do not have the ethical concerns associated with fetal tissue. (Figure 1.11 is an example of one type of pluripotent stem cell.) Animal studies have been successful, but there is concern that the Parkinsonian human brain is more hostile to DA neurons than one finds in the artificially induced animal models. Heck, something had to cause the Parkinson's disease in the first place. Regardless, human studies have commenced again. Stay tuned!

Cell Expansion

The second phase of neuronal growth, often called *synaptogenesis*, describes the extensive growth of axons and dendrites to make synaptic connections—a process that primarily occurs early in life. The tips of axons and dendrites have *growth cones* that appear to reach out with fingerlike structures, *filopodia*, and literally pull the growth cone to its destination. The axons are guided in a specific direction by chemical signals that attract and repel the growth cone, that is, *chemoattractants* and *chemorepellents*.

In a comprehensive postmortem analysis, Huttenlocher determined synaptic density across the life span in two regions of the human brain from 14 individuals. Using an electron microscope and special stains, he counted synaptic connections from thin sections taken from the visual cortex and prefrontal cortex. The results, displayed graphically in Figure 8.7, show that the greatest synaptogenesis takes place shortly after birth and occurs sooner for the visual cortex. Maximum synaptic density is reached before the first year in the visual cortex, but not until 3.5 years in the prefrontal cortex. Synaptogenesis is accompanied by an increase in the size of the nerve cell, presumably to support the increased metabolic needs created by the expanded axons and dendrites. Positron emission tomography scans analyzing regional blood flow in children show a similar pattern: starting low, peaking by the age of 7 and settling to adult vales by adolescence.

Connection Refinement

The third phase of neuronal cell development often referred to as *pruning*, or *synaptic elimination*, entails retraction and elimination of excessive connections. The brain makes many more connections than are needed, and the weak ones (or those not used) regress. As with synaptogenesis, the pruning proceeds at different rates for different regions of the brain, based on the need. For example, sensory

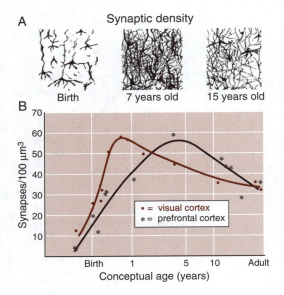

A Synaptic density

Birth   7 years old   15 years old

B

FIGURE 8.7 **A:** Schematic representation of changes in synaptic density. **B:** Measured synaptic densities in visual and prefrontal cortex from 14 individuals who died of nonneurologic diseases. (Adapted from Huttenlocher PR, Dabholkar AS. [1997.] Regional differences in synaptogenesis in human cerebral cortex. *J Comp Neurol*. 387[2]:167–178.)

and motor areas go through refinement before the regions devoted to executive functions. Clearly, moving and seeing are more essential than writing a poem, at least early on in life.

The late and extensive reduction of the frontal cortex correlates with psychological tests measuring improved executive function. It is paradoxical that the maturing process that our adolescents struggle through is actually a refinement and reduction of the gray matter and not growth. Studies suggest adolescents have more gray matter than we do, but we dominate when it comes to wisdom and smarts. The point is this: less is more. This is not the usual pattern in nature. Typically, bigger is better.

Disordered pruning may be the pathologic basis for conditions such as autism and schizophrenia. A consistent finding in patients with autism is greater total brain volume, which is not present at birth but develops during the first few years of life. It has been suggested that this may be due to insufficient pruning. Schizophrenia, on the other hand, is associated with a loss of gray matter, which may be the result of excessive pruning.

One last point about synaptogenesis in adults: Goyal and Raichle performed a mathematical modeling of brain growth and wrote, "Our analysis suggests that modest rates of synaptic growth persist in adulthood, but that this is counterbalanced by increasing rates of synaptic elimination, resulting in stable synaptic number and ongoing synaptic turnover in the human adult cortex." Therefore it may be true that our brains are like a stuffed suitcase. If you put *one more item* in, you will have to remove something to compensate. Darn!

Apoptosis

Programmed cell death, *apoptosis*, is the final phase of the sculpting of the brain. It is called *programmed* because the cells actually carry genetic instructions to self-destruct. Neurotrophins, discussed next, save the neuron by turning off the genetic program. When the intracellular "self-destruct button" has been activated, apoptosis proceeds in a characteristic process: cell shrinkage, fragmentation, and phagocytosis of the cellular remnants. This is distinguished from necrotic cell death, which results from trauma and is characterized by rapid cell membrane lysis.

Modifications of any of these four phases—for example, enhancing neurogenesis or retarding apoptosis—are potential targets for Alzheimer's disease, but nothing has been developed. An alternative area of interest regarding apoptosis is to use this with brain tumors that are notoriously resistant to anticancer treatments, for example, glioblastoma. The hope is to find a way to induce apoptosis in the cancerous cells without affecting healthy tissue.

Brain Imaging Studies

The postmortem studies by Huttenlocher provided an in-depth analysis of synaptic connections but were limited by the total number of brains that he could analyze. Brain imaging technology, on the other hand, allows the noninvasive examination of a larger number of subjects in real time with the potential to be repeated as the subjects age. Unfortunately, brain imaging does not have the resolution to the level of the synapse, so studies follow the trajectory of larger structures, such as gray matter thickness or volume.

The noninvasive magnetic resonance imaging (MRI) technology has allowed extensive studies

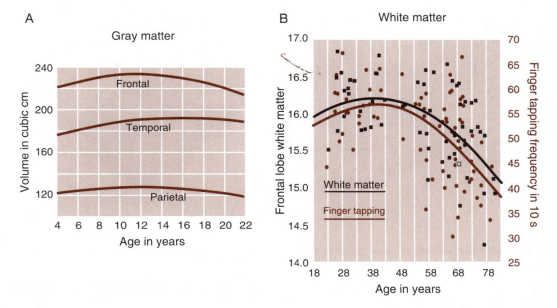

FIGURE 8.8 A: Magnetic resonance imaging analyses from 145 healthy subjects showing the changing gray matter volumes for different regions of the brain for males. **B:** Myelination of the frontal lobes correlates with motor speed and peaks at 39 years of age. **(A:** Adapted with permission from Macmillan Publishers Ltd. Giedd JN, Blumenthal J, Jeffries NO, et al. Brain development during childhood and adolescence: a longitudinal MRI study. *Nat Neurosci*. 1999;2[10]:861–863. Copyright 1999; **B:** Adapted from Bartzokis G, Lu PH, Tingus K, et al. Lifespan trajectory of myelin integrity and maximum motor speed. *Neurobiol Aging*. 2010;31[9]:1554–1562. Copyright 2010 with permission from Elsevier.)

of brain development beginning in childhood and progressing into adulthood. One study, shown in Figure 8.8A, scanned 145 healthy subjects, 99 of whom had at least two scans. Gray matter development proceeded on a trajectory of growth until 10 to 12 years of age followed by a decrease in adolescence—consistent with the pattern of synaptogenesis followed by connection refinement. The age of maximal volume (an indirect measurement of development) varies by brain region.

Figure 8.8B shows MRI results for 72 males between the ages of 23 and 80 years. White matter myelination correlates with high-frequency motor activity. These results have some correlation with peak athletic and academic achievement, showing the importance of white matter integrity in optimum brain performance.

NEUROTROPHIC GROWTH FACTORS

The CNS contains small quantities of *neurotrophic growth factors*, proteins affectionately known as "brain fertilizer." *Rita Levi-Montalcini* and her colleagues in 1952 accidentally discovered the first of this class of proteins now called nerve growth factors (NGFs), trophic factors, or growth factor proteins. They observed sensory nerve cells exploding with growth when cultured next to a mouse

sarcoma. Recognizing the significance of their discovery, they painstakingly isolated the protein and called it *nerve growth factor*. Figure 8.9 shows the profound impact that NGF has on the growth of sensory neurons. Levi-Montalcini was awarded the Nobel Prize in 1986 for this discovery.

Although called NGF—implying that it stimulates all nerve cells—this particular neurotrophin only affects sympathetic neurons and some sensory ganglion cells. Several decades of research have established four principles regarding the cells affected by NGF (Figure 8.10).

1. NGF mediates cell survival.
2. Cells that do not receive enough NGF die.
3. Target organs produce NGF.
4. Specific NGF receptors are present on innervating nerve terminals.

Because NGF is specific for a limited subset of peripheral nerves, it was assumed that there would be a host of other neurotrophic factors following similar rules waiting to be discovered. Unfortunately, the fortuitous discovery of NGF has been slow to replicate. Identifying and purifying factors that are excreted in such minute quantities has turned into an arduous task. Several factors have been discovered and are being studied, such as neurotrophin-3, glial cell line–derived neurotrophin factor, and insulinlike growth factor, to name

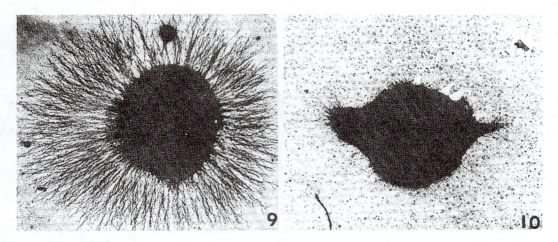

FIGURE 8.9 When exposed to nerve growth factor, these sensory nerves display enthusiastic growth. (From Levi-Montalcini R. The nerve growth factor. *Ann N Y Acad Sci*. 1964;118:149–170.)

a few, but the one that is of most interest to the mental health community is brain-derived neurotrophic factor (BDNF).

The actions of neurotrophins such as BDNF are mediated primarily through Trk (for tyrosine kinase) receptors on the nerve cell membrane. The extracellular portion of the receptor binds with the neurotrophic factor, which in turn initiates an intracellular cascade that leads to gene expression. As yet, there are no small molecule agonists or antagonists for these receptors, which hinders a better understanding (and easier treatment options) of the action of the neurotrophic factors.

The effect of stimulating the Trk receptor is determined by the specific neurotrophic factor, the combination of receptors signaled, and the intracellular pathways expressed in that cell. Disruption of neurotrophic factor signaling is presumably an explanation (and possible treatment) for some neurodegenerative diseases, for example, Huntington's, Parkinson's, and Alzheimer's diseases. Likewise the enduring symptoms resulting from substance abuse may be the result of inappropriate neurotrophic factor synthesis, mediated through epigenetic changes (as we discussed earlier).

CRITICAL PERIODS

As we have said before, genes control development in utero, but the environment influences the direction after birth. Early interactions during the time of great cellular expansion mold the brain's anatomy with an ease and permanence that can never be repeated or completely undone. These stages in development when the environmental input is so crucial to determining the structure of the brain are called *critical periods*.

Language acquisition is a good example of a critical period. Early exposure to native sounds has a lasting impact on speech, which is hard to alter later in life. Johnson and Newport demonstrated this by examining English proficiency in Korean and Chinese speakers who arrived in the United States between the ages of 3 and 39 years. They found that subjects who arrived in the United States before the age of 7 years had equivalent fluency to native speakers, whereas those who arrived after the age of 7 years had a linear decline in performance until puberty (Figure 8.11).

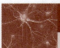

TREATMENT

NEUROTROPHINS

Medicating with neurotrophins or stimulating their increased production is an exciting prospect for future neuropsychiatric treatment. Some studies suggest that this may be the mechanism by which lithium, electroconvulsive therapy, and antidepressants resolve depression. If this is true, future treatments for depression will focus on more effective ways to stimulate growth factors. Other researchers have examined the therapeutic benefits of growth hormones for disorders such as amyotrophic lateral sclerosis and multiple sclerosis. The biggest difficulty is finding effective yet unobtrusive methods to deliver the neurotrophins to the CNS.

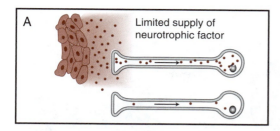

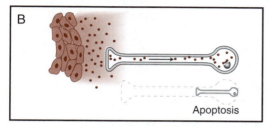

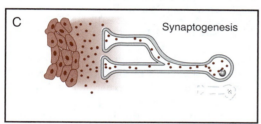

FIGURE 8.10 Neurotrophic factors, such as nerve growth factor, mediate cell proliferation and elimination by promoting cell growth, stimulating synaptogenesis, and preventing apoptosis.

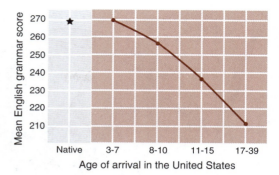

FIGURE 8.11 Language acquisition as measured by English grammar tests for native speakers compared with Korean and Chinese immigrants. (Adapted from Johnson JS, Newport EL. Critical period effects in second language learning: the influence of maturational state on the acquisition of English as a second language. *Cognit Psychol*. 1989;21[1]:60–99. Copyright 1989 with permission from Elsevier.)

The development of the visual cortex provides another example of a critical period. David Hubel and Torstern Wiesel (who received the Nobel Prize for this work) established the importance of normal visual experience early in life for proper development of the visual cortex in cats and monkeys. In a series of experiments, they sutured one eyelid shut in kittens and later monkeys for short lengths of time during various weeks after birth. They established, down to the level of the neuron, the profound effect of visual deprivation at critical periods of development.

Figure 8.12 shows how the experiments by Hubel and Wiesel were conducted. Radioactive proline was injected into an eye where it was absorbed and transported down the axons to the lateral geniculate nucleus (LGN) of the thalamus. Some of the labeled proline that spilled out of the terminal would be taken up by the LGN neurons and transported to the visual cortex. The location of the radioactive molecules can be visualized using autoradiography.

Figure 8.13 shows the results—both real and schematic—of suturing one eye shut for differing periods of time early in life. The autoradiographs in the B row show a normal cat compared with a cat whose eye was closed from 2 weeks until 18 months. This demonstrates—as do the drawings in the C row—how the neurons from the occluded eye regress and the neurons from the good eye grow. The D row shows the terminal branching, *arborization*, of the LGN neurons in the visual cortex for a normal eye and one that was occluded for just 1 week at 30 days of age. Hubel and Wiese have estimated that the critical period for ocular deprivation in a cat is 3 to 4 months.

In humans, the critical period for vision extends up to 5 or 6 years of age. For example, children with congenital cataracts can have substantial and permanent visual deficits if the occluded lens is not corrected early enough. However, adults with cataracts regain their pre-existing visual acuity when the lens is replaced because occlusion past the critical period does not damage the cortex.

Strabismus, often called *lazy eye*, is a misalignment of the eyes because of improper control by the eye muscles. Children with this condition experience double vision. The response of the brain to receiving two images is to suppress the input from one eye. This can result in low acuity or even blindness in the suppressed eye because of developmental impediments during the critical period. One form of treatment is to patch the good eye and force development in the cortical regions connected to the lazy eye.

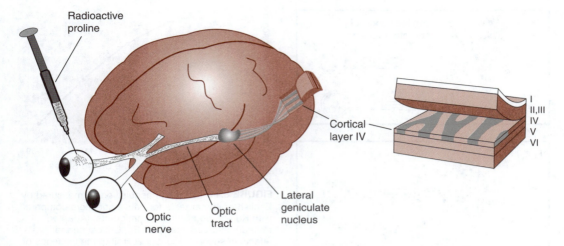

FIGURE 8.12 Injecting radioactive proline into an eye allows visualization of the cortical innervation in layer IV from that eye when the animal is sacrificed several weeks later. (Adapted from Bear MF, Connors BW, Paradiso MA, eds. *Neuroscience: Exploring the Brain*. 4th ed. Baltimore: Lippincott Williams & Wilkins; 2015; and Purves D, Augustine GJ, Fitzpatrick D, et al. *Neuroscience*. Sunderland, MA: Sinauer; 2004, by permission of Oxford University Press, USA.)

DISORDER

PERSONALITY

Extrapolating these studies to behavior, one wonders about critical periods and personality development. Specifically, what about people with severe personality disorders such as borderline personality disorder or antisocial personality disorder? Such troubled people seem to be missing important character traits. Did something fail to develop during an early critical period?

ADULT NEUROPLASTICITY

Plasticity is defined as the capability to be formed or molded. Neuroplasticity describes the brain's ability to adapt to environmental factors that cannot be anticipated by genetic programming. The description of critical periods described above suggests a bleak picture for plasticity in the adult brain, but there is more hope for your old cortex than one might think. For example, the organization of the representation of the sensory input in the cortex (called cortical maps) is continually reshaped by experience.

The work by Michael Merzenich with brain mapping in the 1980s is something that should be included in every clinician's understanding of the brain. Merzenich and colleagues electrically stimulated exposed monkey brains and mapped out the sensory cortex (also called somatosensory cortex) before and after experimental interventions. Before these studies, it had been assumed that the sensory cortex (the body's sensory representations on the brain) was fixed and immutable. By laboriously stimulating and recording, they mapped out the boundaries of the fingers and established that the brain changes in response to input from the digits.

In the first study, they amputated the middle digit from the monkey's right hand and found that the cortex essentially fills the void (Figure 8.14). Neurons deprived of sensory input from the middle finger switch allegiance and respond to stimulation from the closest finger. Similar changes have been observed with humans after medical amputation. For example, the face and hand are topographically close on the sensory cortex, and some patients will "feel" a sensation in their amputated hand, when their face is scratched—a phantom sensation. Functional imaging scans with such patients, performed during facial stimulation, have shown activation of the sensory cortex for both the face and where the lower arm was. It appears that the sensory neurons, like annoying friends, go where they get the most attention.

In a follow-up experiment, Merzenich and colleagues taught the monkeys to rotate a disc using only digits 2, 3, and 4 to receive banana-flavored pellets. After several weeks of practice, the cortical regions (the cortical map) used by fingers 2, 3, and 4 were enlarged (Figure 8.15). Practice literally changes the brain.

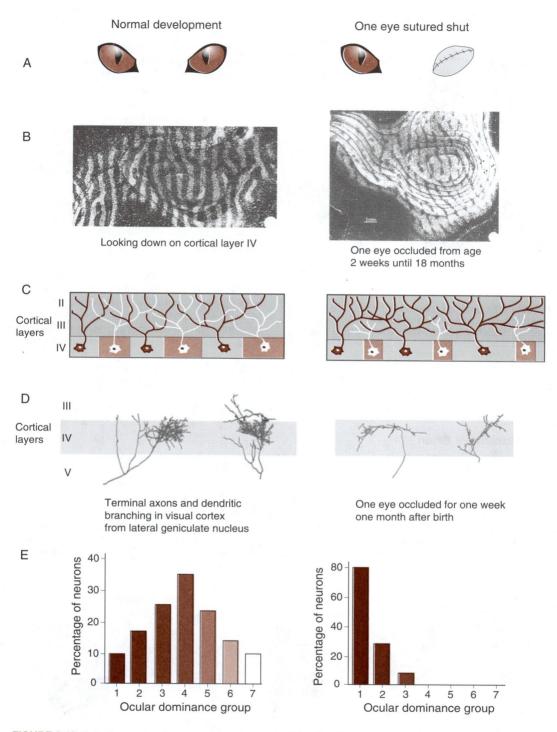

FIGURE 8.13 A–E: Comparing the normal development of the visual cortex on the left with development on the right when one eye has been sutured shut for varying lengths of time. Electrodes inserted horizontal to the cortex show distinctive patterns of ocular dominance depending on which eyes developed properly **(E)**. (**B:** Reprinted by permission from Macmillan Publishers Ltd. Wiesel TN. Postnatal development of the visual cortex and the influence of environment. *Nature*. 1982;299[5884]:583–591. Copyright 1982; **D:** From Antonini A, Stryker MP. Rapid remodeling of axonal arbors in the visual cortex. *Science*. 1993;260[5115]:1819–1821. Reprinted with permission from AAAS.)

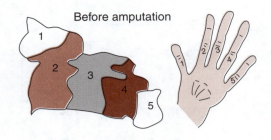

Before amputation

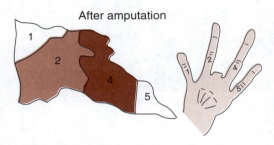

After amputation

FIGURE 8.14 After amputation of a monkey's finger, the cortical neurons reorganize. The neurons formally responding to stimulation of the third finger now respond to stimulation from the second and fourth fingers. Similar "remapping" also occurs in the thalamus. (Adapted from Merzenich MM, Nelson RJ, Stryker MP, et al. Somatosensory cortical map changes following digit amputation in adult monkeys. *J Comp Neurol*. 1984;224[4]:591–605.)

The Musician's Brain

Malcolm Gladwell wrote in his book *Outliers* that to become an expert requires 10,000 hours of practice. If this is true, we would expect there is some correlation between hours practiced, changes in the brain, and the emerging expertise. Indeed, a study of string musicians (violin and guitar) supports this correlation. The researchers measured the magnetic signal (magnetoencephalography) from the fingers of the

left hand (the ones that race up and down the neck of the instrument) and found a greater signal in the sensory cortex for the musicians compared with the musically challenged controls—although there was no difference in the right-hand fingers. Furthermore, the magnitude of the signal had a dose–response relationship—those who had been practicing longest had the greatest signal, particularly for the little finger.

TREATMENT

STROKE

After a stroke, many patients will avoid using the affected limb and preferentially use the intact limb. Functional imaging studies of stroke patients have shown contraction of the cortical representation of the affected limb, which is how the brain responds when it is not used. A new kind of rehabilitation for stroke patients called *constraint-induced movement therapy* corrects this problem and improves function even in chronic conditions. Patients have their good limb restrained with a mitt or harness and are forced to use their impaired limb. Controlled trials have shown this treatment to improve motor skills as well as increase the cortical activity in the affected area. The brain has the capacity to change, but it must be exercised.

Genitalia

A recent study of women who were victims of childhood sexual abuse offers an example of brain plasticity more relevant to mental health… but first, here is a little background. William Penfield was the first to map out the sensory and motor cortex in the human brain—something we'll discuss further

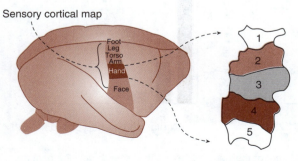

Sensory cortical map

Foot
Leg
Torso
Arm
Hand

Face

Before rotation

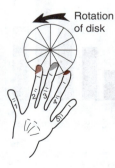

Rotation of disk

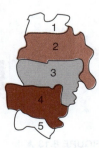

After rotation

FIGURE 8.15 The expansion of cortical representation of the dorsal fingers of a monkey before and after several weeks of controlled hand use. (Adapted from Merzenich MM, Nelson RJ, Stryker MP, et al. Somatosensory cortical map changes following digit amputation in adult monkeys. *J Comp Neurol*. 1984;224[4]:591–605.)

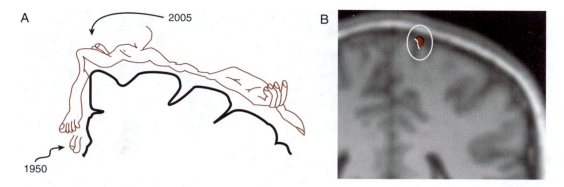

FIGURE 8.16 **A:** The cortical location of the penis seems to have moved in 55 years (not really). **B:** The location of clitoris, on the other hand, was only recently discovered. (Adapted from Michels L, Mehnert W, Boy S, et al. The somatosensory representation of the human clitoris: an fMRI study. *Neuroimage.* 2010;49[1]:177–184. Copyright 2010 with permission from Elsevier.)

in The Electrical Brain chapter. In his famous drawing of the human homunculus in 1938, he politely left out the genitalia (see Figure 10.4B). When asked, he located the genitalia below the toes. Unfortunately, he only identified the genitalia in less than 1% of the subjects he studied—those were more discrete times. More recent studies have placed the penis at the top of the legs— exactly where it should be (Figure 8.16A). Another adventurous group conducted similar studies with women by giving a gentle electrical stimulation to the clitoris while the subject's head was in a scanner (50 Shades of Gray for science?). They located the clitoris sensory cortex in a similar location on the brain as the penis for men (Figure 8.16B).

With this new understanding, a collaborative group from Berlin, Montreal, Miami, and Atlanta recruited women and analyzed cortical thickness— cortical thickness being an indirect assessment of neural development. They found cortical thinning in the region of the genital sensory cortex in women who had experienced childhood sexual abuse. The authors speculated that women who endure sexual abuse at a young age failed to develop normal sensory sensations as a protective response to the aversive experience. An alternative explanation is that individuals who were sexually abused as children are more likely to avoid sexual contact as adults because of the distressful associative memories. If so, the cortical underdevelopment may be a product of infrequent use.

In summary the neuroplastic studies suggest that early experiences are most enduring, but even the late bloomers can change their brains and develop new skills. Clearly, as anyone who has tried to learn a new language, instrument, or sport knows, it requires work and diligence to master the task—or literally to change the brain. Fortunately, it appears that even an old cortex can

adapt. Hubel and Wiesel described a monkey who had one eye occluded between days 21 and 30. Initially the monkey appeared blind in the deprived eye. Remarkably, 4 years later he had an estimated acuity of 20/80 in the bad eye and 20/40 in the normal eye.

Maladaptive Neuroplasticity

Prolonged practice has its dark side. Approximately 1% of professional musicians will develop a condition called *focal dystonia*: loss of control of skilled movements in the performing hand. It is usually a career-ending disorder and is believed to result from maladaptive neuroplasticity stimulated by long hours of repetitive movements. Neuroimaging studies show a fusion of the digital representations in the somatosensory cortex (Figure 8.17). It is almost as though the neurons are attempting to move two fingers when they should be only moving one. Consequently, individual finger movement is no longer possible.

Cellular Changes

The cellular mechanisms that accompany the cortical changes seen with monkeys rotating discs and musicians playing instruments (and hopefully readers of this book) are poorly understood. Some similar processes that may play a role in the dynamics of the neocortex were discussed in the earlier chapters of this book. A good model is long-term potentiation (LTP). Figure 5.8 shows an example of new spine development induced with LTP. Such spine development along with branching of the dendrites is seen with enriched environments (Point of Interest in Chapter 3, Cells and Circuits). It is tempting to speculate that successful learning involves production of growth factor proteins that stimulate arborization of dendrites in the cortex resulting in bigger, bushier neurons.

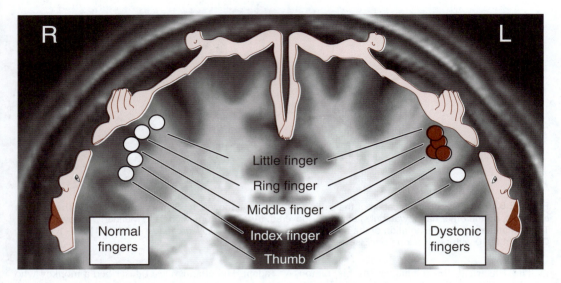

FIGURE 8.17 Functional representation of the fingers from the right and left hands of a musician with focal dystonia of the right hand (left side of the brain). The response from the somatosensory cortex is superimposed on a magnetic resonance imaging scan. Note the fusion of the representations for the fingers from the affected right fingers, which is not seen with the separated fingers from the left hand. The thumb—a digit not requiring as much movement when playing—is unaffected. (Adapted from Elbert T, Candia V, Altenmuller E, et al. Alteration of digital representations in somatosensory cortex in focal hand dystonia. *Neuroreport.* 1998;9[16]:3571–3575.)

Adult Nerve Regeneration

Why is it that the nerves in the peripheral nervous system can regenerate while those in the CNS cannot? Likewise, why can amphibians regrow long nerve connections, but mammals cannot? How come the most complex organ in the universe is less capable of repair? It appears that the brain responds to injuries with actions that are intended to preserve the complex connections, but this ultimately also prevents regeneration.

Oligodendrocytes and astrocytes respond to CNS injury by forming what is called a *glial scar*. This scar is part of the inflammatory response and limits cellular damage by isolating and protecting the injured area. Unfortunately, the glial scar also inhibits growth and prevents regeneration. After a spinal cord injury, the neuronal axons would like to reconnect, but they cannot get through the physical barrier nor can they find their way across the gap. A potential therapeutic solution being researched may be using different glial cells that usher neurons to their proper destination. Such glial cells, called *olfactory ensheathing cells* (OECs), can be found in the olfactory bulb—one of the two locations in the brain where neurogenesis occurs.

A recent operation in Poland suggests that using OECs enables the spinal cord to repair itself. The case involved a man paralyzed from his chest down (T9) after being stabbed in the back in 2010. The corrective procedure performed in 2012 involved two CNS surgeries. The first operation was to open his skull to remove an olfactory bulb so that they could grow OECs. The second operation, 2 weeks later, involved placing peripheral nerve tissue in the spinal gap (as a pathway) and then injecting the OECs into the same space. Many months and a lot of physical therapy later, he has feeling in his legs, has recovered some bowel and bladder function, and can ride a tricycle. This remarkable achievement is extraordinarily expensive and not without risks but shows that a damaged human spinal cord may be capable of repair.

QUESTIONS

1. Brain fertilizer
   a. Apoptosis.
   b. Critical period.
   c. Focal dystonia.
   d. Neurotrophins.

2. Programmed cell death
   a. Apoptosis.
   b. Critical period.
   c. Focal dystonia.
   d. Neurotrophins.

3. Maximum synaptogenesis
   a. Apoptosis.
   b. Critical period.
   c. Focal dystonia.
   d. Neurotrophins.

4. Inappropriate neurogenesis
   a. Apoptosis.
   b. Critical period.
   c. Focal dystonia.
   d. Neurotrophins.

5. Not one of the phases of development
   a. Neurogenesis.
   b. Synaptogenesis.
   c. Neuroplasticity.
   d. Pruning.

6. Factors that do not enhance CNS neurogenesis
   a. Amputation.
   b. Antidepressants.
   c. Enriched environments.
   d. Exercise.

7. Cannot develop from neural stem cells
   a. More neural stem cells.
   b. Oligodendrocytes.
   c. Astrocytes.
   d. Schwann cells.

8. Possible explanation for schizophrenia
   a. Focal dystonia.
   b. Excessive pruning.
   c. Altered neurotrophins.

See Answers section at the end of this book.

CHAPTER 9

Immunity and Inflammation

Up to this point we have discussed a number of mechanisms that may explain how the mentally ill brain is different from the normal brain. The immune system is increasingly being viewed as a possible culprit. The body's reaction to foreign invasion (or mistaken foreign invasion) and the resulting inflammatory response may contribute to the development of some psychiatric disorders.

For a long time there have been indications of subtle links between mental illness and the immune system. The first antidepressants were developed in the 1950s when it was noted that the antituberculous medication *iproniazid* had a positive effect on mood. When treated with this medication, even some terminally ill patients became more cheerful, physically active, and hopeful. Ultimately this antibiotic was refined and transformed into the first effective antidepressant: the monoamine oxidase inhibitors.

In 1929 the Swiss psychiatrist Tramer reported an increase in schizophrenic births during the months from December to May. Tramer noted that children born during the winter/spring months were more likely to develop schizophrenia as adults. It is postulated that the seasonal fluctuation is influenced by exposure to infections during the perinatal period, which are more common during the winter months—more on this topic later in the chapter.

Perhaps the oldest link between infection and psychiatric disorders lies with syphilis. This microbe was the cause of about 20% of the hospitalizations for mental illness at the beginning of the 20th century. In 1910 it was Paul Ehrlich's "magic bullet," compound 606, that became the first effective medication for syphilis—the beginning of psychopharmacology. The microbe that causes syphilis, *Treponema pallidum*, provides an example of the immune response and the problems this response causes.

THE IMMUNE RESPONSE

The body's immune system is poised to recognize and attack foreign invaders—anything that is nonself: splinters, bacteria, Fox News, etc. The attack is conducted by a confusing array of cells and proteins—some of which are standing guard at all times; others of which remain dormant until the alarm is sounded. All the components interact with each other through a litany of signals to rally the defenses when a microscopic terrorist is identified. Likewise the defenses must be turned off when the coast is clear. For the purposes of this book, we can simplify the immune response down to four major components.

1. Cellular—white blood cells (leukocytes)
2. Humoral—antibodies
3. Complement—little torpedoes
4. Cytokines—the molecular signals

All four of these components come into play when the syphilitic bacterium *T. pallidum* invades the body. We will use an infection with syphilis as a case history to illustrate the four components of the immune response.

Syphilis

Syphilis is a sexually transmitted disease caused by the corkscrew-shaped bacterium *T. pallidum* (Figure 9.1). When a contagious individual has sex with an uninfected partner, there is about a 30% chance the disease will be transferred. The body's first line of defense against infection is the skin. *T. pallidum* spirochete penetrates the dermal barrier by twisting through microabrasion.

The body's next line of defense is the complement system (Figure 9.2A). The complement

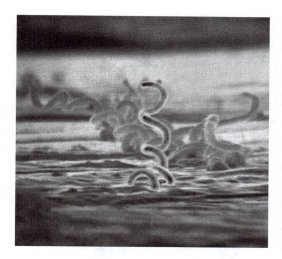

FIGURE 9.1 The bacterium that causes all the problems of syphilis is this annoying spirochete *Treponema pallidum* seen here in an electron micrograph. (From Centers for Disease Control and Prevention, Atlanta, GA.)

system is made up of numerous proteins circulating in the blood poised to coalesce into little torpedoes. When activated by foreign proteins, such as those found on bacteria, the complement molecules lock onto the bacteria. As more and more of these proteins accumulate on the bacteria, the complement can literally drill a hole in the cell wall. This allows fluid to pour in, and the bacteria explode. The trick is to limit the attack to the foreign invaders—to avoid attacking host cells.

Also standing ready to fend off foreign invaders are a variety of white blood cells (leukocytes). Two of these, the macrophage and the neutrophil are frontline defenders. The macrophage patrols the perimeter of the skin and mucous membranes cleaning up debris and searching for bad guys. (They are also one of the cells that will present foreign antigens to T cells to start the production of antibodies.) Neutrophils circulate in the blood ready to come to the aid of defenseless tissue. They aggressively attack *T. pallidum* but generally also make a mess of the healthy tissue. The initial physical sign of syphilis—the chancre that develops on the genitalia at the site of the infection—is in large part due to neutrophils. Pus is predominantly dead neutrophils—suicide bombers at the cellular level.

Inflammation

The inflammatory response is the body's overall reaction to foreign invasion. The signs are swelling, redness, heat, and pain. The mechanisms

that cause the inflammation are engorgement of the blood vessels, movement of fluid into the tissue, and, above all, attraction of leukocytes to the infected area. The signals that start the inflammatory process and coordinate the response are the cytokines (more on the cytokines later in the chapter).

Adaptive Immunity

A large part of the success of the mammalian defense system results from the capacity of the system to proliferate and attack specific and unique molecular features of the invader. This adaptive immunity commences when pieces of the destroyed bacteria are taken to the lymph nodes and presented to T cells—essentially shopped around to find a good match (Figure 9.2B). When a close match is found, the T cells multiply and head off to attack that specific remnant of the invader but not before activating the B cells. The B cells with a similar match will start producing antibodies. Antibodies are the "Y"-shaped proteins that can lock onto the specific foreign molecules of the bacteria, virus, or infected cell. Antibodies attached to a foreign cell serve as a signal to other leukocytes, essentially saying that this cell is ready for demolition (Figure 9.2C).

The important points to grasp are the varied mechanisms the body uses to defend against foreign invasion and the need for numerous checks and balances to keep the response under control, that is, to avoid damaging the host cells. As with any battle, "civilian casualties" are unavoidable. War, even at the microscopic level, is a dirty business.

TREATMENT

VACCINES FOR SUBSTANCE ABUSE?

It is an appealing idea to use vaccines to harness the immune system to combat mental illness. Vaccination is the process by which the body is exposed to just enough of the troubling agent (antigen) so that the immune system will mount an attack the next time the antigen appears. Vaccines that effectively produce antibodies to cocaine, nicotine, and opioids have been developed, thus neutralizing the molecules before they reach the brain. Unfortunately, the vaccines do not reverse the cravings. The determined substance abusers simply smoke more or use more of their addicted substance.

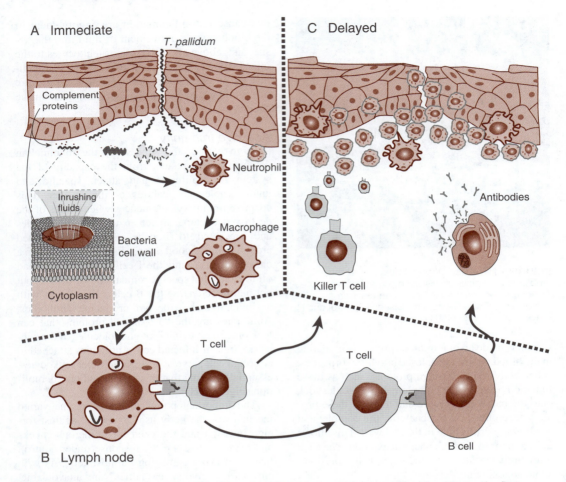

A Immediate

T. pallidum

Complement
proteins

Neutrophil

Inrushing
fluids

Macrophage

Bacteria
cell wall

Cytoplasm

C Delayed

Antibodies

Killer T cell

T cell

T cell

B cell

B Lymph node

FIGURE 9.2 A: When bacteria invade the body, complement, macrophages, and neutrophils are the first defenders. **B:** Antigen-presenting cells take pieces of the bacteria (antigens) to lymph nodes when the B cells and T cells are activated. **C:** T cells and B cells, specifically matched to the antigens of the bacteria, follow the cytokines to the site of the injury.

Syphilis Continued

After the first phases of syphilis, most people enter a latency phase—usually within 6 months. During this phase they do not have signs or symptoms of the illness and are not contagious. However, microbes remain hidden within the body, and laboratory studies are still positive. Remarkably, the *T. pallidum* can quietly live undetected in the host for years. How is this possible?

The best explanation for the ability of *T. pallidum* to hide in plain sight is the relative inertness of its outer membrane. The proteins that protrude through the phospholipid bilayer cell membrane wall (called integral proteins) are few and far between with *T. pallidum*. It is these proteins that killer T cells and antibodies grab when they attack the bacteria. As a comparison, *T. pallidum* has only

1% of the integral proteins found on *Escherichia coli*. Because of this low biochemical exposure, this stealthy naughty bacterium can remain hidden, under the radar so to speak, and not be recognized as different—like little terrorist sleeper cells.

If left untreated, approximately one-third of the people infected with syphilis will cure themselves, another third will remain in the latency phase until they die, and the last third will develop tertiary syphilis—the most serious phase of the infection. Of particular interest for us is neurosyphilis. Neurosyphilis includes inflammation of the meninges, cerebral vasculature, or neural tissue of the brain and/or spinal cord. Although animal studies have shown that *T. pallidum* can find their way to the central nervous system (CNS) within 18 hours after the initial infection, the serious manifestations of neurosyphilis do not develop for 10 to 50 years.

The important point is this: once the immune system catches up with syphilis in the CNS, it is the inflammatory response—not the bacteria per se—that damages the brain. *T. pallidum* does not produce a toxin nor directly attack the cells of the nervous system. It is the overexuberant cellular response to *T. pallidum* that blocks the vascular support and kills the neurons. The military calls this collateral damage. Once the immune system is activated, the progressive neural loss leads to personality changes, psychosis, and dementia as well as paralysis, seizures, and death.

IMMUNITY IN THE BRAIN

The immune response inside the brain is less aggressive than the response normally seen in the rest of the body. Constraining the response is essential because the rejuvenating capacity of the brain is limited and the effects of collateral damage from inflammation are more serious. White blood cells are rarely seen in the CNS. But the brain is not defenseless. Although once thought to be "immune privileged"—that is, able to tolerate the presence of an antigen without eliciting an inflammatory response—the brain is now recognized to have a unique but muted immune response to invaders.

The brain has three layers of protection against foreign invasion:

1. The blood–brain barrier—physical barrier to isolate the brain
2. Microglia—the macrophage of the brain
3. Leukocytes infiltration reserved for serious damage

The distinguishing feature of the CNS immune system is the microglia. The microglia, although considered as nerve cells, actually originate from a different cell line. Neurons, oligodendrocytes, and astrocytes develop from cells of neuroectodermal origin, whereas the microglia come from mesenchymal stem cells (bone, cartilage, and blood cells). Microglia move in and take up residence among the neural cells very early during embryonic development.

Microglia are most closely related to the macrophage and are the central component of the brain's innate immune system. Like the macrophage, microglia are dormant until activated, can migrate to the battle zone, and attempt to gobble up whatever that should not be there. The microglia respond to chemical signals of danger, emit proinflammatory cytokines, and can function as antigen-presenting cells—similar to the macrophage. In addition, microglia can also release cytotoxic substances such as hydrogen peroxide to damage the invader. Unfortunately, the hydrogen peroxide also kills neurons.

Neural Prostheses

The protagonist of the 1970s' television series "The Six Million Dollar Man" was a NASA astronaut whose injured body was rebuilt with mechanical parts. Oh, if only it was this easy. Forty-five years later, researchers are still struggling with the basics. A device that could restore simple movements for people with spinal cord injuries would be of great value to those confined to a wheel chair. Although very much is still in the experimental stages, the goal is to capture the individual's neural signals generated in the motor cortex and turn them into useful movements (Figure 9.3).

Electrodes implanted directly into the gray matter of the motor cortex are an intrusive element needed to determine the person's intentions. The electrode captures the electrical activity as the neurons generate action potentials, and the signals are sent to a computer. The computer—after substantial training—decodes the signals and moves the external device—in this case a mechanical arm. Problems develop as the brain's immune system produces a sustained reaction against the foreign body electrode.

Indwelling Electrodes

The gray matter of the cortex is dense with blood vessels. Invariably, as the electrodes are pushed into the brain, the vasculature is ruptured. This breaches the blood–brain barrier and allows the entry of inflammatory proteins as well as macrophages, neutrophils, and T cells. In short, the wound healing process is initiated and neurons—the ones the electrode needs to record—can be damaged or destroyed. Although the blood-borne inflammatory response is the most serious, microglia and astrocytes become activated regardless of the vascular damage (Figure 9.4).

Microglia, in their resting state, look like stars with an elaborate branching structure. When they sense trouble, they multiply and morph into rounder structures. They also increase their production of cytokines and growth factor proteins. In this activated state they engulf and digest the cellular debris generated by the injury—acting like their macrophage cousins from the periphery.

Astrocytes usually support the neurons and maintain the integrity of the blood–brain barrier. In response to injury they too become activated. Their main function in response to trouble is to isolate

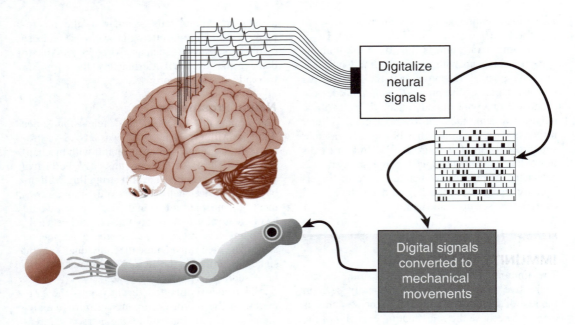

FIGURE 9.3 Electrodes in the motor cortex capture the neural activity of purposeful movement. The signals are digitalized, and the computer learns to turn the impulses into movements of the mechanical arm.

the problem. They produce and release a fibrous substance that plays an essential role in forming a physical barrier around the injury. This barrier is commonly called the glial scar. This is a problem for the whole contraption because the scar impedes contact between neurons and the electrode.

Glial Scar

Reactive gliosis, the formation of the glial scar, helps to isolate the injury, prevent overwhelming inflammation, and limit cellular degradation. The importance of gliosis was established in mice whose astrocytes were depleted. Small stab

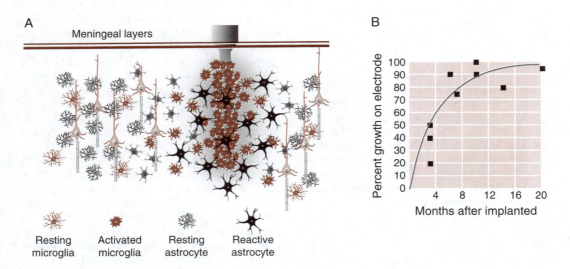

FIGURE 9.4 A: Electrodes implanted in the gray matter elicit an inflammatory response. Activated microglia and astrocytes produce a "scar" that isolates the electrode. **B:** Within 6 months, 75% of the electrode is surrounded by glial cells. (Adapted from Rousche PJ, Normann RA. Chronic recording capability of the Utah Intracortical Electrode Array in cat sensory cortex. *J Neurosci Methods*. 1998;82[1]:1–15. Copyright 1998 with permission from Elsevier.)

wounds in their spinal cords resulted in greater blood–brain barrier disruption, larger leukocyte infiltration, increased neural loss, and more motor deficits than in comparable mice with normal astrocytes. Clearly the glial scar is essential to limiting CNS damage after trauma. Unfortunately, there is a price to pay.

CYTOKINES

Cytokines are known as the "hormones of the immune system." These chemical messengers orchestrate the direction, magnitude, and duration of the inflammatory response. Virtually all the immune cells produce cytokines, although the type and function vary. First discovered in the late 1960s, the number of known cytokines now fills large, small-font charts and tables that most reasonable readers avoid. Suffice it to say that the major cytokines are interferon (IFN), interleukin (IL), and tumor necrosis factor (TNF) although each type has numerous variants designated with numbers or Greek symbols.

Cytokines coordinate the entire response to an infection—from generating a fever to promoting wound healing. However, the primary functions are activating and guiding immune cells. Some of the cytokines activate the white blood cells—inciting the cellular feeding frenzy. Other cytokines, in the presence of an antigen, activate T cells and B cells to multiply and go find the pathogen.

Cytokines play an essential role in guiding the immune cells to the battlefield. Activated cells follow the "scent" of the cytokines to their destination (Figure 9.5). Endothelial cells in the blood vessels respond to cytokines by expressing adhesion molecules that "grab" immune cells floating by in the blood. The cells then transform, squeeze through the blood–brain barrier, and follow the scent of the cytokines to find the pathogen.

An essential feature of fighting any infection is the ability to turn off the inflammation when the job is done to limit injurious side effects. Cytokines are turned off in several ways. First, cytokines have a short half-life and quickly dissipate anyway. Second, production of cytokines is reduced as the offending antigens disappear. Finally, some cytokines are actually anti-inflammatory and are produced to turn down the immune response.

Neural Plasticity

Cytokines have important functions outside their role of coordinating the immune response. Some of the cytokines of the IL-6 family are known to have signaling functions during development of the normal brain and in response to brain injury. Studies have shown these cytokines can

– induce differentiation of neural stem cells
– promote axonal regeneration
– promote maturation and survival of oligodendrocytes
– influence synaptic plasticity

These unexpected discoveries have generated interest in potentially manipulating cytokines to

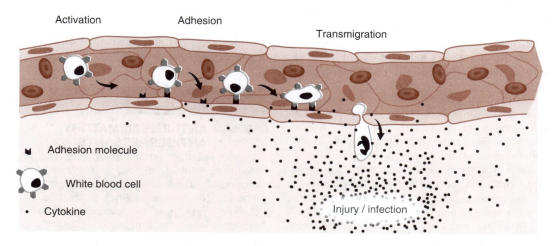

FIGURE 9.5 White blood cells in the capillaries are attracted to the site of an injury. Cytokines released at the injury activate a process that enables leukocytes to adhere to the endothelial cells and then migrate to where they are needed.

prevent illness or promote healing. But it is not easy to determine which cytokines need to be neutralized and which ones need to be enhanced.

Neurogenesis provides an example of the complexity of manipulating cytokines to promote CNS healing. After a stroke, theoretically, it would be beneficial to accelerate neurogenesis. The formation, migration to the site of the injury, and differentiation into functioning neurons hold great potential as a means to help people recover after cerebral ischemia. Unfortunately, the inflammatory response, also occurring after a stroke, blocks neurogenesis. Consequently, controlling the inflammatory response has been one target postulated for enhancing neurogenesis and recovery. But here is where it gets complicated: some of the cytokines (such as IL-4 and IFN-γ) that are also released as part of the inflammatory response actually induce neurogenesis.

Mental Illness

The pathophysiology of most mental disorders remains a mystery. Dysfunctions of the monoamines, the hypothalamic–pituitary–adrenal (HPA) axis, and neurotrophins have been discussed as possible mechanisms. Infections and inflammation may also play a role in the development of psychiatric disorders. The capacity of cytokines to affect neural plasticity may contribute to psychiatric illness as collateral damage from a normal immune reaction or some autoimmune activation. If this mechanism is culpable, it opens a whole new avenue for treatment interventions. The most compelling evidence is found with depression and schizophrenia.

Depression

First, a little background information: when stressed..., say, being chased by a saber-toothed tiger, our brains generate an alarm response and tell the legs to run like the dickens! This includes activating the sympathetic nervous system, pouring out the stress hormones, and (here's the important point) generating an inflammatory response. The brain and body prepare for an assault and ready the immune system to fight pathogens. Raison and Miller have been studying inflammation and depression for several decades and propose that our immune system is more activated than it was in the past, which has resulted in increased occurrence of autoimmune illnesses. Furthermore, an activated immune system leads to "sickness behavior," which looks similar to depression—withdrawal, anhedonia, and fatigue. They believe inflammation leads to or exacerbates depression.

Here is the supporting evidence:

– Proinflammatory cytokines (such as IFN for hepatitis C) can induce mood symptoms that respond to antidepressants.
– Patients with depression have increased expression of cytokines and interleukins.
– Genes implicated in depression are linked with immunity.
– Blocking inflammatory cytokines in patients with medical illnesses such as rheumatoid arthritis and psoriasis can reduce depressive symptoms.
– Inflammatory molecules predict nonresponsiveness to antidepressants.

What about treating depression with anti-inflammatory medication? One would think with all the anti-inflammatory medications on the market (such as prednisone, aspirin, etc.) that some bright clinician would have noted improved mood from one of these medications. The lack of a subtle effect with the prevalent anti-inflammatory medications is a bit disconcerting.

In 2013, Raison et al. published an impressive but disappointing pilot study of an anti-inflammatory medication given to patients with treatment-resistant depression. The active medication, infliximab (Remicade), an inhibitor of the cytokine TNF (with FDA indications for rheumatoid arthritis, psoriasis, and Crohn's disease), was no better than placebo in reducing depressive symptoms. Post hoc analysis found that patients with higher baseline inflammatory markers tended toward a better response to Remicade, which suggests that there may be subgroups of depressive patients who might benefit from anti-inflammatory treatment. However, this study is a big disappointment and suggests inflammation is not an easy target for depression treatment—or may not even be part of the etiology of depression.

TREATMENT

ANTI-INFLAMMATORY ANTIDEPRESSANTS

It turns out that antidepressants as well as the mood stabilizers have anti-inflammatory properties. Bupropion (Wellbutrin) actually inhibits TNF synthesis! What is the effective component of these medications? Increasing monoamines in the synapse or antiinflammation or both?

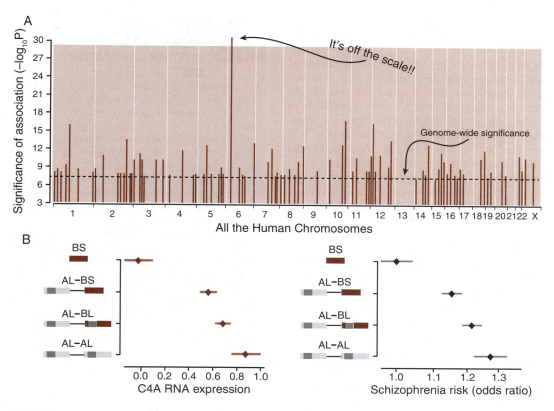

FIGURE 9.6 A: A genome-wide study searching for genes associated with schizophrenia found one region on chromosome 6 that towers above the others. **B:** Different versions of the C4 gene are more expressive of the C4 protein and increase the risk of developing schizophrenia. (**A:** Adapted with permission from Macmillan Publishers Ltd. Schizophrenia Working Group of the Psychiatric Genomics Consortium. Biological insights from 108 schizophrenia-associated genetic loci. *Nature*. 2014;511:421–427. Copyright 2014. **B:** Adapted with permission from Macmillan Publishers Ltd. Sekar A, Bialas AR, de Rivera H, et al. Schizophrenia risk from complex variation of complement component 4. *Nature*. 2016;530:177–183. Copyright 2016.)

Schizophrenia

As we will discuss in the chapter on schizophrenia, the pathophysiology of schizophrenia appears to involve a disruption of neural growth influenced by genetic predisposition and environmental events. It is possible that inflammation is one mechanism that may upset the normal growth of the neurons, which results in schizophrenia. Although Tamer in 1929 was the first to note a relationship between seasonal births and schizophrenia, it was E. Fuller Torrey who has more recently championed the idea of an infectious etiology. In 1973, Dr Torrey published a paper in *Lancet* entitled "Slow and Latent Viruses in Schizophrenia." His theories were not well received at the time. Now there seem to be several articles on the topic every week.

Initially the research focused on finding the specific microbe that might cause schizophrenia—cytomegalovirus or *Toxoplasma*

gondii, for example. In the past decade, as with depression, the focus has shifted to inflammation and cytokines. A meta-analysis of 62 studies comparing cytokine levels in 2,200 schizophrenics and 1,800 healthy controls found an increase in three cytokines and a decrease in one cytokine in the schizophrenic patients. This analysis suggests that inflammation plays a role in maintaining schizophrenia. However, a more convincing explanation may be the disruptive effect the immune system has on the brain during critical developmental spurts.

A study published in 2016 provides the most compelling evidence of a connection between the immune system and schizophrenia. Previously, a genome-wide association study identified a region on chromosome 6 that is strongly associated with schizophrenia (Figure 9.6A). This region is known to facilitate the immune response and surfaces frequently in genetic studies of autoimmune diseases.

Further analysis by the research team at Harvard localized the area of interest for schizophrenia to the C4 gene. Then they analyzed the expression of the different C4 gene in postmortem brain samples from schizophrenic patients and controls. They discovered that versions (alleles) of the gene that expressed more C4 were more likely to cause schizophrenia (Figure 9.6B). In a side study, they were able to establish that the C4 protein is involved with synaptic pruning. Apparently, this immune system protein flags synapses that are destined to be discarded—a process particularly active during adolescence. Too much C4 and the brain is inappropriately thinned—a finding consistent with neuropathology of schizophrenia, but more on that later.

This new information will probably not change how we treat schizophrenia during our careers. However, it implies that at some time in the future, we may be able to reduce the immune response in vulnerable adolescents and *prevent* the development of the disorder. Wouldn't that be wonderful?

Duality of the Inflammatory Response

One gets the impression that if we could just turn off inflammation, we would all live longer, richer, and happier lives. If only it were true. Traumatic brain injury (TBI) provides a good example of the duality of the inflammatory response.

Many people suffer enormous long-term disability after TBI. Increasingly we are recognizing the profound and enduring effects of minor TBI, particularly in soldiers within close proximity to explosions or professional athletes with multiple concussions. Brain damage following trauma is the result of immediate tissue injury from the impact and secondary injury from the inflammatory response. Considerable damage to the neural structures is caused by edema, cytokine release, and leukocyte infiltration after the initial impact.

Studies with animals have established that limiting the inflammatory response can reduce some long-term deficits from TBI. But not all studies are positive. In one interesting study, brain trauma was inflicted on mice genetically engineered not to express TNF-α (knockout mice). Initially the knockout mice showed less behavioral impairment than wild-type mice. However, after several weeks, the knockout mice remained significantly impaired, whereas the wild-type mice recovered. It appears, at least with TNF-α, the inflammatory response also promotes healing. This may be due to the beneficial effects the cytokines have on neural plasticity.

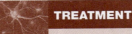

TREATMENT

ANTI-INFLAMMATORY DIET

If one searches "inflammation" on Amazon.com, the screen quickly fills with books extolling the advantages of the anti-inflammatory diet. Is there such a thing? Most people would agree that the Western diet is a catastrophe causing an epidemic of obesity, heart disease, and diabetes. There is substantial evidence that a Mediterranean (Med) diet (rich in fruits and vegetables, nuts, olive oil, legumes, and fish; moderate in alcohol; and low in red meat, processed meat, refined carbohydrates, and whole-fat dairy products) is healthier for the body. A prospective study in Spain found a smaller incidence of depression in subjects with stricter adherence to the Med diet. A study in Scotland found less brain atrophy from the ages of 73 to 76 years for those who adhered more closely to a Med diet. OK, but are the benefits due to anti-inflammatory mechanisms or just better nutrition?

AUTOIMMUNE DISEASE

Multiple sclerosis (MS) is the quintessential autoimmune disease. The immune system is designed to tolerate self and attack foreign bodies. Sometimes mistakes are made. MS patients have T cells that react to a protein in the myelin sheath. In theory, this alone should not be a problem. The T cells are in the periphery, whereas the myelin sheaths are protected behind the blood–brain barrier in the CNS. Additionally, the T cells are no threat as long as they are not activated. But for some people, all these safeguards fail, and the T cells go after the myelin in the CNS.

It is likely that a viral infection initiates the process in genetically vulnerable individuals. A closely matching viral infection activates the aberrant T cells, and the presence of inflammation allows the leukocytes to slip into the CNS where they attack the myelin. The loss of the myelin and axonal damage can result in a variety of unusual symptoms that wax and wane. Before the routine use of brain scans, it was not uncommon for a woman with ambiguous neurologic symptoms to be diagnosed with conversion disorder or hysteria before it was recognized months or years later that she actually had MS (a lesson to remember before

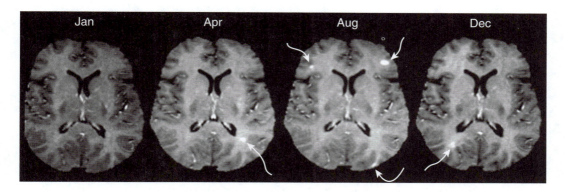

FIGURE 9.7 Serial magnetic resonance imaging scans at the same level for the same patient with multiple sclerosis show how lesions appear and recede over the course of 1 year.

we too quickly diagnose patients with personality, conversion, or factitious disorders).

The development of the MRI has changed the way the illness is diagnosed and managed. The focal demyelination in the white matter is easy to identify on MRI. Furthermore, many lesions are clinically silent—meaning the patient is unaware of the problem because the lesion occurs in an area of the brain that does not produce a physical symptom. Figure 9.7 shows how lesions come and go over several months for one patient.

There seem to be different phases of MS. The first phase is one of demyelination with focal symptoms followed by remyelination and recovery. The second phase is one of increasing and unremitting disability due to axonal loss and whole brain volume shrinkage. How quickly one moves from the relapsing/remitting phase to the secondary progressive phase varies from one person to the next. Of greater relevance to treatment interventions, the first phase appears to have more of an inflammatory component, whereas the secondary progressive phase does not. This becomes apparent in the treatment response.

Prior to 1993, there were no licensed treatments for MS. Now several treatments exist that focus on reducing symptoms (such as unstable bladder or fatigue) or limiting the inflammatory response. Even more exciting are the beta IFNs—naturally occurring cytokines. They have been reported to reduce relapses by 30%. Unfortunately, long-term follow-up suggests that they have limited effect on the only outcome that really matters: advancing disability.

Monoclonal antibodies are a new treatment option for MS. Genetically engineered mice are raised to produce antibodies that target specific molecules on the T cells. When injected, these antibodies latch onto the problematic T-cell molecule,

which results in destruction of the cell and reduced immune cell activity. Is that not incredible? In 2014 the FDA approved the monoclonal antibody alemtuzumab (Lemtrada) for relapsing MS. Lemtrada is more effective than beta IFN and is the first treatment to slow the progression of disability. Unfortunately, Lemtrada does little to affect the illness for those already in the secondary progressive phase—further evidence that the latter phases of MS may have different mechanisms of action.

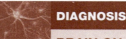

DIAGNOSIS

BRAIN ON FIRE

Susannah Cahalan has written a best-selling account of what she calls her "month of madness." A journalist in her late 20s, she experienced an acute change in personality including psychosis and cognitive impairment that were initially diagnosed as substance abuse, bipolar disorder, or schizophrenia. She was eventually diagnosed with anti–NMDA (*N*-methyl-D-aspartate) receptor encephalitis—an autoimmune disorder directed at the glutamate NMDA receptor—and responded to immune therapies.

NEURAL REGULATION OF IMMUNITY

Until now we have been discussing the effects the immune system has on the brain, but actually the influence is bidirectional. The CNS has the capacity to regulate the immune response as well. Generally speaking, the CNS tends to dampen the

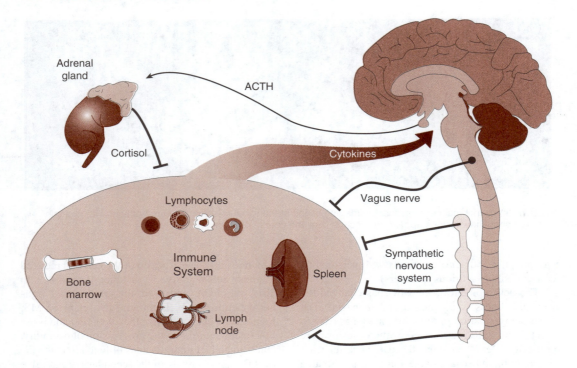

FIGURE 9.8 The central nervous system restrains the immune response by way of the autonomic nervous system and endocrine system. ACTH, adrenocorticotropic hormone. (Adapted with permission from Macmillan Publishers Ltd. Sternberg EM. Neural regulation of innate immunity: a coordinated nonspecific host response to pathogens. *Nat Rev Immunol.* 2006;6:318–328. Copyright 2006.)

immune response to restore homeostasis and prevent excessive inflammation.

The process starts when cytokines are released by white blood cells and travel to the brain in the plasma (Figure 9.8). The CNS responds through the autonomic nervous system (ANS) and endocrine system. The sympathetic and parasympathetic branches of the ANS modulate the immune response through innervation of the individual immune organs such as the spleen and lymph nodes. The endocrine system exerts its control through the release of sex hormones, thyroid hormone, and, most importantly, cortisol.

In 1950 the Nobel Prize was awarded for the discovery of cortisol. Its extraordinary anti-inflammatory properties were quickly recognized and put to use for rheumatoid arthritis and other inflammatory diseases. Endogenous cortisol provides the most powerful feedback loop through which the CNS modulates the inflammatory response. The importance of cortisol to inhibit an excessive immune response has been demonstrated in animal studies. When animals have their adrenal glands removed and then are inoculated with an infectious agent, they show increased mortality from shock. The unrestrained cytokine

and proinflammatory responses overwhelm the animal—too much inflammation is detrimental. One of the jobs of the CNS is to keep the immune response from getting out of control. The brain puts the brakes on the immune response by releasing adrenocorticotropic hormone, which in turn stimulates the adrenal release of cortisol (Figure 9.8).

Stress-Induced Immune Dysfunction

Folk wisdom has long recognized that psychological stress takes a toll on one's physical health. Many years of research supports this belief. Studies with new military recruits, anxious medical students, and caregivers of spouses with Alzheimer's disease have shown the ill effects of stress on the body.

Stress affects the CNS, which in turn alters the signals sent to the body through the endocrine and autonomic systems. Figure 22.2 shows a good example of the endocrine response to the acute stress of learning to parachute. These endocrine and autonomic signals gently suppress the immune response, which in turn puts the subject at a greater risk for illness.

This connection between stress and poor healing is eloquently shown in animal studies. Mice are

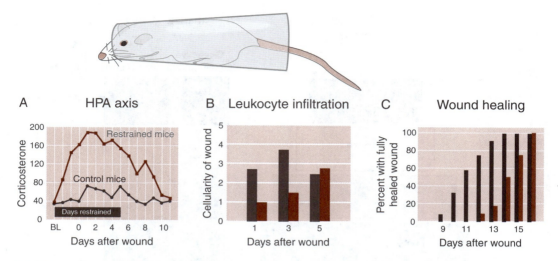

FIGURE 9.9 Mice restrained for 12 hours a night over 8 days show an activated hypothalamic–pituitary–adrenal (HPA) axis **(A)**, poorer cellular response to the wound site **(B)**, and delayed wound healing **(C)**. (Adapted from Padgett DA, Marucha PT, Sheridan JF. Restraint stress slows cutaneous wound healing in mice. *Brain Behav Immun*. 1998;12[1]:64–73. Copyright 1998 with permission from Elsevier.)

stressed by placing them in a restraining tube—overnight, when they are usually most active. In this particular study the mice were restrained for 12 hours a night for 8 days in a row. On the third day a small skin wound was opened. Figure 9.9 shows the results of this study for restrained mice compared with controls. The stressed mice had increased corticosterone (cortisol in a mouse), delayed leukocyte movement into the wound, and delayed wound healing.

Studies with humans have shown similar results—particularly patients with depression. Figure 21.4 shows the increase in cortisol in depressed patients suggesting an activated HPA axis. Furthermore, patients with diabetes, cancer, stroke, and myocardial infarction, who are also depressed, are at a greater risk for death from those diseases than are similar patients without depression. Is the increased mortality secondary to impaired immunity?

Whitehall Study

The Whitehall study is one of those remarkable large epidemiologic studies that established with hard data what previously had been conjectured. The study followed almost 20,000 male British civil servants for 25 years and correlated the employment grade with health. Simply looking at death, there is a dose–response association between employment grade and mortality (Figure 9.10A). A similar pyramid is seen regardless of whether the death is from heart disease, neoplasm, stroke, or respiratory disease. Likewise, in one of the many side studies

that came out of this project, measures of immune status also correlated with employment status. That is, men at the bottom of the employment pyramid had a more activated immune response as measured by C-reactive protein and circulating white blood cells (Figure 9.10B). Men in the lower employment grades were presumably more "stressed out," had poorer health, and showed greater immune activity.

Fatigue

Persistent fatigue is a frequent complaint with a long history. In 1869 the neurologist George Beard named the condition neurasthenia—a term that was in *Diagnostic and Statistical Manual of Mental Disorders II* (DSM-II) in the Neuroses section but was dropped from psychiatric nomenclature in 1980 with the publication of DSM-III.

In the mid-1980s, two practicing internists near Lake Tahoe, Nevada, generated considerable excitement when they reported an epidemic of persistent fatigue associated with elevated titers of the Epstein–Barr virus (EBV). Ultimately, the CDC disproved EBV as a cause of the illness, but this was the start of what became chronic fatigue syndrome.

Chronic fatigue syndrome captured the attention of patients and clinicians. Many patients, who would never agree to see a psychiatrist because of presumed stigma, were thrilled to be treated by infectious disease specialists. Researchers, likewise, raced to find the cause. However, all the findings have remained "soft." Although immunologic abnormalities can be found, they are difficult to reproduce and are not diagnostic.

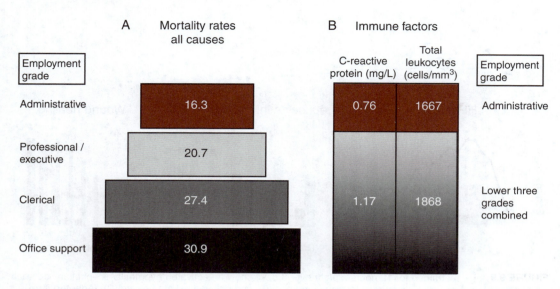

FIGURE 9.10 The Whitehall study showing employment grade correlated with mortality **(A)** and with immune activation **(B)** in British civil servants. Men in upper ranks had lower mortality and a more settled immune system.

Periodically, a new infectious agent theoretically causing chronic fatigue syndrome is identified by one group only to have other laboratories fail to duplicate the results. The XMRV retrovirus is the most recent example.

Many clinicians see chronic fatigue as a psychiatric disorder with similarities to depression. Indeed, antidepressants, cognitive–behavioral therapy, and exercise are effective treatments for depression and chronic fatigue. In general the medical community has gradually placed chronic fatigue back into the psychosomatic category. However, this chapter should attest to the interplay between the infectious/immunologic and the neuro/psychiatric, which raises the question: Is chronic fatigue syndrome a stress-induced immunologic deficiency or a psychiatric disorder caused by an infection? Or are both views partially correct?

QUESTIONS

1. *T. pallidum* damages the brain
   a. Within 18 hours of infection.
   b. By targeting pyramidal neurons in the cortex.
   c. By releasing a toxin.
   d. By inducing an inflammatory response.

2. A cocaine vaccine
   a. Reduces immune activation.
   b. Stimulates anticocaine antibody production in the CNS.
   c. Reduces euphoria.
   d. Stimulates anticocaine leukocytes.

3. Cytokines are involved in all of the following except
   a. Neural plasticity.
   b. Turning off the inflammatory response.
   c. Mental illness.
   d. Identifying *T. pallidum*.

4. All the following are true of MS except
   a. Responds to TNF inhibitors.
   b. Can be confused with hysteria.
   c. Is a T-cell problem.
   d. Induces silent lesions.

5. The CNS reduces the inflammatory response through all of the following except
   a. Parasympathetic nervous system.
   b. Sympathetic nervous system.
   c. Cytokines.
   d. Adrenal gland.

6. An activated immune system
   a. Can be used to diagnose chronic fatigue syndrome.
   b. Complicates neural development.
   c. Occurs in the latent phase of syphilis.
   d. Promotes healing.

See Answers section at the end of this book.

CHAPTER 10

The Electrical Brain

MORE THAN CHEMISTRY

One of our favorite illustrations in this book is Figure 3.9, which highlights the electrochemical configuration of neural communication. Unfortunately, many mental health professionals view psychiatric disorders as exclusively chemical in nature. The term "chemical imbalance" is part of our cultural lexicon, a perspective that misses the rapid electrical signals passed over long distances before any chemicals are released.

Electricity is the currency of the brain. It is not just chemistry—the brain is an electrical organ. This is not new information but rather a different, newer, and more nuanced way to view the brain. The brain uses enough electricity to power the 20 W light in your refrigerator—if it were possible to harness the electricity in your brain. That is a significant amount of electrical energy! Merely keeping our brains running requires about 20% of all the calories we consume and higher amounts when we concentrate (as opposed to watching TV).

We believe the electrical side of the electrochemical signal has been ignored for too long. This chapter was added in the second edition to correct the inequity. Probably the real impetus is not so much an attempt to be fair but our reaction to the explosion of research on the effects of electrical manipulation of the brain, which is now spawning a new generation of treatments.

History of Electrical Stimulation

Before it was possible to produce electricity on demand, the ancient Greeks and Romans reportedly used fish—electric eels or rays—to stimulate the brain as a treatment for intractable headaches. Of course the ancient physicians did not know they were using electricity, and the clinical effectiveness of electrical eels for headaches is unknown. However, it is relevant to note that eNeura Therapeutics has FDA approval for a handheld device that delivers a brief electromagnetic pulse (transcranial magnetic stimulation [TMS]—more on this later) to the back of the head to "short-circuit" an impending migraine. Therefore maybe an electric ray could actually have stopped an ancient headache. (If someone tries out the eel headache therapy, please write us and let us know of the outcome. [We certainly aren't recommending that you try this.])

Luigi Galvani in 18th-century Italy demonstrated that electrical sparks could induce movement in amputated frog's legs. He was the first to propose that the brain generates intrinsic electricity that spreads down through the nerves to the muscles. He believed electricity was the mysterious "vital force" controlling the body. His nephew, Giovanni Aldini (1762 to 1834), spent many years conducting further research and promoting the beliefs of his uncle. Using primitive batteries developed by Volta, Aldini applied electrical stimulation to mammals and, eventually, even humans. He demonstrated throughout Europe—part science, part carnival—the effects of applying electrical stimulation to human cadavers. In London in 1803 at the Royal College of Surgeons, Aldini applied electrical stimulation to a freshly hung criminal and awed his audience with facial and body movements in the deceased human. Aldini's work was an inspiration for Mary Shelley's novel *Frankenstein*.

Of even greater interest were Aldini's efforts to treat the mentally ill with electrical stimulation. He is reported to have treated an Italian farmer suffering from melancholy madness with stimulation applied to the patient's shaved, damp head (Figure 10.1). After several weeks of treatment,

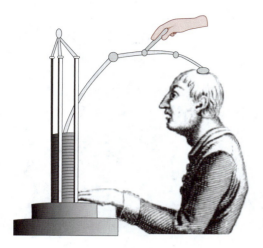

FIGURE 10.1 A patient receiving a crude form of direct current brain stimulation in 1803. Because the brain is an electrochemical organ, it can be changed and manipulated with externally applied electricity. (Adapted from Parent A. Giovanni Aldini: from animal electricity to human brain stimulation. *Can J Neurol Sci*. 2004;31[4]:576–584.)

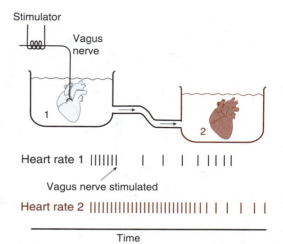

FIGURE 10.2 Otto Loewi's famous experiment establishing that electrical stimulation of the heart from the vagal nerve also produced a chemical.

the patient was well enough to return to his family. Later, Aldini met the famous French psychiatrist Philippe Pinel—the man who removed the chains from the insane—and applied his "galvanic" treatment to several patients at la Salpêtrière Hospital but with limited success. We do not fully understand the doses and actual current that Aldini used, but today a different version of this type of treatment is called transcranial direct current stimulation (tDCS). Although not FDA approved or even in regular use, tDCS is being studied as a possible intervention for Parkinson's disease, tinnitus, poststroke deficits, and, as Aldini demonstrated, melancholy (depression). tDCS involves passing a small (2 mA) direct current through the brain for 20 to 30 minutes. The brain regions under the anode become excited, and it takes less energy for that region to carry out its normal function.

It was Otto Loewi who in 1921 performed the elegant little experiment that proved the electrochemical transmission of nerve impulses. Legend has it that Loewi dreamed of the experiment and, upon awaking early in the morning, rushed down to the laboratory (Figure 10.2). Loewi knew that stimulating the vagus nerve would slow down the rate of a frog heart bathed in Ringer's solution. He then transferred some of that solution to another isolated frog heart and, without electrical stimulation, its rhythm also slowed down—as though its vagal nerve had been stimulated. He concluded that a chemical was excreted from the synapses of the first heart and this chemical could induce

bradycardia in a second heart, thereby establishing that nerves communicated with electricity and chemistry.

In 1939, *Hodgkin* and *Huxley* published the first intracellular recording of an action potential by inserting microelectrodes into the giant axons of squids (Figure 10.3). Before this time, no one had directly measured the electrical charge in an axon as an action potential passed.

Wilder Penfield is another one of the great figures who pioneered the use of electricity to study the brain. Penfield crossed paths with some of the leading neuroscientists in the 20th century. As a Rhodes Scholar, he studied in Sherrington's laboratory at Oxford and later collaborated with Ramón y Cajal in Madrid. However, Penfield was a practicing neurosurgeon in Canada who studied the brain while he was treating patients. He perfected

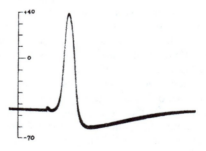

FIGURE 10.3 First-published intracellular recording of an action potential. (Reprinted by permission from Macmillan Publishers Ltd. Hodgkin AL, Huxley AF. Action potentials recorded from inside a nerve fibre. *Nature*. 1939;144:710–711. Copyright 1939.)

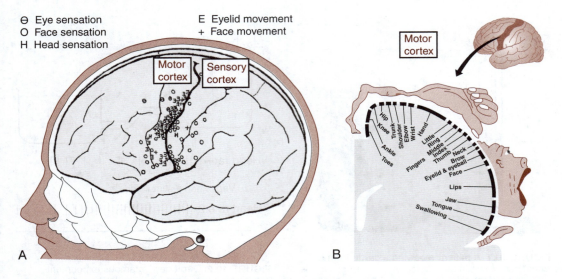

FIGURE 10.4 Actual recordings of sensation and movement for the eyes and face of patients examined by Wilder Penfield **(A)** compared with the cumulative motor homunculus for the average patient **(B)**. (Adapted from Penfield W, Boldrey E. Somatic motor and sensory representation in the cerebral cortex of man as studied by electrical stimulation. *Brain*. 1937;60:389–443, by permission of Oxford University Press.)

what came to be called the Montreal Procedure: the surgical removal of the site of the brain causing intractable seizures—still the most effective treatment for disabling epilepsy.

The unique aspect of the Montreal Procedure was the exploration of the patient's brain while they remained awake. Using local anesthesia, the patient's skull was opened and the brain was exposed. Penfield gently stimulated the cortex with an electrode in the area around the lesion. Patients remained alert so they could identify what they experienced as Penfield applied the electricity. The goal was to identify the pathologic tissue but preserve as much of the healthy brain as possible. (Interested readers can see reenactments on YouTube by searching for "Wilder Penfield.")

While Penfield was treating these patients, he was also mapping out the sensory and motor cortex. For each patient, he would record the location where different body parts were represented on the cortex. For example, Figure 10.4A shows the location of facial and eye sensations and movements for a number of patients. Figure 10.4B shows average location for the motor cortex compiled from data on almost 400 patients over 20 years. We now know that the sensory and motor homunculi are not static but are capable of reorganization after injury or with frequent use as we discussed in Chapter 8, Plasticity and Adult Development.

Penfield is best known in popular culture for awakening memories with electrical stimulation of the temporal lobes. This has led to the perception that memories are a fixed neural network (or an engram), which can be repeatedly elicited when stimulated. The reality is not so impressive. It turns out that only about 8% of people whose temporal lobes were stimulated reported any memory. Of those who did "remember," most reported experiences similar to the aura that preceded their seizure or described something more like a hallucination. Furthermore, modern studies have failed to find clear memories that are reproduced with stimulation. A memory engram remains elusive.

In the late 1930s, around the time Penfield was refining the Montreal Procedure, Ugo Cerletti, an Italian physician, began using electricity to induce seizures as treatment for the seriously mentally ill. Although this may seem like an extreme intervention to us, it was actually a logical step in the progression of physical treatments of mental illness. Psychiatrists had been inducing convulsions with metrazol—a γ-aminobutyric acid (GABA) antagonist that increases neural excitability, but it was difficult to control. Cerletti saw an electrically induced seizure as a cleaner procedure: easier to induce and terminate—no residual metabolite to complicate the recovery. Cerletti's intervention has developed into electroconvulsive therapy (ECT) and remains the most effective acute treatment for depression.

The last historical figure to discuss is Robert Heath, a psychiatrist and neurologist, who in the late 1950s coordinated the placement of electrodes into the brains of patients with serious mental illness. He was influenced by the work of Olds and Milner (see Figure 12.2) and was hoping that small frequent doses of electricity applied directly to deep sectors of the brain might reduce mental suffering. He conceptualized his intervention as an emotional pacemaker. (Interested readers can view actual clips of one patient by searching "Robert Heath" on YouTube.) The results were disappointing, and his approach was controversial. However, Heath's work was the forerunner of deep brain stimulation (DBS), now a common intervention for Parkinson's disease—and something of great interest to many as a possible treatment for intractable depression or other psychiatric disorders.

BIOELECTRICITY

All living cells maintain a negative electrical charge. That is, they are more negative inside relative to the extracellular space. Nerve cells use this property to communicate with one another—a process that through millions of years of evolution has transformed the speed by which biological organisms sense and respond. Without bioelectricity, we would all be slower than slugs.

The negative charge inside a cell is the product of competing forces within the cellular realm. First and foremost the cellular wall creates a boundary that limits the movement of charged substances into or out of the cell. The primary negative charge created in a cell is contained on the negatively charged organic molecules within the cell, e.g., amino acids. These large molecules, too large to escape through the cell wall, provide the bulk of the negative charge inside the cell.

The negative charge inside the cell is reduced by the movement of positive ions, such as potassium (K^+) and sodium (Na^+), into the cell. The positive ions are attracted to the negative charge inside the cell: remember, opposites attract in love and electricity. However, the movement of each ion is different. The K^+ ions flow freely into the cell until they reach a point at which the forces of the *concentration gradient* start to pull some K^+ back into the extracellular space. The propensity of ions to evenly diffuse within a contained space is called the concentration gradient. Ultimately, the amount of K^+ inside the cell is a product of the pull of the *electrostatic forces* into the cell and the push of the concentration gradient back out to the extracellular space.

The Na^+ ions, on the other hand, are actively removed from the intracellular space. Using the *sodium–potassium pump*, the neurons pump out Na^+ ions that have leaked into the cell. Expelling Na^+ ions requires considerable energy, as the ions

must be forced out of the cell against the concentration gradient and against the electrostatic pressure. Running the sodium–potassium pump is one of the primary reasons that the brain is such an energy hog. The final concentrations within and outside the cell are shown as follows. The result is an electrostatic charge of about −60 mV.

	Na^+	K^+	Large Organic Molecules
Intracellular	50	400	Many
Extracellular	440	20	Few

Nerve cells use a rapid and brief change in the polarization as a signal that can be quickly transmitted from one end of the cell to the other. In Chapter 3, Cells and Circuits we briefly described how nerve cells communicate—how the signal from incoming neurons depolarizes or hyperpolarizes the neuron (Figures 3.6 and 3.7)—and when the electrical charge at the axon hillock reaches the threshold (−40 mV), an impulse is sent down the axon (Figure 3.8). We have not discussed the transmission of the electrical impulse down the axon. The voltage-gated channel is the secret, but first a word about normal wave movement.

Usually, waves diminish in size as they move away from the source. Think of throwing a pebble into a pond and watching the waves decay as they spread out. The 2011 tsunami generated waves along the coast of Japan that were estimated to be almost 39 m tall but were only 2 m by the time they reached Hawaii 7 hours later. The action potential, on the other hand, does not diminish in size as it shoots down an axon—the amplitude remains constant.

It is the *voltage-gated sodium channels* that maintain the amplitude of the action potential, which in humans may stretch for over a meter in length. (The recurrent laryngeal nerve in the giraffe, which descends into the thorax before climbing back up the neck to the larynx, may be as long as 15 ft. Fortunately, for the giraffe, the signal at the larynx is just as robust as the one that leaves the brain.) The voltage-gated channel is triggered when it is depolarized—reaches its threshold. It then opens, and ions—in this case Na^+—flood into the axon. This in turn depolarizes the next voltage-gated channels, and the process repeats itself on down the axon (Figure 10.5).

Another trick the brain uses to facilitate rapid transmission to distant sites is to wrap the nerve with swaths of myelin, separated by small gaps called nodes of Ranvier (see Figure 3.10). Remarkably,

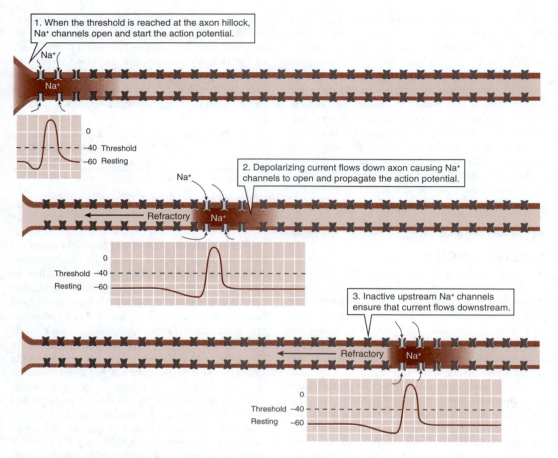

1. When the threshold is reached at the axon hillock, Na⁺ channels open and start the action potential.

Na⁺

Na⁺

0
−40 Threshold
−60 Resting

2. Depolarizing current flows down axon causing Na⁺ channels to open and propagate the action potential.

Na⁺

Refractory   Na⁺

0
Threshold −40
Resting −60

3. Inactive upstream Na⁺ channels ensure that current flows downstream.

Refractory   Na⁺

0
Threshold −40
Resting −60

FIGURE 10.5 The rapid opening and closing of the Na⁺ channels sends an electrical signal down the axon. The refractory period after the passing of an action potential keeps the signal moving in the correct direction. Note that the electrical tracing is proceeding from right to left, which is opposite of how it is usually shown (see Figure 10.3 for comparison).

the electrical signal can skip or jump down the nerve, only depolarizing at the exposed gaps. This is called *salutatory conduction* and is significantly faster than slugging through every Na⁺ channel on a naked neuron. The myelin appears white in typical brain stains and magnetic resonance imaging (MRI) scans (hence white matter) and is what is attacked by the immune system in multiple sclerosis, as we discussed in the last chapter. The images generated by diffusion tensor imaging are of myelin-wrapped axons (see Figure 3.13).

ELECTROENCEPHALOGRAM

Sensitive instruments can detect the electrical signals generated by the nervous system. As early as 1875, recordings captured electrical activity from an exposed monkey brain. However, it was not until 1929 that an Austrian psychiatrist, Hans

Berger, first recorded electrical tracing from the scalp of an awake human. Called electroencephalogram or EEG, Berger was able to show that different states of mind produce different rhythms. The EEG remains a useful tool to analyze sleep and epilepsy.

Synaptic activity at the dendrite generates a tiny electrical charge (Figure 10.6). When thousands of other cells contribute their small voltage, a signal becomes strong enough to be detected by the EEG electrode at the scalp. The EEG measures the sum of the electrical activity from the large pyramidal neurons. When the neurons are firing in unison, large electrical waves are recorded on the EEG. Small waves, typically when one is alert and focused, reflect the chatter of asynchronous neurons. Figure 15.3 shows EEG recordings for different states of consciousness.

EEG recordings are generally made through two-dozen electrodes affixed to the scalp in

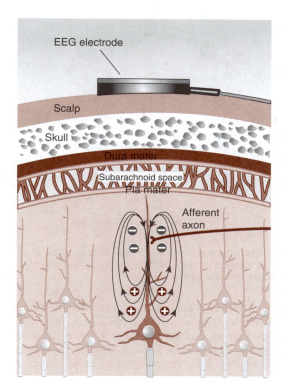

FIGURE 10.6 Signals from afferent neurons (in this example just one afferent neuron) release a neurotransmitter at the synapse. The movement of positive ions into the pyramidal neuron leaves a slightly negative charge in the extracellular fluid. As the current spreads and escapes out of the deeper parts of the neuron, those extracellular sites become slightly positive. The electroencephalogram (EEG) detects the cumulative charge between two scalp electrodes. (Adapted from Bear MF, Connors BW, Paradiso MA, eds. *Neuroscience: Exploring the Brain*. 4th ed. Baltimore: Lippincott Williams & Wilkins; 2015.)

predetermined locations. The electrodes are connected to amplifiers, and continuous recordings are captured between 16 standard electrodes. Small voltage changes are measured between pairs of electrodes. Usually the voltage fluctuations are only a few tens of microvolts in amplitude. During deep sleep and seizure activity, large waves develop. Figure 10.7 shows actual EEG recordings for a patient with absence seizures.

Excessive or Insufficient

In this section of the book, we have been reviewing modulating factors on the brain—hormones, growth factor proteins, immunity, and now electricity. In each case the modulation can be seen as too much or too little, for example, too much cortisol or not enough, excessive or insufficient brain-derived neurotrophic factor, etc. The question

here is: Does this paradigm apply to electricity in the brain?

Excessive Electrical Activity

A seizure is a clear example of excessive electrical activity in the brain. Recognized 3000 years ago by the ancient Babylonians, epilepsy is, by definition, excessive abnormal neuronal electrical activity. The Epilepsy Foundation reports that 3 million Americans have the disorder. There are many different types of seizures, but broadly there are two types: focal seizures—when the electrical activity remains in a limited area of the brain—and generalized seizures—which affect the whole brain.

Every brain has the capacity to have a seizure. Psychiatrists can use ECT to induce a seizure in anyone. Various problems predispose the brain to erupt in a seizure, e.g., fever, trauma, tumors, illicit drug use, and infections, to name a few. But some people appear to have a lower seizure threshold for no obvious reason, and they have spontaneous seizures. Some research suggests abnormalities of neural growth in which abnormal networks connect back on themselves and lead to self-excitation. Other research has identified abnormalities of receptors, in particular the voltage-gated sodium channel, or neurotransmitters, particularly excessive glutamate. Numerous mutations of the sodium channels have been identified that are believed to predispose the cortical neurons to electrical instability and spontaneous activity.

Kindling is a model for seizure activity and epilepsy that is of great interest to biologic psychiatrists. (The concept is similar to the process shown in Figure 5.6.) Repeated subconvulsive stimulation (kindling) of the amygdala or hippocampus with an irritant or stimulant (cocaine) leads over time to an enhanced response and eventually cocaine-induced seizures and then finally spontaneous seizures. Although more theory than fact, this model gives one explanation for the development of some forms of epilepsy or any other neuropsychiatric process where repeated small events or exposure eventually builds to unleash spontaneous pathology.

Some psychiatrists have latched onto the theory of kindling as a model for what might be happening with bipolar and unipolar depression, where first or second affective episodes early in life are often associated with life stresses or triggers, but later episodes appear to be spontaneous and not environmentally triggered. They see the gradual decline in some patients with repeated episodes of the disorder as a kindling process. The effectiveness of the anticonvulsants in mood disorders also

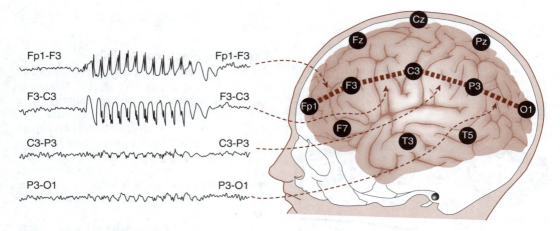

FIGURE 10.7 The electroencephalogram records electrical activity between two electrodes. This example of an absence seizure (also called petit mal seizure) shows just four tracings from the left brain. You do not have to be a neurologist to recognize that the seizure activity emanates from the frontal lobes.

suggests that electrical aberrations may be a driving cause of mood disorders. However, the antidepressants actually lower the seizure threshold. One would think they would exacerbate a mood disorder, instead of improving the mood, if the pathophysiology was solely due to excessive electrical activity.

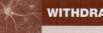

WITHDRAWAL SEIZURES

Alcohol has been used for centuries to calm the brain. Since Librium was introduced in 1960, the benzodiazepines have become popular alternatives for stressed-out people. The brain reacts to the chronic use of sedative hypnotics by decreasing the GABA activity and increasing the excitatory glutamate activity. Sudden withdrawal from alcohol or benzodiazepines unmasks the new balance, which results in too much accelerator and not enough brake. In such an overexcited state, seizures can develop.

Insufficient Electrical Activity

If the epilepsies are a clear example of the brain having too much electrical activity, are there examples where the brain has simply too little electricity? Like a fire that won't light because the wood is damp, are there conditions in which the brain has become too sluggish and the electricity isn't flowing? Certainly it feels this way some mornings!

There are obvious examples of insufficient electrical activity in the brain—coma is one;

intoxication is another. In the intensive care unit when an unresponsive person exists solely on life support, establishing the absence of electrical activity in the brain is used to distinguish brain death from a persistent vegetative state. These are overt examples of insufficient electrical activity associated with significant altered mental status. However, are there conditions we see in mental health that are a product of inadequate electricity in the brain?

The short answer is No! We do not know of any psychiatric disorders that are caused by insufficient electrical activity. Although it appears that some depressive symptoms and the negative signs of schizophrenia, for example, are produced by sluggish electrical connections, in all likelihood the absence of activity is more a product of insufficient neuronal metabolism. However, there is great interest in treatments that can awaken the glutamate neurons. In the next section, we will briefly look at interventions that electrically stimulate the brain as treatment of mental disorders.

STIMULATING THE BRAIN

Selectively stimulating the brain offers the potential to activate the brain using its own method of communication—electrical flow through axons and neurons. Furthermore, because the methods are applied directly to the brain, they do not have systemic side effects found with oral medications, which have to pass through the body before entering the central nervous system. And all this without residue, when the electricity is turned off, there is nothing left to be cleared away.

Interested readers are referred to our other book for an in-depth review of this area, but it is helpful here to outline some of the more important methods. ECT is used to purposefully create a seizure in the prefrontal cortex and is the most effective treatment available for acute depression or mania. It is also used to treat catatonia and can help with Parkinson's symptoms and can even stop status epilepticus. New advances in the type of electricity used (pulse width) and electrode locations have improved outcomes while reducing, but not entirely eliminating, cognitive side effects (see Figure 18.11).

TMS involves placing a small electromagnet on the scalp and turning it rapidly on and off. This creates a powerful, and transient, magnetic field, which travels unimpeded through the scalp and into the brain, inducing an electrical current in brain cells just at the surface of the brain. Repeatedly stimulating the prefrontal cortex every day for 4 to 6 weeks is now an FDA-approved treatment for acute depression. It has also shown promise in treating pain (see Transcranial Magnetic Stimulation, Prefrontal Cortex, and Postoperative Pain box in Chapter 11, Pain).

Vagus nerve stimulation (VNS) involves wrapping an electrode around the vagus nerve in the neck and connecting the nerve to a pacemaker implanted under the skin in the chest. Recent advances have made it possible to noninvasively stimulate the vagus nerve in the neck with a small TMS-like device or to stimulate a sensory branch of the vagus nerve in the ear. Repeated current through the cervical vagus nerve has been shown to treat epilepsy, and the device is approved for medication-resistant epilepsy patients. It is also FDA approved as a long-term treatment for patients with treatment-resistant depression. There has been a recent explosion involving behavioral and therapeutic effects of VNS. In animal models where VNS is active, it reduces the size of a brain stroke or heart attack and even prevents animals from dying of septic shock. It can also abort anaphylaxis, presumably by increasing parasympathetic tone. Perhaps the most exciting VNS advance, however, is that when the vagus is being stimulated, the brain changes gears to "remember" or pay attention to whatever is going on at that moment. Clinical trials in stroke and tinnitus are exploiting this by pairing stoke rehabilitation or auditory tones with VNS.

DBS involves placing a wire directly into the brain through a burr hole in the skull and connecting the wire to small generators implanted in the chest wall. DBS in the basal ganglia can immediately treat tremors in Parkinson's disease and is FDA approved for that indication. There was much excitement about DBS to treat depression, but two large industry-sponsored clinical trials were negative, and the popular press has moved on to other topics. However, research quietly continues with DBS for other neuropsychiatric disorders.

Finally, tDCS, mentioned at the start of this chapter, involves a relatively simple system of passing direct current through discrete brain regions. It is being investigated heavily for a variety of disorders, with no clear therapeutic indications yet—more on this below.

Priming the Pump

A potential emerging use for brain stimulation may be the benefit of adding electrical stimulation to standard treatment. The best example involves the treatment of anomia or aphasia after a stroke. Anomia is impaired word retrieval or, simply, the inability to find the right word. This is a common problem after strokes, and the standard treatment is speech therapy. However, a number of clever researchers have attempted to enhance the treatment by adding electrical stimulation with tDCS to speech therapy. Figure 10.8 illustrates this procedure. Four cathodes and one anode are placed on the brain. The current moves from the cathodes (brown circles) toward the anode (white circle with black outline) (A). Functional MRI shows the activation of the brain during this kind of stimulation (B). In a separate study, 12 patients with chronic anomia from left hemisphere strokes practiced naming different sets of objects with and without electrical stimulation. In this study the stimulation was conducted over the right temporoparietal cortex—an area associated with long-term memory (see Figure 18.8). Both immediately and 2 weeks later, the objects learned with stimulation were more accurately named by the patients. A larger study is currently enrolling patients.

The key feature of using brain stimulation in this manner is that the person must be doing the exercise when the electrical stimulation is added. Simply adding current to the brain is not beneficial. But electrically stimulating the brain while the activity is practiced seems to facilitate learning. Could this intervention expedite acquiring a foreign language? Would psychotherapy be more effective if the brain was mildly stimulated at the same time? It is exciting to envision pairing circuit-specific brain stimulation together with the behavioral therapies that psychiatrists and psychologists have perfected over the decades.

One advantage of tDCS is the simplicity of the procedure. Most new technologies in medical care are expensive and require trained personnel to operate the machinery. tDCS is inexpensive and

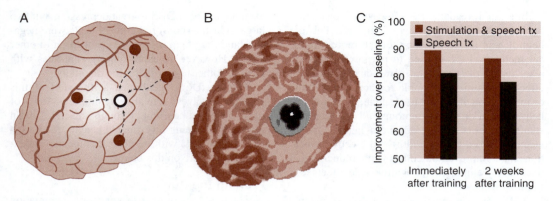

FIGURE 10.8 Electrical stimulation enhances speech therapy. **A:** Schematic of electrode placement. **B:** Functional imaging of actual stimulation. **C:** Stimulation plus speech therapy (tx) improved naming objects in patients with anomia after stroke. (**B:** Adapted from Datta A, et al. Gyri-precise head model of transcranial direct current stimulation: improved spatial focality using a ring electrode versus conventional rectangular pad. *Brain Stimul*. 2009;2[4]:201–207. Copyright 2009 with permission from Elsevier. **C:** Adapted from Flöel A, et al. Short-term anomia training and electrical brain stimulation. *Stroke*. 2011;42:2065–2067.)

easy to use: a few pads and a 9-V battery like the one you have in your smoke detector is all you need. If tDCS can improve learning, we may be on the cusp of a new treatment modality in mental health. Because it is inexpensive and can be sold online, there is a large self-use community using this largely for attempted cognitive or performance enhancement. In fact, following the 2016 Summer Olympics, several US athletes announced that they had used tDCS during their training. We urge extreme caution. Electricity is the currency of the brain, but be careful how you mess with it!!

Consciousness

Let us end this chapter with one of the most important questions regarding the brain. What is consciousness? Is it related to the electrical energy flowing in the brain? Do we have less

electrical activity in the brain when we sleep or are unconscious? The answer is a complicated maybe. In certain stages of sleep, such as rapid eye movement (REM), our brains are just as active as during the day when we are awake. However, in other non-REM stages, it appears as if different parts of the brain isolate themselves from the rest of the brain, and the brain is less connected. When we are unconscious, less electricity is flowing from any given brain region to all others. The brain is compartmentalizing when we are unconscious. This "connectedness as consciousness" theory is being used by some researchers as a way to explain what it means to be conscious (brain regions fully connected and passing electricity freely) or unconscious (brain regions disconnected). Why the brain needs to do this during sleep is still not clear.

QUESTIONS

Match the columns

1. Transcranial direct current stimulation

2. Preserves the action potential

3. Transcranial magnetic stimulation

4. Deep brain stimulation

5. The seizure is the treatment

6. Currency of the brain

7. Insufficient electrical activity

8. Prone to seizure activity

A. FDA indication for depression

B. Electricity

C. Voltage-gated sodium channels

D. Coma

E. 9 V

F. Insufficient GABA

G. Robert Heath

H. Electroconvulsive therapy

See Answers section at this end of this book.

SECTION III

Behaviors

CHAPTER 11

Pain

Pain and pleasure are the major driving forces of human behavior. We will cover pain in this chapter but are ever so looking forward to discussing pleasure in the next chapter.

ACUTE PAIN

Acute pain, as we all have experienced, starts in the periphery, is relayed to the spinal cord, and then passes up to the brain where it produces a negative reaction (Figure 11.1). Pain-producing stimuli are detected by specialized afferent neurons called *nociceptors*. The receptors are free nerve endings—not an identifiable structure as we have for touch and vibration. These cells respond to a broad range of physical and chemical stimuli, but only at intensities that are capable of causing damage.

Peripheral Tissue

The nociceptors in peripheral tissue are activated by injury or tissue damage that results in the release of bradykinins, prostaglandins, and potassium (Figure 11.2). These molecules in turn cause the secretion of substance P from other branches of the axon, which stimulates the release of histamine and promotes vasodilation.

Aδ and C fibers send the signal to the dorsal horn of the spinal cord by way of the dorsal root ganglion. The Aδ fibers are myelinated axons that quickly send the first, sharp signals of pain. The C fibers are unmyelinated and send a slower, dull pain signal (Figure 11.3). It is the duller, slow pain signal of the C fibers that becomes so troublesome in chronic pain conditions (see box).

Spinal Cord

The nociceptive afferent nerve fibers synapse in the dorsal horn of the spinal cord. Information about tissue injury is passed onto the next neurons, which then crosses the contralateral side and ascend to the brain.

The signal can be modified at this point by descending fibers (discussed later) or from simultaneous activity by nonpain neurons (mechanoreceptors: Aβ fibers). The Aβ fibers can dampen the pain signal in the *gate theory of pain*. Figure 11.4 shows how a signal from the larger mechanoreceptor activates an inhibitory interneuron in the dorsal horn, which results in a smaller signal conveyed to the brain. The gate theory explains why rubbing an injury seems to reduce the pain and is the rationale for the use of transcutaneous electrical stimulation.

Ascending Pathways

There are a variety of ways to describe the different nociceptive pathways that ascend to the brain in the spinal cord. Unfortunately, there is no consensus on the proper nomenclature for these tracts, and no two authors seem to use the same terms. Recently, the perception of pain—and the areas participating in the central nervous system (CNS)—has been divided into two prominent domains: *sensory-discriminative* and *affective-motivational*. This dichotomy (summarized in Table 11.1) is a convenient way to understand the ascending pathways.

Sensory-Discriminative

The sensory-discriminative domain encompasses the traditional sensory pathway taught in the first year of medical school. The signal travels up the

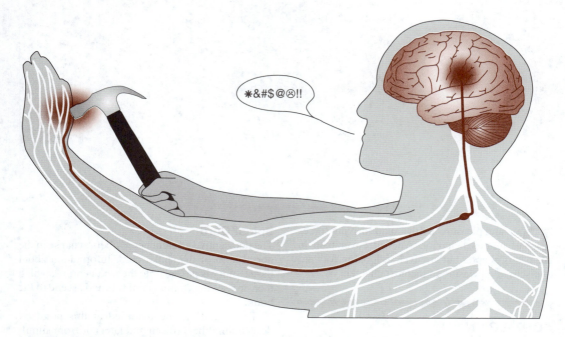

FIGURE 11.1 The somatosensory cortex receives the sensation of pain from the peripheral nerves by way of the spinal cord. (FYI: the signal would terminate in the right somatosensory cortex and not the left, as illustrated above.)

TREATMENT

NEUTRALIZING C FIBERS

The *transient receptor potential vanilloid 1* (TRPV1) receptor found primarily on small diameter sensory neurons, such as C fiber neurons, has become a new target for pain relief.

The TRPV1 receptor responds to a variety of noxious chemical and physical stimuli—including capsaicin, the active component of chili peppers. Animal studies suggest that blocking this receptor reduces the aching quality of chronic pain while preserving the sensations of touch and proprioception. Studies with first-generation oral TRPV1

antagonists have been suspended because of hyperthermia and impaired heat pain sensation. Modified compounds are being tested with the hope that they will preserve the analgesic benefit without the annoying side effects. Topical administration of capsaicin causes an initial stimulation of the TRPV1 receptors, followed by pain reduction. A capsaicin 8% patch (Qutenza) is now available in the United States for neuropathic pain associated with postherpetic neuralgia and appears to provide faster relief than pregabalin (Lyrica).

spinothalamic tract, synapses in the lateral thalamus, and proceeds to the somatosensory cortex. Figure 11.5 is a diagram of this pathway. This type of pain allows the subject to become aware of the location of the pain and answer the question, "where does it hurt?" However, the perception of pain is much more than just identifying the location of a noxious sensation and withdrawing the injured limb.

Affective-Motivational
Other ascending sensory signals communicate the intensity of a noxious stimulus. There are several

tracts that transport these signals, such as the *spinoreticular tract* or the *spinomesencephalic tract*—just to name a few. The important point is that all the signals travel in the anterolateral region of the spinal cord and terminate in different locations such as the reticular formation, periaqueductal gray (PAG) matter, and the amygdala. The rest of the signals synapse in the medial thalamus before proceeding to other areas of the cerebral cortex (Figure 11.6).

The affective-motivational signals communicate the unpleasantness of the sensation and answer the question, "how much does it hurt?" In the cortex,

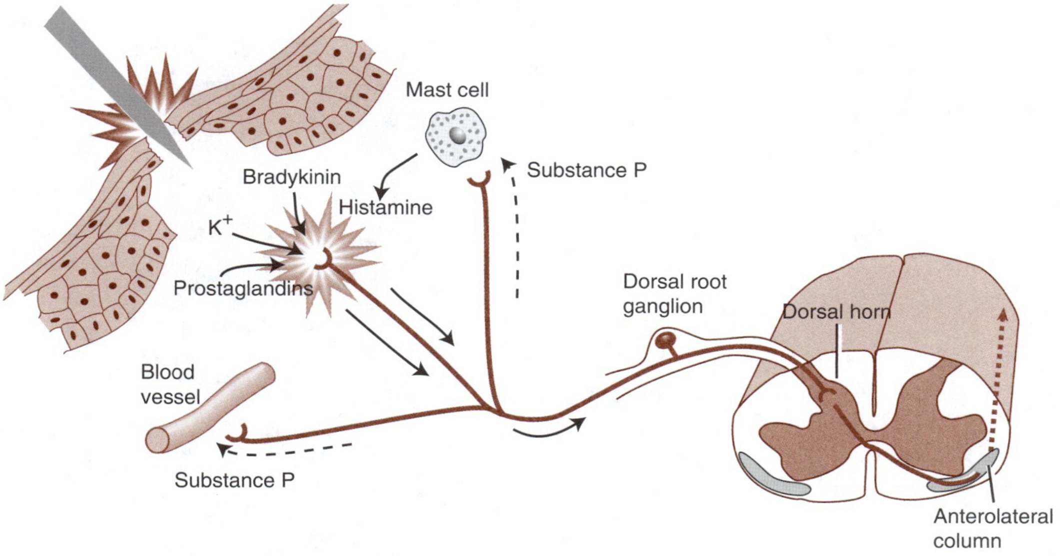

FIGURE 11.2 Peripheral nociceptive responses to acute trauma.

these signals activate areas associated with emotional feelings, such as the anterior cingulate cortex (ACC), insular cortex, and prefrontal cortex—as well as the amygdala. Functional brain imaging studies over the past two decades have documented activity in these areas during pain perception—areas that are typically associated with mood, attention, and fear. Activity in these regions of the brain helps us understand the concomitant depression, hyperfocus, and anxiety we see with patients in pain.

Figure 11.7 shows drawings of some of the areas that become active with acute pain. In this study, subjects were scanned at rest and later with a hot probe (approximately 50°C) applied to the upper right arm. Note the diverse areas that become active with acute pain—thalamus, ACC, prefrontal cortex, and insula, as well as others. The experience of pain is more than just identifying where it hurts.

It is also important to note that some of the activation is on both sides of the brain. This shows that there is more to the processing of pain signals in the CNS than implied by our simplified Figures 11.5 and 11.6.

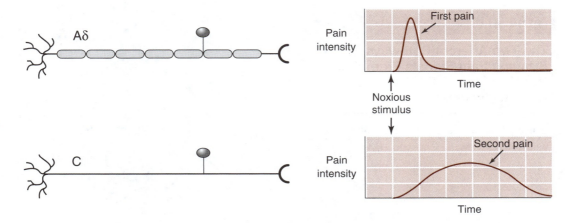

FIGURE 11.3 Aδ and C fibers transmit pain signals at different rates. (Adapted from Bear MF, Connors BW, Paradiso MA, eds. *Neuroscience: Exploring the Brain*. 4th ed. Baltimore: Lippincott Williams & Wilkins; 2015.)

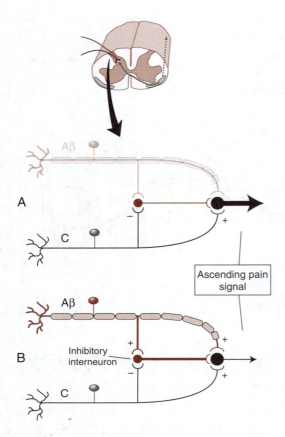

FIGURE 11.4 Gate theory of pain in the dorsal horn of the spinal cord. **A:** Without input from Aβ fibers a large signal is transmitted to the brain. **B:** A smaller signal is transmitted with input from Aβ fibers.

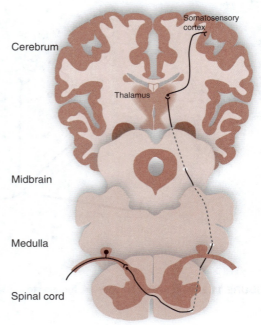

FIGURE 11.5 Spinothalamic tract transmitting the sensory-discriminative pain signal from the periphery to the somatosensory cortex.

TABLE 11.1

The Two Afferent Pathways Bringing Pain Signals From the Periphery to the Central Nervous System

Sensory-Discriminative	Affective-Motivational
Where does it hurt?	How much does it hurt?
Lateral thalamus	Medial thalamus
Somatosensory cortex	Anterior cingulate cortex, insular cortex, prefrontal cortex, and amygdala

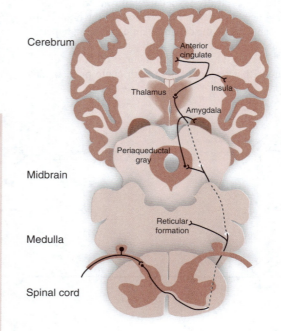

FIGURE 11.6 Affective-motivational pain tracts.

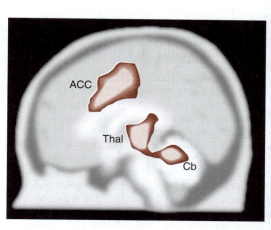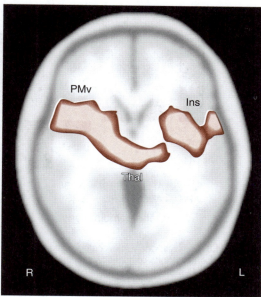

FIGURE 11.7 Positron emission tomography scans showing activity in the brain with acute pain. ACC, anterior cingulate cortex; Cb, cerebellum; Ins, insula; PMv, ventral premotor cortex; Thal, thalamus. (Data from Coghill RC, Sang CN, Maisog JM, et al. Pain intensity processing within the human brain: a bilateral, distributed mechanism. *J Neurophysiol.* 1999;82[4]:1934–1943.)

CONGENITAL INSENSITIVITY TO PAIN

Congenital insensitivity to pain, a term used to describe rare genetic conditions in which people lack the ability to sense pain, initially sounds like a blessing but is actually a nightmare. Individuals with this condition fail to identify or respond to noxious, injuring stimuli and suffer excessive burns, fractures, and soft tissue damage. Ultimately the unrecognized injuries and secondary complications lead to an early death.

The spectrum of congenital insensitivity to pain provides an example of the distinction between sensory and affective components of pain. Subjects with frank congenital insensitivity to pain are without the peripheral Aδ and C fibers. These patients lack the sensory-discriminative as well as affective components of pain and are the most at risk for harm and premature death.

A milder condition, termed *congenital indifference to pain*, is found in individuals who can distinguish sharp and dull pain but are indifferent to the sensation. They lack the emotional responses and normal withdrawal movements; they can feel the pain but are not concerned. Subjects with this disorder have normal peripheral nerve fibers but seem to have an as yet unidentified central impairment of the affective-motivational component of pain.

Congenital insensitivity to pain with anhidrosis is a specific rare autosomal recessive disorder characterized by absence of pain (along with inability to sweat, unexplained episodes of fever, and mental retardation). Patients with this condition have a mutation in the gene for the Trk receptor—the receptor that binds with nerve growth factor. As we saw in Chapter 8, Plasticity and Adult Development, nerves need nerve growth factor proteins to survive. Cells lacking the receptor are unable to incorporate the growth factor and wither away (or fail to develop). Such a patient lacks pain fibers and does not experience pain.

Pain Tolerance Spectrum

People have different abilities to tolerate pain. This has been shown in multiple psychological studies and observed by most of us in our clinical population. Brain imaging studies have documented that subjects with less pain tolerance have greater activation of the cortical areas discussed earlier (ACC, insular cortex, and prefrontal cortex, along with the somatosensory cortex).

Genetic factors undoubtedly play a role in the spectrum of pain tolerance. A study reported in 2005 examined pain tolerance in 202 women and genetic variants for the gene encoding for catecholamine-*O*-methyltransferase (COMT), an enzyme involved in the regulation of catecholamines and enkephalins. After initially measuring

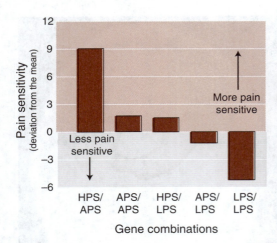

FIGURE 11.8 Pain responsiveness categorized by three major combinations of genetic variations for the catecholamine-*O*-methyltransferase enzyme. Subjects with the low pain sensitivity (LPS) variation were 2.3 times less likely to develop temporomandibular joint disorder. APS, average pain sensitivity; HPS, high pain sensitivity. (Adapted from Diatchenko L, Slade GD, Nackley AG, et al. Genetic basis for individual variations in pain perception and the development of a chronic pain condition. *Hum Mol Genet*. 2005;14[1]:135–143, by permission of Oxford University Press.)

pain tolerance with a noxious thermal stimulus, the researchers assessed the genetic makeup of each participant. They found that three genetic variants for COMT accounted for 11% of the variation in pain perception (a large percentage in genetic studies). Figure 11.8 shows how five different combinations of these genetic variants accounted for differing pain responsiveness. Further studies by this same research group examined patients in the emergency department after a motor vehicle accident. They found that those with the pain-vulnerable genes were more likely to report neck pain, headaches, and dizziness.

One wonders whether subjects who excel at physically demanding professions are more tolerant to pain than those of us with more sedentary jobs. Legend has it that Edward Villella, the famous American dancer, had his feet X-rayed in his 30s and discovered nine old fractures of which he was unaware. Ostensibly, what would have crippled us was just an aching foot to Villella. A recent meta-analysis of studies of pain perception in athletes found increased pain tolerance compared with healthy controls. The authors concluded that "regular physical activity is associated with specific alterations in pain perception," a finding that supports therapeutic exercise as an important ingredient for reducing pain. However, it is possible that individuals who are successful in physically demanding professions were born wired for

better tolerance to pain—along with being stronger, more coordinated, and driven to succeed.

DISORDER

SCHIZOPHRENIA

There is a long history dating back to Kraepelin and Bleuler of observing increased pain tolerance in patients with schizophrenia. Since then, surgeons and internists have written anecdotal reports of patients with schizophrenia who appear to experience little pain despite suffering from extremely painful physical conditions. It is not clear if the pain tolerance is a consequence of the illness, the psychotropic medications, or simply a lack of affect i.e., the patient feels the pain but fails to express it appropriately.

Hooley and Delgado sought to avoid these complicating factors by measuring pain sensitivity in the relatives of patients with schizophrenia. They found that subjects with a family history of schizophrenia showed elevated pain thresholds and tolerance. Of interest, the pain correlated with measures of self-referential thinking, magical ideation, and perceptual disturbances. The pathology of this aberrant pain sensitivity is unknown but may be part of the genetic makeup of schizophrenia.

DESCENDING PATHWAYS AND OPIOIDS

The discovery of the opioid-mediated pain modulation circuits is one of the great stories in neuroscience. In the late 1960s it became apparent that the brain exerts a top-down control of pain. A big break came in 1969 with the discovery that electrical stimulation of the *periaqueductal gray*, the gray matter surrounding the third ventricle and the cerebral aqueduct in the midbrain, induces analgesia. Reynolds implanted electrodes in the PAG of rats and performed abdominal surgery without problems when the electrodes were stimulated. Although the animals did not respond to the pain, they were able to move about the cage (before and after surgery) and displayed a startle response to visual or auditory stimuli even while the electrodes were active.

Subsequent work has led to a detailed knowledge of the descending pain-modulating circuits. Figure 11.9 shows a drawing of the important features of these pathways. Input from the prefrontal areas of the anterior cingulate and insular cortex as well as the hypothalamus and amygdala converge on the PAG.

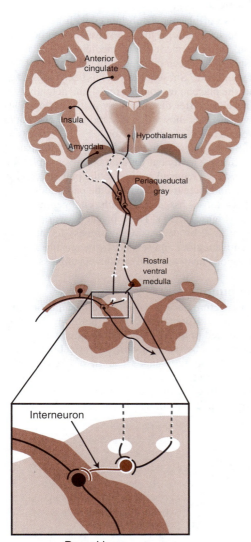

FIGURE 11.9 Descending pain-modulating pathways that enable the brain to inhibit the intensity of the ascending pain signals.

The PAG does not send neurons directly onto the dorsal horn but rather projects by way of intermediary nuclei such as the *rostral ventral medulla* (RVM). Other serotonergic and noradrenergic neurons (not shown) also project down onto the afferent pain neurons. The end result is inhibition and diminution of the pain signal that is sent up the ascending anterolateral tracts to the brain.

Opium

It is likely that opium was used as early as 4000 BC by the ancient Sumerians. By the 17th century, the therapeutic value of opium was well known.

Morphine was first isolated in 1806 and codeine in 1832. Heroin was introduced to medicine in 1896—and marketed as a nonaddictive. The uses and abuses of opium and its analogues have permeated most cultures of the world.

By the mid-1960s it was known that microinjections of morphine into the PAG or the dorsal horn produced a powerful analgesia and that the opioid antagonist naloxone could block this effect. Furthermore, transection of the axons from the RVM reduces the morphine-induced analgesia. Yet it was unknown how morphine relieved pain.

Opioid Receptors

The discovery of the opioid receptors was a major breakthrough in understanding the pain modulatory system. Three major classes of opioid receptors have been identified: μ (mu), δ (delta), and κ (kappa). However, most of the focus has been on the μ receptor because its activation is required for most analgesics. Indeed the affinity that a medication has for the μ receptor correlates with its potency as an analgesic. *Naloxone* also binds with the μ receptor and acts as the quintessential antagonist for it blocks activation and can precipitate withdrawal.

The opioid receptors are concentrated in the PAG, RVM, and dorsal horn—areas well known for pain modulation. However, the receptor can be found throughout the body, including intestines, muscles, and joints, which helps explain the benefits as well as typical side effects associated with opioids, such as constipation and respiratory depression.

For centuries, opioids have been used to boost mood and reduce anxiety, although with troubling addictive sequela. With the advent of the antidepressants in the 1950s, the "opium cure" was largely abandoned. However, recent attention has returned to the opioid receptor as a novel focus for psychiatric problems. Studies with buprenorphine and methadone have shown rapid and positive effects for treatment-resistant depression, but again with concerns about abuse. Some argue that the rapid antidepressant effects of ketamine are due to its opioid effects.

Animal studies and preliminary studies with humans suggest that blocking the κ receptor may improve mood and treat substance abuse. The challenge is to block the κ receptor without stimulating the μ receptor—the receptor most closely associated with euphoria and abuse. ALKS-5461 is a medication that is a combination of *buprenorphine* (stimulates the μ receptor and blocks the κ receptor) and *samidorphan* (blocks the μ receptor as well as the κ receptor), which is being studied as a supplemental treatment for persistent depression and cocaine dependency. People who know this medication say it improves mood *without* the potential for addiction (they actually say that). Studies are under way.

Endogenous Opioids

Clearly, animals did not evolve a receptor so that drug abusers could enjoy heroin. In the mid-1970s the race was on to find the neurotransmitter that the body produces to activate the opioid receptor. The result was the discovery of the β-endorphin, enkephalins, and dynorphins: the three major classes of endogenous opioid peptides. The genes for these peptides are active throughout the CNS.

Figure 11.10 shows an example from the dorsal horn of the enkephalins and the μ receptors working together to decrease the pain signal sent to the brain. Note that the μ receptors are on both the presynaptic and the postsynaptic neurons.

POINT OF INTEREST

β-Endorphin is derived from a larger precursor molecule called *proopiomelanocortin* (POMC), found primarily in the pituitary (see Figure 16.13). POMC contains other biologically active peptides, including adrenocorticotropic hormone (ACTH). Consequently, the stress response includes the release of ACTH as well as β-endorphin into the bloodstream. One wonders about the evolutionary advantage of the simultaneous synthesis and release of these two neuropeptides.

Placebo

The use of placebos, substances with no intrinsic therapeutic value, is the oldest treatment known to man. In the modern era of medicine, the placebo response has been equated with the statement "all in your head." Subsequently, it has been recognized that the placebo response is real—and actually is in our heads. After the discovery of the endogenous opioid, it was shown that placebo anesthesia could even be reversed with naloxone.

Brain imaging studies of subjects anticipating an effective treatment for pain but given a placebo have shown reduced activity in the pain perception areas and increased activity in the pain modulation areas—those associated with endogenous opioids (Figure 11.11). Thus, placebos work in two ways: first, by decreasing awareness in the pain-sensitive regions and second, by increasing activity in regions involved with top-down suppression.

Acupuncture

Acupuncture has been used for thousands of years in China, Korea, and Japan but only recently introduced to the West. The healing power of acupuncture is believed to work by reestablishing the proper "energy balance" in disordered organs. The treatment is conducted by inserting a needle into specific locations along meridians established through ancient clinical experience. The lack of

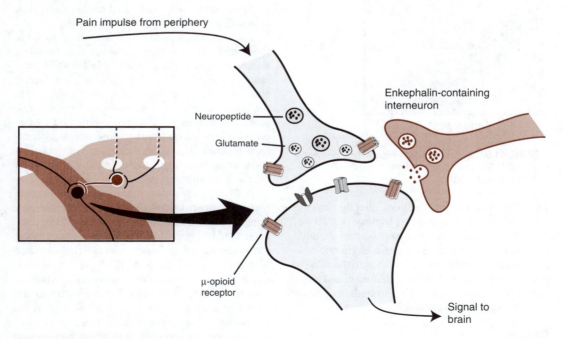

FIGURE 11.10 Descending pathways stimulate an interneuron in the dorsal horn to release enkephalins that activate the μ receptors. The effect on the presynaptic neuron is to decrease the release of glutamate and neuropeptides. With the postsynaptic neuron, stimulation of the μ receptors hyperpolarizes the membrane. These two actions result in a smaller signal coming out of the dorsal horn.

Placebo-induced decrease

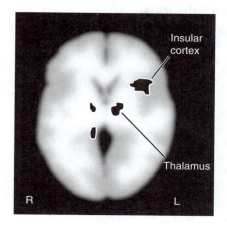

Placebo-induced activation

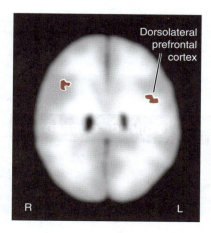

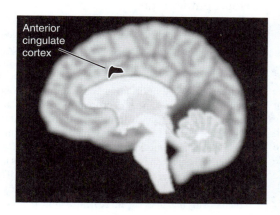

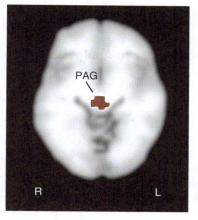

■ Decreased activity in pain-
sensitive regions

■ Increased activity in
pain-suppressing regions

FIGURE 11.11 The brain imaging studies of the placebo response showing two aspects to the brain's reaction. On the left, control minus placebo shows decreased activity in those areas that perceive pain. On the right, placebo minus control shows increased activity in areas that suppress pain from the top down. PAG, periaqueductal gray matter. (Adapted from Wager TD, Rilling JK, Smith EE, et al. Placebo-induced changes in fMRI in the anticipation and experience of pain. *Science*. 2004;303[5661]:1162–1167. Reprinted with permission from AAAS.)

scientific correlation or good clinical trials can be troubling to those of us who subscribe to a Western orientation of physiology and illness.

One of the difficulties in conducting good clinical trials with acupuncture is separating the specific effect of stimulating the acupoints from the placebo effect. A study in London sought to overcome this problem by including two placebo arms along with active acupuncture treatment. The first placebo treatment was with a blunt needle, and the patients were aware they were being given an "inert" treatment. The second placebo arm intervention used what can best be described as a "stage needle"—when poked, the

needle retracted into the handle, giving the appearance that the skin had been pierced. Surprisingly, few of the subjects were aware of the difference between the "stage needle" and real acupuncture.

While these patients—all with osteoarthritis—were being poked, they also had their heads in a positron emission tomography (PET) scanner. The results showed that areas of the brain associated with top-down modulation of pain—DLPFC, ACC, and midbrain—were active with "stage needles" as well as real needles. Only the ipsilateral insula was solely activated by real acupuncture. These results suggest that acupuncture works by way of a large placebo response and also a distinct, but as yet unknown, unique physiologic effect.

A recent meta-analysis of acupuncture for chronic low-back pain encapsulates our belief about acupuncture treatment. Acupuncture plus standard care was more effective than standard care alone. However, sham acupuncture was just as effective as real acupuncture.

POINT OF CORRECTION

In earlier editions of this book we included a sidebar about acupuncture activating the occipital cortex when a needle is inserted in the "visual meridian" in the *foot*. It seemed too good to be true, and indeed it was. The authors issued a retraction of their findings. Oops!

Stress-Induced Analgesia

Perhaps the most impressive demonstration of top-down modulation of pain is the extreme analgesia shown by individuals at times of stress, for example, the athlete or performing artist who does not appreciate the pain until much later. The classic example was described by Beecher regarding men wounded in battle during the Second World War. He examined 215 men brought to a forward hospital with serious injuries: long bone fractures, penetrating wounds, etc. He found that only 25%, on being directly questioned regarding pain relief, said their pain was severe enough to want morphine. Beecher believed the relief the men experienced, when taken from the battle and brought to a safe location, blocked the pain.

The modern belief is that stress stimulates opioid-dependent pathways that inhibit the pain signal. However, a group at the University of Georgia has revealed a role for the endocannabinoids in stress-induced analgesia independent of the opioid pathways. Several endocannabinoids rapidly accumulate in the PAG in the midbrain with stress. The group in Georgia demonstrated that stress-induced analgesia in rats could be inhibited with endocannabinoid blockers. Their results suggest that higher cortical regions such as the amygdala release endocannabinoids into the PAG during stressful times to suppress pain perception. We appreciate the brain's wisdom in using several mechanisms (endocannabinoids and opioids) to put pain on hold when other more pressing tasks are at hand.

CHRONIC PAIN

Until the past century, pain was thought to be produced by a passive, direct transmission system from peripheral receptors to the cortex. This is called *nociceptive pain*, and examples include acute trauma, arthritis, and tumor invasion. There is a thriving medical industry based on locating and correcting the source of the nociceptive pain for patients who are suffering. Unfortunately, most evaluations fail to turn up a cause that explains the pain. One reason is that the traditional model of pain fails to take into account changes in the nerves. Clearly, many patients in pain—particularly chronic, persistent pain—have developed autonomous, maladaptive pain perception independent of tissue damage.

Neuropathic Pain

Neuropathic pain is a heterogeneous term used to describe pain that arises from an injured nerve—either centrally or peripherally, e.g., postherpetic neuralgia, diabetic neuropathy, and phantom limb. The distinction between neuropathic and nociceptive pain is important when choosing proper treatment. For instance, neuropathic pain may not respond as well to nonsteroidal anti-inflammatory agents, or opioids, and is better managed with antidepressants and anticonvulsants.

Neuropathic pain is frequently persistent, does not resolve with time, and is resistant to treatment. The pain often disables patients. The pathophysiologic mechanisms that underlie these neuropathic pain conditions are beginning to be teased out. One promising area of research is looking at the role of neurotrophic factors in the development of pathologic pain states.

As we discussed in previous chapters, tissue injury induces an inflammatory response, which recruits immune cells that release cytokines. The cytokines are literally toxic to the sensory neurons. For example, inflammation interrupts the retrograde transport of neurotrophins from the periphery back to the cell body, where it is needed to maintain normal cell functioning. One neurotrophic factor in particular (glial cell line–derived neurotrophic factor [GDNF]) has been identified as a possible target. Several studies have shown that exogenous GDNF can prevent the development of experimental neuropathic pain.

Pain Memory

A striking example of the brain's elaboration of pain without sensory input can be found in patients after limb amputation. Many will continue to experience pain from lesions that existed on the limb before the surgery—what some call pain memory. For example, a person with an ulcer on the foot at the time of the operation will still feel the presence of the ulcer many months after the limb has been removed.

Several clever clinicians have shown that sufficient local anesthesia of the affected limb several days before the amputation significantly reduces the incidence of pain memories. These results suggest that pain has an enduring effect on the brain, which can be attenuated with appropriate treatment.

Gray Matter Loss

A study in 2004 at Northwestern University demonstrated structural changes in the CNS with chronic pain. Apkarian et al. scanned 26 patients with chronic back pain and compared the results with age-matched controls. They found a 5% to 11% loss of gray matter in the dorsolateral prefrontal cortex (DLPFC) in patients with chronic back pain. Subsequently, a number of studies have found a pattern of gray matter thinning (cingulate cortex, orbitofrontal cortex, insula, and thalamus, as well as DLPFC) in a variety of chronic pain syndromes, e.g., migraine, phantom pain, fibromyalgia, etc.

What causes the gray matter loss with chronic pain? There has been speculation about cellular atrophy or loss due to damaging effects of the pain experience or toxic mechanisms from pain medications. Some wonder if the gray matter loss explains why some people develop chronic pain. Others have postulated that the gray matter changes might be reversible if the pain is treated. A group in Hamburg, Germany, chose to test this theory and prospectively studied 20 patients with chronic hip pain, before and after total hip replacement—a procedure that is almost 90% curable. Before surgery the subjects had gray matter loss in the ACC, insula, DLPFC, and orbitofrontal cortex compared with a control group. After surgery, when the patients were pain free, they had gray matter increases in nearly the same areas as well as the motor cortex (Figure 11.12). The authors concluded the results "suggest that

chronic nociceptive input and motor impairment in these patients leads to altered processing in cortical regions and consequently structural brain changes which are in principle reversible." This is another example of the remarkable plasticity of the brain.

Unexplained Chronic Pain

Twenty years ago, opioids were primarily used for acute pain or those with terminal illnesses. Then in the late 1990s there came a push from the pharmaceutical industry, pain specialists, advocacy groups, and even the government for physicians to be more aggressive in treating nonmalignant chronic pain. In brief, it has been a disaster. Americans account for the lion's share of opioid consumption in the world, and yet there are more people in pain than ever before. Abuse and diversion have sky rocketed. Opioid overdose deaths have quadrupled since 1999. Furthermore, once people get on opioids, it is very difficult to get them off.

The most troubling aspect about extended opioid treatment is the possibility that chronic use of opioids might not be beneficial and might even make pain worse.

1. Evidence for long-term use of opioids for nonmalignant chronic pain is almost nonexistent.
2. Tolerance to analgesic and euphoric effects develops quickly, which requires dose escalation. (However, tolerance for respiratory depression develops slower, which explains why dose escalation by well-meaning prescribers can precipitate an overdose.)
3. Clinicians are recognizing what is called opioid-induced hyperalgesia—a phenomenon in which patients on long-term use of opioids become increasingly sensitive to painful stimuli.
4. Animal studies have produced troubling findings.

Peter Grace and colleagues at the University of Colorado studied the enduring effects of morphine

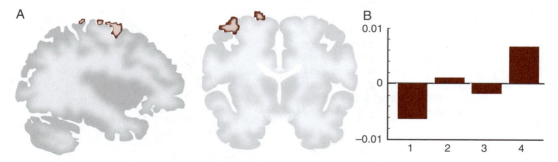

FIGURE 11.12 A: Gray matter thickness at the areas in brown (part of the motor cortex) increased with pain relief. **B:** Data showing the thickening gray matter in the weeks and months after total hip replacement. (Adapted from Rodriguez-Raecke R, et al. Structural brain changes in chronic pain reflect probably neither damage nor atrophy. *PLoS One.* 2013;8[2]:e54475. © 2013 Rodriguez-Raecke, et al.)

treatment on subsequent painful tolerance in rats. First, they inflicted a constriction injury on the sciatic nerve—considered an animal model of neuropathic pain. After 10 days, the rats were given 5 days of morphine or saline. Then their reactions to painful stimuli were assessed over the next 13 weeks. Figure 11.13A shows that the rats treated with morphine experienced more pain as measured by their reactions to noxious mechanical stimuli. The authors found evidence that the persistent pain sensitivity induced by the morphine is caused by an inflammatory response (cytokines) mediated by spinal microglia, which may explain how acute pain can transition into chronic pain.

In a follow-up study, Grace and colleagues blocked the inflammatory response with naloxone. Naloxone comes in two versions—the same chemical structure but mirror images of each other—sort of a left and right version. The "normal" naloxone (also called Narcan) blocks the opioid receptors and is given in opioid overdoses. The more precise name for this medication is (−)-naloxone. Its sister molecule, called (+)-naloxone, amazingly has no affinity for the opioid receptors but blocks TLR4 receptors—the receptor that mediates the inflammatory response induced by opioids. With this in mind

Grace et al. injected (+)-naloxone into rats sensitized by morphine treatment, which reversed opioid-induced sensitization (Figure 11.13B). Although such an intervention would not stop addiction, because it does not block the euphoric effects, TLR4 blockers if given with opioid treatment might reduce the development of chronic pain conditions.

Safer Treatments

The "promised land" in pain management is an analgesic as effective as morphine but devoid of narcotic side effects or addictive potential. There are a few prospects on the horizon. One approach is to find a molecule with restricted activation of the μ receptor. It turns out that when morphine couples with μ receptors, it triggers two signaling cascades: G protein and β-arrestin. These have different effects. The G protein cascade produces more pain relief, whereas the β-arrestin cascade produces the side effects. Two compounds (affectionately called PZM21 and TRV130) bind with the μ opioid receptor but trigger the G protein signaling without β-arrestin activation. In animal studies, these compounds appear to relieve pain as effectively as morphine with less constipation, less respiratory depression, and with no more abuse potential than saline.

TMS, PFC, AND POSTOPERATIVE PAIN

Transcranial magnetic stimulation (TMS) is a noninvasive procedure that can stimulate the cerebral cortex. The PFC has been implicated as a region that modulates pain tolerance. A clever collaboration between anesthesiology and psychiatry shows that activation of the PFC with TMS can decrease pain perception.

Patients undergoing gastric bypass surgery were randomized to receive 20 minutes of either active or sham TMS immediately after surgery. Total morphine administered by patient-controlled analgesia pumps was tracked as an indirect measurement of pain. Remarkably, one session of TMS applied to the left PFC greatly reduced the total morphine self-administered by the patients (see figure). Although not practical for chronic pain, further studies with TMS have shown some positive results for patients with fibromyalgia.

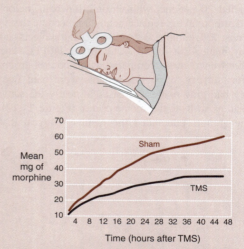

(Adapted from Borckardt JJ, Weinstein M, Reeves ST, et al. Postoperative left prefrontal repetitive transcranial magnetic stimulation reduces patient-controlled analgesia use. *Anesthesiology.* 2006;105[3]:557–562.)

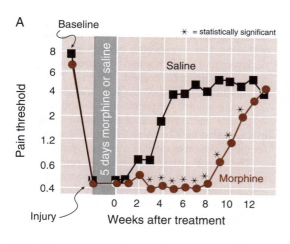
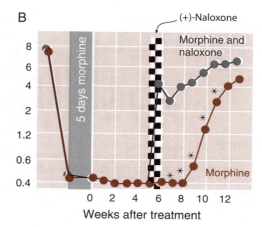

FIGURE 11.13 A: Rats given morphine endure a lower pain threshold months after treatment. **B:** (+)-Naloxone reverses the sensitizing effects of morphine. (Adapted from Grace PM, et al. Morphine paradoxically prolongs neuropathic pain in rats by amplifying spinal NLRP3 inflammasome activation. *Proc Natl Acad Sci U S A.* 2016;113[24]:E3411–E3450.)

DEPRESSION AND ANTIDEPRESSANTS

There is a long and well-documented correlation between depression and pain. Patients with chronic pain have a high incidence of depression, and patients with depression have an increased expression of painful physical symptoms. Recently, studies have shown that patients with depression and pain are less likely to achieve remission of their depression.

Antidepressants have been shown to be effective in decreasing pain for low-back pain, diabetic neuropathy, postherpetic neuralgia, fibromyalgia, and migraines. Traditionally, tricyclics were used, but with the development of cleaner medications, other agents were tried. Of interest, the selective serotonin reuptake inhibitors (SSRIs) have been disappointing—often not separating from placebo in controlled trials. It appears that only agents that inhibit the reuptake of norepinephrine as well as serotonin are effective for pain reduction. The newer agents that tout a dual mechanism of action (venlafaxine and duloxetine) have been shown to reduce neuropathic pain. Duloxetine even has an FDA indication for peripheral diabetic neuropathy.

How do the antidepressants decrease pain? One possibility could be the beneficial effect of correcting the mood. Yet SSRIs give disappointing results. Likewise, patients without depression will show some pain reduction. Another possibility is the enhancement of the descending pathways. Some of the fibers projecting from the brain stem down onto the dorsal horn of the spinal cord are serotonergic and noradrenergic. More action from these neurons would further dampen the signals from the periphery.

A final possibility for understanding the effectiveness of antidepressants for pain is a cortical mechanism. PET scans of both depressed patients and patients with pain show decreased activity in the prefrontal cortex and increased activity in the insula and ACC. It is possible that antidepressants moderate the pain perception by correcting the cortical imbalance associated with depression and pain.

Epidemic of Unexplained Pain

Let us not forget that pain is highly influenced by one's psychosocial expectations. A good example is the epidemic of vague upper limb pain from Australia called *repetitive strain injury* (RSI). This condition was attributed to repetitive keyboard movements by telegraphists but failed to follow the usual medical model. Reports in the medical literature and sensational media coverage as well as union and legal advocacy produced a dramatic increase in reports of RSI (Figure 11.14). The complaints peaked in 1984 and then declined, as the condition came to be perceived as psychosomatic, and the courts went against the litigants. Similar epidemics have occurred in the United Kingdom and Japan.

Another classic study analyzed the development of late whiplash syndrome in Lithuania—a country where few drivers have car insurance or seek legal

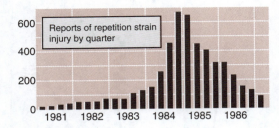

FIGURE 11.14 A psychosomatic pain epidemic. The graph shows reports of repetition strain injury at Telecom in Australia by quarter. (Adapted from Hocking B. Epidemiological aspects of "repetition strain injury" in Telecom Australia. *Med J Aust.* 1987;147[5]:218–222. © Copyright 1987 *The Medical Journal of Australia*—reproduced with permission.)

compensation after an accident. The authors questioned the subjects involved in known rear-end car collisions, 1 to 3 years after the accident, regarding neck pain and headaches and compared their symptoms with matched control subjects. There was no significant difference between the groups. The authors concluded, "expectation of disability, a family history, and attribution of preexisting symptoms to the trauma may be more important determinants for the evolution of the late whiplash syndrome."

The important point is that the perception of pain is a product of the brain's abstraction and elaboration of sensory input. Many factors affect that process—not just nociceptive signals from the periphery.

QUESTIONS

1. Slow aching pain signals
   a. Aδ fibers.
   b. Aβ fibers.
   c. C fibers.
   d. D fibers.

2. Simultaneous input from these nerve fibers explains the inhibitory effect of the gate theory of pain
   a. Aδ fibers.
   b. Aβ fibers.
   c. C fibers.
   d. D fibers.

3. Not associated with the affective-motivational pathways of pain
   a. Somatosensory cortex.
   b. "How much does it hurt?"
   c. Medial thalamus.
   d. Anterior cingulate and insular cortex.

4. Condition associated with increased pain tolerance
   a. Depression.
   b. Anxiety.
   c. Fibromyalgia.
   d. Schizophrenia.

5. Not part of the descending pathways of pain
   a. Periaqueductal gray.
   b. Dorsal horn.
   c. Spinothalamic tract.
   d. Rostral ventral medulla.

6. The primary opioid receptor
   a. β receptor.
   b. δ receptor.
   c. κ receptor.
   d. μ receptor.

7. Unlikely explanation for chronic persistent pain
   a. Genetic predisposition.
   b. Extinguished placebo response.
   c. Changes in the gray matter.
   d. Damaged nerves.

8. Lacks significant analgesic effects
   a. Selective serotonin reuptake inhibitors.
   b. Opioids.
   c. Nonsteroidal anti-inflammatory drugs.
   d. Anticonvulsants.

See Answers section at the end of this book.

CHAPTER 12

Pleasure

SEEKING PLEASURE

Voluntary and unconscious behavior in animals is motivated by the avoidance of pain and the pursuit of pleasure. In this chapter we will focus on the neuronal mechanisms that guide our choices toward stimuli that give a little reward to the brain.

Our existence—as individuals and as a species—is dependent on using the five senses to recognize and pursue actions necessary for survival. The motivation to pursue a beneficial act is driven in part by giving the brain a brief squirt of euphoria. This reward system has evolved over millions of years to enable an individual to sort through a variety of stimuli and choose the ones that are most appropriate.

The orbital aspect of the prefrontal cortex (PFC) is known to play a critical role in goal-directed behavior. Figure 12.1 shows that the relative appeal for an item can be recognized in the brain even down to the level of a single neuron. In this study, electrodes placed in a single neuron in the orbitofrontal cortex registered different levels of activity based on the appeal of the food. A raisin generated the largest signal and was the most desired object; cereal was the least active and least desired, although, frankly, we would have preferred the apple.

Many of our patients, family, and friends struggle with problems that they have created by pursuing the wrong rewards. Clearly, the addicted individual has lost control over his or her choices but what about the promiscuous college student, the young adult who accumulates excessive debt on new credit cards, or the author who surfs the Internet instead of writing? These people are choosing pleasurable activities that are not to their benefit and are even harmful. Remarkably, all our joys, the good ones and the wrong ones, funnel into the same neural mechanisms.

The problems are related to the sensitivity of our reward system. We are built for acquiring rewards that were historically in short supply. Now with the extraordinary success of the human race and industrialized civilization, we are exposed to abundance beyond what our wiring has evolved to handle. Junk food, pornography, and shopping malls as well as alcohol, stimulants, and opioids usurp the mechanisms developed to enhance the survival of the hunter-gatherer in all of us.

DISORDER

MARITAL CONFLICT

Disparity in the pursuit of joy is a major source of conflict in most relationships. Married couples frequently argue about sex, money, and how to spend leisure time. With each conflict, one partner wants to spend more time and money involved in some activity. For example, he wants to golf and buy a big boat for fishing; she wants to vacation with her family and fix up the house. He wants more sex; she wants more romance. Different joys bring discord.

Happiness

There is clinical evidence to suggest that one's level of happiness remains remarkably fixed. For example, the person winning a lottery or the one suffering the loss of a limb tends to revert to their preexisting level of happiness after a period of exultation or depression. It seems that happiness is hardwired and closely fluctuates around a genetic "set point" for each person. Unfortunately, there is surprisingly little neuroscience insight on this topic.

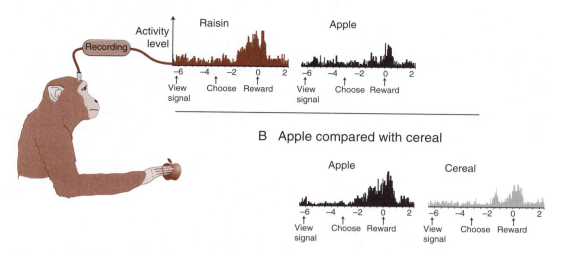

FIGURE 12.1 A monkey is taught to view a signal, make a choice, and be rewarded with a designated food morsel. **A:** The activity in an individual neuron in the orbitofrontal cortex when the monkey is offered a reward of either a raisin or an apple. **B:** Rewarded with either an apple or cereal. The size of the signal is believed to represent the motivational value, i.e., raisin > apple; apple > cereal. (Adapted from Macmillan Publishers Ltd. Tremblay L, Schultz W. Relative reward preference in primate orbitofrontal cortex. *Nature*. 1999;398[6729]:704–708. Copyright 1999.)

ANATOMY OF REWARD

Pursuing a reward can be conceptualized as a ball rolling downhill. Animals will gravitate toward the most enjoyable activity the way a ball rolls to the lowest point. It seemingly happens without effort. However, although we cannot visualize the force of gravity pulling on a moving ball, we continue to tease out the neuroanatomy of the mammalian reward system.

The initial studies came in the mid-1950s when Olds and Milner accidentally discovered that a rat would seek to continue stimulation from a thin electrode implanted in certain parts of its brain. Figure 12.2 shows the relative placement of an electrode in a rat's skull and the apparatus that Olds and

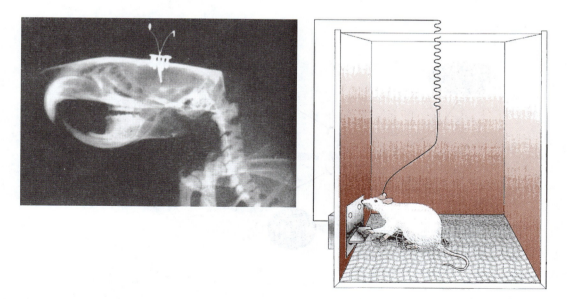

FIGURE 12.2 An X-ray showing the placement of an electrode through the skull into the brain of a rat. On the right, when the rat presses the lever, it receives a mild stimulus—which can be highly motivating. (From Olds J. Pleasure centers in the brain. *Sci Am*. 1956;195:105–112.)

Milner used to study the animals' inclination for self-stimulation. Remarkably, the rats exceeded all expectations in what they were willing to sacrifice to receive stimulation. Depending on where the electrode was placed, they would press the lever up to 5000 times in an hour, choose stimulation over food even when starving, and cross an electrified grid for a chance to press the lever.

Fifty years of research has established that the mesolimbic dopamine (DA) system, including the ventral tegmental area (VTA) and nucleus accumbens (NAc) (also called the *ventral striatum*), is the central structure of reward. These old but effective nuclei lie at the base of the brain (Figure 12.3) and are the structures that were being indirectly stimulated in the Olds and Milner experiments. The NAc and VTA receive signals from a multitude of sources—the most prominent of which are the PFC, amygdala, and hippocampus. It is significant that input to the NAc and VTA originates from areas involved in attention, executive decisions, and emotional memories—areas that help the brain negotiate the path to the rewards.

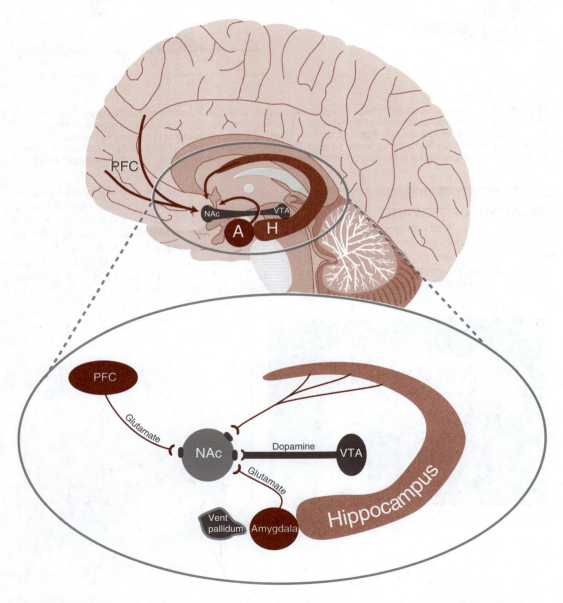

FIGURE 12.3 The anatomy of pleasure and reward is mediated in the nucleus accumbens (NAc) with input from a variety of structures, only a few of which are shown here. PFC, prefrontal cortex; VTA, ventral tegmental area.

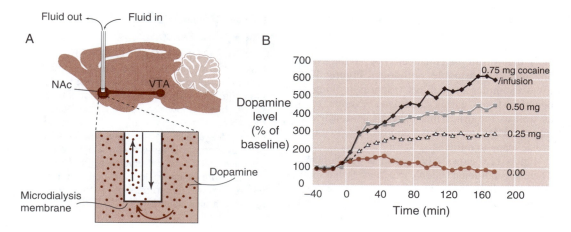

FIGURE 12.4 Using microdialysis in rats **(A)**, Pettit and Justice found that increasing self-administered doses of cocaine resulted in greater extracellular dopamine at the nucleus accumbens (NAc) **(B)**. VTA, ventral tegmental area. (Adapted from Pettit HO, Justice Jr JB. Effect of dose on cocaine self-administration behavior and dopamine levels in the nucleus accumbens. *Brain Res*. 1991;539[1]:94–102. Copyright 1991 with permission from Elsevier.)

Converging lines of evidence have shown that DA is the primary neurotransmitter that modulates the reward system. Using an implanted microdialysis apparatus, Pettit and Justice were able to regularly sample DA concentration at the NAc. They found a correlation between the amounts of cocaine a rat would self-administer and the extracellular DA at the NAc (Figure 12.4). Alternatively, blocking the effect of cocaine either with a DA antagonist (e.g., haloperidol) or lesioning the dopaminergic cells in the NAc eliminated the self-administration and drug-seeking behavior.

Brain Imaging

Brain-imaging studies with human volunteers have further established the link between DA and reward. Volkow administered IV methylphenidate (MPH) (Ritalin) and established a correlation between the dose of the medication and the occupancy of the DA transporter (stimulants work in part by blocking the DA reuptake pump). Additionally, by asking the participant how they felt, a correlation between feeling "high" and the occupancy of the DA transporter was established (Figure 12.5).

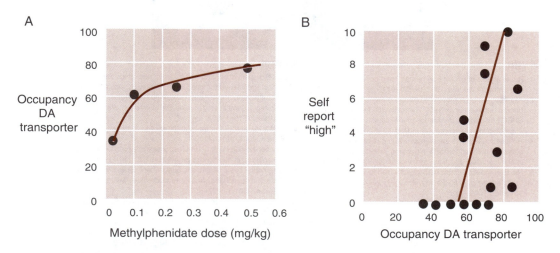

FIGURE 12.5 Methylphenidate (MPH) and occupancy of the dopamine (DA) reuptake transporter. Higher doses of MPH result in increased occupancy of the DA transporter **(A)**, which results in increased DA available to the nucleus accumbens and—at strong enough levels—feeling "high" **(B)**. (Adapted from Volkow ND, Fowler JS, Wang GJ, et al. Role of dopamine in the therapeutic and reinforcing effects of methylphenidate in humans: results from imaging studies. *Eur Neuropsychopharmacol*. 2002;12[6]:557–566. Copyright 2002 with permission from Elsevier.)

Creative studies with functional imaging scanners have shown that it is not just drugs of abuse (such as amphetamines, alcohol, nicotine, etc.) that result in enhanced DA at the NAc, but many pleasurable activities. Figure 12.6 gives examples of feelings (such as looking at beautiful faces, eating chocolate, revenge, etc.) as well as the drugs that have all demonstrated increased DA at the NAc and/or VTA in functional scans in humans.

Figure 12.6 shows only the studies with humans. There are additional hedonic experiences that show similar findings with animals. For example, sexual behavior, violence, opioids, and marijuana all increase DA at the NAc in animals. Furthermore,

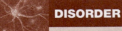

DISORDER

COMPLICATED GRIEF

It is not uncommon to see patients who are experiencing prolonged and unabated grief after the loss of a loved one. Functional brain scans have shown persistent activation of the NAc in patients with such complicated grief: more activity in the NAc correlated with greater yearning when viewing a picture of the deceased. This report suggests that unsuccessful adaptation to loss is complicated by the reward of remembering—even when the memory is also painful.

Drugs

1. Cocaine
2. Alcohol
3. Amphetamines
4. Methylphenidate
5. Nicotine

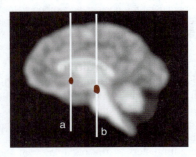

Feelings

6. Romantic love
7. Listening to music
8. Humor
9. Expectation of $$$
10. Inflicting punishment
11. Looking at beautiful faces
12. Social cooperation
13. Eating chocolate
14. Talking about yourself

a. Nucleus accumbens   b. Ventral tegmental area

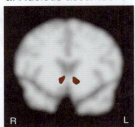   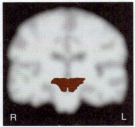

Drugs

1. Acute effects of cocaine on human brain activity and emotion. *Neuron.* 1997;19:591–611.
2. Alcohol promotes dopamine release in the human nucleus accumbens. *Synapse.* 2003;49:226–231.
3. SPECT imaging of striatal dopamine release after amphetamine challenge. *J Nuc Med.* 1995;36:1182–1190.
4. Role of dopamine in the therapeutic and reinforcing effects of methylphenidate in humans: results from imaging studies. *Eur Neuropsychophar.* 2002;12:557–566.
5. Nicotine-induced limbic cortical activation in the human brain: a functional MRI study. *Am J Psych.* 1998;155:1009–1015.

Feelings

6. Reward, motivation, and emotion systems associated with early-stage intense romantic love. *J Neurophysiol.* 2005;94:327–337.
7. Intensely pleasurable responses to music correlate with activity in brain regions implicated in reward and emotion. *Proc Natl Acad Sci U S A.* 2001;98:11818–11823.
8. Humor modulates the mesolimbic reward centers. *Neuron.* 2003;40:1041–1048.
9. Functional imaging of neural responses to expectancy and experience of monetary gains and losses. *Neuron.* 2001;30:619–639.
10. The neural basis of altruistic punishment. *Science.* 2004;305:1254–1258.
11. Beautiful faces have variable reward value: fMRI and behavioral evidence. *Neuron.* 2001;32:537–551.
12. A neural basis for social cooperation. *Neuron.* 2002;35:395–405.
13. Changes in brain activity related to eating chocolate. *Brain.* 2001;124:1720–1733.
14. Disclosing information about the self is intrinsically rewarding. *Proc Natl Acad Sci U S A.* 2012;109:8038–8043.

FIGURE 12.6 Drugs of abuse and pleasant feelings light up the mesolimbic dopamine pathway (either the NAc and/or the VTA) in functional imaging studies in humans. The studies documenting these findings are listed at the bottom of the figure.

we can speculate that other pleasurable behaviors—those that would be difficult to investigate in a scanner, such as shopping, gambling, extreme sports, and defeating one's arch enemy—also may deliver a splash of DA to the NAc. The key point is this: Behaviors that people enjoy seem to precipitate an increase in the DA produced at the NAc.

One particularly interesting study conducted at the primate laboratory at Wake Forest University looked at the effect of social rank on DA in monkeys. The monkeys were initially housed individually and scanned for dopamine D_2 receptors, which were found to be similar for all monkeys. Next they were housed together in groups of four. After 3 months, the researchers determined who were the dominant and subordinate monkeys and then rescanned them. The results are shown in Figure 12.7. Note that the dominant monkey now has significantly greater dopamine D_2 receptors in the striatum—an area that includes the NAc.

The researchers also allowed the monkeys to self-administer different doses of cocaine. The graph on the right of Figure 12.7 shows that the dominant monkeys gave themselves less cocaine than the subordinates at different strengths of the drug. This suggests that the "good feelings" that come from being the alpha monkey buffer against seeking external sources of reward. This provides some insight into the correlation between increased substance abuse and lower socioeconomic status.

Amygdala

The amygdala, along with the frontal cortex, also influences the mesolimbic DA system. Although better known for its role in fear and avoidance, the amygdala plays a role in evaluating pleasures. The point being, the amygdala is critically involved in the process of acquiring and retaining lasting memories of emotional experiences whether they are pleasurable or traumatic. Studies have shown correlations between the activation of the amygdala during emotionally arousing events and subsequent recall. It is not known if the memories are actually stored in the amygdala or recalled from the cortex by the amygdala.

The process of associating emotional memories with particular events—a special song, helicopters flying overhead, or the smell of a cigarette—is classic conditioning. A demonstration of the

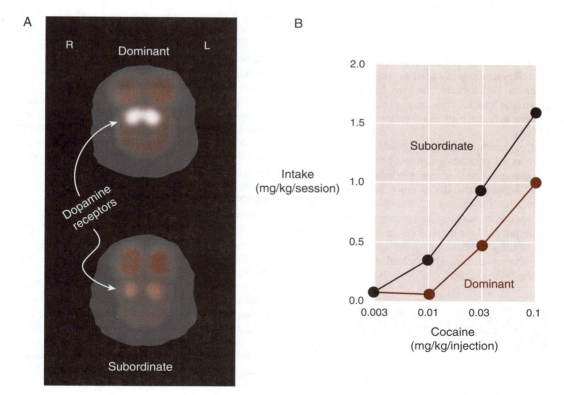

FIGURE 12.7 A: Drawings of positron emission tomography scans showing the prevalence of dopamine D_2 receptors for monkeys after establishing social hierarchy. **B:** The graph shows that the dominant monkey always self-administered less cocaine at different strengths of the drug compared with the subordinate monkey. (Adapted with permission from Macmillan Publishers Ltd. Morgan D, Grant KA, Gage HD, et al. Social dominance in monkeys: dopamine D_2 receptors and cocaine self-administration. *Nat Neurosci*. 2002;5[2]:169–174. Copyright 2002.)

role of the amygdala and seeking pleasure can be shown when a rat is conditioned to associate a sound or light with pressing a lever and receiving cocaine. When the cocaine ceases to be delivered, the rat will almost completely stop pressing the lever—extinguishing the behavior. Later if the rat hears the conditioned sound or sees the light, it will resume pressing the lever as long as its amygdala is intact. A rat without an amygdala will fail to resume pressing the lever when stimulated with the tone or light. Clearly, the amygdala is essential to remembering the associations.

The Pursuit of Pleasure

People spend time doing what they enjoy. "Time sure flies when you're having fun" is the old saying. The propensity to get "lost" in an activity and lose track of time is a feature of rewarding activities—and something that can be a source of frustration for friends and family who do not enjoy the same activity.

The brain has several internal clocks. The suprachiasmatic nucleus and circadian rhythm are the most renowned internal clocks and will be covered in Chapter 15, Sleep. However, there are lesser-known circuits to manage milliseconds, which are essential for sports, dancing, music, and speech. Of relevance to this chapter, these circuits use DA and to some extent activate the VTA. Studies with rodents have found that D_2 agonists, such as methamphetamine, accelerate the internal clock, whereas D_2 blockers, such as haloperidol, slow down the clock. This may explain why people inaccurately estimate the duration of a pleasurable activity.

People who have the propensity to enjoy work have an adapted advantage over those who do not. We can imagine that nature selects for individuals who possess the traits to enjoy activities that are beneficial, for example, hunting and gathering as well as communicating and planning. Alternatively, some people lose themselves in activities that are not healthy and continue to pursue them in spite of negative outcomes. This behavior and the effects on the brain are the focus of the next section.

POINT OF INTEREST

Albert Einstein is reported to have described his theory of relativity as such: "Put your hand on a hot stove for a minute, and it seems like an hour. Sit with a pretty girl for an hour, and it seems like a minute." Einstein eloquently described how our perception of the passage of time is affected by our feelings of pain and pleasure.

REWARD = WANTING AND LIKING

There has been a change in the conceptualization of pleasure since the first edition of this book. Previously it was assumed that activation of the DA neurons at the NAc was a pleasurable experience. Now the thinking is that mesolimbic DA pathway is more about craving (or wanting) and it is the activation of opioid receptors in a few regions of the brain that facilitates the *real* pleasure (or liking). Several lines of evidence support this new assessment.

Dopamine Is Wanting

First of all, DA is activating, and energy is what animals need to pursue a goal. The best example is the medications that tweak the DA receptor—the stimulants: amphetamine, MPH, etc.—affectionately called Speed on the streets. Also, wanting is not enjoying. For example, almost everyone wants more money and will work hard to get it, but accumulating money per se does not feel good although it can be used to purchase items that do. Furthermore, rats deficient in DA (or depleted of DA neurons) will not eat even in the presence of palatable food. But if scrumptious rat morsels are put in their mouths, they display the usual signs of a pleasurable response—tongue thrusting and paw licks. In other words they enjoy the food, but they simply have no motivation to even make a call for takeout. Finally, patients with Parkinson's disease (PD), who have extensive destruction of DA neurons, still experience pleasure. And, on the other hand, some PD patients will develop addictive behaviors (such as gambling, shopping, drugs, etc.) when treated with DA agonists but typically do not report intense pleasure.

Opioids Bring the Joy

Pleasure is a calming experience—think of the relaxing, serene quality of an orgasm. The substances we associate with calming are γ-aminobutyric acid (GABA), the endocannabinoids, and the opioids. All appear to be involved with the euphoric sensation, but several lines of evidence point to opioids as the major currency of pleasure. Experimentally in humans, naloxone (the μ receptor blocker) will reduce subjective pleasure at orgasm. Likewise, naltrexone (a longer-acting μ blocker) will blunt the joy of alcohol and morphine but not affect the cravings. Cocaine addicts will report that when deep into their addiction, they no longer enjoy the cocaine although they cannot quit. It is presumed that the addicts are driven by the mesolimbic DA pathway but no longer receive a little squirt of endogenous opioids. Is this what happens when we experience "buyer's remorse"? We cannot resist the urge to make the purchase but then fail to experience any euphoria when the transaction is complete.

Hedonic hot spots in the brain also support an opioid mechanism for pleasure. Hot spot is the term used to describe areas in the brain that enhance liking—what might be called pleasure centers. Kent Berridge and his group at the University of Michigan are probably the leaders in identifying and understanding hot spots. To do this, they experimentally stimulate a rat brain in conjunction with a pleasurable taste and observe the reaction. For example, a rat given sucrose will respond with expressions believed to convey "liking" such as lip smacking (similar facial reactions are seen in orangutans and human babies). Microinjections of opioids in the medial shell of the NAc in combination with oral sucrose will induce amplified liking reactions in a rat, e.g., more tongue thrusts. Using this system of study, a small number of hedonic hot spots have been identified in the brain, including parts of the orbitofrontal cortex, amygdala, NAc, and ventral pallidum.

Not all hot spots are essential to experience pleasure. The orbitofrontal cortex and NAc can be removed without the loss of hedonic pleasure. For example, lobotomy patients or patients with large PFC lesions still retain the capacity to experience pleasure although they are cognitively impaired. Only the ventral pallidum appears to be essential for pleasure. Destruction of the ventral pallidum uniquely results in loss of hedonic pleasure—sort of where the buck stops.

With this new conceptualization of reward (that wanting and liking are different mechanisms), Berridge and Kringelbach reexamined the original experiments by Olds and Milner. They found studies showing electrical self-stimulation increases dopamine at the NAc, establishing a similar mechanism to cocaine administration as shown in Figure 12.4. Likewise, they demonstrated that self-stimulating rats would eat four times more than normal but fail to display amplified "liking" and actually showed signs of disgust. In a review of Robert Heath's studies with electrical stimulation in humans (Chapter 10, The Electrical Brain), they point out that the patients never showed signs of pleasure nor emitted blissful statements.

Deep brain stimulation (DBS) is the modern application of electrical stimulation and is approved for treatment of PD. Some experimental trials with DBS have placed the electrode at the NAc for conditions such as treatment-resistant depression and chronic pain. Some patients have developed addictive behaviors but do not report pleasurable feelings. In short, Berridge and Kringelbach propose that the electrical stimulation seen in rats and humans will increase reward-seeking behavior,

which may give the appearance of pleasure but without actually amplifying liking.

In reality, there is probably considerable overlap between wanting and liking. It is never as simple as one neurotransmitter correlating with one feeling. Most likely, stimulating the mesolimbic DA pathway does result in some semblance of pleasure.

Habituation

We have our strongest responses to positive, novel rewards. Unfortunately, as time goes on, we adapt to most pleasurable experiences. In the literature this is called habituation. Clark and his group in Germany asked about life satisfaction for 20 years (over 120,000 contacts) and looked at changes around important events, such as the birth of a child or divorce. Figure 12.8A shows the changes around marriage for women. We all think we'll live happily ever after, but in reality there is an attenuation of the joy. Clark concludes that "life is to some extent typified by a hedonic treadmill." Darn!

The neuroscientists have shown what this looks like in the brain. Rats equipped with cannulas at the NAc that measure DA levels were evaluated when

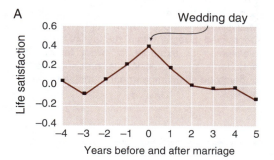

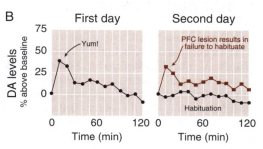

FIGURE 12.8 Habituation. **A:** Life satisfaction before and after marriage. **B:** Rats given chocolate will have a jump in the dopamine (DA) at the nucleus accumbens, which will habituate by the second day, unless they have lesions of the DA neurons in the prefrontal cortex (PFC). (**A:** Adapted from Clark AE, et al. [2008.] Lags and leads in life satisfaction: a test of the baseline hypothesis. *Econ J.* 118:F222–F243. **B:** From Bimpisidis Z, et al. [2013.] Lesion of medial prefrontal dopamine terminals abolishes habituation of accumbens shell dopamine responsiveness to taste stimuli. *Eur J Neurosci.* 37:613–622.)

they were given a dollop of chocolate. Figure 12.8B showed the jump in DA on the first day. The graphs for the second day make two points. First, by the second day, chocolate wasn't near as stimulating. Second, rats that had lesions of the DA neurons in the PFC failed to habituate. The authors called this "excessive motivation for inappropriate actions," which may be a fancy way of saying that people with frontal lobe damage have a difficult time with impulse control.

In other studies, Di Chiara has shown that habituation does *not* occur with cocaine. Not only is the increase stronger in magnitude (up to 400% over baseline compared with 150% for chocolate) but also does not attenuate like the natural reinforcers. Day after day, rats will have a spike in DA at the NAc when given cocaine, which explains why cocaine is so addictive.

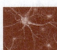

DISORDER

ANHEDONIA

It is tempting to conceptualize the anhedonia of depression as impairment in the capacity to savor pleasure—as though depression is in part a deficit in the reward mechanism. Closer analysis does not support this hypothesis. Depressed people retain the ability to enjoy pleasures, for example, a sweet taste. The anhedonia of depression is probably better understood as an impairment of motivation and energy.

ADDICTIONS CHANGE THE BRAIN

Most of the pleasurable activities that we are wired to pursue occur in nature in limited supply, making it hard to overindulge. Modern life, however, is full of many temptations that activate the mesolimbic pathway. Drugs of abuse, in particular, overwhelm and fundamentally alter the neurons that were never intended to experience such supraphysiologic levels of neurotransmitters. Addictions entail the persistent, destructive, and uncontrollable behaviors that involve obtaining the object of desire.

One simple definition of an addiction is the continued pursuit of a substance or activity in spite of negative consequences. This could apply to gambling, sex, alcohol, smoking, food, and even work. All these activities result in increased DA at the NAc. We will focus in this section on drugs of abuse and the changes they cause in the addicted brain. Figure 12.9 shows the location of several commonly abused drugs.

Some drugs have direct effects on the mesolimbic pathway, whereas others work indirectly. The stimulants and nicotine result in increased DA at the NAc. The opioids, alcohol, and phencyclidine (PCP) (and to some extent nicotine) suppress the inhibitory neurons that modulate the NAc and VTA. With less inhibition, more DA is released to the NAc.

Drug use occurs along a continuum—from casual use to dominating one's life. Addictions result from a combination of genes and environment and develop over time. But once addicted, the drugs alter the architecture of the brain. Tolerance and withdrawal are two clinical manifestations of the changes that occur to the addicted brain. Other clinical examples that show the effects of persistent abuse are as follows:

1. Depression and anhedonia when not using
2. Less responsive to natural rewards
3. The capacity to relapse even many years after abstinence

Global Impairments

One of the most consistently reproducible findings in the addictions field is the reduction in brain volume in chronic alcoholics. Studies have shown decreased total volume and gray matter, particularly in the frontal lobes. These findings co-occur with declines in cognition and memory. Alcoholics evaluated after a period of sobriety show some recovery of tissue volume, whereas those who continue to drink show further reductions.

Recent research has established cigarette smoking as a confounding variable in brain volume reductions and cognitive decline. One study compared intelligence as measured by IQ in 172 men (Figure 12.10). Alcoholism and smoking were independent risk factors for reductions in IQ. In follow-up studies, this same group found that alcoholism correlated with a broad range of impairment in executive function while smoking affected measures that emphasize response speed. It is not known if smoking has a direct neurotoxic effect on cognition or an indirect effect from cardiovascular or pulmonary damage. Interestingly, smokers report that a cigarette enhances their attention, and in studies, nicotine acutely improves cognitive performance. Yet the long-term effect on cognition is detrimental.

Dopamine Receptors

The stimulants work by blocking the DA reuptake pump as well as increasing the release of DA, which results in more DA available to stimulate the NAc. Using positron emission tomography (PET) scans, Volkow has shown decreased D_2 receptors in cocaine addicts during withdrawal (Figure 12.11),

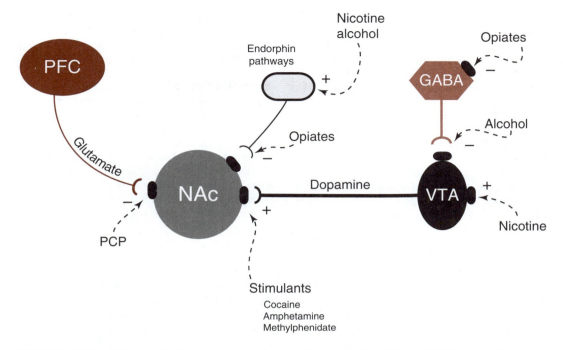

FIGURE 12.9 Possible sites of action by drugs of abuse on the mesolimbic pathway. GABA, γ-aminobutyric acid; NAc, nucleus accumbens; PCP, phencyclidine; PFC, prefrontal cortex; VTA, ventral tegmental area.

which persisted even when tested 3 to 4 months after detoxification. Similar findings have been demonstrated in subjects withdrawn from heroin, methamphetamine, and alcohol. These results suggest that excessive use of hedonic substances results in downregulation of the D_2 receptor (although we cannot be sure they were not this way before the addictions). This may explain the development of tolerance and need for the addict to take

"more." Likewise, this helps us understand why the abstinent user has difficulty experiencing pleasure with the natural joys of life.

Craving and the Frontal Cortex

The addict is someone who has moved from getting high to getting hooked. They are haunted by persistent, intrusive thoughts about their drug and intensely desire to obtain more. They have lost

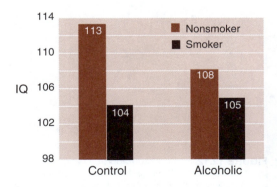

FIGURE 12.10 IQ is independently reduced in subjects with heavy alcohol or cigarette use. (Adapted from Glass JM, Adams KM, Nigg JT, et al. Smoking is associated with neurocognitive deficits in alcoholism. *Drug Alcohol Depend*. 2005;82[2]: 119–126. Copyright 2005 with permission from Elsevier.)

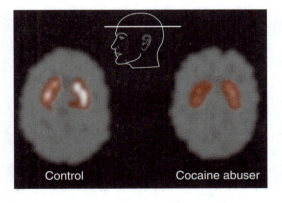

FIGURE 12.11 Horizontal positron emission tomography scans at the level of the striatum. The cocaine abuser has less D_2 receptor binding compared with the control. (Adapted with permission from Macmillan Publishers Ltd. Volkow ND, Li TK. Drug addiction: the neurobiology of behaviour gone awry. *Nat Rev Neurosci*. 2004;5[12]:963–970. Copyright 2004.)

control. In the literature and on the street, this is called *craving*.

As with obsessions, the PFC has been identified as the source of craving. Functional imaging studies have shown enhanced activity in the PFC, particularly the orbitofrontal cortex and dorsolateral PFC, when addicts are presented with drug-related cues. For example, when cocaine addicts are shown pictures of white powder, it will light up their frontal lobes and they report "drug craving." It is noteworthy that the activity in the PFC correlates with the intensity of self-reported craving.

We discussed in the first section of this chapter the important role the PFC plays in making choices (Figure 12.1). An essential feature of addictions is the inability to make good choices. This problem can be demonstrated in the relative activity of the PFC when addicts are shown various film clips.

In one important study, cocaine users were shown video clips of men smoking crack, sexually explicit scenes, and scenes of nature while in a functional brain scanner. Compared with the controls, the cocaine users showed increased activation in the frontal cortex while viewing videos of men smoking crack but not when shown sexually explicit content. The authors concluded that the drug abusers had developed a heightened response to stimuli associated with drug use but blunted response to other rewarding stimuli (Table 12.1).

The persistence of cravings and the susceptibility to lose control even after years of abstinence suggest long-term changes in the neurons of the PFC. Several findings with rats suggest that the glutamatergic projections from the PFC to the NAc (Figure 12.3) may be the culprit. The important findings are as follows:

1. Inactivation of the PFC prevents relapse.
2. Glutamate receptor blockade at the NAc prevents relapse.
3. Increased glutamate is released in the NAc during relapse.

These results not only point to the glutamatergic projections as a source of craving but also suggest a possible site to intervene for preventing relapse.

Synaptic Remodeling

The fact that drug-induced adaptations are so permanent suggests that the drugs fundamentally alter the organization of the neuronal circuits and synaptic connectivity. In a series of experiments, Robinson et al. at the University of Michigan have studied the effects of amphetamine, cocaine, and morphine on the structure of pyramidal cells in various parts of the brain. Figure 12.12 is a great picture of a pyramidal neuron from the parietal cortex.

The dendritic spines on the neuron are the postsynaptic receptors for input from other neurons. Presumably, changes in the number of spines reflect changes in the number of synapses on the neuron. In different experiments, Robinson et al. have shown that amphetamine and cocaine will increase the number of spines, whereas morphine results in a decrease. Figure 12.13 shows

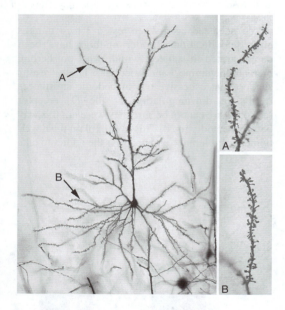

FIGURE 12.12 Photomicrograph of a Golgi-stained pyramidal cell from the parietal cortex. Multiple photographs at different focal planes were merged together to create this composite. The inserts on the right are from the apical **(A)** and basilar **(B)** regions. (From Kolb B, Gorny G, Li Y, et al. Amphetamine or cocaine limits the ability of later experience to promote structural plasticity in the neocortex and nucleus accumbens. *Proc Natl Acad Sci U S A.* 2003;100[18]:10523–10528. Copyright [2003] National Academy of Sciences, U.S.A.)

TABLE 12.1

Reaction by Cocaine Users to Different Stimuli

Drug-Related Cues	Natural Reinforcing Stimuli
Overrespond	Underrespond
Craving	Lack of interest
Increased activity in prefrontal cortex	Hypometabolism in prefrontal cortex

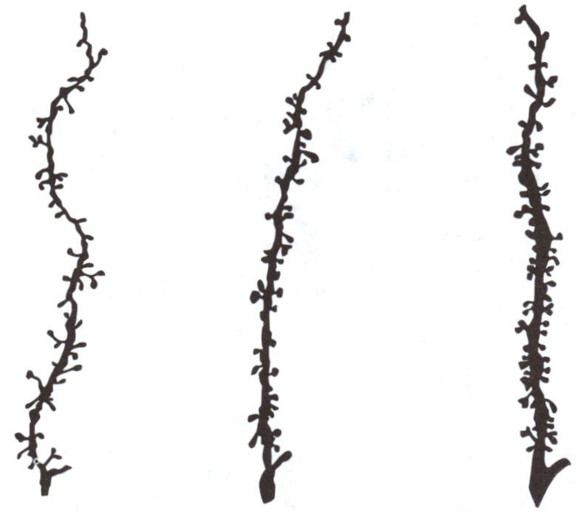

Morphine   Saline   Amphetamine

FIGURE 12.13 Changes in dendritic spines in the nucleus accumbens from rats exposed to morphine, saline, and amphetamine. Morphine decreases the number of spines, whereas amphetamine induces an increase. (Data from Robinson and Kolb, 1997, and Robinson et al., 2002.)

drawings of neurons from the NAc in rats exposed to morphine, saline, and amphetamine. One can see that these drugs (and presumably other substances of abuse) induce lasting changes to the brain by altering the morphology of the neural cells.

Molecular Changes

Nestler et al. at the University of Texas Southwestern Medical Center examined the molecular changes that underlie the long-term plasticity of addiction. As we discussed in Chapter 5, Receptors and Signaling the Nucleus, changes in the neuronal architecture are driven by gene expression. Nestler et al. identified two transcription factors in the NAc that contribute to gene expression and the resulting protein synthesis in the addicted state.

Cyclic adenosine monophosphate response element–binding protein (CREB) is a transcription factor that is activated by increased DA concentrations during drug binges. CREB in turn promotes the production of proteins that dampen the reward circuitry and induce tolerance. The dampening effects stimulated by CREB are believed to be one of the reasons drug users need to take more of their substance to get the same effect. CREB may also mediate the depression and anhedonia felt by the addicts when unable to get drugs.

However, CREB is only part of the story. It is switched off within days of stopping drug use, yet the addict remains vulnerable to relapse for a long time. δ-FosB is another transcription factor that may explain the lasting effects of drug abuse. Unlike CREB, δ-FosB accumulates in the cells of the NAc and is remarkably stable. It remains active in the cells for weeks and months after drugs have been stopped. This kind of enduring molecular change shows why addicts are susceptible to relapse even after years of abstinence.

Relapse

There are three well-known causes for relapsing:

1. Even a minimal use of the drug or a similar drug
2. Exposure to cues associated with drug use
3. Stress

All three causes result in increased release of DA at the NAc, which seems to impair the addict's will to abstain.

The effects of stress on the mesolimbic DA system are mediated in part through the hypothalamic–pituitary–adrenal (HPA) axis. It appears that corticotropin-releasing factor (CRF) and cortisol stimulate the release of DA. Studies with rats have shown that a stressor, such as a foot shock, stimulates the HPA axis as well as reinstates drug-seeking behavior. Different studies have shown that the reinstatement for heroin, cocaine, and alcohol can be blocked by the administration of a CRF antagonist.

Developmental Disorder?

It is readily apparent that our joys and pleasures change as we age. A latency-age boy is not the least bit interested in sex, but a few years later as an adolescent he is bubbling over with sexual excitement. The old saying, "the difference between men and boys is the price of their toys," describes the development of new sources of pleasure as men age. Changes in the brain most likely accompany the maturing of what we enjoy.

Adolescence is a time characterized by high levels of risk-taking and impulsivity. This can be seen as enhanced approach behavior and reduced harm-avoidance behavior—or too much accelerator and not enough brake. In simple terms, the role of the NAc is to enhance approach behavior, whereas the role of the amygdala is to warn animals to avoid negative situations. A study looking at the activity in these brain areas during reward and loss, with adolescents and adults, sheds some light on this topic.

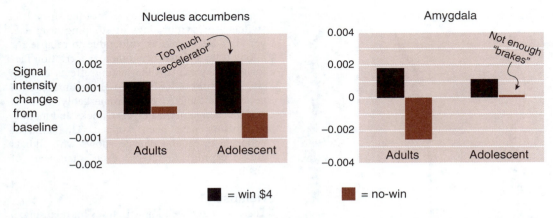

FIGURE 12.14 Activation in the nucleus accumbens and amygdala is different for adults and adolescents when they win or fail to win during a game with financial reward. (Adapted from Ernst M, Nelson EE, Jazbec S, et al. Amygdala and nucleus accumbens in responses to receipt and omission of gains in adults and adolescents. *NeuroImage.* 2005;25[4]:1279–1291. Copyright 2005 with permission from Elsevier. https://doi.org/10.1016/j.neuroimage.2004.12.038.)

Ernst et al. examined the activity of the NAc and amygdala in adolescents and adults while they were playing a game with a monetary reward. The subjects could win $4 if they made a correct choice. The authors looked at the relative activity of the NAc and amygdala when the subjects won compared with when they lost. Finally, they compared the regional activity for the adults and adolescents. The results (Figure 12.14) show that all subjects had enhanced activity when they won and less when they did not. However, the adolescents showed greater activity in the NAc when winning and less decrease in the amygdala when losing. Specifically, the results verify that the adolescent brain is different—more inclined to approach and less inclined for restraint.

The government restricts the use of legally available habit-forming substances and activities to adults, for example, nicotine, alcohol, and gambling. There are many reasons for this policy, but in part it is driven by the belief that early exposure to these hedonic pleasures increases the risk of addiction. With nicotine, there is some evidence that early exposure increases the likelihood of developing an addiction as an adult.

Epidemiologic studies of adolescents suggest that smoking at a younger age leads to increased addiction to cigarettes. A study with rats has shown that early exposure has lasting effects when compared with later exposure. Exposure to nicotine during the period that corresponds with preadolescence, but not as a postadolescent, increased the self-administration of nicotine as adults. Additionally, the adult rats exposed to nicotine at the younger age had greater expression of the nicotine receptor.

Adolescence is a time of great risk-taking and novelty seeking. Unfortunately, many addictions commence during this period. It appears that early use is genetically predetermined and socially triggered (hanging around with the wrong crowd). Either way, studies suggest that keeping our adolescents involved in wholesome activities—such as sports, art, camping, and so on—may keep them away from drugs and alcohol until their developing brains are more immune to the damaging effects of hedonic substances.

Treatment

Without a doubt, successful abstinence is most effective when the subject is motivated to stay clean, almost regardless of the treatment approach. An analysis of three psychological treatments for substance abuse demonstrated that all were equally effective. The most important factor was the subjects' desire to abstain.

Medications to treat addictions are helpful but not robustly effective. We are still unable to restore the addicted brain to its preexisting condition. Pharmacologic treatments generally fall into two categories. The first category is those interventions that interfere with the reinforcing action of the drugs of abuse, for example, naltrexone. The second category is those agents that mimic the action of the abused substance, for example, methadone. Neither of these treatments cures the underlying central nervous system alterations but can help in keeping a substance abuser clean.

Most problematic for the recovering addict is the intense craving that leads to relapse. Some addicts even report craving dreams during withdrawal. Efforts are under way to find medications that will decrease the thoughts and desires stimulated by memories of drug use. Much of the focus has been on agents that affect glu-tamate and GABA, but as yet no substantial interventions have been discovered. The challenge is to selectively eliminate the craving for drugs without affecting interest in the natural reinforcing stimuli.

Are Stimulant Medications Neurotoxic?

The diagnosis and treatment of attention deficit hyperactivity disorder (ADHD) has increased dramatically over the past decade—what we call *the other epidemic*. Psychostimulants such as MPH and amphetamine remain the most effective and widespread pharmacologic interventions for ADHD. These medications are potent inhibitors for the DA reuptake transporter and result in increased DA stimulation of postsynaptic neurons.

The psychostimulants are effective in improving attention and reducing impulsivity, but the long-term effects are not well studied. A meta-analysis of stimulant therapy and substance abuse shows that the medications did not promote substance abuse later and may even decrease the potential. However, we have seen in this review that other substances that increase DA at the NAc result in changes in the molecular and structural character of neurons. It is unknown if such changes occur with sustained use of the psychostimulants. This has become a particular concern because ADHD is likely overdiagnosed in the United States. Additionally, more patients are staying on more medication for more years than ever before.

Several studies with MPH in rodents have shown persistent neural effects after the treatment is terminated. A compelling study by Kolb et al. found that exposure to amphetamine has enduring impairments on the development of dendritic branching and spine formation 3 months after stopping the medication. A recent study with MPH in mice showed loss of DA neurons in the substantia nigra. This is of concern because a retrospective analysis out of Utah found tripling of the risk for PD in methamphetamine abusers.

Another concern is the effect the psychostimulants might have on the developing brain of children and adolescents. A group from Israel, again using rats, demonstrated alterations in nerve growth proteins such as brain-derived neurotrophic factors in the frontal cortex after chronic early MPH treatment. A group at Drexel University assessed the effect of 3 weeks of MPH administration on electrical activity on individual pyramidal neurons from the PFC. They found MPH-reduced electrical activity in the neurons was dose dependent and persisted for 10 weeks after stopping the medication (Figure 12.15). Finally, in a behavioral study, adult rats showed signs of reduced responsiveness to normal stimuli and increased reactions to aversive situations after early MPH treatment. All these studies raise concerns, but they are conducted on rodents, use high doses of the medications, and administer the medication by injection. It is difficult to estimate the clinical significance to humans.

A recent study out of the National Center for Toxicological Research is the sort of study we need to see more often. This group gave rhesus monkeys oral doses of MPH twice a day at doses equivalent to human plasma levels for 7 years. Then they conducted micro-PET scans when the animals were off the medication for 3 days. They found less metabolic activity in the cerebellum and PFC of the treated monkeys compared with that in the controls.

While we must be cautious when we extrapolate from animal studies to humans, we must also be vigilant about avoiding harmful treatments. The

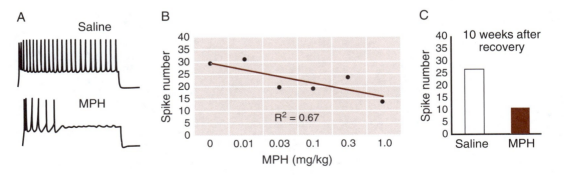

FIGURE 12.15 A: Suppression of layer 5 pyramidal neurons in juvenile rat prefrontal cortex on methylphenidate (MPH). **B:** Decreased neuron excitability with increasing doses of MPH. **C:** Neuronal excitability remains depressed 10 weeks after stopping MPH treatment. (Adapted from Urban KR et al. Distinct age-dependent effects of methylphenidate on developing and adult prefrontal neurons. *Biol Psychiatry*. 2012;72:880–888. Copyright 2012 with permission from Elsevier. https://doi.org/10.1016/j.biopsych.2012.04.018.)

history of medicine is replete with interventions that initially seemed safe, only to show problems later. Our understanding of DA receptor antagonism shows that supraphysiologic doses, as one gets with cocaine, can result in detrimental changes to the neurons. The long-term effects of smaller, controlled doses with stimulant medications, especially after years of prolonged exposure, remain unknown. (More on this topic in Chapter 20, Attention.)

CONCLUSION

The good news—we are designed to experience pleasure. The bad news—pleasure is supposed to wane. We are only meant to feel satisfied for a short period. We are wired to "lead lives of quiet desperation." People satisfied with their accomplishments fall behind. Some of the patients we see, particularly the chronic schizophrenic and seriously depressed, are cursed with a lack of motivation and joy. They are unable to work toward a goal that will be rewarding and bring them pleasure.

Likewise we frequently deal with patients who create havoc in their lives through their excessive pursuit of pleasurable substances and activities. An understanding of the neuroscience of pleasure helps us conceptualize that these patients fail to find joy in alternative, natural reinforcers. Our task is to assist them in developing healthy activities that will stimulate the mesolimbic cortical pathway but not alter the chemical or cellular substrate.

QUESTIONS

1. Cocaine induces craving by
   a. Inhibiting GABA.
   b. Stimulating GABA.
   c. Inhibiting DA reuptake.
   d. Stimulating DA reuptake.

2. Heroin induces craving by
   a. Inhibiting GABA.
   b. Stimulating GABA.
   c. Inhibiting DA reuptake.
   d. Stimulating DA reuptake.

3. Microdialysis allows
   a. Pharmacologic stimulation at precise locations.
   b. The development of conditioned behaviors.
   c. Biopsy of cellular tissue.
   d. Continuous sampling of extracellular fluid.

4. Pleasurable feelings include all of the following except
   a. Increased DA at the NAc.
   b. DA receptor antagonism.
   c. Increased activity of the VTA.
   d. μ receptor stimulation.

5. All of the following are involved with the development of tolerance except
   a. Activation of the PFC.
   b. Habituation.
   c. Downregulation of DA receptors.
   d. Accumulation of inhibitor transcription factors.

6. All of the following are involved with craving except
   a. Hypometabolism of the PFC to natural stimuli.
   b. Hypermetabolism of the PFC with drug cues.
   c. Enhanced GABA activation.
   d. Glutamatergic activation of the NAc.

7. The alpha monkey has
   a. Increased glutamatergic activation of the NAc.
   b. Increased frontal lobe metabolism.
   c. Greater propensity to self-administer stimulants.
   d. Increased DA receptors.

8. Enhanced transmission of all of the following can result in relapse except
   a. γ-Aminobutyric acid.
   b. Glutamate.
   c. Dopamine.
   d. Corticotropin-releasing hormone.

9. All of the following result in increased spine formation in rats except
   a. D-Amphetamine.
   b. Heroin.
   c. Methylphenidate.
   d. Cocaine.

See Answers section at the end of this book.

CHAPTER 13

Appetite

SET POINT

In spite of great fluctuation in the quantity and frequency of eating, our brain is remarkably adept at balancing energy expenditure and energy intake. Social factors, emotions, and time of day, as well as taste, satiety, and personal habits, influence our eating patterns, yet we maintain a reasonably stable body weight month after month. This is referred to as *energy homeostasis* or simply a metabolic "set point." It is as though the brain has a "thermostat" for body size.

Evidence of a set point comes from a variety of sources. If a rat is deprived of food, then, when offered a normal diet, it will overeat for a short period and return its body weight to its preexisting level. Likewise, after being force-fed to increase body weight, it will limit its food intake to return to normal weight (Figure 13.1). The brain and body work in harmony to keep the body weight at a specific point.

The human corollary to this is the disturbingly low success rates that people have with most diets. In a review of long-term efficacy of dietary treatment interventions for obesity, Ayyad and Anderson found that only 15% of the patients fulfilled at least one of the criteria for success 5 years after the study. Unfortunately, most people who diet will slowly return to their preexisting weight within 1 year.

Several lines of research suggest that the set point is genetically controlled. Adoption studies provide a unique way to separate the effects of genetics from environment on body weight by comparing children with their biologic parents and with the parents from the house in which they were raised. In an analysis of Danish adoptees, Stunkard et al. found a strong relation between the weight class of the adoptees and the body mass of the biologic parents, and no correlation between the weight class of the adoptees and their adopted parents, suggesting that genetic makeup, not environment, is a major determining factor in one's body weight.

Yet obesity was a rare condition 50 years ago. Clearly, our genes have not evolved in half a century. There must be other explanations for the significant change in body weight that is occurring in first-world nations. The Pima Indians of Mexico and Arizona provide some insight on this issue.

The Pima Indians separated into two tribes approximately 700 to 1000 years ago—one tribe remained in Mexico and the other settled in what is now Arizona. In spite of their similar genetic makeup, they have significantly different average body weights. The Arizona Indians have a high prevalence of obesity and non–insulin-dependent diabetes mellitus, whereas their Mexican relatives are not overweight and have less diabetes. The difference can be best explained by understanding the divergent lifestyles these two populations developed.

The Mexican Pima Indians have remained in the mountains, continuing a traditional rural lifestyle. They expend considerable physical energy working in the farms and eating a diet high in starch and fiber. The Arizona Indians on the other hand were forced to move on to reservations where they now lead more leisurely lives and eat a diet high in fat and sugar.

The Pima Indians' obesity problem has been attributed to a "thrifty gene"—a gene that promotes saving and storing calories. Two thousand years ago, such a genetic predisposition would enhance survival for those struggling with the fluctuations of prosperity and famine. However, with

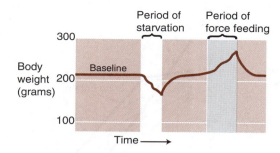

FIGURE 13.1 A rat will return its body weight to its preintervention weight when allowed to eat a regular diet. (Adapted from Keesey RE, Boyle PC. Effects of quinine adulteration upon body weight of LH-lesioned and intact male rats. *J Comp Physiol Psychol*. 1973;84[1]:38–46.)

plentiful high-caloric, highly palatable food, the "thrifty gene" promotes accumulation and storage beyond what is healthy. Therefore the weight problem is genetic but influenced by what is available in the environment.

One of the mechanisms the brain uses to return body weight to its baseline set point became apparent in the Minnesota Starvation Experiment. This was an experiment conducted with conscientious objectors in Minnesota toward the end of the Second World War to prepare the military for the starving civilians in Europe.

Participants were subjected to a semistarvation diet for 6 months with the goal of losing approximately 25% of their weight. From our perspective, one of the more interesting symptoms these men quickly experienced was an obsession with food. Not unlike the cravings discussed in the previous chapter, food became the principal topic of their thoughts, conversation, and daydreams. Reading cookbooks and collecting recipes suddenly were of great interest. Eating, either mentioned in a book or displayed in a movie, was the cue that put the men at heightened risk for breaking their diet. The urge to eat was so powerful that the researchers established a buddy system so that participants would not be tempted to cheat when away from the dorm. Clearly, their brains were focusing on what the body needed.

In addition to increasing hunger, the brain has another way to maintain a stable body weight. First, let's agree that energy-in (e.g., food) equals energy-out (e.g., heat, work, etc.), otherwise we would gain or lose weight. Not rocket science. Energy-out, or what is called total energy expenditure, is made up of resting metabolic rate (RMR) (calories burned at rest—sometimes called the

basal metabolic rate) and physical activity. The body and brain conspire to adjust the RMR in relation to caloric intake. That is, if we eat more, the RMR is turned up, and if we diet, the RMR is turned down.

OK, so when we diet, the total energy expenditure decreases—that is, the body burns less calories, which in part is due to the reduced metabolic requirements of the smaller fat cells. Unfortunately, the brain further turns down the energy expenditure. The difference between the expected RMR and what is actually found is called the metabolic adaptation. For example, in the Minnesota Starvation Experiment, metabolic adaptation accounted for about 35% more reduction in energy expenditure than that expected from fat cell loss.

Nowhere is this shown more clearly than with a follow-up study of contestants from the eighth season of The Biggest Loser. (It's come to this—we're citing reality TV!) Kevin Hall and his colleagues at the NIH assessed 14 of the 16 participants at baseline, at the completion of the competition (30 weeks), and 6 years later. Of the 14 contestants, 13 regained weight in the follow-up, and 4 were heavier than they were before the show. And here's the real jip—almost all of the contestants are burning less energy at rest (RMR) 6 years after the completion of the show (Figure 13.2). And worse, they still struggled with frequent hunger. Therefore in spite of eating less and exercising more—and having a healthier body—their brains have turned *down* their resting metabolism and turned *up* their food cravings. It's not fair!

One last point before we discuss the brain mechanisms that maintain the "set point." Energy expenditure changes over the life span—another great frustration for many of us. Figure 13.3 shows a cross-sectional analysis of total energy expenditure, RMR, and weight. As you can see, the problems start in the 30s. The question for us is: How does the brain manage all this?

HOMEOSTATIC MECHANISMS

The key point is that despite large day-to-day fluctuations in food intake and energy expenditure, our weight remains within a relatively narrow range. This is accomplished through feedback loops between the brain and the body. Brain lesion and stimulation studies in the 1940s identified the hypothalamus as a major center controlling food intake. Although the initial studies

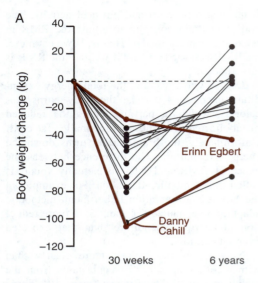

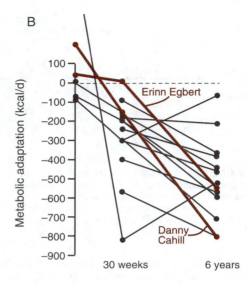

FIGURE 13.2 A: Danny Cahill dropped 239 pounds and won the eighth season of the "Biggest Loser," but Erinn Egbert was the only contestant who weighed less 6 years later. **B:** Cahill regained 100 pounds in 6 years but had a slower metabolism and remained hungry. (Adapted from Fothergill E, et al. [2016.] Persistent metabolic adaptation 6 years after "The Biggest Loser" competition. *Obesity.* 24:1612–1619.)

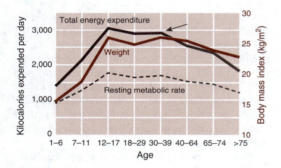

FIGURE 13.3 A cross section of average energy expenditure and weight from 2 to 95 years. (Adapted from Manini TM. Energy expenditure and aging. *Aging Res Rev.* 2010;9[1]:1–11. Copyright 2010 with permission from Elsevier. https://doi.org/10.1016/j.arr.2009.08.002.)

turned out to be overly simplified, the hypothalamus remains an important command center for weight maintenance.

But what are the signals the brain receives and sends? It would be ideal to understand these signals, as they may provide opportunities for interventions to stem the obesity epidemic. In a nutshell, they are hormones and the autonomic nervous system (ANS). The best way to understand the current conceptualization of the central nervous system's (CNS's) homeostatic mechanisms is to separate the short-term signals from the long-term ones.

Short-Term Signals

The short-term signals tend to affect meal size rather than overall energy storage. The signals comprise nutrients and gut hormones in the circulation as well as afferent signals sent up the vagus nerve. These signals to the brain result in the sensation of satiety but do not produce sustained alteration in body adiposity.

Nutrients

Glucose is the primary nutrient that mediates satiety. Hypoglycemia increases hunger sensations and stimulates eating. Glucose infusions will decrease food intake. Other nutrients in the systemic circulation, such as fats and amino acids, play a real but limited role in signaling to the brain the effects of a recent meal. High levels of these nutrients tell the brain to stop eating, but the brakes are insufficient when the individual has been starving.

Mechanoreceptors

The physical presence of food in the stomach and upper small intestine activates mechanoreceptors. The stomach wall is innervated with stretch receptors that increase in activity in proportion to the volume in the stomach. We usually think of the vagus as a conduit from the brain to the gut, but as much as 80% of the neural traffic is flowing in the opposite direction (see Figure 2.10). The vagus nerve transmits signals about gastric distension to the hindbrain.

Gut Hormones

Numerous gut hormones are involved in food intake regulation. The most widely studied hormone is *cholecystokinin* (CCK). CCK is released from endocrine cells in the mucosal layer of the small intestine in response to fats and proteins. CCK inhibits further food intake through several mechanisms, such as stimulating the vagus nerve and inhibiting gastric emptying. Additionally, there are CCK receptors in the brain. The injection of CCK directly into the ventricles will inhibit eating. CCK appears to have central and peripheral mechanisms to put the brake on a meal.

Although CCK will limit food intake, its long-term administration does not induce significant weight loss. In studies with rats, the repeated administration of CCK resulted in smaller but more frequent meals. Thus, the overall energy balance was not altered. Figure 13.4 summarizes the short-term signals regulating food intake.

There are many other gut hormones that also inhibit eating, e.g., glucagonlike peptide-1 (GLP-1) and peptide tyrosine–tyrosine. *Ghrelin* is of most interest as it is the only gut hormone that stimulates

hunger. Produced in the stomach, fasting increases the levels of ghrelin, which then fall after a meal. Peripheral and central administration of ghrelin increases food intake. In contrast to CCK, there is some evidence that ghrelin has long-term effects on weight and may be a potential culprit in obesity. Some studies suggest that reduced ghrelin production is one of the reasons gastric bypass surgery is so effective.

The Joy of Eating

Eating is more than just sustenance; it is one of the great pleasures of life. The perception of pleasure that we get from some foods is most likely an adaptation that enhanced the survival of our ancestors during lean times. However, with the abundance of inexpensive highly palatable refined foods, genes that favored sweet foods cause us to overeat.

Certain foods increase dopamine at the nucleus accumbens (see Figure 12.6). Additionally, the endogenous opioids appear to be more active during a good meal. Other evidence suggests that eating is a highly valued pleasure, which can resemble an addiction. For example, obese individuals have reduced D_2 receptors in the striatum and display activation of the orbitofrontal cortex when craving for food. Clearly, dopamine and the endogenous opioids are signals that influence energy consumption.

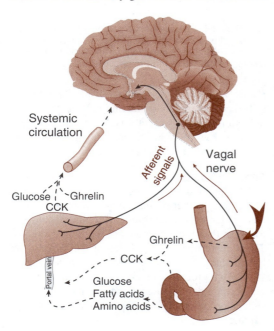

Systemic circulation

Afferent signals

Vagal nerve

Glucose Ghrelin
CCK

Portal vein

Ghrelin

CCK

Glucose
Fatty acids
Amino acids

FIGURE 13.4 Short-term signals from the intestines (hormones in the circulation and stimulation of the vagus nerve) signal to the brain that the body is full. (For now, ignore the *arrow* pointing to the vagus nerve at the stomach.) CCK, cholecystokinin. (Adapted from Havel PJ. Peripheral signals conveying metabolic information to the brain: short-term and long-term regulation of food intake and energy homeostasis. *Exp Biol Med.* 2001;226[11]:963–977.)

DISORDERS

YOUR GRANDFATHER'S DIET

A remarkable study from an isolated community in Sweden has shown that a man's risk of death from cardiovascular disease and diabetes is affected by his grandfather's diet during his grandfather's slow growth period—ages of 9 to 12 years for boys. Using records of harvest success or failure during the 19th century, researchers found increased risk of heart disease and diabetes if the grandfather lived through bountiful harvests during his slow growth period. Alternatively, grandfathers who grew up during times of famine sired grandchildren who lived longer. The mechanism, derived in part from rodent studies, is believed to be transgenerational epigenetic inheritance.

Long-Term Signals

Long-term signals tell the brain about overall energy storage, not just the caloric content of the recent meal. In the 1950s, it was suggested that adipose tissue releases a hormone that signals the hypothalamus about the current state of energy storage. Termed an *adiposity signal*, the elusive hormone must have three traits:

- Circulate in the blood in proportion to the amount of stored fat.
- Cross the blood–brain barrier and stimulate specific receptors in the brain.
- Produce changes in caloric intake and energy expenditure when levels of the hormone fluctuate.

Leptin

It was not until the discovery of *leptin* in 1994 that the first adiposity signal was identified. The mutant ob/ob mice (ob = obese) have an alternation in one gene, which results in hyperphagia and weight gain of three to five times the normal. Identifying the locus of the genetic defect allowed the cloning of the protein that the ob/ob mice were missing: leptin.

Leptin is primarily produced in white fat cells and circulates in direct proportion to the total fat load. The largest concentration of leptin receptors is found in the arcuate nucleus of the hypothalamus. Mice lacking leptin are obese. When given exogenous leptin, they decrease food intake and lose weight (Figure 13.5). Leptin appears to be a hormone that tells the brain, "I'm full." In The Biggest Loser study, leptin averaged 41 ng/mL at the start of the competition, 2.5 ng/mL after 30 weeks of rigorous dieting/exercise and remained low 6 years later at 28 ng/mL. In other words the leptin was still telling the brain, "I'm not full yet!"

Other hormones have been proposed as adiposity signals, the most prominent of which is *insulin*. The role of insulin is complicated because its primary function is to enhance glucose intake into

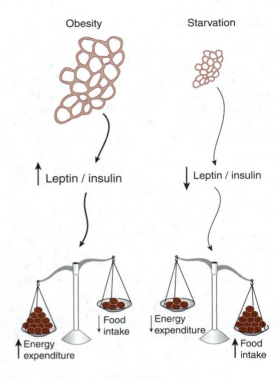

FIGURE 13.6 Adipose tissue secretes hormones in proportion to the total fat stored. The hormones in turn affect energy expenditure and food intake in relation to their levels in the circulation.

muscle and adipose tissues. Yet insulin secretion is influenced by total body fat and in turn can elicit a reduction in body weight. Insulin appears to work in parallel with leptin. Figure 13.6 shows a schematic representation of these adiposity signals.

Arcuate Nucleus

The hypothalamus is at the heart of the regulation of the body's energy metabolism. It is no wonder that the largest concentration of leptin receptors is found in the arcuate nucleus of the hypothalamus. The arcuate nucleus is located at the base of the hypothalamus next to the third ventricle (Figure 13.7). Two groups of neurons have been identified within the arcuate nucleus that mediate the leptin signal: proopiomelanocortin (POMC) and neuropeptide Y (NPY).

Proopiomelanocortin

The POMC neurons put the brakes on eating. The POMC neuropeptide is cleaved to produce α-melanocyte–stimulating hormone (α-MSH), which is a potent suppressor of food intake. The effects of α-MSH are mediated through the melanocortin (MC) receptors, particularly MC3R and MC4R, which are strongly expressed in the hypothalamus.

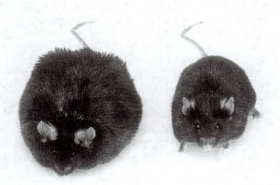

FIGURE 13.5 Two ob/ob mice, both of which are missing the gene to produce leptin. The mouse on the right has received daily leptin injections for 4.5 weeks and weighs about half as much as the mouse on the left. (From Amgen Inc., Thousand Oaks, California. Photo by John Sholtis.)

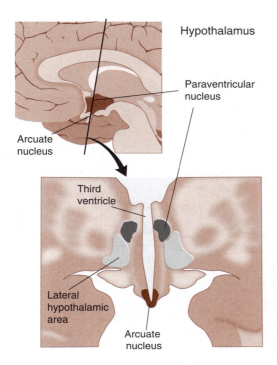

Hypothalamus

Paraventricular nucleus

Arcuate nucleus

Third ventricle

Lateral hypothalamic area

Arcuate nucleus

FIGURE 13.7 Two sections of the brain showing the location of the arcuate nucleus within the hypothalamus along with two other important nuclei for the control of energy balance.

High levels of leptin as well as other circulating hormones will stimulate the POMC neurons. Conversely, low levels of leptin inhibit the POMC neurons. Thus, POMC neurons and α-MSH are directly responsive to circulating hormones that signal an excess of adipose tissue.

Neuropeptide Y

The NPY neurons work to increase food intake and decrease energy expenditure. The NPY neurons express a peptide called *agouti-related peptide* (AGRP), which is an antagonist at the MC4 receptor. Consequently, activation of the NPY neurons blocks the effects of α-MSH and the POMC neurons. The role of NPY neurons and AGRP in the accumulation of calories has been demonstrated in many experimental conditions:

1. Stimulation of the NPY neurons increases food intake.
2. Increased expression of AGRP results in increased food intake (see Figure 6.10).
3. During starvation, there is increased activation of the NPY neurons and increased expression of AGRP.
4. Leptin inhibits the NPY neurons and AGRP expression.

Thus, there is an accelerator and brake relationship between the NPY neurons and the POMC neurons that respond to signals from the body about the long-term status of energy storage (Figure 13.8). Of particular relevance to the current epidemic of obesity is the unequal relationship between each set of neurons. Although they provide equal stimulation of the downstream effort neurons, only the NPY neurons directly inhibit the POMC neurons. The POMC neurons do not inhibit the NPY neurons. Consequently, there appears to be a slightly greater emphasis on the accumulation of calories. In other words, the accelerator is stronger than the brake, which, from an evolutionary perspective, would seem to enhance survival in times of low food supply or famine.

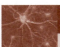

DISORDER

STRESS

Many patients will report that food is a source of comfort when they are "stressed out." Several lines of evidence suggest there may be a correlation between the hypothalamic–pituitary–adrenal axis and the ability to resist the pleasures of food:

1. Childhood stress is associated with increased weight problems in adolescence and adulthood.
2. Corticotropin-releasing hormone and cortisol stimulate the release of dopamine at the nucleus accumbens, which makes it harder to resist temptations.
3. Glucocorticoids increase fat deposits.
4. Stressed rats given access to sweet water have lower glucocorticoid levels.

Downstream Targets

The downstream effects of the arcuate neurons are numerous and largely remain mysterious. Two important sites are the paraventricular nucleus (PVN) and the lateral hypothalamic (LH) area, also shown in Figure 13.7. The POMC and NPY neurons project in parallel to these sites with corresponding activation and deactivation, depending on the short-term and long-term signals from the periphery.

The effects of the hunger and satiety signals are carried out by three systems: the cerebral cortex (behavior), the endocrine system, and the ANS. The PVN affects the output of the endocrine system and the ANS—both of which affect energy expenditure. The LH communicates with the cerebral cortex, which in turn modulates food-seeking

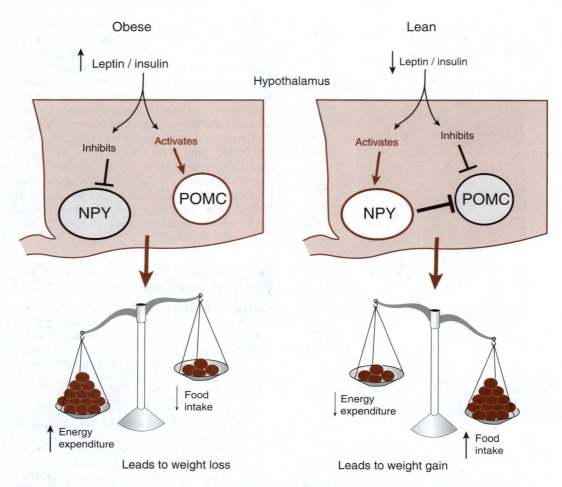

FIGURE 13.8 The presence or absence of adiposity signals, such as leptin and insulin, has opposite effects on the NPY and POMC neurons. In turn, the activation of the NPY and POMC neurons has different effects on energy balance and body weight. NPY, neuropeptide Y; POMC, proopiomelanocortin.

behavior. This simplified analysis of the downstream effects of signals from the body is shown in Figure 13.9.

POINT OF INTEREST

Smoking has one legitimate virtue: appetite suppression. Smokers are generally thinner and typically gain about 10 pounds when they cease smoking. Nicotine binds with a subunit of the nicotine acetylcholine receptors on the POMC neurons. This activates the POMC neurons, which leads to reduced food intake and weight loss. This receptor subunit may be accessible to pharmacologic manipulation turning on the one benefit of smoking without the toxic effects.

Endocannabinoids

It has been known for a long time that marijuana stimulates appetite. The naughty boys at our colleges called it *the munchies*. Stimulation of the cannabinoid receptor by the main active component of marijuana, Δ^9-THC (tetrahydrocannabinol), is believed to induce this behavior. Clinicians have successfully used this effect when treating anorexic conditions such as AIDS-related wasting syndrome. With animals it has been found that the endocannabinoid system is activated with short-term fasting or the presentation of palatable food, thereby enhancing appetite.

The cannabinoid (CB_1) receptor is involved with regulation of food intake at several levels. First, it increases the motivation to seek and consume palatable food possibly by interactions with the mesolimbic pathways. Studies with rodents

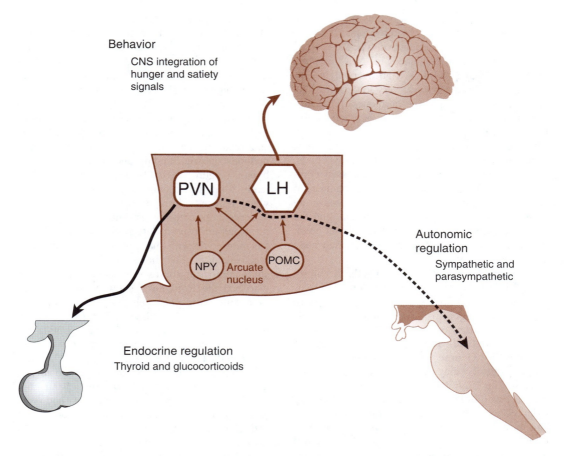

FIGURE 13.9 The PVN and lateral hypothalamus (along with others) influence the three major effort pathways so that the body can maintain a stable energy balance. CNS, central nervous system; LH, lateral hypothalamic; NPY, neuropeptide Y; POMC, proopiomelanocortin; PVN, paraventricular nucleus.

show that endocannabinoids enhance the release of dopamine at the nucleus accumbens and may synergize the effects of the opioids.

The endocannabinoid system also stimulates food consumption in the hypothalamus. Studies have shown that endocannabinoid levels are the highest in the hypothalamus with fasting and lowest when eating. Additionally, the endocannabinoids appear to work in concert with the neurohormones such as leptin and ghrelin to control appetite. The ultimate effect may be through the CB$_1$ receptors at the PVN and lateral hypothalamus. One of the most exciting but disappointing developments in the treatment of obesity was the CB$_1$ receptor blocker rimonabant (the antimunchie pill). Rimonabant induced about 10 pounds of weight loss but also led to the emergence of anxiety, depression, and suicidal thinking. The FDA rejected the medication, and it was withdrawn in Europe.

EATING DISORDERS

Obesity

It is estimated that a third of the adults in the United States are obese. Most disturbing is the rapid rise in childhood obesity. Clearly, diet and exercise are first-line interventions for this condition, but these efforts are a constant uphill battle against a genetic set point that favors rich, sweet food that historically was in short supply.

After the discovery of leptin, there was great excitement about the prospect of a treatment for obesity. Leptin was shown to reduce obesity in genetically leptin-deficient humans and rodents (Figure 13.5). Unfortunately, the magnitude of weight loss in most obese humans who received exogenous leptin in studies has been modest. In actuality, most obese people have high levels of circulating leptin but for some reason fail to respond to the signal. This has generated speculation that obesity may be associated with, or even caused by, a resistance to leptin, as is seen with insulin resistance in type 2 diabetes.

A recent study published in *New England Journal of Medicine* followed 50 overweight subjects enrolled in a 10-week, very-low-calorie diet and followed the appetite hormones. The subjects lost weight and kept much of it off at follow-up a year later. However, leptin, peptide YY, CCK, and insulin remained below baseline levels. Furthermore, ghrelin, gastric inhibitory polypeptide, and pancreatic polypeptide were increased compared with baseline…, and the subjects continued to be hungry. In other words the brain receives an array of signals, some that push and some that pull the brain and body to return to the metabolic set point. And worse, the signals do not readjust to a new body size, even after a year.

Why can't we find a pill that tells the brain, "I'm full"? It is not for lack of trying. The fen-phen debacle (fenfluramine/phentermine)—with its modest weight loss and potential for pulmonary hypertension or valvular disease—has spooked the field. Table 13.1 is a partial list compiled by George Bray of medications used to treat obesity that developed significant side effects. The FDA has approved a few medications for weight loss, but their benefits only range from 3% to 9% reduction in average weight loss, and they do not directly block the appetite hormones. Attempts to fool the brain by manipulating these appetite hormones (such as leptin, ghrelin, CCK, etc.) to facilitate weight loss have not been successful.

TABLE 13.1

Drug Treatments for Obesity with Serious Adverse Effects

Year	Drug	Toxic Effect
1892	Thyroid	Hyperthyroid
1932	Dinitrophenol	Cataracts/neuropathy
1937	Amphetamine	Addiction/psychosis
1968	Rainbow pills	Death—arrhythmias
1971	Aminorex	Pulmonary HTN
1997	Fen/Phen	Valvulopathy
1998	Phenylpropanolamine	Stroke/death
2009	Rimonabant	Depression/suicidality
2011	Sibutramine	Cardiovascular risk

Gastric Bypass Surgery

One success during the past decade has been gastric bypass surgery. Also called bariatric surgery, it is clearly the most effective treatment for morbid obesity. Many patients not only lose substantial weight but also can be cured of secondary problems such as diabetes and sleep apnea. Unfortunately, many patients also experience indigestion, abdominal pain, dumping syndrome, and food intolerance as a result of the surgery. There are two primary methods: gastric banding and Roux-en-Y gastric bypass (Figure 13.10). Both procedures mechanically limit the amount of food in the stomach, which reduces caloric intake.

Recent research suggests that one of the reasons the Roux-en-Y procedure may be more effective has more to do with changes in gut hormones than mechanical effects. In a small nonrandomized study comparing the two procedures, the patients who had the Roux-en-Y showed greater weight loss along with greater changes in gut hormones (Figure 13.10). Not shown in the figure are the other hormones such as GLP-1 and peptide YY, which also showed significant differences at 1 year between the two procedures.

A separate study by a different group investigated brain activation before and after a Roux-en-Y bypass. Subjects were cued with auditory and visual representations of food while a functional magnetic resonance imaging (MRI) followed their brain response. As expected, the food cues activated the reward pathways discussed in the previous chapter. Remarkably, after the surgery, the reward pathway activation was significantly reduced in response to food cues. In other words, the subjects had less food cravings after the bypass surgery.

Taken together, these studies suggest that Roux-en-Y procedure dampens numerous hormones and neurotransmitters that mediate the neural response to food. Maybe one reason why it is so hard to find a pill that reduces appetite is because one molecule cannot replicate the panoply of hormones released by the gastrointestinal tract that regulate the body's energy balance.

One last point about bariatric surgery: Mental health problems are common in the morbidly obese, and because of this, most centers include mental health evaluations as part of the workup before surgery. One would think that mental health would improve after successful surgery and weight loss, but a recent study in Canada suggests otherwise. They followed over 8,000 patients and looked at emergency department visits for suicide attempts 3 years before and after surgery. Remarkably, they found a 50% increase in suicide attempts (from 2.3 per 1,000

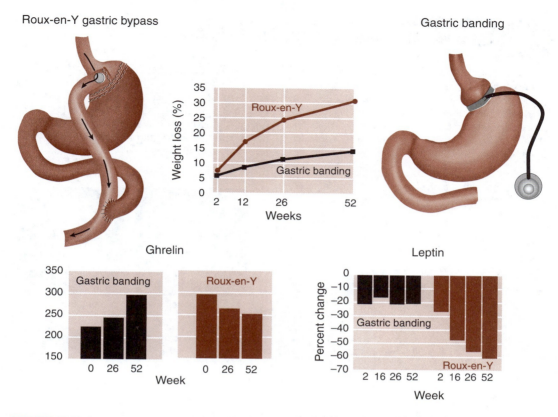

FIGURE 13.10 The superiority of Roux-en-Y gastric bypass surgery to produce substantial weight loss that may be due to changes in hormones that regulate appetite. (Adapted with permission from Macmillan Publishers Ltd. Korner J, Inabnet W, Febres G, et al. Prospective study of gut hormone and metabolic changes after adjustable gastric banding and Roux-en-Y grastric bypass. *Int J Obesity*. 2009;33:786–795. Copyright 2009.)

patient years to 3.6) after the procedure. The authors speculate that changes in appetite hormones may affect mental health as well as body size—feeling empty while feeling full, if you will.

Vagus Nerve Stimulation

The vagus nerve transmits information to the brain about hunger and satiety. Vagus nerve stimulation (VNS), the little pacemaker for the vagus nerve, is now FDA approved as a way to treat morbid obesity. Attached laparoscopically to the vagus fibers as they exit the stomach (about where the big arrow is pointing at the stomach in Figure 13.4), VNS sends intermittent impulses to the brain that appear to mimic some of the messages sent by a satiated stomach. Recent studies have demonstrated significant weight loss, which did not return as long as the stimulator was pulsing. Even better, the complications from VNS appear significantly less than in gastric bypass

surgery. Controlled studies to compare the two procedures are needed.

Purging

It is tempting to speculate that patients with anorexia and bulimia have set points that favor lean body mass, in other words, some pathology in their hypothalamus. However, most of the studies point to the involvement of other areas of the brain. Specifically, the symptoms of anxiety, perfectionism, and obsessions about body image are more consistent with disorders in the prefrontal cortex and amygdala. Likewise, eating disorder patients who have lost significant weight experience food cravings similar to what the men in the Minnesota Starvation Experiment experienced. Finally, the neuropeptide and neuroendocrine alterations present when patients are restricting return to normal levels when the patients recover. Eating disorder patients struggle with a drive to be thin, but this is not likely to be caused by pathologic appetite signals.

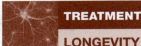

TREATMENT

LONGEVITY

Caloric restriction (CR) is the most reproducible intervention to extend life. Rhesus monkeys whose caloric intake is restricted by 30% live longer. The figures (A) show the survival curves for age-related mortality and overall mortality for the monkeys with CR compared with controls. The CR monkeys have less diabetes, cancer, and cardiovascular disease. Furthermore, MRIs show that CR monkeys have more brain volume and less CNS fluid (B). CR appears to prevent cell loss and brain atrophy associated with aging. Although beneficial, it is unlikely humans can muster the self-control to use CR to prevent age-related CNS decline.

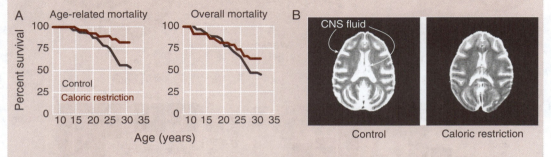

(Adapted from Colman RJ, et al. Caloric restriction delays disease onset and mortality in rhesus monkeys. *Science*. 2009;325:201–204. Reprinted with permission from AAAS.)

PSYCHIATRIC MEDICATIONS

Weight gain is one of the most difficult side effects associated with psychiatric treatment and often a reason that patients stop effective treatments. Surprisingly little is known about the mechanism of this problem. The new antipsychotic agents have been of particular concern. The FDA has required all manufacturers to include black box warnings documenting concerns about weight gain as well as the development of diabetes and hypercholesterolemia.

Although the mechanisms of the weight gain remain a mystery, one compelling study examined the affinity for various receptors (such as serotonergic, adrenergic, dopaminergic, histaminergic, and muscarinic) compared with reports of short-term weight gain. They determined that the strongest correlation for gaining weight is with H_1 histamine receptor activity ($r = -0.72$). Table 13.2 shows the relative risk of weight gain from the second-generation antipsychotic agents, as determined by a consensus group that included the American Diabetes Association and the American Psychiatric Association (as well as others), compared with the H_1 affinity.

The histamine neurons are known to be involved with energy homeostasis—an effect enhanced by modafinil. Additionally, centrally administered histamine increases the activity of leptin in rodents. Inversely, the blocking effect of the antihistamines may result in weight gain through decreased energy metabolism as well as increased appetite. However, diphenhydramine (Benadryl) is considered weight neutral, so there must be more than

TABLE 13.2

The Relation Between Risk of Weight Gain with Second-Generation Antipsychotic Agents and Affinity for the H_1 Histamine Receptor

	Weight Gain	Amount of Drug Needed to Block H_1 Histamine
Clozapine	+++	1.2
Olanzapine	+++	2
Quetiapine	++	11
Risperidone	++	15
Aripiprazole	+/–	29.7
Ziprasidone	+/–	43

just H_1 affinity causing the weight problems associated with antipsychotic medications.

Patients on antidepressants or mood stabilizers are also often caught between maintaining an ideal body size and the negative consequences of effective treatment. Long-term studies find weight gain and increased risk of diabetes mellitus in patients treated with these medications. What could be causing this? One theory is that patients are regaining the weight they lost before starting treatment. More likely explanations are that psychiatric mediations increase food craving or reduce RMR. Unfortunately, there is scant evidence to identify a specific mechanism.

Few psychiatric medications induce weight loss. Bupropion and topiramate have demonstrated beneficial effects on weight and are included in two of the new FDA-approved diet pills (Contrave: bupropion and naltrexone, Qsymia: topiramate and phentermine). Amphetamines were the original "diet pills" and were freely prescribed in the 1950s and 1960s. In the early 1970s, because of problems with addiction and occasional psychosis, the government deemed this class of medications Schedule II and required new studies to establish effectiveness. These steps, for all intents and purposes, shut down the use of stimulants as diet pills. More recently the quick removal of dexfenfluramine (Redux) in the 1990s and the massive lawsuits that followed portend further research with stimulants for weight control.

The mechanism by which stimulants induce weight loss is not as straightforward as one would expect. These medications—affectionately called "speed" and "uppers" on the street—actually reduce motor activity: *the paradoxical effect.* Figure 13.11 documents this effect in a group of boys with no behavioral or learning difficulties and an average IQ of 130. Motor activity was measured by a little sensor the children wore around their ankles during a 2-hour test period. The graph shows that, with few exceptions, the boys had reduced motor activity while on amphetamines. (Some clinicians incorrectly interpret this normal response to stimulants as an indication that the subject has attention deficit hyperactivity disorder.)

A more recent study analyzed resting energy expenditure (see Figure 13.3) in 14 normal men and women given methylphenidate. Subjects received 0.5 mg/kg of methylphenidate or placebo in a blinded, crossover study. While on the methylphenidate, the resting energy of the subjects increased by 7%. Other studies with humans have consistently shown decreased caloric intake while on stimulants. Subjects appear to consume a normal quantity when eating, but eat less frequently.

The stimulants appear to increase energy expenditure and reduce energy intake—which on the surface is exactly what we want. Unfortunately,

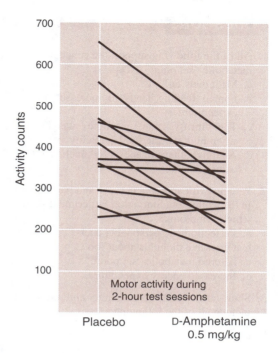

FIGURE 13.11 Physical activity in normal prepubertal boys decreased when they were on amphetamines compared with placebo. (Adapted from Rapoport JL, Buchsbaum MS, Zahn TP, et al. Dextroamphetamine: cognitive and behavioral effects in normal prepubertal boys. *Science*. 1978;199[4328]:560–563. Reprinted with permission from AAAS.)

the stimulants also have a host of adverse CNS effects, but the real problem may have more to do with lack of long-term effectiveness. Nicolas Rasmussen, author of *On Speed: The Many Lives of Amphetamine*, wrote us that amphetamines only suppress appetite in the short term and then, because of tolerance, need to be increased to maintain weight control. He went on to say that the pharmaceutical companies had negative long-term studies, conducted after Second World War, but hid the results.

TREATMENT

NUTRITION AND MENTAL HEALTH

There is a growing body of evidence correlating nutrition and mental health. Separate studies in the United Kingdom, Spain, and Australia have shown that increased consumption of a Western diet (such as processed food, refined grains, and sugary products) is associated with more depressive symptoms. Although unproven as a therapeutic intervention, maybe a healthy diet rich in fruits and vegetables should be a prescription we give to every patient.

QUESTIONS

1. All of the following support the concept of a metabolic "set point" except
   a. Most diets fail.
   b. Forced feeding leads to increased energy expenditure.
   c. The "thrifty gene" promotes weight gain when high-caloric food is readily available.
   d. Adaptive thermogenesis is unchanged by caloric intake.

2. Patients with anorexia nervosa and participants in the Minnesota Starvation Experiment share which symptoms?
   a. Perfectionistic personality traits.
   b. Obsessive thoughts about food.
   c. Altered metabolic "set point."
   d. Increased energy expenditure.

3. Short-term signals about hunger and satiety include all of the following except
   a. Leptin.
   b. CCK.
   c. Glucose.
   d. Ghrelin.

4. Adiposity signals must be able to do all of the following except
   a. Cross the blood–brain barrier.
   b. Change in relation to amount of stored fat.
   c. Alter afferent signals from the vagus nerve.
   d. Inhibit or enhance caloric intake.

5. The largest concentration of leptin receptors are in the
   a. Amygdala.
   b. Arcuate nucleus.
   c. Adrenal cortex.
   d. Anterior corticospinal tract.

6. The AGRP does which of the following?
   a. It is an antagonist at the MC4 receptor and stimulates eating.
   b. It is an antagonist at the MC4 receptor and inhibits intake
   c. It is an agonist at the MC4 receptor and stimulates eating.
   d. It is an agonist at the MC4 receptor and inhibits intake.

7. The MC system
   a. Has been implicated as a cause of anorexia nervosa.
   b. Stimulates foraging for food.
   c. Potentiates the endocannabinoid receptor.
   d. Suppresses food intake.

8. The effects of the brain's assessment of caloric needs are carried out by all of the following except
   a. Endocrine hormones.
   b. Changes in behavior.
   c. Modulation of the "set point."
   d. Alterations in the ANS.

See Answers section at the end of this book.

CHAPTER 14

Anger and Aggression

DIAGNOSIS

Anger and aggression are fundamental reactions throughout the animal kingdom. Defending against intruders and hunting for the next meal are traits that were essential for the survival of our ancestors. However, some individuals are too aggressive. We all know a few dogs (and relatives for that matter) that are easily agitated and quick to bite. Animals and people with this tendency are a significant social problem.

Terms such as *road rage*, *spouse abuse*, and *mass shootings* are all too common in our daily papers. Yet the *Diagnostic and Statistical Manual* (DSM) does not include a category for inappropriate anger. It has been suggested this is because men created DSM and they do not see anger as a problem. (PMS, on the other hand, now *that's* a disorder!)

The absence of a diagnostic category is clinically relevant. For example, a small Danish pharmaceutical company in the 1970s was pursuing a treatment for aggression, called *serenics*. In spite of promising results, the company shelved the medication when it became clear the US Food and Drug Administration would not approve the medication because aggression is not a specific disorder. Consequently, although psychologists and other counselors provide treatment for "anger management," there is no sanctioned pharmacologic intervention for excessive anger and irritability.

Aggression is clearly influenced by one's culture and upbringing. Violence on TV and early physical abuse increase the likelihood a person will be aggressive. Alternatively, the context in which an assault occurs determines the appropriateness of the aggression. For example, fighting on the ice at hockey games is accepted, but fighting in the stands is not. These are issues beyond the scope of this text. We are interested in the processes in the brain that generate or fail to impede violence toward another.

Two Kinds of Aggression

Working with cats, Flynn at Yale and Siegel at University of Medicine and Dentistry of New Jersey identified two types of aggressive behavior. One is more predatory—similar to hunting—the cat quietly and calmly stalks its prey. The other type of aggression is defensive. The cat becomes agitated and makes a big display of its feelings, in part to avoid a fight, but is also ready to respond if provoked. In the cat, these different responses can be elicited by electrical stimulation of different regions of the hypothalamus.

MECHANISMS IN THE BRAIN

Hypothalamus

In a series of experiments over many years, Flynn and Siegel placed electrodes into the hypothalamus of cats and searched for the regions that would, with stimulation, elicit aggression. Remarkably, they found separate regions that elicited the different aggressive behaviors. Figure 14.1 shows the location of the hypothalamus and the two general areas (lateral and medial) on either side of the third ventricle that correspond with predatory and defensive aggression.

Figure 14.2 shows an example of predatory aggression elicited in a cat by stimulation of the *lateral hypothalamus*. Quiet, stealthy circling of the rodent precedes the bite to the back of the neck. It is worth noting that the researchers used cats in these experiments that would not bite the rat prior to the hypothalamic stimulation.

Figure 14.3 shows the defensive type of aggressive behavior induced by stimulating the *medial hypothalamus*. In this case the cat becomes aroused (such as high sympathetic tone, increased heart rate, dilated pupils, etc.) and displays hostile behavior (such as hissing, growling, arching back, piloerection, etc.). The different features of each kind of aggression are summarized in Table 14.1.

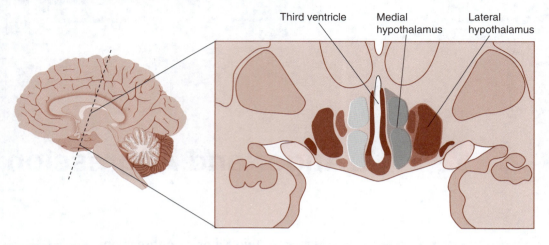

FIGURE 14.1 The medial and lateral regions of the hypothalamus.

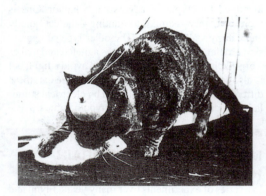

FIGURE 14.2 Predatory attack (quiet bite) of a rat induced by stimulating the lateral hypothalamus. (From Flynn JP. The neural basis of aggression in cats. In: Glass DC, ed. *Neurophysiology and Emotion*. New York: Rockefeller University Press; 1967.)

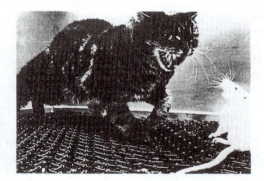

FIGURE 14.3 Defensive attack elicited by stimulating the medial hypothalamus. (From Flynn JP. The neural basis of aggression in cats. In: Glass DC, ed. *Neurophysiology and Emotion*. New York: Rockefeller University Press; 1967.)

TABLE 14.1

The Different Features of Predatory and Defensive Aggression

	Predatory Aggression	**Defensive Aggression**
CNS location	Lateral hypothalamus	Medial hypothalamus
Sympathetic tone	Calm	Autonomic arousal
Behavior	Stealthy movement, bite to back of rat's neck	Hissing, arching back, paw swipe, piloerection
Evolutionary function	Hunting	Protection
Quality	Hidden, premeditated	Overt, reactive

CNS, central nervous system.

The two pathways and subsequent behavior elicited in the cat also describe the two basic kinds of aggression seen in humans. Analysis of playground behavior, spousal abuse, and serial killers supports the dichotomy of a reactive/impulsive/defensive type of aggression and a stealthy/premeditated/hunting type of aggression, although a combination of the two types is commonly found in any specific aggressive act.

The Research Domain Criteria includes a third classification of aggression called *frustrative nonreward*—withdrawal or prevention of a reward. An example of this appeared recently in our local paper. Apparently, one of the most likely times a prison corrections officer will be assaulted by an inmate is when the officer has confiscated a cell phone. We will not be covering that type of aggression in this chapter, in part because there is little neuroscience on the topic and in part because it is probably better placed in Chapter 12, Pleasure.

Frontal Cortex

Random acts of aggression are a problem for any species. The brain has mechanisms to modify aggressive behavior either by putting on brakes or applying an accelerator. The frontal cortex is well known for controlling impulsive behavior. Impairment of the frontal cortex is the equivalent of taking off the brakes on impulses. The most famous example of this is Phineas Gage. Gage was a foreman at a railroad construction company in Vermont in 1848. A tamping iron was blown through his left frontal skull when a spark inadvertently ignited explosive powder.

Gage's skull has been preserved, and Figure 14.4 shows a reconstruction of the path the tamping iron took through his skull. Remarkably, he recovered, was out of bed within a month, and lived another 12 years. However, his personality had drastically changed. Prior to the accident he had been efficient, balanced, and responsible; then he was fitful, impulsive, unfocused, and easily agitated.

If we imagine that the frontal cortex applies the brakes to the array of primitive impulses that arise from the subcortical brain, then we can see how taking the brakes off (due to a poorly functioning frontal cortex) allows the expression of feelings that would normally be withheld. Specifically, a poorly functioning frontal cortex allows more aggressive impulses to be expressed. A healthy, active frontal cortex in general says, "Stop!"

Experiments out of Siegel's laboratory provide more evidence of the important role the frontal cortex plays in restraining aggression. In this study a cat has one electrode in its lateral hypothalamus and one in the lateral aspect of its frontal cortex. What is being measured is the time until the cat

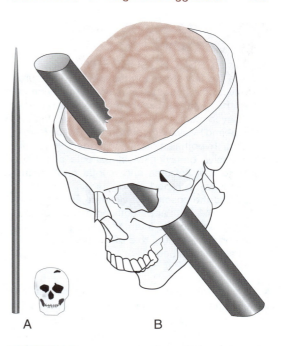

A   B

FIGURE 14.4 A: The skull of Phineas Gage and the tampering iron that exploded through his head in 1848. **B:** Drawing of a computerized reconstruction of the path the rod took through his skull and brain. The damage involved both left and right prefrontal cortices. (Adapted from Damasio H, Grabowski T, Frank R, et al. The return of Phineas Gage: clues about the brain from the skull of a famous patient. *Science.* 1994;264:1102–1105. Reprinted with permission from AAAS.)

attacks the rat after stimulation of the electrodes. With just hypothalamic stimulation, the cat only waits approximately 12 seconds before attacking. However, with stimulation of both the hypothalamus and the frontal cortex, the time to attack is doubled (Figure 14.5). This study was repeated with many cats with electrodes in a variety of locations in the frontal cortex with similar results. Clearly, the frontal cortex has an inhibitory effect on aggressive expressions, but there is no one specific location in the prefrontal cortex (PFC) that controls impulses.

DISORDER

HEAD TRAUMA

Garfman and colleagues queried the family of 279 Vietnam veterans, who sustained penetrating head injuries in the war, about aggressive behavior. Those with frontal lobe injuries had more aggressive displays compared with controls: verbal as well as physical, but mostly verbal. Those with injuries to the ventral medial PFC (often called orbital PFC) had the most.

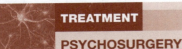

PSYCHOSURGERY

There are few studies in the medical literature involving the hypothalamus and aggression in humans, with the exception of a few reports of psychosurgery. For example, in Japan, Sano and Mayanagi performed 60 postero-medial hypothalamotomies in the 1960s for aggressive behavior. Most patients also had a history of seizures and mental retardation. In a follow-up report conducted in 1987, they reported the absence of violence and aggression in 78%, with apparently normal endocrine function. Although a drastic procedure, this supports the central role of the hypothalamus and aggressive behavior.

Frontal lobe dysfunction is one of the most consistent findings with humans and violence. With the advent of neuroimaging capabilities, many researchers have looked at activity in the PFC in men with violent histories. In a review of the literature on the topic, Brower and Price concluded that significant frontal lobe dysfunction is associated with aggressive dyscontrol—in particular, impulsive aggressive behavior.

A study of convicted murderers by Adrian Raine and his colleagues provides further insight on this topic. Raine separated a group of murderers who committed planned, predatory violence from those

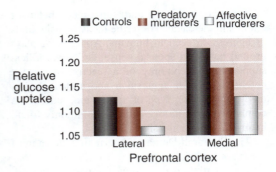

FIGURE 14.6 The relative activity in the lateral and medial aspects of the prefrontal cortex of predatory and affective murderers compared with normal controls. (Adapted from Raine A, Meloy JR, Bihrle S, et al. [1998.] Reduced prefrontal and increased subcortical brain functioning assessed using positron emission tomography in predatory and affective murderers. *Behav Sci Law*. 16[3]:319–332.)

who perpetrated affective, impulsive violence. Positron emission tomography scans were conducted on these subjects along with normal controls, examining the activity in the frontal cortex. The results are shown in Figure 14.6. Both groups of murderers had less activity in the PFC compared with controls, but the impulsive, affective group had the least. One wishes there was a way for men in prison to exercise and strengthen their frontal cortex as much as they exercise their biceps.

VIOLENCE AND AGE

The incidence of violent crime rises rapidly until the ages of 18 to 22 years and then gradually declines over the next three decades. The very young and very old are the least violent (although often the most cranky). There are many sociocultural variables that contribute to the violent trend, but the delay in the maturing of the PFC, riding atop a fully developed physical body, provides the best explanation.

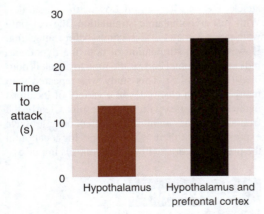

FIGURE 14.5 The time it takes for a cat to attack a rat after the hypothalamus is stimulated is greatly increased when the frontal cortex is simultaneously stimulated. (Adapted from Siegel A, Edinger H, Dotto M. Effects of electrical stimulation of the lateral aspect of the prefrontal cortex upon attack behavior in cats. *Brain Res*. 1975;93:473–484. Copyright 1975 with permission from Elsevier.)

Amygdala

There is conflicting information about the role of the amygdala and aggressive behavior. Although better known for being activated during fearful situations, the amygdala may have a broader function in processing emotional stimuli. Early studies with monkeys showed that bilateral removal of the amygdala produced an animal that was placid—neither frightened nor aggressive. This is called the *Klüver–Bucy syndrome*, after the two researchers who performed the experiments. This and other research studies suggest that the amygdala is instrumental in recognizing whether a stimulus is threatening and that an overactive amygdala can lead to excessive defensive aggression.

There are reports in the literature of bilateral amygdalotomies for untreatable aggression in humans. Some of the reports are disturbingly optimistic. A group from India reported on 481 cases, stating that 70% showed excellent or moderate improvement after 5 years (remember the Prefrontal Lobotomy for another example of psychosurgery hyperbole). A report about two cases from Georgia in 1998 provides a more balanced assessment. Two individuals who were essentially institutionalized because of aggressive behavior received amygdalotomies after years of failed medical therapies. The procedures resulted in reductions but not elimination of the assaultive behavior. The authors concluded that the procedure produced a "taming effect," which they attributed to reduced perceptions of threats. Removing the amygdala decreased false perceptions and reduced reactive aggression. Other research suggests that the amygdala is *underactive* in those with aggressive problems.

Work by Siegel with his cats may shed light on the conflicting data about the role of the amygdala with aggressive behavior. We must remember that the amygdala is not just one organ, but made up of multiple nuclei. Siegel found with cats that stimulating the lateral and central groups facilitates predatory attacks and suppressed defensive rage. Conversely, stimulation of the medial aspect of the basal complex has just the opposite effect. This subtle difference within the amygdala would be hard to identify in humans with current imaging technology. The amygdala may be overactive with different subtypes of aggression and underactive with others. Alternatively, it could be that different nuclei are activated for the different types of aggression.

An old case recently came to our attention that emphasizes the points of this section. Charles Whitman was described as an intelligent, loyal young man who was leading an uneventful life until he started to struggle with episodes of anger in his early 20s. In March 1966, he sought psychiatric help at the University of Texas medical center, but failed to return after the initial, psychoanalytic evaluation. In August, after killing his mother and wife—whom he professed to love—he climbed up the tower at the University of Texas and shot 48 people, killing 16. At autopsy a walnut-sized glioblastoma was discovered beneath the thalamus pressing on the hypothalamus. The tumor also extended into the temporal lobe and was compressing the amygdala.

It is impossible to identify what caused the emergence of Whitman's unimaginable violence. He was abusing amphetamines (Dexedrine) at the time of the shooting and was raised in a dysfunctional family with an abusive father. However, it is likely that some of the murderous rage resulted from the tumor's compression of the hypothalamus and amygdala.

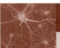

TREATMENT

INTERMITTENT EXPLOSIVE DISORDER

There is no FDA-approved treatment for anger, but medications and cognitive behavioral therapy can reduce violence. Emil Coccaro suggests a stepwise approach for treating intermittent explosive disorder. Start with a selective serotonin reuptake inhibitor (SSRI). For resistant patients, try phenytoin or oxcarbazepine/ carbamazepine. If that fails, try lamotrigine, topiramate, valproate, or lithium. Antipsychotics can help in some, but not with others.

HORMONES AND NEUROPEPTIDES

Testosterone

Everyone "knows" that testosterone stimulates aggression. Males fight more than females. It seems like a "no-brainer." Fortunately, the role of testosterone in aggression is not as simple as it first seems.

In 1849, Arnold Adolph Berthold, a German physician, conducted an experiment that is considered the first formal study of endocrinology (Figure 14.7). With this elegant little study he demonstrated the importance of a substance from the testes (later discovered to be testosterone) and aggressive behavior.

Berthold knew that male chicks grow into roosters with typical secondary sexual characteristics displaying sexual and aggressive behavior. In the experiment, Berthold removed the testes from chicks, which curtailed their normal development and eliminated sexual and aggressive behavior. In a second group he reimplanted the testes into the abdominal cavity. If the testes could establish a blood supply, the chick would develop into a normal rooster with the usual sexual and aggressive tendencies. Berthold concluded that the testes release a substance that affected male body structures and behaviors.

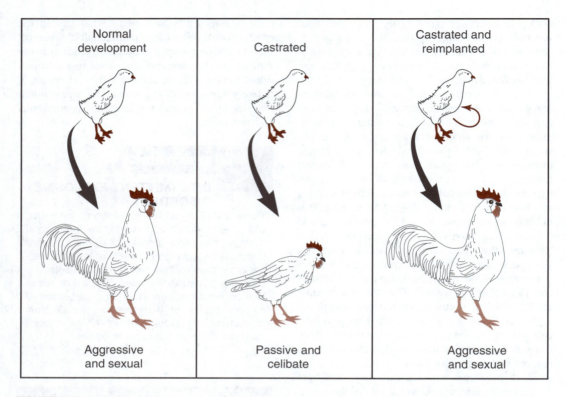

FIGURE 14.7 Berthold established in 1849 that a substance in the testes was necessary for the development of male behavior and body structure. (Adapted from Rosenzweig MR, Breedlove SM, Watson NV. *Biological Psychology*. 4th ed. Sunderland, MA: Sinauer; 2004, by permission of Oxford University Press, USA.)

Research with laboratory animals in the years since Berthold has consistently demonstrated similar correlations between testosterone and aggressive behavior. A good example by Wagner et al. shows the effect of castration on bite attacks on an inanimate target for adult male mice (Figure 14.8). Before castration and with testosterone replacement the male mice will frequently bite the

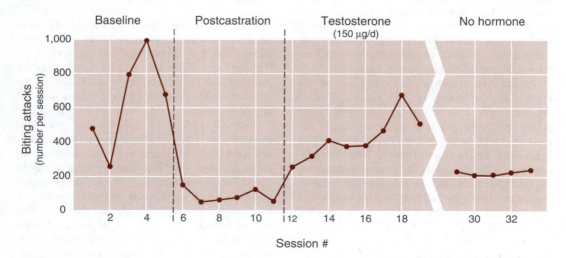

FIGURE 14.8 Baseline bite attacks for male mice are markedly diminished with castration. This effect can be reversed temporally with testosterone replacement. (Adapted from Wagner GC, Beuving LJ, Hutchinson RR. [1980.] The effects of gonadal hormone manipulations on aggressive target-biting in mice. *Aggr Behav*. 6:1–7.)

target. However, in the absence of the hormone, bite attacks drop close to the frequency seen with females.

For humans, it is not so easy to establish a direct link between plasma testosterone and magnitude of hostility. Conflicting results are found throughout the literature. It is hard to establish cause and effect. For example, a popular study is to compare testosterone levels in male prisoners with their crimes. As expected, the more aggressive prisoners have higher levels of testosterone, but so do the socially dominant, nonaggressive inmates. A study with baboons sheds light on this issue. The researchers followed changing social rank for 125 adult males from five social groups over 9 years. Simultaneously, they collected fecal samples to measure testosterone as well as glucocorticoid (stress hormone). Their results are shown in Figure 14.9. It appears that plasma testosterone rises as one ascends the social ladder. The inverse is true for the glucocorticoids except for the highest-ranking male. (Sapolsky, in an editorial on this article, expressed sympathy for the poor CEO (alpha male) who, although at the top of the pyramid, is more stressed than his immediate subordinate.)

Another popular belief is that exogenous steroids that some athletes take to enhance performance increase aggression in most men: "roid rage." This too is murky. In the best study of the effects of supraphysiologic doses of testosterone on normal men, Tricker et al. found no difference in anger for those on either testosterone or placebo, as noted by the spouse or by self-report after 10 weeks. Likewise, studies of sexual predators treated with antiandrogens have demonstrated remarkable decreases in libido but with little change in aggression.

It appears that testosterone, besides its physical effects on sexual characteristics, has behavioral effects that might best be described under the umbrella of dominance behavior. That is, a display of behaviors to achieve and maintain a higher social status. There are a host of behaviors such as staring, tone of voice, cajoling, projecting confidence, and monopolizing the conversation that can advance ones social position. These behaviors, what we sometimes call "mojo," might be enhanced by testosterone. This is in stark contrast to the traditional view of testosterone as a hormone that incites antisocial, egotistical, and even aggressive behaviors.

Vasopressin

Vasopressin, better known as an *antidiuretic hormone* for its physiologic effect on water retention and bedwetting, is increasingly recognized as playing an important role in social attachment. Many neuropeptides have multiple functions in the brain: both physical and behavioral. We are only beginning to understand the role of vasopressin in the aggressive behaviors. When given to hamsters, rats, and voles, for example, vasopressin will increase aggressive display. Alternatively, vasopressin receptor blockers will decrease aggression.

A remarkable study by Coccaro et al. looked at cerebrospinal fluid (CSF) vasopressin and aggression in 26 subjects with personality disorders. They found a positive correlation between CSF vasopressin and a life history of aggression against other people. That is, higher levels of CSF vasopressin correlated with more frequent aggressive acts. Vasopressin has broader effects on social connectedness than just aggression and we see this peptide again in Chapter 17, Social Attachment. This may be a neuropeptide with a bright future in mental health treatment.

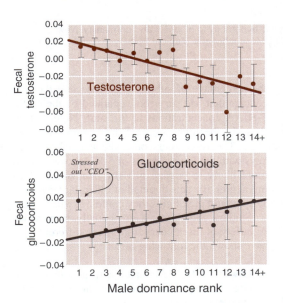

FIGURE 14.9 Testosterone levels rise as baboons ascend in social rank. Glucocorticoids, with the exception of the alpha man, descend with rank. (Adapted from Gesquiere LR, Learn NH, Simao CM, et al. Life at the top: stress in wild male baboons. *Science*. 2011;333:357–360. Reprinted with permission from AAAS.)

SEROTONIN

There is actually a more robust association between low serotonin and aggression than between low serotonin and depression. Because there is no feasible way to directly measure serotonin in humans or animals, most studies examine the correlation between violence and CSF 5-hydroxyindoleacetic acid (5-HIAA), a metabolite of serotonin.

ATTENTION DEFICIT HYPERACTIVITY DISORDER

Attention deficit hyperactivity disorder (ADHD) is correlated with criminal behavior. Small studies have shown reduction in conduct problems for patients treated with ADHD medication. In a large study that could only be conducted in a Scandinavian country, Swedish researchers identified over 25,000 patients with ADHD and matched them with the Prescribed Drug Register and National Crime Register over 4 years. As shown in the graph, the researchers found an inverse relationship between ADHD medication use and criminal activity. Of interest, nonstimulant medications were as effective as the stimulant medications. It is likely that the medications reduce impulsiveness and its complications. Raine has noted that all the medications raise the heart rate and wonders if this side effect reduces the low arousal, and desire for stimulation, found in violent people.

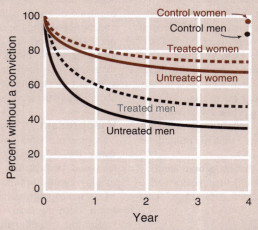

(From Lichtenstein P, et al. Medication for attention deficit-hyperactivity disorder and criminality. *New Engl J Med*. 2012;367[21]:2006–2014. Copyright © 2012 Massachusetts Medical Society. Reprinted with permission from Massachusetts Medical Society.)

Studies with monkeys have found high rates of wounding, violence, and inappropriate aggression in subjects with low CSF 5-HIAA. Analysis of these monkeys has shown that they are not necessarily uniformly more aggressive. However, they are more likely to engage in rough interactions that escalate into unrestrained aggression with a high probability of injury. This behavioral trait can be viewed as poor impulse control, which could underlie the aggressive tendency.

One group has studied the relationship between 5-HIAA and violence in a longitudinal study of free-ranging rhesus monkeys secluded on a small island on the coast of South Carolina. The researchers captured 49 two-year-old males and measured their CSF 5-HIAA. Two years is the age for a monkey that corresponds to middle to late childhood in humans and is a particularly dangerous age for male monkeys. This is a phase of life when males move from their group of origin to a new social group. The monkeys were followed for up to for 4 years.

By the time most of the subjects had reached young adulthood, 11 had died. Figure 14.10 shows the percentage of subjects that died and the percentage that had survived, separated by their CSF 5-HIAA concentrations at the start. Note that all those in the high concentration group were still alive. The researchers observed that those monkeys with the lowest levels of 5-HIAA were much more likely to engage in risky behavior, including aggressive acts directed at older, larger males. They would pick fights they could not win.

Studies with humans are equally impressive. A variety of researchers from many different sites have shown the following results:

1. Lower 5-HIAA correlates with greater suicide intent and higher lethality in those who have attempted suicide.
2. 5-HIAA levels show an inverse correlation with lifetime histories of aggression.
3. Low 5-HIAA levels predict recidivism for violent offenders.
4. Acute tryptophan depletion, which causes a transient decline in brain serotonin, will result in increased irritability and aggression.

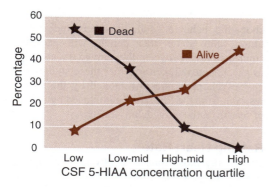

FIGURE 14.10 The percentage of 2-year-old monkeys that are still alive after 4 years, separated by the metabolite of serotonin (5-HIAA) in the cerebrospinal fluid (CSF). (Data from Higley JD, Mehlman PT, Higley SB, et al. Excessive mortality in young free-ranging male nonhuman primates with low CSF 5-hydroxyindoleacetic acid concentrations. *Arch Gen Psychiatry*. 1996;53[6]:537–543.)

Most relevant for the practicing clinician are the studies with SSRIs and aggression. Several double-blind, placebo-controlled studies have found reduced aggression with SSRIs in patients with personality disorders, autism, schizophrenia, and dementia. Although there are no medications with FDA approval for treating aggression, a serotonin reuptake inhibitor might not be a bad place to start.

THE PSYCHOPATH

Being violent is not the same as being cruel or mean. Violence in defense of oneself or one's family is not considered a crime, especially not in South Carolina! Alternatively, there are many examples of violence that seem to have no purpose other than inflicting emotional or physical pain. Furthermore, people can be mean and spiteful without being violent.

Psychopathy is the closest definition we have in psychiatry to understand wicked behavior. It is not included in the DSM. The Psychopathy Checklist-Revised created by Robert Hare provides the best definition of psychopathy and is made up of two factors. The first factor includes impulsive aggression and a wide variety of offenses, which correlates closely with antisocial personality disorder in the DSM.

The other factor defines the emotional shallowness of the psychopath: superficial, egotistical, lack of remorse, lack of empathy, and manipulative. This factor has a smaller correlation with antisocial personality disorder and more closely resembles what popular culture considers evil and sadistic. Serial killers are an extreme example. The core symptoms tend to persist as the subject ages, although the impulsive, aggressive factor decreases with maturity. The older psychopath is no more empathetic or remorseful, but less likely to be violent.

TREATMENT

LITHIUM

One of the most unique treatment studies for aggressive behavior was conducted in a prison in Connecticut in the 1970s. They randomly assigned volunteers with a history of violence to receive lithium or placebo. The exclusion of inmates with psychosis was the only psychiatric criterion applied to this study. The number of infractions reported by the institutional staff that was blind to the treatment administered served as the measure of response. The figure shows the results.

Although the study has methodological problems (small *n*, high dropout rate for those on lithium), it nonetheless demonstrates the powerful effect that lithium has on violent behavior. This is consistent with lithium's well-documented capacity to decrease suicide—which can be considered violence against oneself. More recent studies have shown small correlations between suicide as well as violence and lithium concentrations in the groundwater.

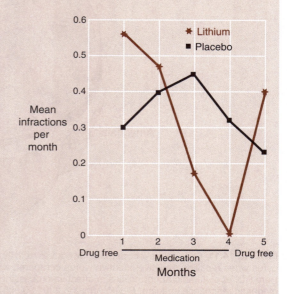

Psychopaths are a whirlwind of chaos and anguish for those around them. However, they are blasé about the turmoil they create and lack insight into their role in the mess. They may represent a little less than 1% of the population but are a huge financial drain on society. In 2011, Kiehl estimated that psychopaths are responsible for $460 billion per year in criminal social costs. Hare has suggested that the psychopath lacks some internal control. Raine has described them as broken brains. What's going on in the brain?

Prefrontal Cortex and Amygdala

Frontal lobe impairments are a consistent finding in psychopaths—particularly the orbital frontal PFC. But, as noted before, psychopaths have less activity in the PFC compared with controls but more found for offenders with reactive aggression (Figure 14.6). The amygdala is another area of interest in psychopaths—it seems to be small and underactive. An fMRI study conducted by Kiehl and Hare with psychopaths recalling negatively charged words found reduced activity in the amygdala and cingulate gyrus compared with controls (Figure 14.11). A recent study by Raine on a group of 56 men at 26 years found that a smaller amygdala volume correlated with a history of aggression and psychopathy from childhood to adulthood. Prospectively followed for another 3 years, a small

amygdala predicted violence, aggression, and psychopathic behavior. Finally, other studies have found white matter tract deficits with decreased connectedness between the amygdala and PFC in psychopaths. Taken together these studies suggest psychopaths are disinhibited by the lack of restraint from the PFC and emboldened by the lack of fear from the amygdala.

Resting Heart Rate

One of the most consistent physiologic findings in psychiatry is the correlation between low resting heart rate and aggressive behavior in children. Furthermore, a low heart rate in a child is predictive of future criminal behavior independent of all other psychological variables. Some people speculate that the low heart rate reflects a fearless, low arousal, stimulus-seeking temperament. A fascinating study from Europe supports this conclusion.

The study is based on Pavlovian (classical) conditioning. When presented repeatedly with a neutral stimulus followed by an aversive stimulus, most people will show some anxiety when seeing the neutral stimulus in anticipation of what will follow. Birbaumer et al. scanned 10 criminal psychopaths out on bail and 10 healthy controls repeatedly presented with neutral pictures followed by a painful stimulus. The controls showed increased activity in areas underlying conditioned

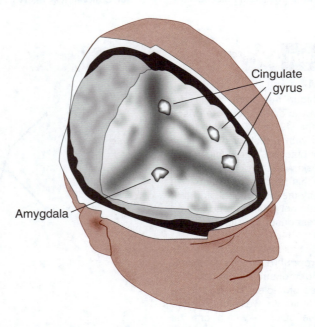

FIGURE 14.11 Criminal psychopaths showed less activity in the amygdala along with parts of the cingulate gyrus when recalling negative affective words compared with controls. (Adapted from Kiehl KA, Smith AM, Hare RD, et al. Limbic abnormalities in affective processing by criminal psychopaths as revealed by functional magnetic resonance imaging. *Biol Psychiatry*. 2001;50[9]:677–684. Copyright 2001 with permission from Elsevier.)

fear response: amygdala, orbitofrontal cortex, insula, and anterior cingulate (Figure 14.12). Remarkably, the psychopaths showed almost no activity in these areas. This disconnect between emotion and cognition may be the neural basis for the cold, detached demeanor of psychopaths.

The Pleasure of Violence

The lack of fear alone does not seem sufficient for some of the cruel actions perpetrated by psychopaths. Many people can use their fearless temperament to help others. For example, decorated bomb-disposal operators have been shown to have unusually low heart rates during experimental simulations. We can imagine that other high-stress professions are overrepresented with individuals who are innately calm: firefighters, air-traffic controllers, trauma surgeons, etc. Something else is needed to understand the behavior of the psychopath. A study with rats suggests another neurologic abnormality that may help us understand the behavior of psychopaths.

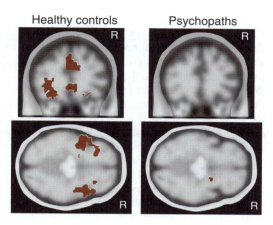

Healthy controls   Psychopaths

FIGURE 14.12 Healthy controls show a robust fear response in anticipation of an adverse stimulus. Psychopaths fail to develop a similar fear. (Data from Birbaumer N, Veit R, Lotze M, et al. Deficient fear conditioning in psychopathy: a functional magnetic resonance imaging study. *Arch Gen Psychiatry.* 2005;62[7]:799–805.)

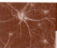

DISORDER

TEMPORAL LOBE EPILEPSY

There is a subgroup of patients with temporal lobe epilepsy who have aggressive outbursts between seizures. Some have attributed this to an interictal syndrome often called *episodic dyscontrol*. However, many of these patients have alternative explanations for their aggression, for example, low IQ, antisocial personality disorder, etc. The concept remains controversial but may apply to a few patients with seizure disorder.

More appealing is the prospect that patients with aggressive outbursts may be having unrecognized subclinical temporal lobe seizures. Unfortunately, this has been difficult to substantiate. However, the anticonvulsants do show some positive effects as treatment for aggression, although the benefits are primarily limited to those with impulsive aggressive acts rather than premeditated acts.

this book, etc. It seems logical that violence induces a spritz of dopamine at the nucleus accumbens.

The missing study is shown in Figure 14.13. In this experiment, male rats were implanted with micropipettes that sampled the extracellular concentration of dopamine at the nucleus accumbens every 10 minutes. The sampling was done during an aggressive encounter with a naive male intruder in which two to six bites and at least 140 seconds of aggressive behavior were displayed by the rat under study. The graph shows that dopamine significantly rose above baseline for up to 60 minutes after the encounter. The thrill of victory?

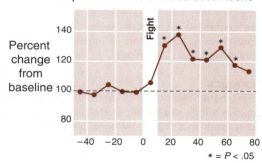

Dopamine at the nucleus accumbens

*= P < .05

FIGURE 14.13 Increase in dopamine at the nucleus accumbens following an aggressive encounter with another rat. (Adapted with permission of Society for Neuroscience from van Erp AM, Miczek KA. Aggressive behavior, increased accumbal dopamine, and decreased cortical serotonin in rats. *J Neurosci.* 2000;20:9320–9325.)

First, we must acknowledge that many people enjoy violence. One has to only look at what is popular at the movies, in video games, and on the news to recognize that blood sells. Second, as we described in Chapter 12, Pleasure, the nucleus accumbens lights up with dopamine during pleasurable activities: cocaine, sex, gambling, reading

In his book, *The Anatomy of Violence*, Adrian Raine reviewed some of the human evidence showing differences in reward-seeking behavior and neuroanatomy for psychopaths. First, psychopaths are driven by reward-seeking behavior—sex, drugs, money, etc. Raine puts it this way, "When there is a chance of getting the goods, they seem to go all out – even at the risk of negative consequences." Psychopaths are not good at delaying gratification or knowing when to stop.

Imaging studies of psychopaths consistently, but not always, find abnormalities in the reward centers. Structural imaging has shown the striatum (which contains the nucleus accumbens) to be 10% larger in psychopaths compared with controls. Functional imaging studies show a disturbing increase in activity in the striatum when psychopaths are contemplating pain in others, for example, during a game when retaliating against a partner after being slighted, or when viewing pictures of other people in painful situations. The Germans have a word for this: *schadenfreude*—pleasure derived from the misfortune of others. To some extent we all have this, but the psychopath has more.

Unfortunately, there is very little we can do for the psychopaths. Medications do not help and psychotherapy may make the condition worse as it appears that the little devils learn in psychotherapy to improve their ability to *pretend* to be empathetic, and hence become more deceptive. One possible approach is intervening early. Calwell and Van Rybroek reviewed the literature and found a "handful of treatment programs" for violent adolescents that were effective in reducing recidivism. Most were not. The effective programs had results such as recidivism of 50% in the treatment group and 75% in the control group over 2 years. The common characteristics were comprehensive programs that viewed violence as a social problem and relied on systems theory interventions. Unfortunately, not the sort of intensive treatment state governments like to fund.

Genetics

In his book, Adrian Raine starts the chapter on genetics with a story about Jeffrey Landrigan who never knew his father and was put up for adoption by his mother at 8 months. Fortunately, he was taken in by a wholesome family and raised in a nurturing environment. However, within a short time he became aggressive, destructive, and deceitful. His first arrest was at the age of 11 years. His first murder occurred when he was 20 years old and his second at 27 years. It was when he was on death row in Arizona that another inmate recognized a physical similarity between Jeffrey and Darrel Hill, an inmate on death row in Arkansas. It turned out that Darrel was Jeffrey's biological father. He too was a career criminal and had killed twice. Furthermore, Darrel's father (Jeffrey's grandfather) had a long criminal history and was shot to death by police in a car chase after a robbery. This case is an impressive example of the power of genes.

It has long been recognized that violence travels in families, but it can be difficult to separate the effects of environment from genes. In a twin study, Laura Baker out of Raine's laboratory, followed a group of 9- to 10-year-old twins using multiple informants to assess behavior. They calculated that antisocial behavior has a heritability of 96%—which ranks right up there with schizophrenia and bipolar disorder. Genome-wide studies of large samples have not yet been possible, but individual genes have been identified—and even given names, for example, the MAOA low-activity genotype dubbed the *Warrior Gene*. (Oh, please!) The consensus is that individual genes by themselves have low predictive value. However, the risk of violence increases when social deprivation (such as poverty, maternal hostility, low education, etc.) and environmental factors (such as head trauma, substance abuse, etc.) are added to "aggressive" genes. Jeffrey Landrigan's case shows that sometimes bad genes overpower a good environment.

SUMMARY

OK, let's return to where we started this chapter—two kinds of aggression: predatory and defensive. This dichotomy was defined in the 1960s with brain stimulation of the hypothalamus in cats. After 50 years and tens of thousands of brain imaging studies, we can update this model in humans. But first let's remember, aggression is heterogeneous and no two studies are the same. Most discouraging is that few studies compare the three main groups: aggressive psychopaths, nonpsychopathic aggression, and normal controls. Therefore we are making sweeping generalizations with only moderate consensus.

Defensive/reactive/impulsive aggression is characterized as a hot subcortical activation with not enough cortical constraint. The imaging studies consistently show reduced prefrontal gray matter—particularly the orbital PFC (sometime referred to as the ventral medial PFC) in subjects exhibiting defensive aggression. The heat comes from enhanced amygdala responses. Too much passion and not enough brakes.

Predatory/psychopathic aggression also comes about with impaired orbital PFC, but not to the extreme seen in the reactive group—sort of in between. The amygdala, on the other hand, is smaller and shows a blunted response—cold rather than hot. Likewise, the resting heart rate is reduced suggesting diminished autonomic arousal. Finally, predatory aggression appears to generate a little squirt of dopamine in the nucleus accumbens, which provides a different kind of passion—the enjoyment of others suffering. Yuck!

POINT OF INTEREST

One gets the impression with all the press about mass shootings that the United States is on the brink of Armageddon. However, violence has actually dropped in the past 25 years according to the FBI report Crime in the United States. The figure shows the national trend as well as the decline in two sample states. Some have suggested that this is due to the drop in environmental lead levels—lead being one of the heavy metals associated with aggressive behavior. Others have suggested the drop in violence is due to increased incarceration of the bad guys. Still others believe this is another example the world is becoming more civilized. Whatever the cause, it's a reason to be optimistic. We appear to be moving in the correct direction. Who knew?

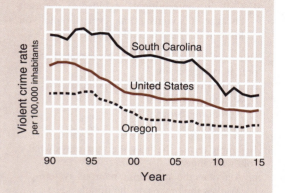

QUESTIONS

1. When dealing with a patient with an anger problem and trying to make the right diagnosis, which of the following do you not do?
   a. Refuse to treat him because there is no DSM diagnosis for anger.
   b. Call it a variation of bipolar disorder.
   c. Call it a wastebasket term, such as depression not otherwise specified (NOS) or anxiety NOS.
   d. Call it intermittent explosive disorder because it sounds good, even though you know it does not actually apply.

2. Which of the following is not associated with predatory aggression?
   a. Activation of the lateral hypothalamus.
   b. Stealthy movement.
   c. Autonomic arousal.
   d. Premeditated.

3. In simple terms, the frontal cortex plays what role with anger?
   a. Activates the autonomic neurons system.
   b. Applies the brakes on the impulses.
   c. Modulates the nucleus accumbens.
   d. Activates the lateral hypothalamus.

4. All of the following apply to the amygdala and aggression, except
   a. Klüver–Bucy syndrome.
   b. Shows less activity with criminal psychopaths.
   c. Different nuclei could be activated with different subtypes of aggression.
   d. Facilitates the expression of the serotonin receptor.

5. Testosterone
   a. Is the primary cause of fighting.
   b. Increases plasma levels for the loser.
   c. May show a better correlation with social dominance.
   d. Stimulates overt hostility in weight lifters.

6. All of the following statements about low CSF concentration of the serotonin metabolite 5-HIAA are true, except
   a. Common with major depression.
   b. Correlates with greater lifetime history of aggression.
   c. Predicts relapse for criminal offenders.
   d. Associated with greater suicide intent.

7. The psychopath can be conceptualized as having all of the following, except
   a. Low resting heart rate.
   b. Activated frontal cortex.
   c. Hypofunctioning amygdala.
   d. Increased activity at the nucleus accumbens.

See Answers section at the end of this book.

CHAPTER 15

Sleep

NORMAL SLEEP

Sleep remains a mystery. We spend roughly a third of our lives in this suspended state. All mammals sleep, as does most of the animal kingdom. Even the fruit fly sleeps—although not enough. Most people look forward to sleeping, especially if they have been deprived of sleep. Without enough sleep, people function as poorly as if they are drunk. Significant sleep deprivation will cause psychosis and physical problems. What is this all about?

The average length of sleep is approximately 7.5 hours per night (Figure 15.1). Remarkably, some people, called *nonsomniacs*, require much less. Meddis studied a retired nurse who was happily functioning on an hour of sleep a night. She reported that she had needed little sleep all her life. When studied in Meddis's sleep laboratory, she did not sleep the first night and then slept, on average, only 67 minutes for each of the remaining four nights. She did not complain of being tired or wanting more sleep. (As an aside, some in the psychiatric community might diagnose this woman with a bipolar spectrum disorder, although her condition appears to be a variant of sleep need.)

Most people show deterioration in performance when deprived of sleep. Figure 15.2 shows the results of neurobehavioral tasks for subjects deprived of differing amounts of sleep. One group was totally sleep deprived for 3 days, two other groups were restricted to 6 or 4 hours of sleep per night for 14 days, and the control group got 8 hours of sleep per night. Figure 15.2A shows the effects of sleep restriction on a sustained attention task; Figure 15.2B shows the effects on a test of memory. Sleep deprivation takes a big toll on performance. Of interest, the subjects were largely unaware of their impairments—a finding that is not uncommon when cognition declines, e.g., intoxication and dementia.

We often wonder what price we pay for our modern sleep habits. Long-term shift work, for example, has a detrimental impact on physical health problems as well as the brain. A recent examination of workers employed in rotating shift work for over 10 years found they had lower cognitive and memory scores compared with day workers. This was the equivalent of 6.5 years of age-related cognitive decline.

However, it appears that our modern sleep patterns, for most people, are more similar to what our hunter–gatherer ancestors experienced than we might imagine. Yetish et al. studied sleep patterns in three preindustrial societies in Africa and South America. These are societies without electricity or caffeine. In spite of this, adults slept only an average of 5.7 to 7.1 hours a night. They went to sleep about 3 hours after sunset and were up before sunrise. In general, they slept an hour longer in the winter than in the summer, and there was very little napping. Sounds like the pattern of a hardworking stockbroker on Wall Street, except without the cocaine!

Stages of Sleep

For centuries, sleep had been considered a passive, uniform process that simply restored the body. That changed in 1953 when Nathaniel Kleitman and Eugene Aserinsky examined electroencephalographic (EEG) recordings from sleeping healthy subjects. They discovered that sleep comprises different stages that repeat in characteristic patterns throughout the night. They identified the three states of consciousness as awake, non–rapid eye movement (non-REM) sleep, and rapid eye movement (REM) sleep. Non-REM sleep has been further subdivided into four stages.

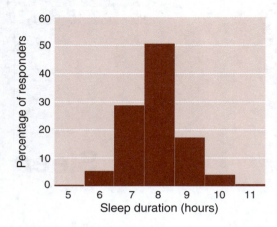

FIGURE 15.1 Self-reported average duration of sleep from 8,070 adults submitted through a smartphone app. (Data from Walch OJ, et al. A global quantification of "normal" sleep schedules using smartphone data. *Sci Adv.* 2016;2:e1501705.)

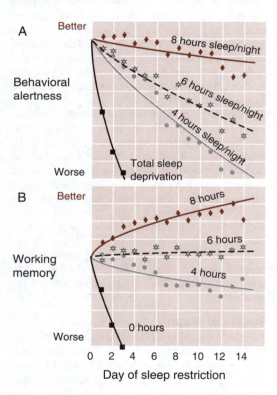

FIGURE 15.2 The effects of total sleep deprivation for 3 days and chronic sleep restriction for 14 days are measured with neurobehavioral tasks. The psychomotor vigilance task **(A)** measures alertness and attention. The digit symbol substitution task **(B)** measures working memory. (Adapted from Van Dongen HP, Maislin G, Mullington JM, et al. The cumulative cost of additional wakefulness: dose-response effects on neurobehavioral functions and sleep physiology from chronic sleep restriction and total sleep deprivation. *Sleep.* 2003;26[2]:117–126, by permission of Oxford University Press.)

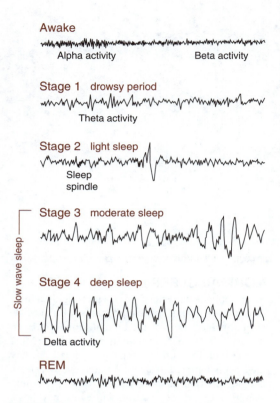

FIGURE 15.3 Characteristic electroencephalographic rhythms during the stages of consciousness. REM, rapid eye movement. (Adapted from Horne JA. *Why We Sleep: The Functions of Sleep in Humans and Other Mammals.* Oxford: Oxford University Press; 1988, by permission of Oxford University Press.)

Electroencephalographic Patterns

Figure 15.3 shows the characteristic EEG patterns during the different stages of sleep. From an awake state to the deepest sleep of stage 4, there is a progression of decreasing frequency and increasing amplitude of the EEG activity. Stage 1 sleep, also called the *drowsy period*, is so light that most people when awoken from this stage will say that they were not asleep. Stage 2 sleep shows the development of sleep spindles, which are periodic bursts of activity resulting from interactions between the thalamus and the cortex. Stages 3 and 4 sleep, also called *slow wave sleep* (SWS), are the deepest stages of sleep characterized by the development of delta waves. REM sleep is the most unusual finding that Kleitman and Aserinsky discovered. In REM sleep, the EEG activity is remarkably similar to that of the awake state, but the body or at least the major muscles are paralyzed.

In a typical night, a person cycles through five episodes of non-REM/REM activity (Figure 15.4A). The first REM episode occurs after

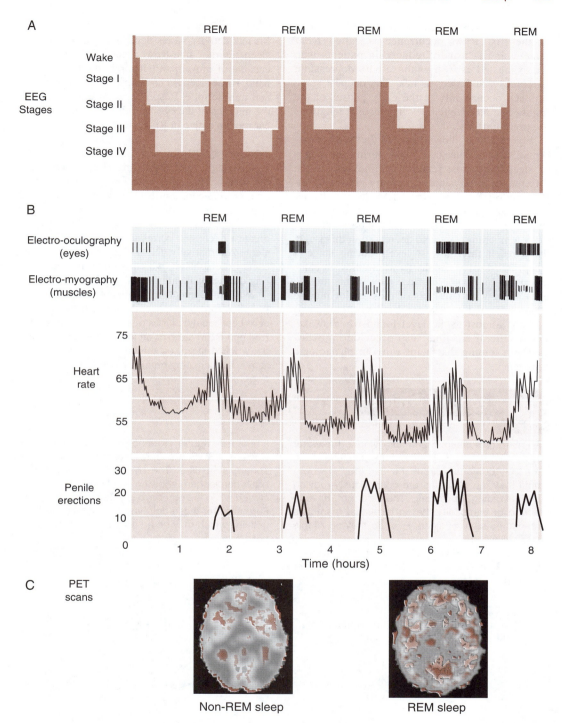

FIGURE 15.4 Physiologic changes in a healthy volunteer during 8 hours of sleep. EEG, electroencephalograph; REM, rapid eye movement. (**A** and **B:** Adapted from Purves D, et al. *Neuroscience*. 3rd ed. Sunderland, MA: Sinauer; 2004, by permission of Oxford University Press, USA. **C:** Adapted with permission from Macmillan Publishers Ltd. Buchsbaum MS, et al. Positron emission tomography with deoxyglucose-F18 imaging of sleep. *Neuropsychopharmacology*. 2001;25:S50–S56. Copyright 2001.)

approximately 90 minutes of sleep. The time to the first REM occurrence is called *REM latency* and is usually reduced in patients who are exhausted as well as those with depression, narcolepsy, and sleep apnea. The deepest stage of sleep occurs only in the early phases of the night. The REM episodes increase in length as the night unfolds.

Figure 15.4B shows some of the other physiologic changes that take place during the stages of sleep. The most remarkable findings are the differences in physiologic activity between non-REM and REM sleep. Non-REM sleep is characterized by limited eye movement and a decrease in muscle tone and heart rate. Metabolic rate and body temperature are also decreased in this stage. They reach their lowest levels during stage 4 sleep. REM sleep, as the name implies, is characterized by rapid, darting movements of the eyes along with paralysis of most major muscle groups. Heart rate and respirations (not shown) increase almost to the level found when awake. Penile/clitoral erections also occur during REM sleep—a finding that helps rule out physiologic impotence.

Muscle Tone

Muscle activity varies depending on the phase of sleep. During non-REM sleep, the muscles are capable of movement but rarely do. On the other hand, REM sleep is characterized by a loss of skeletal muscle tone. Respiratory muscles along with the muscles of the eyes and the tiny muscles of the ear remain active in REM sleep.

Brain Imaging

Brain imaging studies during sleep reveal a pattern that is consistent with EEG findings. During non-REM sleep, positron emission tomography (PET) studies show decreased cerebral blood flow and energy metabolism (Figure 15.4C). The greatest decreases correlate with greater depth of sleep. Alternatively, REM sleep shows a cerebral energy metabolism, which is equal to that occurring during awakening.

William Dement, a prominent sleep researcher from Stanford, has eloquently summarized the difference between the phases of sleep. He has characterized non-REM sleep as an idling brain in a movable body. REM sleep, on the other hand, describes an active, hallucinating brain in a paralyzed body.

POINT OF INTEREST

All mammals sleep. Mammals living in the water are able to sleep but still must regularly surface for air. Additionally, from the day they are born until they die, dolphins are continuously moving and avoiding obstacles. They do not have a period of immobility that in terrestrial mammals marks the state of sleep. How do they do all this and still sleep?

Studies of EEG tracings of the bottlenose dolphin show that they rest one hemisphere at a time (see figure). Note how the large amplitude waves of SWS are only present in one hemisphere at a time. The eye contralateral to the brain hemisphere showing slow waves is usually closed while the other eye is almost always open. Furthermore, these dolphins do not display REM activity, which may be an adaptation so they can keep moving.

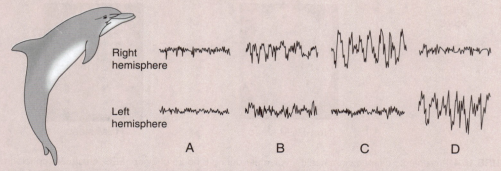

Electroencephalographic tracings from bottlenose dolphins. (Adapted from Mujhametov LM. Sleep in marine mammals. In: Borbely AA, ed. 1984 and Purves D, Augustine GJ, Fitzpatrick D, et al. eds. *Neuroscience*. 3rd ed. Sunderland, MA: Sinauer; 2004, by permission of Oxford University Press, USA.)

DISORDERS

SLEEPWALKING AND NIGHT TERRORS

Approximately 40% of people are *sleepwalkers* as children, although few are sleepwalkers as adults. This behavior usually occurs in the first stage-4 non-REM period of the night. In a typical episode, the child's eyes will be open and the child will avoid obstacles when moving about the room or house. The cognition is clouded, and the child will usually have no memory of the event. The best intervention is to gently guide the sleepwalker back to bed.

Night terrors are characterized by extreme terror and an inability to be awakened. Typically occurring in children between the ages of 4 and 7 years, this condition only affects approximately 3% of the population. As with sleepwalking, it develops in the deep stages of non-REM sleep. Night terrors are not to be confused with nightmares, which are vivid dreams during REM sleep.

The child appears in a state of panic, may even scream and cry. Fortunately, the child usually returns to sleep in 10 to 20 minutes, and little is remembered the next day. The greatest toll may be on the parents who have to comfort the frightened child. The best intervention is support.

Changes with Aging

Total sleep duration and the proportions of time spent in various stages change as people age. Figure 15.5 shows the duration of sleep across the life span. Neonates (on the left of the figure) spend most of their time sleeping, with a large percentage of that time in REM sleep. Some have suggested that REM serves a developmental purpose and this is why neonates and young children require so much time in this phase.

On the right side of Figure 15.5 is a meta-analysis of sleep duration from childhood to old age. Note the gradual reduction in the deepest stages of sleep and the increase in awakening after sleep onset as people age. Dissatisfaction with sleep is a common complaint in the elderly, and the reason for these complaints can be seen in the figure.

Dreaming

Historically it was believed that dreaming is limited to REM sleep. A thorough analysis of what people are experiencing at different stages of consciousness reveals that dreams occur in all stages of sleep, but the content varies. Researchers gave college students a pager and instructed them to sleep with a special nightcap that recorded eye and head movement (see Figure 15.6A). The students were considered to be in non-REM sleep when there was an absence of eye movement. REM sleep was defined as rapid eye movements without head movement. The students dictated what they were doing, thinking, and feeling when they were paged or spontaneously awoke.

The results showed that the subjects had dreams at all stages of sleep; however, the nature of dreams was different. In non-REM sleep the dreams were more of thoughts—as though the person is solving a problem. In REM sleep the dreams are illogic, bizarre, and even hallucinatory. Figure 15.6B shows the decrease in thoughts as the subject goes from an awake state to REM sleep and the corresponding marked increase in hallucinations.

Robert Sapolsky asked an interesting question about dreaming: why are dreams dreamlike? He asserts that activity in the prefrontal cortex decreases dramatically in REM sleep, which in turn removes the brakes on the lower brain centers, e.g., amygdala, hippocampus, etc. Consequently, "the limbic system is disinhibited and runs wild, and you have dreamlike content in your dreams."

NEURONAL CIRCUITS

Until the 1940s, sleep was generally conceptualized as the body's reaction to the lack of stimulation, that is, the brain passively turns "off" when there is no input. We now know that sleep is an active process initiated and terminated by different regions of the brain.

Suprachiasmatic Nucleus

The master clock of the brain is the suprachiasmatic nucleus (SCN) located in the anterior hypothalamus (Figure 15.7). The SCN orchestrates circadian rhythms throughout the brain

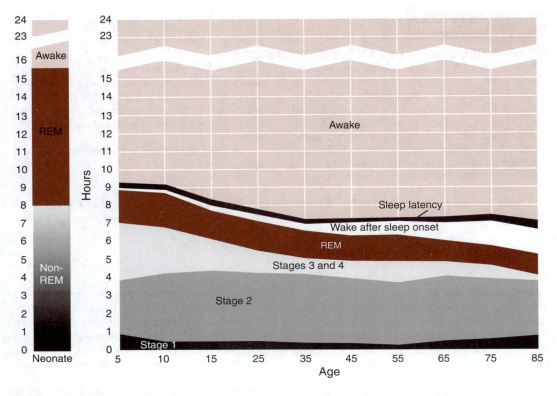

FIGURE 15.5 Sleep duration across the life span. Neonates are shown on the left, and on the right is a meta-analysis of sleep parameters in healthy individuals across the life span. REM, rapid eye movement. (Adapted from Ohayon MM, Carskadon MA, Guilleminault C, et al. Meta-analysis of quantitative sleep parameters from childhood to old age in healthy individuals: developing normative sleep values across the human life span. *Sleep*. 2004;27[7]:1255–1273.)

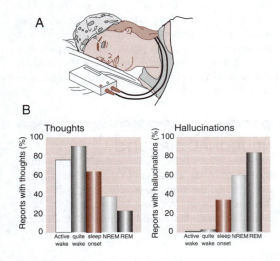

FIGURE 15.6 A special home-based sleep monitoring system **(A)** allows researchers to correlate dream content with the stage of consciousness **(B)**. NREM, non–rapid eye movement; REM, rapid eye movement. (Adapted from Fosse R, Stickgold R, Hobson JA. Brain-mind states: reciprocal variation in thoughts and hallucinations. *Psychol Sci*. 2001;12[1]:30–36.)

and body. The SCN is synchronized (entrained) by signals from the retina, which are activated by inputs from the sun. When humans are prevented from receiving cues about the solar day (such as living in a cave for weeks), the 24-hour sleep–wake cycle will gradually increase to approximately 26 hours—a condition that is called *free-running*.

The SCN is made up of some of the smallest neurons in the brain and has a volume that is approximately 0.3 mm³. Output from the SCN synchronizes other cellular oscillators throughout the brain and body. Studies with hamsters have established the crucial role this tiny collection of neurons plays in the regulation of sleep–wake cycles. Figure 15.8A shows how recordings of the time a hamster spends on the running wheel can be used to establish its circadian rhythm. When the SCN is ablated, the 24-hour rhythm is lost and no regular pattern can be identified. If the hamster receives a transplant from a strain of mutant hamsters with a 22-hour circadian rhythm, the foreign rhythm becomes established.

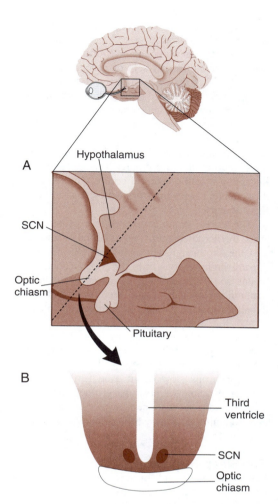

FIGURE 15.7 A sagittal view **(A)** and frontal view **(B)** of the human suprachiasmatic nucleus (SCN). (Adapted from Bear MF, Connors BW, Paradiso MA, eds. *Neuroscience: Exploring the Brain*. 4th ed. Baltimore: Lippincott Williams & Wilkins; 2015.)

TREATMENT

MELATONIN

Under normal circumstances, the SCN is reset each day by signals of light from the retina. However, melatonin secreted during the dark cycle from the pineal gland can also entrain the SCN. This justifies the use of melatonin to promote sleep in those with delayed sleep onset or to reset the internal clock that is disrupted with jet lag. Studies with melatonin agents have been effective, although less robust than we might hope. Success with melatonin requires proper timing of administration. Taking a dose at the wrong time will not only be ineffective but can make things worse!

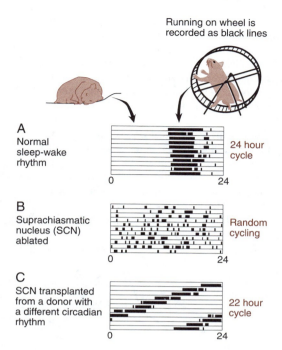

Running on wheel is recorded as black lines

A Normal sleep-wake rhythm — 24 hour cycle

B Suprachiasmatic nucleus (SCN) ablated — Random cycling

C SCN transplanted from a donor with a different circadian rhythm — 22 hour cycle

FIGURE 15.8 A usual 24-hour circadian rhythm **(A)**. Lack of rhythm after the suprachiasmatic nucleus (SCN) is destroyed **(B)**. New 22-hour rhythm after transplantation of SCN from hamster with genetically different rhythms **(C)**. (Adapted from Ralph MR, Lehman MN. Transplantation: a new tool in the analysis of the mammalian hypothalamic circadian pacemaker. *Trends Neurosci*. 1991;14[8]:362–366. Copyright 1991 with permission from Elsevier.)

Molecular Mechanisms

Work with fruit flies and mice has begun to tease out the molecular mechanisms that control circadian rhythm. Although all the details remain to be worked out, the basic mechanism is becoming clear. The cell produces two proteins: CLOCK and BMAL1. These proteins bind together to form a dimer, which then activates the transcription of other proteins, called *PER* (*Period*) and *CRY* (*Cryptochrome*). PER and CRY form a dimer that inhibits the transcription of CLOCK and BMAL1, providing a negative feedback loop.

The buildup and breakdown of these proteins take 24 hours. Figure 15.9 shows the daily fluctuation in the proteins PER and CRY from a mouse SCN. Note the 6-hour lag between the buildup of the messenger RNA (gene expression) and the production of the proteins. Although the functions of PER and CRY remain to be elucidated, this molecular mechanism is believed to drive the 24-hour cycling of the SCN.

An area of great interest involves the genes that control these proteins in humans and their role with sleep disorders. For example, mutations of CLOCK and PER have been found in some individuals with delayed or advanced sleep phase syndromes. Additionally, of great interest to us, is the question of damaged *clock* genes and psychiatric disorders. Clearly, sleep impairments have a strong correlation with psychiatric disorders, but as yet there is only limited evidence implicating *clock* genes as the culprits.

Ascending Arousal Systems

In 1949, the Italian neurophysiologists Horace Magoun and Giuseppe Moruzzi discovered the first circuits governing sleep and wakefulness. They found that stimulating a group of neurons in the midline of the brain stem aroused a sleeping animal. Likewise, lesions of this region resulted in

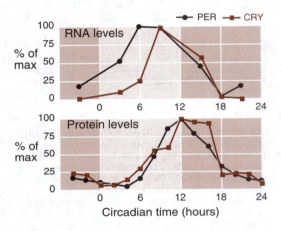

FIGURE 15.9 Fluctuations of gene expression and protein levels in the mouse suprachiasmatic nucleus (SCN). These proteins are believed to be the molecular signal of circadian rhythm. (Adapted with permission from Macmillan Publishers Ltd. Pace-Schott EF, Hobson JA. The neurobiology of sleep: genetics, cellular physiology and subcortical networks. *Nat Rev Neurosci.* 2002;3[8]:591–605. Copyright 2002.)

persistent sleep. They called this region the *reticular activating system.*

It is likely that Magoun and Moruzzi were stimulating many different sets of ascending arousal neurons during their experiments. A further study in the intervening years has identified several of the important nuclei and neurotransmitters. One group is the cholinergic neurons with cell bodies located near the pons–midbrain junction. These neurons project to the thalamus and activate the thalamic relay neurons that are crucial for transmission of information to the cerebral cortex. Stimulation of these nuclei causes high-frequency, low-amplitude EEG activity.

The second group comprises four neuronal systems: the noradrenergic neurons of the locus coeruleus, the serotonergic neurons of the raphe nuclei, the dopaminergic neurons from the periaqueductal gray matter, and the histaminergic neurons in the tuberomammillary nucleus. These neurons project to the hypothalamus and throughout the cerebral cortex.

All five neuronal systems are active during arousal and quiescent during non-REM sleep. However, the cholinergic neurons resume their activity during REM sleep while the monoaminergic neurons slow down even further. This is another example of how wakefulness and REM sleep (conditions that seem so similar) are different. A summary of these arousal networks is given in Table 15.1.

The Sleep Switch

In general, most people experience a relatively rapid transition from arousal to asleep or vice versa. This transition can be conceptualized as the flipping of a switch. The closest approximation to a "sleep switch" in the brain is the ventrolateral preoptic nucleus (VLPO). The VLPO has projections to the

TABLE 15.1

A Summary of the Major Neuronal Systems That Mediate Arousal and Comprise the Ascending Reticular Activating System

Neurotransmitter	Cell Bodies	Projections	Active During
Cholinergic	Nuclei of pons–midbrain junction	Thalamus	Awake and rapid eye movement
Noradrenergic	Locus coeruleus	–	–
Dopaminergic	Periaqueductal gray matter	Hypothalamus and cerebral cortex	Awake
Serotonergic	Raphe nuclei	–	–
Histaminergic	Tuberomammillary nucleus	–	–

main components of the ascending arousal system as shown in Table 15.1. The VLPO is inhibitory and primarily active during sleep. In other words, an active VLPO induces sleep by putting the brakes on the arousal nuclei. People with damage to their VLPO experience chronic insomnia.

Conversely, the VLPO must be inhibited so that people can wake up. Indeed, the VLPO receives inputs from the monoaminergic neurons—the very neurons that it inhibits. Therefore the "sleep switch" has mutually inhibitory elements in which activity from one side shuts down the other side and disinhibits its own actions. This helps explain the relatively abrupt change from awake to asleep that occurs in most mammals (Figure 15.10).

Narcolepsy

A problem with such a switch is that rapid, unwanted transitions from one state to another can occur when it is unstable. Presumably this is the mechanism of narcolepsy. Attacks of irresistible sleepiness as well as episodes of physical collapse and loss of muscle tone during emotional situations (*cataplexy*) characterize narcolepsy. In 2000, it was discovered that patients with narcolepsy have few orexin neurons in

the hypothalamus (Figure 15.11). Orexin neurons (also called *hypocretin*) are mainly active during wakefulness and reinforce the arousal system.

It appears that patients with narcolepsy have lost the stabilizing influence of the orexin neurons and can abruptly switch from one state of consciousness to another. In other words they have a floppy "sleep switch." Patients with narcolepsy do not sleep more than normal individuals; they just take more naps during the day and are awaken more frequently during the night.

TREATMENT

NARCOLEPSY

Amphetamines were first used in 1937 as a treatment for narcolepsy and remain popular. More recently, modafinil, an agent with minimal potential for abuse and a different mechanism of action, has become the first-line treatment for patients with the disorder. Modafinil works by indirectly activating the histamine network—the opposite effect of an antihistamine. Although effective for excessive daytime sleepiness, modafinil has limited benefits for cataplexy. Some clinicians add a tricyclic antidepressant or a newer antidepressant with dual action to decrease cataplectic attacks. Such a combination will affect histamine, serotonin, and norepinephrine—all components of the "sleep switch."

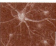

DISORDER

OBESITY

A recent analysis of more than 1,000 volunteers found a U-shaped curvilinear association between sleep duration and body mass. Subjects who slept, on average, 7.7 hours per night had the lowest weight, whereas those sleeping for more or less time were heavier. The authors suggest the cause may be due to changes in hormones regulating appetite, such as leptin and ghrelin.

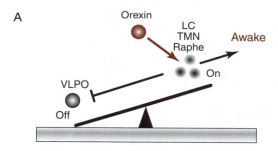

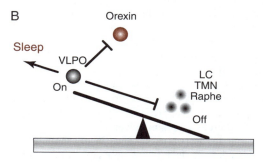

FIGURE 15.10 A schematic diagram of the "sleep switch." **A:** Locus coeruleus (LC), tuberomammillary nucleus (TMN), and raphe nuclei in the awake state are stabilized by the orexin neurons. They also inhibit the VLPO. **B:** In the sleep state, the VLPO inhibits the orexin neurons as well as the LC, TMN, and raphe nuclei. VLPO, ventrolateral preoptic nucleus. (Adapted with permission from Macmillan Publishers Ltd. Saper CB, Scammell TE, Lu J. Hypothalamic regulation of sleep and circadian rhythms. *Nature.* 2005;437[7063]:1257–1263. Copyright 2005.)

Normal   Narcoleptic

FIGURE 15.11 Neuronal degeneration of orexin neurons in lateral hypothalamus of a patient with narcolepsy compared with a control. (Courtesy of Jerome Siegel.)

The link between SCN and the "sleep switch" is more confusing than one might expect. SCN actually has few direct projections to the VLPO and orexin neurons. There appears to be a third system: the dorsomedial nucleus of the hypothalamus (DMH). Why might the brain have evolved a three-stage pathway for control of sleep? Well, the SCN is always active during the light cycle and the VLPO is always active during sleep. Without an intermediate step, nocturnal animals could not sleep during the day.

The DMH receives projections from the SCN and sends projections to the VLPO. However, the DMH appears to do more than just relay signals from one nucleus to another. There are many factors that influence the sleep–wake cycle: hunger, stress, and sleep debt—not just the cycle of the sun. In turn, many physiologic functions are affected by the DMH: eating, temperature, and corticosteroid cycles, as well as sleep and arousal. The three-stage pathway allows greater integration of multiple factors and greater flexibility in behavioral response.

WHY DO WE SLEEP?

Life is competitive. However, when we sleep, we can neither advance our position nor protect ourselves or our families. From this perspective, sleep is a costly process. Therefore it must be important for us to pay such a high price. Allan Rechtschaffen put it nicely when he said, "If sleep doesn't serve an absolutely vital function, it is the biggest mistake evolution ever made."

A rat deprived of sleep will die faster than if deprived of food. Humans with fatal familial insomnia, an inherited disease that develops in middle age and results in degeneration of the thalamus, usually die within 24 months (although there may be other reasons for death). Humans forced to remain awake will pursue sleep with a vigor that rivals sex and food. When allowed to sleep, they will make up for the loss by sleeping deeper and longer—called *sleep rebound*. Clearly, something essential happens when we sleep, and most of us suffer when we are shortchanged. But what is this?

The primary proposals for the function of sleep fall into two groups: the *restorative* and the *information-processing*. Both theories sound important and are not mutually exclusive.

RESTORATIVE

It has been proposed that animals have a *homeostatic sleep drive*, which would be a second mechanism that works in synch with our circadian rhythm. It is postulated that there is some "vital energy" that needs to be restored each day—or inversely some "toxin" that needs to be cleared while we sleep for us to function effectively when awake. However, no one has identified a neural mechanism to explain the sleep drive—no depletion of a neuropeptide that needs to be restored or buildup of an annoying enzyme that needs to be removed. As yet, we can only postulate as to why animals not only need sleep but also become unconscious and vulnerable when in such a state.

Energy Conservation
Sleep may be a form of energy conservation across the 24-hour day, the way hibernation conserves energy through winter. An animal that is protected in a warm location minimizes the energy expenditure that will later need to be replaced. However, conserving energy does not explain the drive to sleep or sleep rebound.

Immune Function
Putting a patient to bed may be the oldest effective treatment offered by mothers and physicians. Although likely not the primary purpose of sleeping, there is substantial evidence that sleeping affects the immune system. We all know that we should sleep when fighting an infection: somehow sleep helps our immune system battle the invaders. Likewise, it is clear that our defenses are not as robust following sleep loss.

Reparative
Comparing sleep duration across species sheds some light on the function of sleep. One established relationship in biology is the inverse correlation between body mass and metabolic rate; that is, smaller animals have higher metabolic rates and a higher metabolic rate means greater metabolic activity in the brain. Greater activity in the brain means greater metabolic by-products. Small animals with higher metabolic rates tend to sleep longer. For example, bats and opossums sleep approximately 18 to 20 hours per day, whereas elephants sleep as little as 2 hours a night in short bursts—and (in one naturalistic study) did not sleep for 46 hours at a time roughly once a week.

A high metabolic rate results in increased oxidative stress produced from the mitochondria. Higher rates of oxidative stress have been linked to aging, arthritis, and dementia in the mouse. Sleep may be the time that the brain "cleans up" and repairs the damage that accumulated during the day.

Siegel et al. have shown that sleep deprivation in rats results in increased oxidative stress, which can be reversed with sleep. Additionally, they have shown tissue damage in the brain stem, hippocampus, and hypothalamus with sleep deprivation. Siegel believes that wakefulness produces a gradual toxic state that is corrected with sufficient sleep. Animals with a higher metabolic rate require greater sleep amounts to repair the more extensive wear and tear on their neurons during arousal.

Glymphatic System

In the body, the lymphatic system is a network of vessels that clear molecular debris and fight infection. Recently a system somewhat similar has been discovered in the brain. It is called *glymphatic* because of the glial channels that regulate fluid flow and its clearance function that is lymphaticlike. The system works when cerebrospinal fluid (CSF) moves from the arteries, through the glial channels on the blood–brain barrier, then through the brain tissue, and out the veins, taking molecular waste products in the flow. Nedergaard called this the "garbage truck of the brain."

Nedergaard speculated that the brain could not process information during the day at the same time it was collecting garbage, so to speak, that they likely occur at different times. Her laboratory has been able to show, by examining a live mouse awake and asleep, that more CSF flowed into the brain during sleep. They measured a 60% increase in the glial channels during sleep. Furthermore, they injected beta-amyloid proteins (infamously associated with Alzheimer's disease) into the mouse brains and showed they were cleared twice as fast during sleep. Some have referred to this function as a "nightly brain washing" and wonder if it is impaired in people who develop dementia.

INFORMATION PROCESSING

Development

Some have speculated that sleep serves to establish brain connections during the critical periods of development. For example, all the twitching that infants exhibit during sleep may serve to help babies get control of their muscles. If this theory is true, then it would explain why we sleep most when young and less as we age. Additionally, species that are more mature at birth (e.g., those that can thermoregulate and ambulate) have sleep durations close to adult levels.

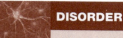

DISORDER

DREAM ENACTMENT

In the REM state the mind is active, but the body is virtually paralyzed. We dream, but we only move our eyes. Unfortunately, some people lose the ability to induce muscle paralysis—a condition called *REM sleep behavior disorder*. Often this condition precedes by many years the emergence of a neurodegenerative disorder such as Parkinson's disease.

Patients who fail to suppress muscle tone during REM sleep are condemned to act out their dreams. Such patients thrash about in bed and frequently hurt themselves or their partners. In some cases it even gets violent. In cats a similar condition has been elicited with small lesions of the pons just above the locus coeruleus. In humans it has been harder to find a specific lesion. It is presumed that some subtle disruption of the balance between atonic and motor generation may be occurring in the spinal cord, brain stem, or even higher cortical areas.

Frank and his group have conducted studies that suggest sleep enhances the plasticity of the developing cortex. We discussed the devastating effects that occluding an eye at critical periods has on normal development in Chapter 8, Plasticity and Adult Development. Frank and his group took this research one step further. They occluded an eye of 1-month-old cats for 6 hours. Then one group was allowed to sleep for 6 hours, and the other group was kept awake in darkness for an equal amount of time. Both groups were anesthetized, and their visual cortex was probed. Electrodes inserted almost parallel to the visual cortex recorded activity from different locations while a light shone in the cat's eyes.

The results are shown in Figure 15.12. Compare these results with the studies shown in Figure 8.13. Note that the cats that were allowed to sleep developed the typical pattern of unilateral ocular dominance. That is, the opened eye dominates the neurons in the visual cortex. The cats that did not sleep maintained a more even distribution of ocular dominance. This research suggests that the effects of occluding an eye are not fully processed until the animal is asleep; to put this in another way, the changes in the brain that develop with experience are imprinted during sleep.

Taken together, these observations suggest that sleep is a crucial ingredient for the developing brain. However, Siegel has noted an almost complete absence of sleep for dolphin mothers and

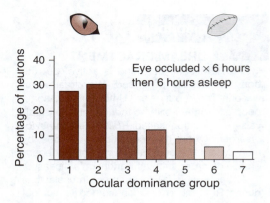

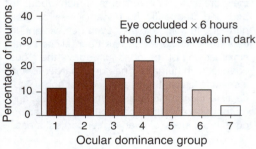

FIGURE 15.12 The effects of sleep and sleep deprivation on ocular dominance plasticity during the critical period of visual development in 1-month-old cats. (Adapted from Frank MG, Issa NP, Stryker MP. Sleep enhances plasticity in the developing visual cortex. *Neuron.* 2001;30[1]:275–287. Copyright 2001 with permission from Elsevier.)

their newborns after birth. The calf will gradually increase its sleep to adult amounts over a period of months. This is the opposite of what is seen with terrestrial mammals, which suggests that sleep is either not essential for normal development or dolphins have adapted alternative mechanisms.

Neurogenesis

A group at the University of California, Los Angeles (UCLA), examined the effects of sleep deprivation on neurogenesis. Adult rats were deprived of sleep for 4 days and then examined for new cells in the dentate gyrus of the hippocampus. There was a 68% reduction in new cells in the sleep-deprived group compared with the controls. Stress hormones did not mediate the change as the serum corticosterone levels were not significantly different in the two groups.

Memory Consolidation

The idea that sleep improves the consolidation of memories has been debated and studied for more than 80 years. There is still no consensus. The underlying hypothesis proposes that information acquired during the day is reviewed and strengthened during sleep. Many different experimental designs have shown that memory for procedures or the ability to recognize patterns improves after sleeping—or even just napping during the day. However, memories for facts (declarative memory) do not seem to improve with sleep. So, the relationship between sleep and memory may depend on the material learned.

It was discovered in the 1970s that some neurons in the rat hippocampus fire when the animal is in a specific location or moving toward that location. These cells were called *place cells.* It was subsequently shown that specific patterns of activity by the place cells during the day were reactivated during non-REM sleep that night. That is, the synchronicity established between hippocampal cells and cortical neurons when the rat is running from place to place is repeated again when the animal sleeps. This suggests that the hippocampus revisits the events of the day "off-line" and possibly orchestrates the consolidation of memories to long-term cortical stores.

Pierre Maquet et al. in Belgium has taken this one step further and used functional imaging studies to look at the activity in the human hippocampus the night after learning a new task. Participants were instructed to memorize the route through a complicated virtual town. It was observed that regions of the hippocampus that were active during the task were reactivated during subsequent non-REM sleep. Of particular interest, everyone improved on the task the following day. However, those with the greatest activity expressed during SWS also showed the greatest improvement navigating the virtual town the following day (Figure 15.13).

Pruning

We know the brain is continuously remodeling and changing—way more than we ever imagined. It is reasonable that these changes continue while we sleep but may serve a different purpose. Work from the University of Wisconsin by Tononi and Cirelli has produced studies with mice that suggest we sleep to forget... sort of.

First, let's remember that the ability to adapt to a changing environment (or worse, a new operating system) requires a mechanism for the brain to change—which we believe is embodied in spine formation and elimination. In 2011, Tononi and Cirelli's laboratory literally cut a window in the brains of mice and observed synaptogenesis and pruning of spines on the same neuron when awake and asleep. With painstaking analysis, they found that the spines are growing and shrinking all the time. However, there is a net gain of cortical spines

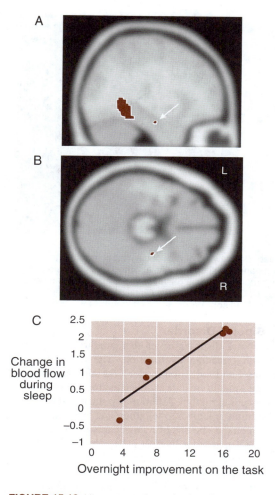

FIGURE 15.13 Hippocampal reactivation during non–rapid eye movement sleep and memory consolidation. The sagittal **(A)** and horizontal **(B)** sections show the areas of the right hippocampus that were reactivated during sleep and correlated with improved scores on the task **(C)**. (Adapted from Peigneux P, Laureys S, Fuchs S, et al. Are spatial memories strengthened in the human hippocampus during slow wave sleep? *Neuron.* 2004;44[3]:535–545. Copyright 2004 with permission from Elsevier.)

during waking hours and a net loss during sleep. Figure 15.14A shows the loss of a spine after 6 to 8 hours of sleep. It appears that the number of spines (which correlates with the number of synapses) increases when we are waking and learning but decreases when we sleep. The researchers make an important point: the overall spine density remains the same. That is, we cannot build new connections without removing some. We have to make space in the closet for new items, if you will.

In a follow-up study, this research group observed almost 7,000 synapses in mouse motor and sensory neurons while asleep and awake. They measured the synaptic connections and discovered an almost 20% shrinkage in the connection at the synapse between spines and the terminal axon synapse after sleeping (Figure 15.14B). However, this was only observed in the smaller, thinner spines and spared in the larger ones. Tononi and Cirelli call this "smart forgetting." Figure 15.14C is a 3D electron micrograph of a dendrite that shows small and large spines. The authors believe we strengthen synaptic connections during the day through experience but weaken and even remove irrelevant connections as a way to maintain homeostasis in the brain.

In conclusion, sleep appears to serve a number of functions none of which explains the irresistible urge to lie down on a couch after a heinous night on call. And furthermore, why do we have to be unconscious when we sleep?

MOOD DISORDERS

There is a long-standing suspicion that mood disorders are initiated or at least maintained by circadian dysfunction. Several lines of evidence suggest this to be true for depression. For example:

1. Depression has a diurnal variation—worse in the morning.
2. Insomnia is one of the most common complaints.
3. Insomnia resolves with effective treatment.
4. Sleep deprivation is an effective, although short-lived, antidepressant.

Seasonal Affective Disorder

Seasonal affective disorder (SAD), also called *winter depression*, is most suggestive of circadian changes affecting mood. Many mammals display seasonal fluctuations in behavior that are regulated by the change in day length. Hibernation may be the extreme form of this seasonal change. Humans with SAD develop symptoms of depression in the winter, along with weight gain, increased sleep, and decreased activity. This array of symptoms resembles changes seen in animals preparing to hibernate.

The changes in daylight hours are transmitted from the retina to the SCN. The SCN activates the paraventricular nucleus of the hypothalamus, which indirectly (by way of the sympathetic nervous system) inhibits the pineal gland. When the SCN is inactive during darkness, the inhibition is reduced, and the pineal gland secretes melatonin. In other words, melatonin is secreted during the night when the "brakes" are off. The duration of

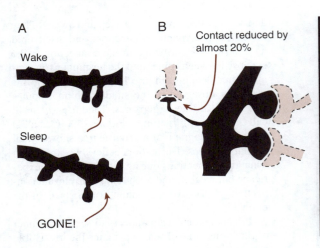

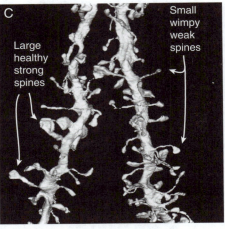

FIGURE 15.14 A: The loss of a spine after a period of sleep. **B:** Drawing of reduced synaptic contact in small spines after sleep. **C:** 3D electron micrograph showing large and small spines. (**A:** Adapted by permission from Macmillan Publishers Ltd. Maret S, et al. Sleep and waking modulate spine turnover in the adolescent mouse cortex. *Nat Neurosci*. 2011;11:1418–1420. Copyright 2011. **C:** Courtesy of Chiara Cirelli, Wisconsin Center for Sleep and Consciousness, University of Wisconsin-Madison, Madison, WI.)

elevated nightly melatonin provides every tissue with information about the time of day and time of year. Some have called the pineal gland both a *clock* and a *calendar*. For example, animals that hibernate, such as the Syrian hamster, produce more melatonin in winter and less in summer.

Analysis of melatonin secretion in 55 patients with SAD in summer and winter found that patients with SAD had nocturnal secretion of melatonin longer in winter than in summer but with no seasonal change for the healthy volunteers. Other research has found that early morning light therapy for patients with SAD improved their mood and produced phase advances of the melatonin rhythm. In total, these results suggest that the neural circuits that mediate season change in mammals may be impaired in patients with SAD.

Bipolar Disorder

Bipolar disorder is another condition associated with circadian dysfunction. The delay in sleep onset and reduction in sleep duration accompanying a manic episode are clear examples of disrupted circadian rhythm. Additionally, the mood stabilizer lithium is known to lengthen the circadian period, which may be one of its mechanisms of action.

Of particular interest is the predictive value of sleep disruption and mania. It is well known that a decreasing need to sleep can precede a manic episode. Wehr et al. believe that individuals with bipolar disorder are predisposed to exacerbations of the illness when sleep deprived. Because manic behavior interferes with sleep and sleep deprivation makes mania worse, a vicious downward cycle can be established. They describe a highly educated, successful individual who developed

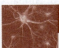

DISORDER

HYPERAROUSAL

Trouble in sleeping is a common complaint. Some patients cannot turn off the arousal networks at bedtime. Patients with anxiety disorders, attention deficit hyperactivity disorder, and hyperthymic temperament will often complain that they cannot stop thinking when trying to sleep. Patients who abuse alcohol, opioids, and marijuana often use the substance as a hypnotic and frequently show rebound insomnia when substance free. Furthermore,

insomnia is a risk factor for relapse with recovered alcoholics.

A neuroimaging study of patients with insomnia showed greater global cerebral metabolism while awake and asleep compared with controls. Additionally, the patients showed a smaller decline in relative metabolism from waking to sleep states in some of the structures discussed earlier, for example, ascending reticular activating system and hypothalamus.

bipolar disorder in his mid-40s. Despite aggressive pharmacologic management, he cycled between depression and mania every 6 to 8 weeks. He also showed great fluctuations in his sleep–wake phases across these cycles.

The clinicians interupted the cycling by encouraging the subject to remain at bed rest in a dark room for 14 hours each night. This was later tapered to 10 hours per night. Remarkably, his mood and sleep stabilized. Periods of hyperactivity and hypoactivity were greatly reduced. The effects were still present after 1 year. It is worth noting that he remained on divalproex sodium and sertraline. The authors believe that "dark therapy" synchronized and stabilized the circadian rhythms. Subsequently a randomized controlled study showed positive results but is not an easy treatment to coordinate.

More recently a group in Norway has been studying blue-blocking glasses (also called orange-tinted glasses). This treatment is based on the finding that blue light–sensitive photoreceptors in the eye are responsible for communicating with the master clock: the SCN. Blocking blue light inhibits signals to the SCN, which creates virtual darkness in the brain, synchronizes circadian rhythms, and restores normal melatonin levels. A small randomized placebo-controlled trial found that the addition of blue-blocking glasses to usual care was significantly more effective at reducing manic symptoms than usual care and placebo.

Treating Insomnia

Insomnia is generally a long-term problem. Hypnotic medications are not without risk. Nonpharmacologic interventions, such as cognitive behavior therapy (CBT) and stimulus control, are as effective as medications, show enduring benefits, and have no side effects. The American College of Physicians now recommends CBT should be the first-line interventions, particularly for the young and middle aged.

The evolution of sleep medications is a story of searching for agents with shorter duration, more specific mechanisms of action, and less potential for abuse. Alcohol is perhaps the oldest sleep medicine. Chloral hydrate, first synthesized in 1832, was the first medication specifically indicated for insomnia. The development of barbiturates in the early 1900s brought a new class of agents that were widely used for 50 years. The introduction of benzodiazepines in the 1960s provided a treatment that was effective and safer.

As shown in Figure 5.3, benzodiazepines work by sensitizing the γ-aminobutyric acid (GABA) receptor, which in turn increases the movement of negatively charged chloride ions into the cell and ultimately enhances the activity of the GABA neurons. More GABA activity means more inhibition of the central nervous system.

There are two benzodiazepine receptor subtypes on the GABA receptor. The traditional benzodiazepines bind to both, but the newer agents (zolpidem, zaleplon, and eszopiclone) bind to just one subunit. This subunit mediates the sedating and amnesic effects, but not the anxiolytic, or myorelaxation. Whether this selective binding translates into fewer side effects remains to be determined. The newest sleep aid is suvorexant that works by inhibiting the wakefulness-promoting orexin neurons. This is an entirely new mechanism of action for treatment of insomnia, and it remains to be seen how this fits in with the other treatments.

The chronic use of sleep aids for insomnia remains controversial. Some epidemiologic data have documented increased mortality with chronic hypnotic use, presumably due to residual cognitive impairment the following day. Fortunately, a placebo-controlled study with eszopiclone demonstrated enduring benefits for sleep and improved functional status during the day for the 6 months of the trial. However, many patients, once started on a sleeping pill, will take something for years. We still do not know if such treatment is beneficial in the long run.

QUESTIONS

1. Which do you typically see in stage 2 of sleep?
   a. Sleep spindles.
   b. Alpha waves.
   c. Delta activity.
   d. Slow wave sleep.

2. REM latency is decreased in all of the following except
   a. Depression.
   b. Generalized anxiety.
   c. Narcolepsy.
   d. Sleep apnea.

3. Which of the following is true?
   a. The average length of sleep is 8 hours/night.
   b. The deepest sleep occurs in the latter third of the night.
   c. Muscle tone increases during REM sleep.
   d. PET scans show decreased cerebral blood flow during SWS.

4. Which of the following is true about dolphin sleep?
   a. They never show REM sleep.
   b. New born calves sleep the most during the neonatal period.
   c. They close their eyes and navigate by echolocation.
   d. They sleep on the surface, so they can breathe.

5. All of the following are true regarding sleep and aging except
   a. We sleep less as we age.
   b. Arousal after sleep onset increases with age.
   c. REM sleep increases in the latter part of life.
   d. SWS decreases with aging.

6. Which of the following is active during the night in humans?
   a. The SCN.
   b. Orexin neurons.
   c. The VLPO.
   d. Tuberomammillary nucleus.

7. Which of the following systems is active during arousal and REM sleep?
   a. Noradrenergic.
   b. Dopaminergic.
   c. Histaminergic.
   d. Cholinergic.

8. Possible functions for sleep include all of the following expect
   a. Memory consolidation.
   b. Energy conversation.
   c. Neurotransmitter reaccumulation.
   d. Metabolic restoration.

See Answers section at the end of this book.

CHAPTER 16

Sex and the Brain

SEXUAL DIMORPHISM

Humans are sexually dimorphic (*di*, "two"; *morph*, "type"). That is, we come in two styles. How one conceptualizes these differences depends on one's perspective. Table 16.1 summarizes the major categories of sexual dimorphism. In this chapter, we will focus on how the hormones change the morphology of the brain and how this affects behavior and sexuality.

Pink and Blue

In general, men and women behave differently and enjoy different activities. The etiology of this difference remains a hotly debated topic. Is it nature or nurture—genetic or environmental? With humans, it is almost impossible to tease out these opposing causes. The signals a baby receives about its sexual identity start early—in the nursery. Typically, boys favor construction and transportation toys. Girls show less rough physical play and prefer toys such as dolls. Is this a product of learned gender social roles or something more innately wired in the brain?

A study with vervet monkeys suggests that the choices of toys children make to play with are more ingrained than some might think. Monkeys in large cages at the Los Angeles (UCLA) Primate Laboratory, University of California, were allowed 5 minutes of exposure to individual toys classified as "masculine" (police car and ball) or "feminine" (doll and pot). The amount of time they were in direct contact with each of the toys was recorded. Figure 16.1 shows a female monkey and a male monkey playing with the toys and the percent time that each gender spent in contact with the toys. These results show that even nonhuman primates, who are not exposed to social pressure regarding toy preference, will choose gender-specific toys. (Although why a pot would be feminine for a monkey who's never seen a kitchen remains a mystery to us.)

If we remember the important role of pleasure in determining behavioral preferences, we can speculate that the monkeys spend more time with the toys they enjoy. Likewise, we can speculate that the association between an object and pleasure is hardwired in the brain. Furthermore, some of this "wiring" must have arisen early in human evolution before the emergence of our hominid ancestors.

The Boy Who Was Raised as a Girl

One of the more remarkable stories of sexually dimorphic behavior involves a tragic story of a boy raised as a girl. David was 8 months old in 1966 when his entire penis was accidentally burned beyond repair during a routine circumcision. Dr John Money, a psychologist at Johns Hopkins Hospital with an expertise in sexual reassignment, convinced the family to proceed with surgical sex change and raise the boy as a girl. Dr Money believed that sexual identity/orientation developed after 18 months of age and children could adapt to a new sexual identity if the procedure was started early enough. David provided an ideal case study as he had an identical twin brother with a normal penis.

Amazingly, Dr Money reported in the medical literature that the reassignment was a success, but it was in actuality a disaster. David, whose name was changed to Brenda, did not want to wear dresses or play with dolls. She preferred to play with guns and cars. She could beat up her brother and throw a ball like a boy. Worst of all, this unusual behavior was not well received at school. She was relentlessly teased for her masculine traits. Brenda was shunned by the girls and not accepted by the boys.

By the time Brenda was 14 years old, she was still unaware of the sexual reassignment and remained distressed. A local psychiatrist who was treating Brenda convinced the parents to reveal the truth. Brenda

TABLE 16.1

Different Ways of Conceptualizing Sexual Dimorphism

Perspective	Example
Chromosomal	XX, XY
Gonadal	Ovaries, testes
Hormonal	Estrogen, androgens
Morphologic	Genitalia, body size, body shape
Behavioral	Nurturing, aggressive, hunter, gatherer, etc.
Sexual	Identity, orientation, preference

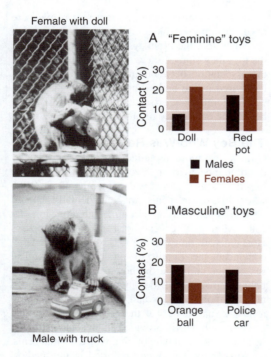

Female with doll

A "Feminine" toys

Male with truck

B "Masculine" toys

FIGURE 16.1 Female vervet monkeys spent more time in contact with "feminine" toys **(A)**, whereas males spent more time with "masculine" toys **(B)**. (From Alexander GM, Hines M. Sex differences in response to children's toys in nonhuman primates [*Cercopithecus aethiops sabaeus*]. *Evol Hum Behav*. 2002;23[6]:467–479. Copyright 2002 with permission from Elsevier.)

recalls her reaction, "Suddenly it all made sense why I felt the way I did. I wasn't some sort of weirdo."

David immediately decided to revert to his genetic sex. Within several months he began going out in public as a boy. He stopped estrogen and started testosterone. He had bilateral mastectomies and several

operations to rebuild male genitalia. In his 20s he married, but was unable to have children. Worse, he battled with depression and the demons from this childhood experience. In May 2005, at the age of 38 he killed himself.

The significant point about this case is that in spite of being raised as a girl, estrogen hormones, and the absence of testosterone, David continued to have male pattern psychosocial and psychosexual development. Larger case studies are consistent with David's experience. One analysis of XY individuals assigned female roles at birth because of a severe pelvic defect (cloacal exstrophy) found that all showed masculine tendencies. Slightly more than half chose to declare themselves male when older. These studies suggest that something durable happens in utero that determines sexual identity/orientation.

Environment

It would be naive to dismiss the significance of environment on sexually stereotypical behaviors. History is replete with examples of men and women showing varying amounts of masculine and feminine behavior that are clearly molded by shifts in social norms. Kim Wallen reviewed 30 years of research with rhesus monkeys and attempted to separate hormonal and social influences. For example, rough-and-tumble play is one of the most robust sexually dimorphic behaviors. Juvenile males wrestle more frequently than females in almost every rearing condition. However, if reared in a group with only males, the males actually engage in less rough-and-tumble play (suggesting that the presence of females stimulates males to play). Likewise, mounting behavior is seen more with males than females. However, when reared in isolated, same-sex environments, males display less mounting while females display more.

Rust et al. looked at gender development in preschool children and the effect of an older sibling. They discovered that having an older brother was associated with greater masculine and less feminine behavior in boys and girls. However, boys with older sisters were more feminine but not less masculine, whereas girls with older sisters were less masculine but not more feminine.

Together, these studies suggest interplay between hormones and the environment. That is, biologic factors predispose individuals to engage in specific behaviors, which can be modified by social experience.

HORMONES

Figure 14.7 showed the classic experiment by Berthold who was the first to establish that the testes contain a substance that controls the development of male secondary sexual characteristics. In Chapter 7, Hormones and the Brain, we discussed the relationship between the cortex, hypothalamus, pituitary gland, and end organ. Briefly, with input from the cortex, the hypothalamus produces gonadotropin-releasing hormone (GnRH), which in turn stimulates the anterior pituitary gland to produce luteinizing hormone (LH) and follicle-stimulating hormone (FSH). LH and FSH stimulate the gonads to produce the sex hormones.

GONADS

The gonads (ovaries and testes) serve two major functions. First, they produce eggs or sperms to pass on DNA to the next generation. Second, they produce the sex hormones that not only promote the development of secondary sexual characteristics but also drive the behavior that increases the chances of an egg and sperm meeting.

Cholesterol is the precursor of all steroid hormones. Figure 7.7 shows the three major steroids synthesized from cholesterol: glucocorticoids, mineralocorticoids, and the sex steroids. The sex steroids are synthesized in the adrenals or gonads. Because the steroid hormones are lipid soluble and can easily pass through the cell walls, they are released as they are synthesized.

Testosterone, as shown in Figure 16.2, is converted into 17β-estradiol (E2) and an androgen, 5α-dihydrotestosterone. (An androgen is a generic term for a hormone that stimulates or maintains male characteristics.) Amazingly, much of the androgen effects in the brain are actually implemented by E2. For example, an injection of estrogen to a newborn rat is more masculinizing than an injection of testosterone.

Why do the maternal estrogens not masculinize all fetuses? One of the functions of α-fetoprotein during pregnancy is to bind with maternal estrogens, which are then cleared through the placenta. This protein, which does not bind testosterone effectively, prevents estrogens from reaching the brain.

We have discussed in other chapters how the sex steroids can work directly on synaptic receptors or indirectly through gene transcription (see Figures 5.3, 7.1, and 7.3). These different effects are summarized in Figure 16.3. The direct effects are fast, whereas the indirect effects take longer to transpire. Because the sex hormones can influence neural function, they are sometimes called *neurosteroids* in neuroscience literature.

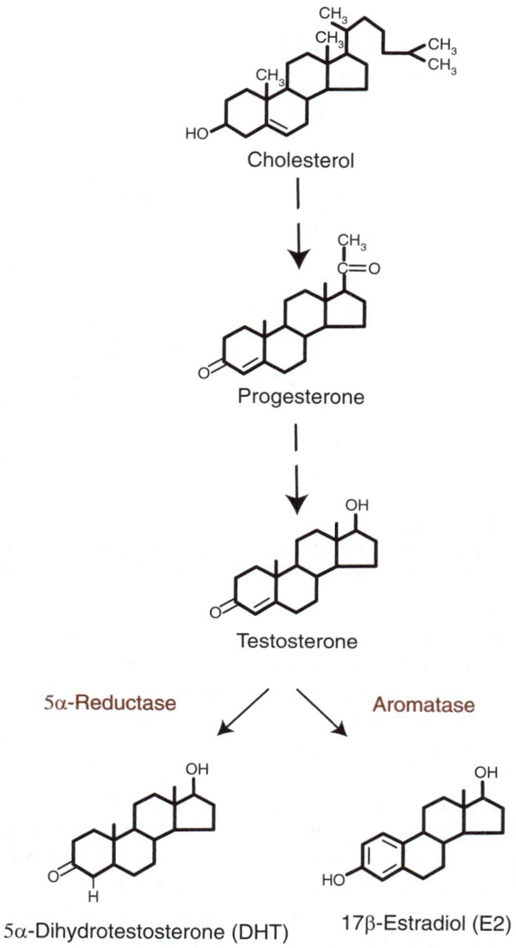

FIGURE 16.2 The sex hormones are synthesized from cholesterol. Testosterone serves as a prohormone for 17β-estradiol.

Differentiation and Activation

The development of sexual dimorphism is dependent on the sex hormones. The presence of testosterone at critical periods of time both masculinizes and defeminizes the brain. Likewise, the absence of testosterone feminizes and demasculinizes the brain. William C. Young et al. published in 1959 a classic paper that rivals Berthold's work with roosters in helping us understand the fundamental principles of hormones and behavior.

To understand Young's study, it is important to be aware of the different sexual postures males and females display at appropriate times. Female rodents will stand immobile and arch their backs: *lordosis*. Males will *mount* such a receptive female. Females and males rarely (although not completely) exhibit the opposite behavior. Researchers use the presence or absence of lordosis and mounting as expressions of sexual behavior. For example, castration of a

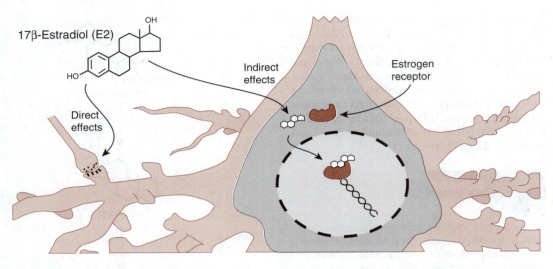

17β-Estradiol (E2)

Indirect effects

Estrogen receptor

Direct effects

FIGURE 16.3 Steroids can directly affect transmitter synthesis/release or postsynaptic transmitter receptors. They can also indirectly influence gene transcription. (Adapted from Bear MF, Connors BW, Paradiso MA, eds. *Neuroscience: Exploring the Brain*. 4th ed. Baltimore: Lippincott Williams & Wilkins; 2015.)

male stops his mounting behavior. But this can be reinstated with injections of testosterone.

Young's group sought to understand the effects of early and late exposure to sex hormones on sexual behavior. Their experiment, which is shown in Figure 16.4, started with injecting testosterone in a pregnant female guinea pig. Their first observation (not shown in the figure) was that female pups exposed to high doses of androgens in utero were born with masculinized external genitalia.

The rest of the study focused on the female pups, which were allowed to mature and were then spayed. Later they were all given estrogen and progesterone to stimulate female sexual behavior. Each was paired with a normal male guinea pig. Some time later, the procedure was reversed. All were injected with testosterone and paired with a receptive female. The results were striking. The females exposed to testosterone in utero failed to display lordosis when given estrogen and progesterone. However, they would mount other females when given testosterone. The control group displayed the opposite behavior.

This elegant experiment established a clear distinction between the differentiating effects of sex hormones during development and the activating effects during adulthood. The females exposed to testosterone in utero had alterations in the organization of their brains that prevented the normal activation by female sex hormones as an adult.

Human Congenital Anomalies

Occasionally, people are born with genetic alterations that give us insight into the differentiation and activation of human sexual dimorphism. One such condition is *congenital adrenal hyperplasia*.

Children with this condition are exposed to excessive androgens because of overactive fetal adrenal glands. Paradoxically, the condition is caused by an impaired ability of the fetal adrenal gland to produce cortisol. Because the pituitary fails to receive the appropriate negative feedback, it continues to secrete adrenocorticotropic hormone (ACTH), which in turn induces hyperplasia of the androgen-producing cells of the adrenal cortex.

As we might predict from Young's studies with guinea pigs, human males are unaffected by the exposure to excess adrenal androgens in utero. Females, on the other hand, are born with masculinized external genitalia. Additionally, the females tend to exhibit more rough-and-tumble play as children. As adults, they have an increased tendency to prefer other females as partners.

An extraordinary condition in men provides a different example of anomalous sexual development. *Androgen insensitivity syndrome* (AIS) is a condition in which XY (male) individuals are born as normal-appearing females. The problem is caused by a mutation in the androgen receptor. These individuals produce testosterone, but the cells are unable to recognize it. Consequently, there is no activation of the genes necessary for male characteristics.

These individuals are born looking like normal little girls and are raised as such (Figure 16.5). Typically, the problem is only recognized when they fail to menstruate in adolescence. Unfortunately, they are unable to conceive as they have failed to develop uteri, fallopian tubes, and ovaries. However, their behavior is

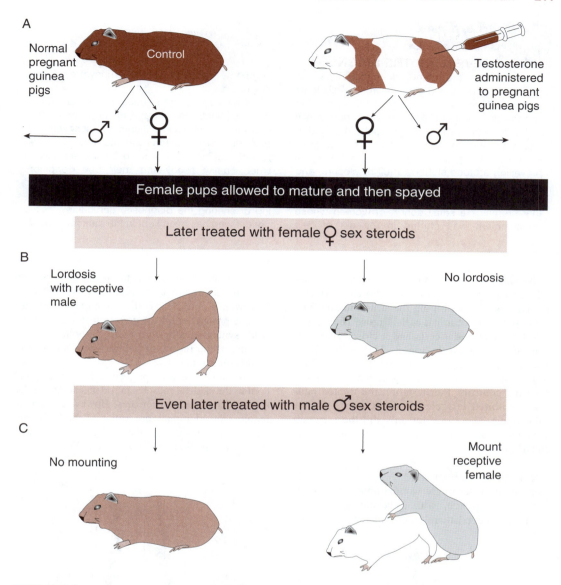

FIGURE 16.4 Guinea pigs exposed to testosterone in utero **(A)** fail to show feminine sexual behavior **(B)** when given female sex hormones and instead act like males **(C)** when given testosterone.

unequivocally feminine. Hines et al. examined the psychological development of 22 XY individuals with complete AIS compared with 22 XX normal controls and found no differences on any measure of psychological outcome. They concluded that these results argue against the need for ovaries and two X chromosomes in the development of traditional feminine behavior. Likewise, it reinforces the importance of the androgen receptor in masculine development. It is an interesting thought that all humans (both men and women) would develop into women unless other hormones intervene. The default model for mankind is a woman!

NEURONAL CIRCUITRY

Nerve Growth

Gonadal steroids grow more than just testes and breasts—they also cause selective neuronal growth. As shown in Figure 16.3, gonadal steroids stimulate gene expression through the androgen and estrogen receptors. These receptors, once bound with the hormone, also function as transcription factors, which, in turn, stimulate gene transcription and protein synthesis. Ultimately, the gonadal steroids can affect nerve volume, dendritic length, spine density, and synaptic connectivity.

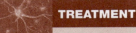

TREATMENT

REVEALING THE DIAGNOSIS

In the 1950s the standard practice was to withhold the actual diagnosis from individuals with AIS. They were told that childbearing was impossible but not told they were genetically male. It was believed that such information would produce psychiatric disorders and possibly even thoughts of suicide. In the 1990s the prevailing attitude shifted to full disclosure, and now it is the standard practice to reveal all the details to patients with this disorder. However, there remains a small cohort of women whose management was started in the era of less autonomy and who are still unaware of their diagnosis.

Many patients can sense when the truth is being withheld. In this age of the Internet, it is possible for curious patients to discover their own diagnosis. Some patients have avoided further medical care or even committed suicide when finally discovering their true condition. When confronted with such a patient, clinicians struggle with the appropriate manner and timing of sharing the diagnosis, particularly with a patient who has been kept in the dark for so long.

Woolley et al. demonstrated this effect by administering estradiol or placebo to ovariectomized rats and examining the structure and function of the hippocampal cells. Figure 16.6 shows two CA1 pyramidal cells and a closer examination of their dendritic spines. The estradiol-exposed neurons had 22% more spines and 30% more *N*-methyl-D-aspartate glutamate receptors than the controls. Furthermore, the treated neurons exhibited less electrical resistance to cellular input. Therefore not only did the estrogen change the structure of the neuron but also the function.

Growth Factor Proteins

The astute reader might wonder about the role of growth factor proteins with sex hormones and nerve plasticity. Indeed there is considerable evidence linking gonadal steroids with growth factors such as brain-derived neurotrophic factors (BDNFs). However, it is unclear if the sex hormones stimulate the production of the growth factor protein, or work synergistically with them, or both. A study looking at the rat motor neuron sheds some light on this question.

The motor neurons projecting from the spinal cord to the skeletal muscles in rodents are generally similar for males and females. However, the male requires the additional innervation of the *bulbocavernosus* muscles around the penis, which are necessary for erections and copulation (Figure 16.7).

FIGURE 16.5 This person with complete androgen insensitivity syndrome has an XY genotype but has developed unambiguous feminine characteristics. (Courtesy of John Money.)

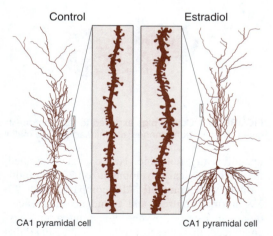

Control   Estradiol

CA1 pyramidal cell   CA1 pyramidal cell

FIGURE 16.6 Ovariectomized rats treated with estradiol display greater spine formation on CA1 pyramidal cells from the hippocampus. (Data from Woolley CS, Weiland NG, McEwen BS, et al. Estradiol increases the sensitivity of hippocampal CA1 pyramidal cells to NMDA receptor-mediated synaptic input: correlation with dendritic spine density. *J Neurosci*. 1997;17[5]:1848–1859.)

A

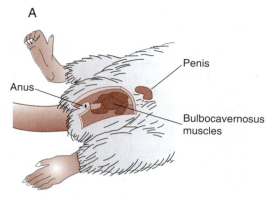

Penis

Anus

Bulbocavernosus muscles

B   Cross section of lumbar spinal cord
Female   Male

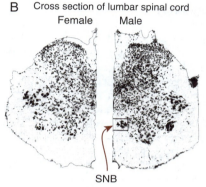

SNB

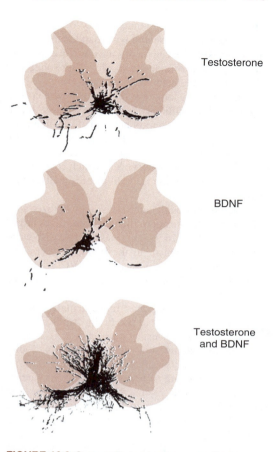

Testosterone

BDNF

Testosterone and BDNF

FIGURE 16.7 A: The male rat has bulbocavernosus muscles that are needed to control the penis for copulation. **B:** Cross sections of the female and male lumbar spinal cord show the presence of the spinal nucleus of the bulbocavernosus (SNB) for the male but not the female. (**A:** Data from Breedlove SM, Arnold AP. Hormonal control of a developing neuromuscular system. II. Sensitive periods for the androgen-induced masculinization of the rat SNB. *J Neurosci.* 1983;3[2]:424–432.)

FIGURE 16.8 Composite lumbar cross sections showing the extent of spinal nucleus of the bulbocavernosus motor neurons that remain 1 month after surgical excision. Testosterone plus brain-derived neurotrophic factor (BDNF) preserved more of the motor neurons than either alone. (Adapted from Yang LY, Verhovshek T, Sengelaub DR. BDNF and androgen interact in the maintenance of dendritic morphology in a sexually dimorphic rat spinal nucleus. *Endocrinology.* 2004;145[1]:161–168, by permission of Oxford University Press.)

Consequently, the motor neurons in the lumbar region of the spinal cord of the male rat (collectively called the *spinal nucleus of the bulbocavernosus* [SNB]) are approximately four times larger than those in the female. These motor neurons regress in the female shortly after birth. Similar regression occurs with castrated males, although androgen treatment will preserve the motor neurons.

The dendrites of the motor neurons have extensive branching that makes connections spanning several spinal segments. Cutting the SNB motor neurons results in regression of the dendrites. Previous research has shown that testosterone or BDNF can limit the dendritic regression.

Yang et al. took this a step further. They cut the SNB motor neurons in castrated males. Then they put BDNF over the cut axons or administered testosterone, or both, in different groups of rats. A

month later the motor neurons were injected with a marker that allows visualization of the dendrites and axons after the animal is sacrificed. Figure 16.8 shows computer-generated composite sections marking the presence of the SNB motor neurons for the three groups of rats. The BDNF plus testosterone group preserved substantially more dendritic branching than seen with either alone (similar to what would be seen in a normal control). This suggests that BDNF and testosterone act synergistically to maintain the SNB motor neuron morphology.

Songbirds

The study of the sexually dimorphic brain structures of the songbirds is one of the great discoveries of neuroscience—one that transformed our recognition of the dynamic quality of the brain. The leader in this research is Fernando Nottebohm at the Rockefeller University in New York. He and others wanted to understand why male songbirds sing and females seldom do.

They initially looked at the syrinx (vocal cords) trying to find differences, without success. Later they focused on the neuronal mechanisms that control singing: the high vocal center (HVC), robust nucleus (RA), and area X. These nuclei send projections to the cranial nerve XII, which controls the syrinx. Lesions of the HVC bilaterally will silence a bird.

The breakthrough came when they realized that the song nuclei are approximately three times larger in males (Figure 16.9). This was the first discovery of sexual dimorphism in the brain. Furthermore, they showed that the size of the HVC correlates with the number of song syllables a male canary sings.

Their next finding has fundamentally altered the way we think about the brain. Adult canaries change their songs every year, which is accomplished by adding new syllable types and discarding others. Remarkably, this occurs through the birth and death of neurons in the song nuclei. Nottebohm et al. were the first to show that working neurons develop in adult warm-blooded vertebrates—an idea that received a cool reception when first presented in 1984.

The reason to discuss this topic in the current chapter is the fact that much of the differences in the male canaries' nuclei and song production are controlled by testosterone. Evidence to support this includes the following:

1. The nuclei of the adult song system have high concentrations of testosterone.
2. Adult males with higher testosterone sing more than the adults with less testosterone.
3. Females given testosterone will sing more and show increased volume of their HVC and RA.
4. Drops in testosterone levels at the end of the breeding season correspond with the death of HVC neurons.

Pregnancy

"During pregnancy, there are unparalleled surges of sex steroid hormones, including, for instance, an increase in progesterone of 10- to 15-fold relative to luteal phase levels and a flood of estrogens that typically exceeds the estrogen exposure of a woman's entire nonpregnant life." This hormonal deluge leads to well-known physical changes, but what effect does it have on the brain? Animal studies have shown a number of neural changes, which appear to persist beyond the pregnancy. In Chapter 8, Plasticity and Adult Development, we discussed the remarkable changes that occur in the adolescent brain as a result of the initiation of sex hormone production. We believe the teen brain is cleaned up and refined to make it more efficient, which ultimately leads to a shrinking of the now more specialized gray matter.

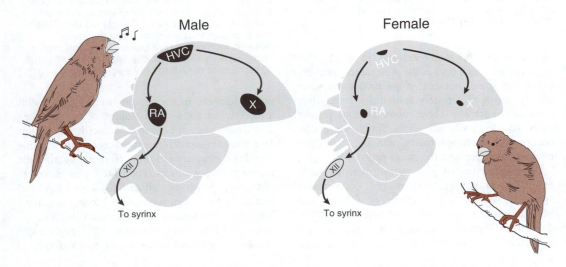

FIGURE 16.9 The difference in the song nuclei in canaries explains why males sing but females rarely do. HVC, high vocal center; RA, robust nucleus. (Adapted from Nottebohm F. [2004.] The road we travelled: discovery, choreography, and significance of brain replaceable neurons. *Ann N Y Acad Sci*. 1016:628–658.)

A research team at the University of Barcelona performed brain scans on first-time mothers before and after pregnancy and compared them with a nulliparous control group (not borne offspring) and fathers. They found that pregnancy resulted in significant reductions in gray matter in parts of the frontal, temporal, and parietal lobes. Remarkably, the changes were so unique and substantial that the researchers were able to separate the new mothers from the nulliparous based on their MRI scans. Furthermore, gray matter changes correlated with psychological measures of mother–infant attachment. (It seems perplexing that gray matter reduction would *enhance* anything, but this is probably an example of improved efficiency—sort of like exercising and losing weight.) In follow-up studies they also showed that the same regions of gray matter loss lit up in fMRI scans when the mothers looked at pictures of their child. Finally, repeated scans 2 years after delivery showed that the gray matter changes remained.

Taken together, these results suggest the pregnant brain undergoes remodeling and refinement to better handle the new role of mothering an infant—a finding that is consistent with an evolutionary perspective on what is best for infant survival. By the way, the father's brain did not change at all, but no one was amazed.

SEXUAL INTEREST

Although most people have sexual interest directed toward age-appropriate members of the opposite sex of the same species, not everyone does. It is generally believed that one's sexual focus is something we are born with ("hardwired"), not something we develop through life experiences. The race is on to identify the variants in the brain that explain differences in sexual orientation and identity. A good place to start is the hypothalamus.

The hypothalamus is instrumental in regulating the release of sex hormones. Specifically, the anterior aspect of the hypothalamus is known to control a wide variety of mating behaviors: desire, sexual behavior, and parenting. Lesions in this area can lead to alterations in sexual behavior. The *preoptic area* (POA) in the rat is an area where significant differences between the sexes are found (see Figure 2.9). In the male rat the POA is five to seven times larger than that in the female. The difference is so prominent that it can be accurately identified with the naked eye. This region of the POA is called the *sexually dimorphic nucleus of the preoptic area* (SDN-POA). Female rats given androgens will develop an SDN-POA approximately the size of that of a male. As with the SNB motor neurons, it appears that the androgens preserve the nerve cells, which otherwise waste away.

Humans

Allen et al. examined the anterior aspect of the hypothalamus in a postmortem analysis of 22 human brains: half of each sex. They focused their attention on an area that is the human equivalent of the rat SDN-POA. They identified four cell groupings within the anterior hypothalamus, which they called the *interstitial nuclei of the anterior hypothalamus* (INAH). They numbered the INAH from 1 to 4 and reported that INAH-2 and INAH-3 are approximately twice as large in males compared with females. Figure 16.10 shows actual comparative micrographs through the INAH of males and females—the differences are subtle.

Homosexual Males

Simon LeVay took this work one step further and compared the INAH for females, heterosexual males, and homosexual males. He confirmed the work by Allen et al. that is, two of the four interstitial nuclei are sexually dimorphic. However, even more interesting, he found that INAH-3 was twice as large in heterosexual men as it was in homosexual men. Although this provides compelling evidence that sexual orientation is "hardwired," we must be cautious for there could be other explanations. For example, almost all of the homosexual men died of AIDS, whereas only approximately one-third of the heterosexual men did. Likewise, there was considerable overlap in the size of the nuclei between groups, implying that it is impossible to predict the sexual orientation of any individual based on the measurement of his INAH-3.

Other researchers have addressed this topic in different species. Approximately 8% of the domestic male sheep display sexual preference for other males. A group in Oregon identified a cluster of cells within the POA of the anterior hypothalamus (analogues to the INAH) that is significantly larger in rams than ewes. They compared these nuclei for rams with different sexual preferences and found they were twice as large in heterosexual rams as it was in homosexual rams. Hence, an animal model that is consistent with the work by LeVay.

Transgender

A group in Amsterdam (the capital of the sex trade industry) examined the INAH-3 from brains of

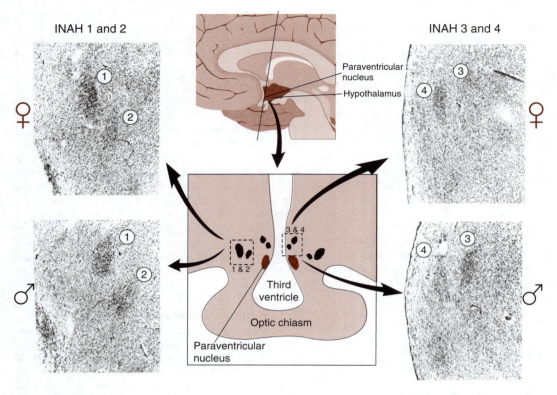

FIGURE 16.10 Representative micrographs showing the interstitial nuclei of the anterior hypothalamus (INAH) for women **(top)** and men **(bottom)**. Note that INAH numbers 2 and 3 are less distinct in the women micrographs. (Data from Allen LS, Hines M, Shryne JE, et al. Two sexually dimorphic cell groups in the human brain. *J Neurosci.* 1989;9[2]:497–506.)

individuals with and without gonadotropin hormones compared with those of male-to-female transsexual individuals who completed sex-reassignment surgery. The volume of the INAH-3 was larger in the males compared with females and transsexual subjects. It is tempting to say that the transsexuals have a brain that falls between male and female, but we know hormones affect the brain, so castration and/or supplemental hormones likely altered the brain architecture in the subjects in this study (Figure 16.11).

More recently there has been interest in imaging the brains of transgender people before hormone therapy searching for differences before the treatment. The studies are small, have not been replicated, and do not provide results that are intuitively meaningful, for example, small gray matter differences. Finding differences may be difficult in part because of the number of sexual possibilities, e.g., male-to-female homosexual compared with male-to-female heterosexual compared with heterosexual men and homosexual men... and that's just for XY.

Pedophilia

James Cantor, a psychologist at the University of Toronto has said, "pedophilia is something that we are essentially born with, does not appear to change over time and it's as core to our being as any sexual orientation is." Cantor and others are searching to identify the neural correlates of immature sexual preference. MRI scans show subtle frontal lobe deficits, which suggests problems with impulse control. But this is nonspecific and fails to shed light on the underlying problem. More recently, fMRI scans have identified a visual network that processes sexual preference. This network includes the inferior occipital gyrus, fusiform gyrus, and ventral lateral prefrontal cortex and lights up when looking at faces of one's sexual interest. For example, heterosexual men show greater activity in the network when looking at adult women, whereas pedophilic homosexual men display more activity when looking at boys. Although interesting, this is no better than asking the subjects who they prefer before putting their head in a scanner. We still don't know which "wires are crossed" in pedophilia.

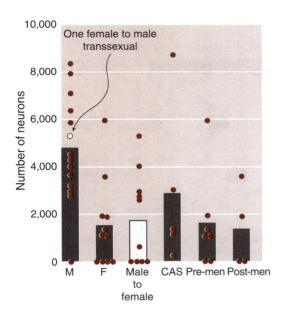

FIGURE 16.11 Postmortem analysis of the number of neurons in the INAH-3 nucleus for males (M), females (F), male-to-female transsexuals, and castrated males due to prostate cancer (CAS). All the women are separated by menopausal status in the last two bars. One female-to-male transsexual is included with the males. (Adapted from Garcia-Falgueras A, Swaab DF. A sex difference in the hypothalamic uncinate nucleus: relationship to gender identity. *Brain*. 2008;131:3132–3146, by permission of Oxford University Press.)

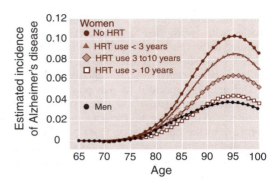

FIGURE 16.12 A prediction of the incidence of Alzheimer's disease calculated from data collected about men and women over 3 years shows the beneficial effects of sex hormones. HRT, hormone replacement therapy. (Data from Zandi PP, Carlson MC, Plassman BL, et al. HRT and incidence of Alzheimer's disease in older women: the Cache County Study. *JAMA*. 2002;288[17]:2123–2129.)

PSYCHIATRIC DISORDERS

Cognitive Decline

There is evidence that estrogens (and presumably testosterone) are neuroprotective. Figure 16.6 shows the robust increase in spine formation that can be induced by estrogen in hippocampal neurons. Presumably, such an arborization of the neurons enhances neural connections. Research with rodents and nonhuman primates demonstrates beneficial effects of estrogen on cognition. Observational studies in humans suggest that hormone replacement protects against the development of Alzheimer's disease, although there are other risks of continued hormone replacement.

Figure 16.12 is an example of one such observational study with humans. This was a study of more than 3,000 elderly people from one county in Utah. The objective was to test for the development of Alzheimer's disease and see if a history of hormone replacement therapy (HRT) was protective. Note that the men (who presumably maintain adequate levels of sex hormones) fare better than the women in terms of developing Alzheimer's disease. Likewise, the women who took HRT displayed a dose–response

effect. That is, the longer a woman took HRT, the less likely she was to develop Alzheimer's disease.

Unfortunately, clinical trials of HRT and cognition have been disappointing. In 2014, Victor Henderson from Stanford University reviewed the literature on Alzheimer's disease and hormone therapy. He concluded that estrogen initiated in women with dementia due to Alzheimer's disease shows "no important cognitive benefits." Additionally, initiation of estrogen and progesterone to women 65 years or older *increased* the risk of dementia. The only possible benefits have been found when HRT was initiated in younger postmenopausal women. "Observational studies… imply that midlife hormone therapy could indeed reduce Alzheimer's risk." Therefore if estrogen is neuroprotective, it likely needs to be started around the time of menopause.

Sexual Dysfunction

A survey of adults between the ages of 18 and 59 years in the United States found a high prevalence of sexual dysfunction: 31% for men and 43% for women. The most common complaint for men was premature ejaculation, whereas for women it was lack of interest. There are pharmacologic interventions available for premature ejaculation. For example, the selective serotonin reuptake inhibitors make it harder to have an orgasm, although they are not approved by US Food and Drug Administration (FDA) for this indication.

Lack of interest in sex, on the other hand, is a difficult nut to crack, so to speak. Certainly the qualities of the relationship, secondary medical conditions, and the presence of other psychiatric disorders have strong influences on the joy of sex. However, some women find sex boring, or worse annoying. As many as one in three women never or infrequently achieve orgasm during intercourse—one in five with masturbation. Studies with twins show a genetic component to orgasmic ability. Estimated heritability for difficulty achieving orgasm during intercourse is 34%—on par with anxiety and depressive disorders (see Table 6.1).

Dopaminergic mechanisms may play a large role in modulating sexual drive and orgasmic quality. As we discussed in Chapter 12, Pleasure, the dopamine pathways to the nucleus accumbens are active in motivated behavior. Dopamine agonists such as the stimulant medications and cocaine are anecdotally reported to enhance human sexual behavior. More recently, genetic studies have shown that different genotypes of the dopamine D4 receptor correlate more or less closely with sexual desire and arousal. This suggests that biology as well as environmental signals (in close proximity to finding Mr or Miss Right) interact to determine the sexual experience.

The prospect of giving a woman a medication to enhance sexual desire, although of interest to the pharmaceutical industry and feared by domineering fathers everywhere, has a long and disappointing history. The phosphodiesterase-5 inhibitors (e.g., Viagra) have been tested in large trials for female sexual dysfunction and failed to enhance interest any more than placebo. The testosterone patch, although effective for some patients, failed to win FDA approval because of safety concerns.

Recent research suggests that α-melanocyte-stimulating hormone (α-MSH) may be, what some call, a genuine aphrodisiac. We mentioned in Chapter 11, Pain, that a large precursor neuropeptide in the pituitary gland, proopiomelanocortin (POMC), is cleaved to form active neuropeptides, which include ACTH, β-endorphin, and α-MSH (see Figure 16.13). α-MSH is the peptide that also causes the skin to darken in patients with Addison's disease and also suppresses appetite. The story is told that a company was testing a melanocortin product as a possible tanning agent that did not require sun exposure. During early testing the medication triggered erections in most of the men. *Eureka!* Subsequently, a peptide analogue of α-MSH called *bremelanotide* (a melanocortin receptor agonist) was developed for further study.

Research with animals has shown that bremelanotide enhances female sexual solicitation in rats. The female rats became overtly flirtatious in a rodent sort of way—even climbing through little holes in the walls to get to the males. A study with married women in Iran (of all places) using an intranasal spray to administer the medication reported greater intercourse satisfaction in those receiving the active medication. Unfortunately, testing has been halted because of increased blood pressure in a few subjects. The company is considering subcutaneous administration as a means to eliminate the hypertensive adverse effect.

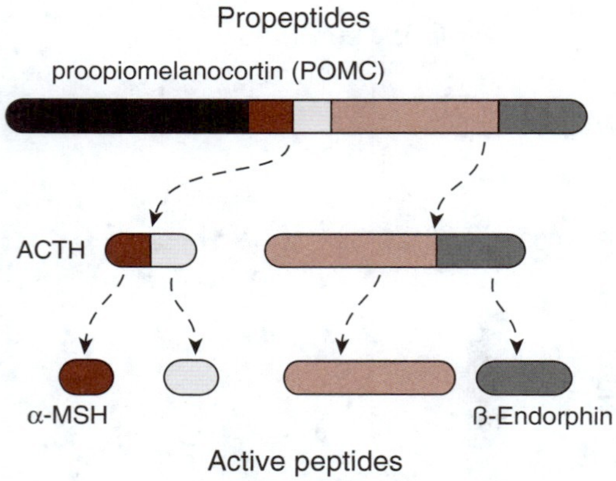

Propeptides

proopiomelanocortin (POMC)

ACTH

α-MSH   ß-Endorphin

Active peptides

FIGURE 16.13 The propeptide proopiomelanocortin is produced in the pituitary gland where it is cleaved to smaller active peptides such as adrenocorticotropic hormone (ACTH), α-melanocyte-stimulating hormone (α-MSH), and β-endorphin.

It is not clear why the pituitary neuropeptide α-MSH enhances sexual interest. Studies in which the medication was injected directly into a female rat's lateral ventricles increased solicitations establishing that its effects are mediated centrally. Additionally, α-MSH activated the Fos proteins (markers of gene expression) in the POA of the hypothalamus as well as the nucleus accumbens—areas that would be consistent with sexual pleasure.

The newest, and the only medication to receive FDA approval for hypoactive sexual desire disorder, is flibanserin (Addyi), which is believed to increase dopamine and norepinephrine in the prefrontal cortex. Initially developed as an antidepressant, it was ineffective at improving mood but appeared to enhance libido in women. Since then, clinical trials in women with hypoactive sexual desire have established statistically significant improved sexual satisfaction. It remains to be seen if this translates into clinical utility. It takes several weeks before it is effective and even then only increases satisfying sexual encounters by one every 2 months. Sales have not been impressive. Skeptics think this is because it is contraindicated with alcohol. An unqualified pink Viagra continues to elude us.

Mood Disorders

The lifetime prevalence of mood disorders in women is approximately twice that of men. Although the cause of this difference remains undetermined, one possible explanation is the sex hormones—or more specifically, the fluctuation in sex hormones. Figure 16.14 shows the alterations in estrogen levels for a hypothetical woman across her life span. The times of greatest risk for mood disturbances are during times

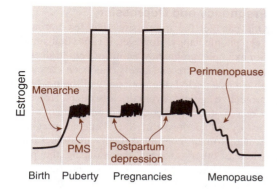

FIGURE 16.14 Estrogen levels fluctuate for women from puberty to menopause. The times of greatest vulnerability for depression occur when estrogen levels are changing. (Adapted from Stahl SM. *Essential Psychopharmacology: Neuroscientific Basis of Practical Applications*. 2nd ed. New York: Cambridge University Press; 2000.)

of fluctuating estrogen levels: menarche, premenstrual syndrome, postpartum, and perimenopausal.

The correlation between dropping sex hormones and depressive symptoms is not limited to women. The difference is the fluctuations. Men typically have stable testosterone levels. However, when testosterone drops, psychiatric symptoms become more prevalent. In one Veterans Administration (VA) study, the researchers followed up the testosterone level and emergence of depressive illness in men older than 45 years for 2 years. They found that 22% of the hypogonadal men (total testosterone <200 ng/dL) experienced depression, whereas only 7% of the eugonadal men did. Another group looked at the emergence of psychiatric symptoms in men treated for prostate cancer with GnRH agonists (see sidebar), which causes testosterone to plummet. They reported significant increases in anxiety and depression while the testosterone was low.

TREATMENT

GONADOTROPIN-RELEASING HORMONE AGONIST

Clinicians can override the pulsatile nature of a releasing hormone to effectively shut down production of the sex hormones and treat problems such as endometriosis, prostate cancer, and early-onset puberty.

This treatment has also been used with sex offenders as a form of "chemical castration." In this process, a long-acting GnRH agonist, leuprolide (Lupron Depot), inhibits the release of LH and FSH, although it stimulates the receptor. This effect is achieved because the continuous stimulation—in contrast to the usual intermittent stimulation—causes the desensitization of receptors in the pituitary. As a result, LH and FSH are not produced, which subsequently reduces the production of sex hormones.

Some of the most convincing data regarding the effects of sex hormones on mood have been treatment studies. Both with men and women, positive results have been shown for improving mood when sex hormones were administered. Figure 16.15 shows two representative studies. These studies have many differences, but they both reveal less depression with sex hormones.

The study on the left is with perimenopausal women who have mild or moderate depressive symptoms. One group was given placebo and the other estradiol. No antidepressants were used. The graph on the right was a study with men. All the men had failed antidepressant therapy and had low or borderline testosterone levels. Everyone remained on this antidepressant while half the group also received supplemental testosterone gel.

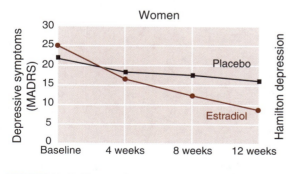

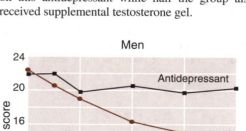

FIGURE 16.15 Two studies highlighting the mood-altering effects of sex hormones for women and men with sluggish gonads. (*Left:* Data from Soares CN, Almeida OP, Joffe H, et al. Efficacy of estradiol for the treatment of depressive disorders in perimenopausal women: a double-blind, randomized, placebo-controlled trial. *Arch Gen Psychiatry*. 2001;58[6]:529–534. *Right:* Adapted from Pope Jr HG, Cohane GH, Kanayama G, et al. Testosterone gel supplementation for men with refractory depression: a randomized, placebo-controlled trial. *Am J Psychiatry*. 2003;160[1]:105–111. Reprinted with permission from the *American Journal of Psychiatry* [Copyright © 2003]. American Psychiatric Association. All Rights Reserved.)

Both of these are small studies and need to be repeated with larger numbers. Likewise, it is important to remember that hormone replacement is not without significant risks. However, the studies demonstrate the powerful effects sex hormones can have on mood.

Traumatic Brain Injury

Traumatic brain injury (TBI) is increasingly recognized as more than just short-term confusion. Soldiers and football players are reporting enduring problems from the cortical bruising and microscopic tears the brain sustains when it is rattled around inside the hard skull. Memory, cognition, and impulse control in many cases never return to baseline. Although there is currently no medical treatment for TBI, progesterone, often thought of as the "pregnancy hormone," has garnered considerable interest. Studies with animals and small human studies suggested that progesterone, administered shortly after the head injury, might have nurturing properties that enable the brain to repair more effectively. Unfortunately, a large, multicenter trial (PROTECT III) failed to show any benefit for progesterone over placebo. The authors concluded, "The PROTECT III trail joins a growing list of negative or inconclusive trials in the arduous search for a treatment for TBI." At this point, if this was an e-mail, we'd insert an emoji sad face.

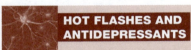

HOT FLASHES AND ANTIDEPRESSANTS

Some women want treatment for the hot flashes associated with menopause but do not want HRT. The newer antidepressants have been shown to have some benefit. In the best study, the researchers felt that venlafaxine was clearly superior to placebo but not as effective as estrogen. Their study stands as further evidence that mood and gonadal steroids are linked in ways that we are only beginning to understand.

Pregnancy and Depression

One can get the impression that sex hormones keep people happy. However, it is not that simple. For example, pregnancy, a time of very high estrogen and progesterone levels, has been conceptualized as a period of emotional well-being—even protective against psychiatric disorders. However, a recent study was conducted on women with a history of depression who became pregnant. Some women continued their antidepressants, whereas others stopped them during the pregnancy. The relapse rates for depression during the pregnancy were 26% for those still on their medication and 68% for those who discontinued their antidepressants.

Clearly, pregnancy is not protective against depression for women with a history of depression. Some think the high levels of progesterone during pregnancy may have negative effects on mood. Others speculated about the negative effects of low BDNF during pregnancy. More research is needed to understand this paradoxical finding.

SUMMARY

The sex hormones are not just for fostering the procreation of the species. One focus of this chapter has been on the nourishing capacity the neurosteroids have on the brain cells and subsequently on behavior and emotions. European physicians are more familiar with this body of research and are more comfortable using small doses of hormone replacement to optimize the treatment of mental problems—a perspective we may embrace as the gonads of the baby boomers languish.

QUESTIONS

1. Female gonadal steroids include all of the following except
   a. Testosterone.
   b. Estradiol.
   c. Progesterone.
   d. Gonadotropin-releasing hormone.

2. Many of the androgen effects in the brain are triggered by
   a. 17β-Estradiol.
   b. 5α-Dihydrotestosterone.
   c. Aromatase.
   d. α-Fetoprotein.

3. Which rat will display lordosis when primed with estrogens and progesterones and paired with a sexually active male?
   a. Males of normal pregnancies.
   b. Males exposed to androgens in utero.
   c. Females of normal pregnancies.
   d. Females exposed to androgens in utero.

4. Known effects of female sex hormones include all of the following except
   a. Increased spine formation.
   b. Decreased risk of stroke.
   c. Increase GABA inhibition.
   d. Gene transcription.

5. Evidence of sexual dimorphism in the vertebrate CNS include all of the following except
   a. Spinal nucleus of the bulbocavernosus.
   b. The robust nucleus.
   c. Sexually dimorphic nucleus of the preoptic area.
   d. Paraventricular nucleus.

6. Some research suggests which area is smaller in homosexual men compared with heterosexual men?
   a. Interstitial nucleus of the anterior hypothalamus-1.
   b. Interstitial nucleus of the anterior hypothalamus-2.
   c. Interstitial nucleus of the anterior hypothalamus-3.
   d. Interstitial nucleus of the anterior hypothalamus-4.

7. The propeptide POMC is cleaved into all the following active peptides except
   a. Δ-Fos.
   b. Adrenocorticotropic hormone.
   c. α-Melanocyte-stimulating hormone.
   d. β-Endorphin.

8. Evidence of the importance of sex hormones and mood includes all of the following expect
   a. Premenstrual syndrome.
   b. Athletes on anabolic steroids.
   c. Chemical castration for prostate cancer.
   d. Randomized controlled trials.

See Answers section at the end of this book.

CHAPTER 17

Social Attachment

PARENTAL BEHAVIOR

The goal of reproduction is successful offspring. Parents want offspring who can survive the rigors of the world and produce their own descendants. Many animals produce offspring that require sustained assistance to successfully reach maturity. The particular actions that parents undertake to ensure the growth and survival of their offspring constitute *parental behavior*.

The extent of parental behavior in the animal kingdom occurs along a spectrum ranging from none to helicopter parents. Female salmons lay hundreds of eggs to be fertilized and then swim away. Humans are at the other end of the spectrum—investing many years and enormous resources—hoping to be surrounded by their loving children until the very end.

Females in the animal kingdom do most of the parenting, although there are some exceptions. It is generally believed that males seek to fertilize as many eggs as possible, whereas females seek to successfully raise the few they sire. Parental behavior constitutes any behavior that the parent does for the offspring. For example, a pregnant dog will build a nest a day or two before giving birth. After the delivery, she will lick them clean, eat the placentas, feed them, and keep them warm (and for all this she is called a bitch). Additionally, she will aggressively defend the pups against any suspicious intruders.

The demand to behave like a mother develops rather abruptly. An inexperienced mother must immediately perform a full range of new behaviors without much room for error. How does this happen? Well, as we saw in the last chapter, pregnancy changes the brain. Terkel and Rosenblatt established that there must be something in the blood that induces maternal behavior. They transfused blood from a female rat that had just delivered to a virgin rat (Figure 17.1). Within 24 hours, the virgin rat was displaying maternal behavior.

Hormones

Biologic endocrinologists have spent considerable time and energy trying to tease out the maternal molecules. Although they have gotten close, there is still no definitive concoction of hormones that will immediately trigger maternal behavior in a nulliparous (virgin) rat. The leading culprits are estrogen, progesterone, and prolactin. An important ingredient appears to be the changing levels of the hormones. In Figure 17.2, note how the progesterone drops while the estrogen and prolactin rise in a rat just before delivery.

Oxytocin also plays some important role. Traditionally we conceptualize oxytocin as the neuropeptide released from the posterior pituitary into general circulation, which leads to uterine contractions and milk "let down" (see Figure 7.4). Recent research has found receptors for oxytocin within the brain, establishing central actions for this neuropeptide. Indeed, injecting oxytocin directly into the lateral ventricles in a rat will induce maternal behavior in a hormone-primed virgin rat. More recently, it has been shown that oxytocin levels in the paraventricular nucleus (PVN) increase with maternal aggression. Likewise, infusion of synthetic oxytocin into the PVN also increases maternal aggression toward an intruder.

Further complicating this picture is the fact that hormones facilitate maternal behavior but are not required for it. Nulliparous rats will initially avoid new pups placed in their cage. However, if exposed over a series of days (1 hour each day), they will respond maternally to the pups within 5 to 6 days. Pregnant rats will show similar avoidance until after they have delivered. Then they will quickly display maternal behavior to any pup for the rest of their lives, proving that "once a mother, always a mother" (Figure 17.3).

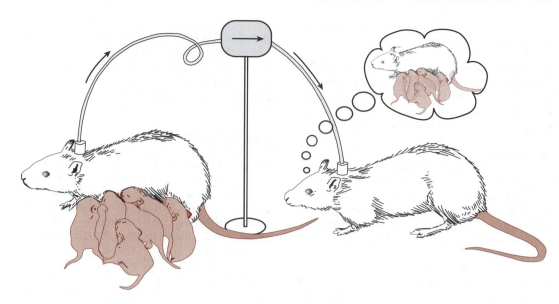

FIGURE 17.1 When nulliparous rats are transfused with blood from a new mother, they will display maternal behavior within 24 hours. (Adapted from Nelson RJ. *An Introduction to Behavioral Endocrinology*. 3rd ed. Sunderland, MA: Sinauer; 2005, by permission of Oxford University Press, USA.)

The Brain

Taken together, these studies suggest that the hormonal fluctuations late in pregnancy act on the brain to decrease fear or aversion and increase attraction toward infants. Because maternal behavior persists once it is established, it is likely that the experience permanently changes some regions in the brain. An area that has been intensely studied is the one that we discussed in the previous chapter: the preoptic area (POA) located in the anterior hypothalamus.

The POA is rich in estrogen, progesterone, prolactin, and oxytocin receptors, all of which increase during gestation. Lesions of the POA will disrupt maternal behavior. The POA appears to be a region that receives olfactory and somatosensory input and has projections to midbrain and brain stem nuclei. Numan and Sheehan describe an elegant experiment that demonstrates the central role of the POA in maternal behavior. Postpartum rats were exposed to either pups or candy for 2 hours. Then their brains were analyzed for the presence

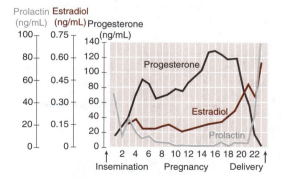

FIGURE 17.2 Blood levels of progesterone, estradiol, and prolactin in the pregnant rat. The changes that occur prior to delivery may influence maternal behavior. (Adapted from Rosenblatt JS, Siegel HI, Mayer AD. Progress in the study of maternal behavior in the rat: hormonal, nonhormonal, sensory, and developmental aspects. *Adv Study Behavior*. 1979;10:225–311. Copyright 1979 with permission from Elsevier.)

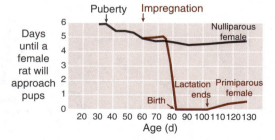

FIGURE 17.3 Female rats initially avoid pups. Several days of exposure are required for a nulliparous rat to display maternal behavior. Pregnant rats act similarly until after they deliver. (Adapted from Bridges RS. Endocrine regulation of parental behavior in rodents. In: Krasnegor NA, Bridges RS, eds. *Mammalian Parenting: Biochemical, Neurobiological and Behavioral Determinants*. New York: Oxford University Press; 1990, by permission of Oxford University Press, USA.)

of the transcription factor Fos. (Fos is used as a general marker of gene expression.)

Figure 17.4 shows the results of the study. This is a slice through the forebrain, which includes the anterior hypothalamus on either side of the ventricle. (For a human comparison, see Figure 16.10.) Note the increased activation in the POA as well as other regions for the rat exposed to pups.

Dopamine

Up to this point, we have stressed the importance of gonadal steroids and neuropeptides in the development of maternal behavior, but the neurotransmitter dopamine also appears to play an important role. We discussed in Chapter 12, Pleasure, the neuroanatomy of wanting and liking: the activation of the orbitofrontal cortex (OFC) and the ventral tegmental/nucleus accumbens area (see Figure 12.3). As might be expected, these areas are active in mothers.

One study scanned new mothers while they were looking at pictures of their own child and pictures of unfamiliar children. The mothers showed greater activation of the OFC when viewing their own child. With rats, researchers have found that mother rats will press a bar for access to pups the way they will press a bar for amphetamines or electrical stimulation. Additionally, pup exposure increases the release of dopamine at the nucleus accumbens. Alternatively, dopamine blockers will impair maternal behavior (see box). These studies give some neurobiologic explanations for the "joys of motherhood."

Licking and Grooming

This brings us to a series of studies from Michael Meaney's laboratory when he was at McGill University, which are important neuroscience studies for mental health professionals. Their studies tie together maternal behavior with lasting effects on the offspring's behavior, hypothalamic–pituitary–adrenal (HPA) axis, and even their DNA.

The story starts in the 1960s when researchers noted that pups "handled" once a day during the first weeks of life showed a reduced adrenocorticotropic hormone and corticosterone response to stress. Later it was established that it was not the "handling" per se that produced this effect, but the mother's increased licking of the pups when they were returned to the nest. The mothers were simply

---

SCHIZOPHRENIA AND DOPAMINE BLOCKERS

Mothers who suffer from schizophrenia are known to be less involved with their children. They are generally more remote and less responsive during mother–infant play. This could be an example of the negative symptoms of the disorder. Worse yet, the problem might be exacerbated by the medications used to treat the patients.

Li et al. looked at the effect of injections of haloperidol, risperidone, and quetiapine on maternal behavior in rats. The antipsychotic medications inhibited maternal behaviors, such as nest building, pup licking, and pup retrieval. The figure shows the results for pup retrieval. Shortly after the injections, mothers failed to retrieve their own pups. Such studies suggest caution when treating human mothers with antipsychotic agents.

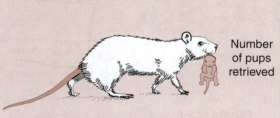

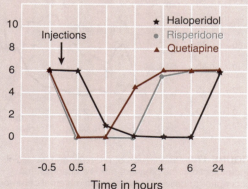

Antipsychotic medications disrupt a mother rat's tendency to retrieve her pups. (**Left:** Adapted from Nelson RJ. *An Introduction to Behavioral Endocrinology.* 3rd ed. Sunderland, MA: Sinauer; 2005, by permission of Oxford University Press, USA.)

trying to get the human odor off their pups, and this extra attention to the pups resulted in their improved response to stress when they grew up to be adults.

Meaney discovered naturally occurring strains of rats that licked and groomed their pups at different rates. This particular behavior occurs when the mother rat enters the nest and gathers her pups around her for nursing. She will intermittently lick and groom the pups as they nurse. Meaney named one group the high lick and groom (high L and G) mothers and the other the low lick and groom (low L and G) mothers.

In a flurry of experiments in Meaney's laboratory, it was established that high L and G mothers produced offspring with subtle but significantly different brains. After 20 minutes of restraint (very stressful for a rodent), the rats from high L and G mothers secrete less corticosterone (Figure 17.5A). They also produce less corticotropin-releasing hormone messenger RNA (CRH-mRNA) in the hypothalamus (Figure 17.5B). Additionally, the amount of maternal licking and grooming correlates with the number of glucocorticoid receptors (GRs) in the hippocampus (Figure 17.5C). They literally produce more GRs as a result of enhanced gene expression.

In summary, a mother's increased attention enhances the sensitivity of the HPA axis most likely by turning on the appropriate DNA. Offspring of attentive high-licking mothers demonstrate greater feedback to the hypothalamus by way of the increased GRs, which inhibits CRH production and corticosterone release. Perhaps most significant, the pups from a high L and G mother show a greater willingness to explore novel environments as adults and demonstrate enhanced resilience under duress.

Trading Places

In a follow-up study, Meaney et al. switched some of the mothers and pups. That is, pups from high L and G mothers were raised by low L and G mothers and vice versa. The results were stunning and show how behaviors and patterns emerge from combinations of genetic predisposition and environment. Figure 17.6 shows the behavior of the adopted female rats raised by high L and G mothers once they matured. They were more inclined to explore an open area and provided greater licking and grooming to their own pups. Note how the determining factor is not just the genetic makeup, but also the nurturing behavior of the mother that raised them. In other words, a low L and G female will become a high L and G mother if she is raised by a high

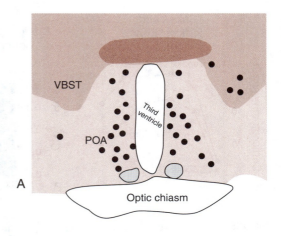

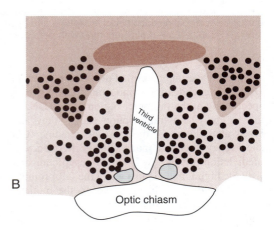

FIGURE 17.4 Hypothalamic region of postpartum rats exposed to candy **(A)** or newborn pups **(B)**. Each dot represents five cells labeled with Fos activity—a measure of gene expression. POA, preoptic area; VBST, ventral bed nucleus of the terminalis. (Adapted from Numan M, Sheehan TP. [1997.] Neuroanatomical circuitry for mammalian maternal behavior. *Ann N Y Acad Sci*. 807:101–125.)

L and G mother. Therefore behavioral traits can be passed from generation to generation, but it is not always genetic—it can be epigenetic.

Effect on the DNA

Meaney and his group have taken this line of research to the next level by searching for epigenetic mechanisms that can explain the enduring effects the mother's behavior has on the pups. Briefly, epigenetic molecular attachments on the DNA (see Figures 6.7 and 6.8) affect gene expression, which in turn alters the proteins produced—in this case the GR.

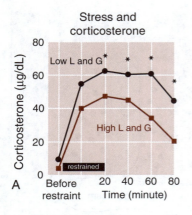

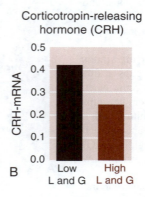

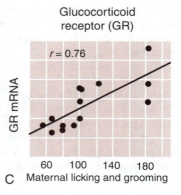

FIGURE 17.5 Rats raised by a mother with a high frequency of licking and grooming behavior show a more modest corticosterone release in response to stress **(A)**, less corticotropin-releasing hormone messenger RNA (CRH-mRNA) **(B)**, and greater glucocorticoid receptors (GRs) in the hippocampus. **C:** The correlation between GRs and licking and grooming by the mother. (Adapted from Liu D, Diorio J, Tannenbaum B, et al. Maternal care, hippocampal glucocorticoid receptors, and hypothalamic-pituitary-adrenal responses to stress. *Science.* 1997;277[5332]:1659–1662. Reprinted with permission from AAAS.)

Meaney's group identified the section of the rat DNA that encodes for hippocampal GR. Looking specifically at the promoter region of this DNA— the region where transcription starts—they analyzed methylation of the cytosine–guanine (CG) sites. They found a much greater frequency of methylation for the low L and G group compared with the high L and G pups along the GR promoter gene (Figure 17.7). In other words, the mother's attentive behavior reduced the methylation of the gene and allowed for greater production of the GR, which in turn made the rats more resilient. This is an excellent example of the neuroscience model (see Figure 6.12) showing how environment, gene expression, and brain development affect behavior.

The researchers conducted a follow-up study with their rats that is almost unbelievable. They administered directly into the cerebral ventricles an inhibitor (trichostatin A) that results in demethylation of the DNA (Figure 17.8A). These rats displayed less methylation of their DNA and, consequently, greater numbers of GRs. Furthermore, when stressed, these animals showed a modest HPA response (Figure 17.8B); that is, their corticosterone levels become indistinguishable from those of rats raised by a high L and G mother.

The implications from these studies are profound. We can now trace the effects of a mother's behavior down to the offspring's DNA. Furthermore, if we can find ways to cleanse the DNA, we might be able to correct psychiatric problems, not just treat symptoms. However, it is important to note that although demethylation may be the treatment of the future, it is not without

risks. Some cancers are believed to result from demethylation of growth-promoting genes—genes we do not want to inadvertently turn on.

What about in humans? Meaney and his colleagues recently analyzed the human equivalent of the promoter region of the glucocorticoid gene in cells from the hippocampus in a postmortem study of human brains. They compared suicide victims with a history of childhood abuse with two control groups both without a history of abuse—a control suicide group and a control sudden death, nonsuicide group. The suicide victims with a history of abuse had greater methylation of the GR gene compared with the nonabused controls. Additionally, as would be predicted, the messenger RNA transcribed from the GR gene was reduced in the subjects with a history of abuse. The human findings are consistent with the rat studies.

PAIR BONDING

The attraction between men and women is a special form of social attachment. In the short term, it is required for sexual reproduction; in the long run, bonded parents coordinate the rearing and protection of the offspring. Surprisingly, monogamous pair bonds are rare among mammals: approximately 5%. Monogamy is much more common among birds. The unusual bonding and rebonding that is common with humans might be best described as serial monogamy. The question for us: what parts of the brain drive the affiliation of men and women, or homosexual couples?

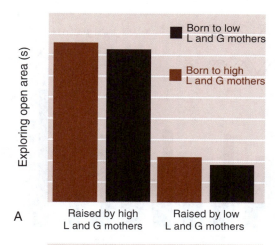

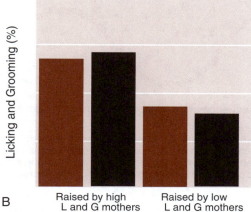

FIGURE 17.6 Female rats raised by mothers who were high lickers (L) and groomers (G) are less anxious in an open area **(A)** and are more likely to be high lickers and groomers when raising their own pups **(B)**—regardless of their genetic lineage. (Adapted from Francis D, Diorio J, Liu D, et al. Nongenomic transmission across generations of maternal behavior and stress responses in the rat. *Science*. 1999;286[5442]:1155–1158. Reprinted with permission from AAAS.)

Romantic Love and Dopamine

Romantic love is a universal human experience. The feeling of attraction that one person may feel for another can be intense, all-consuming, and difficult to control. A person in love feels euphoric. A spurned lover is despondent and even violent. The obsessional thinking and the willingness to "cross mountains" to be with a lover suggest the activation of the brains reward system (see Figure 12.6) when one is in love.

Anthropologist Helen Fisher at Rutgers University has spent her career studying the science of love. She and her colleagues scanned the brains of people who were "intensely in love."

During the magnetic resonance imaging (MRI) examination, subjects were alternatively shown pictures of their beloved or a neutral individual and the differences were measured. As expected, the images of the object of one's affection lit up the ventral tegmental area (VTA) (Figure 17.9A). The VTA is a dopamine-rich area with projections to the nucleus accumbens. These are the subcortical regions that mediate motivation and reward.

Another area activated in the study was the caudate nucleus (CN) (Figure 17.9B). This area is also active in obsessive–compulsive disorder. In the Fisher's study, activity in the CN correlated with the total score on a test of the subject's feelings: the Passionate Love Scale. Therefore, in simple terms, we can conceptualize love as both an addiction and an obsession.

Growth Factors

A group in Italy—a country that knows a thing or two about romance—studied growth factors in subjects who had recently fallen in love. They speculated that nerve growth factors (NGFs) might be activated when people experience romantic feelings. They drew blood from subjects who fell recently "in love" and couples in long-lasting relationships. They measured the values of four growth factors. Only one—NGF—was significantly higher in the subjects recently in love. Moreover, there was a positive correlation between the level of NGF and the subject's score on the Passionate Love Scale.

Of particular interest, the researchers reexamined the levels of NGF a year or two later in the subjects in love. They found that the levels of NGF had dropped back to the levels seen in the control group (Figure 17.10). This is the neuroendocrine equivalent of what we all know: the honeymoon does not last (see Figure 12.8A). It is another example that the brain does not tolerate euphoria for too long. However, if the pleasure wanes, why do we stay in a relationship? In addition to psychological and practical answers, it may be that other neuropeptides kick in. Work with voles may shed some light on this.

Vasopressin

The vole is a rodent that looks like a plump mouse, but is related to the lemming. They are common in the grassy fields of North America. Voles are relevant to our discussion because of their diversity in forming pair bonds. For example, the *prairie vole* will form enduring pair bonds and mutually care for the offspring. In nature, most prairie voles that lose a mate never take on another partner. The closely related *meadow (mountain, montagne) vole*, on the other hand, is socially promiscuous and does not display biparental care.

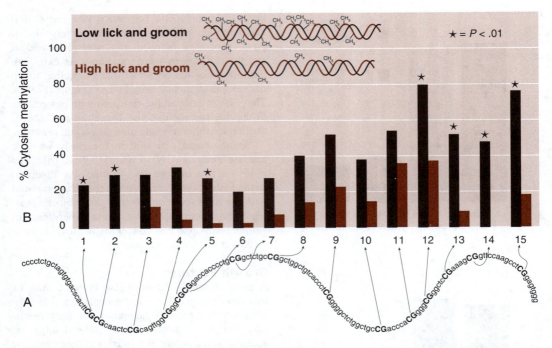

CG sites along a single strand of the DNA sequence of the glucocorticoid receptor gene

FIGURE 17.7 The presence of methyl groups attached to cytosine–guanine (CG) sites was assessed along the DNA of the rat glucocorticoid receptor **(A)**. Pups from mothers who were high lickers and groomers had significantly less methylation of this section of DNA **(B)**. (Adapted with permission from Macmillan Publishers Ltd. Weaver IC, Cervoni N, Champagne FA, et al. Epigenetic programming by maternal behavior. *Nat Neurosci.* 2004;7[8]:847–854. Copyright 2004.)

In the laboratory, researchers have observed that prairie vole males prefer to spend time next to their partners, called *huddling* (see Figure 17.11A). The meadow vole, on the other hand, is more independent. With the proper arrangements, this behavior can be measured and quantitated (Figure 17.11B).

Vasopressin has emerged as a critical neuro-peptide mediating the pair bond formation in male voles. Infusion of vasopressin into the male cerebral ventricles accelerated pair bond formation. Likewise, infusion of a vasopressin antagonist prevents pair bond formation. Furthermore,

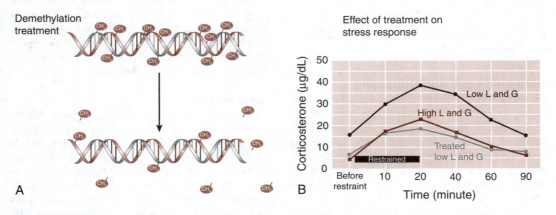

FIGURE 17.8 Trichostatin A can remove the methyl groups from DNA **(A)**. Rats from low lick and groom mothers who have been treated with the Trichostatin A display a normal hypothalamic–pituitary–adrenal response to stress **(B)**. (B: Adapted with permission from Macmillan Publishers Ltd. Weaver IC, Cervoni N, Champagne FA, et al. Epigenetic programming by maternal behavior. *Nat Neurosci.* 2004;7[8]:847–854. Copyright 2004.)

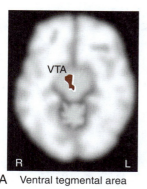
A Ventral tegmental area

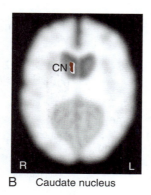
B Caudate nucleus

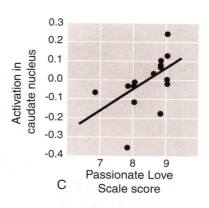
C

FIGURE 17.9 Subjects intensely in love show activity in the ventral tegmental area (VTA) and caudate nucleus (CN) when looking at pictures of their lover **(A** and **B)**. Activity in the CN correlated with scores on the Passionate Love Scale **(C)**. (Adapted from Aron A, Fisher H, Mashek DJ, et al. Reward, motivation, and emotion systems associated with early-stage intense romantic love. *J Neurophysiol*. 2005;94[1]:327–337.)

differences in expressions of the vasopressin receptor can be demonstrated in the two species of voles (Figure 17.11C). The prairie vole has significantly more receptors in the ventral pallidum (VP).

In a study that seems like something out of a science fiction novel, Young et al. have increased partner preference in meadow voles. They used a viral vector to transplant into the VP of meadow voles the segment of DNA that encodes for the vasopressin receptor. This resulted in increased expression of vasopressin receptors. The usually solitary meadow voles now were huddling with their partners. In essence, they changed an uncommitted promiscuous male into a monogamous family man. (Won't the social conservatives be thrilled?)

With human men, we know that the endurance of pair bonding runs in families. In some families the men partner up for life, whereas in other families, the men act more like meadow voles. The role of VP in marital commitment is of great interest, but few studies have addressed the issue. One report in 2008 looked at variations of the vasopressin receptor 1a gene in over 500 pairs of Swedish twins, all of whom were married or living with a partner. Everyone answered a questionnaire on the quality of their relationship, which generated a score from 0 to 66 for each person—66 being marital bliss. Men, but not women, with one particular allele (called 334) had lower scores on the Partner Bonding Scale as measured by self-report as well as their wives' score. The results were small but statistically significant and suggest, as with the voles, that the neuropeptide vasopressin influences pair bonding duration in humans. However, a larger analysis of Finnish twins and their siblings found an association between vasopressin genes and infidelity in women, but not in men.

Oxytocin

Oxytocin and vasopressin are remarkably similar in structure and size (Figure 17.12A). The body and brain, fortunately, recognize the subtle differences and produce distinct responses to these messengers. They are synthesized in the

FIGURE 17.10 Nerve growth factor (NGF) in subjects in long-lasting relationships, subjects actively "in love," and these same subjects a year or two later. The hearts on the NGF molecule are the authors' license.

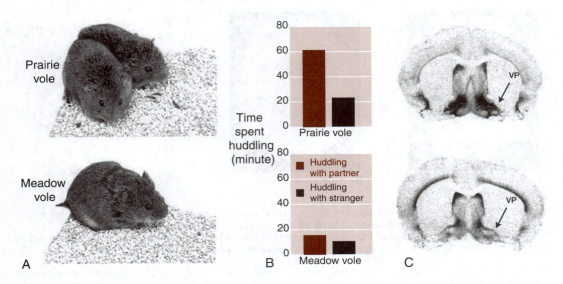

FIGURE 17.11 The male prairie vole will spend more time huddling with his partner than does the meadow vole **(A** and **B)**. The difference in vasopressin receptors (*dark areas* in **C**) in the ventral pallidum (VP) may explain the difference in this behavior. (Reprinted by permission from Macmillan Publishers Ltd. Lim MM, Wang Z, Olazabal DE, et al. Enhanced partner preference in a promiscuous species by manipulating the expression of a single gene. *Nature*. 2004;429:754–757. Copyright 2004.)

hypothalamus and permeate out into the body and brain by three mechanisms. The best known of these is the release of the molecules into the general circulation from the posterior pituitary (Figure 17.12B). Additionally, the molecules are released from the dendrites of the neurons and diffuse throughout the brain (dashed arrows). Finally, small neurons project from the hypothalamus to areas such as the anterior cingulate, nucleus accumbens, and amygdala, as well as

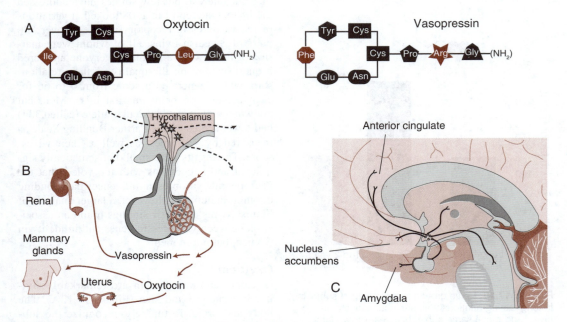

FIGURE 17.12 Oxytocin and vasopressin **(A)** are proteins with just a few different amino acids. These neuropeptides are excreted into the pituitary circulation **(B)**, diffused into the brain from the dendrites of the cells **(B)**, and released by small neurons at several locations around the brain **(C)**.

others (Figure 17.12C). The essential point is that oxytocin and vasopressin are hormones as well as neurotransmitters with diverse methods of transmission and effects on physiology and behavior.

In the lay press, oxytocin is affectionately called the "cuddle hormone" because oxytocin levels are elevated with childbirth, breast-feeding, and an orgasm—all circumstances in which a women is prone to bond with another human. In one frequently cited study, that may be the source of the "cuddle hormone" term, oxytocin significantly jumped in women after 10 minutes of "warm contact" with her spouse or partner, but did not change in men (Figure 17.13). Subsequent research using intranasal oxytocin (because it cannot be administered orally) has shown that intranasal oxytocin may do the following:

- Improve positive communication between couples
- Increase trusting behavior and produce more positive responses from fathers toward toddlers
- In general, enhance emotional recognition and responsiveness to others

Brain imaging studies suggest that oxytocin may, in part, improve social interactions by dampening the amygdala/cingulate circuit—a circuit known to be activated in fearful situations. It might be that trust and social comfort are increased through less social anxiety.

Enduring Bonds

A simple understanding of human male–female affiliation proposes that it all starts with dopamine and the pleasure centers of the brain. We speculate that other neuroendocrine systems such as oxytocin

and vasopressin may then take over to ensure enduring pair bond formation once "the thrill is gone." Although there are no data to support this as yet, twin studies suggest monogamy has biologic roots. We wonder if those individuals who are prone to stay in one relationship are genetically more endowed with the neuropeptides of attachment.

TEND-AND-BEFRIEND

Fight-or-flight has been the prevailing model to describe the mammalian response to stress. That is, stress causes a hormonal cascade that produces secretion of catecholamines and the organism either fights or retreats. Taylor has proposed that this model is male centric and does not describe how females cope in difficult times. Taylor believes females respond to stress by nurturing others and enhancing their social network, which she calls "tend-and-befriend." Although the neuroendocrine mechanisms are the same, the behavior is different. In fact, the gender difference in affiliation is one of the most robust findings in human behavioral research.

Engh et al. provide an example from a free-ranging troop of baboons in Africa that they followed. They have observed and recorded grooming behavior among the females. They found that females who lost a close relative experienced a significant increase in glucocorticoid levels after the death. However, they did not experience a decrease in their grooming although they had lost their close partner. Instead, other associations were established and the rate of grooming remained stable. The authors speculated that this social networking might modulate the stress response.

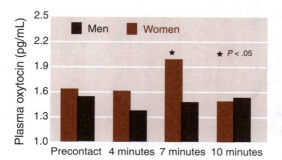

FIGURE 17.13 Oxytocin levels increase in women 7 minutes after cuddling with their partner. (Adapted from Grewen KM, Girdler SS, Amico J, et al. Effects of partner support on resting oxytocin, cortisol, norepinephrine, and blood pressure before and after warm partner contact. *Psychosom Med.* 2005;67:531–538.)

DISCONNECTED

Affiliation and pair bonding are on one end of the social attachment spectrum. On the other end are those individuals who are isolated and disconnected—individuals who are aloof, distant, and fail to derive pleasure from social interactions. The Unabomber is an extreme example of this sort of person. A graduate of Harvard, with a PhD in mathematics, he lived alone for 16 years in a 10 ft by 12 ft cabin in the woods of Montana without electricity or plumbing. A psychiatrist conducting a court evaluation of the Unabomber gave him a provisional diagnosis of schizophrenia.

The schizophrenic spectrum disorders include the following:

- Schizotypal personality disorder
- Schizoid personality disorder
- Delusional disorder
- Schizoaffective disorder
- Schizophrenia

These comprise a large percentage of the cases of socially disconnected individuals seen in most clinical practices. The impairment in social skills these individuals have, part of the negative signs of schizophrenia, is possibly the most troubling aspect of the illness for unaffected family members—something is missing and no treatment will bring it all back. Very little is known about the neuroanatomic deficits that contribute to the social aspect of the illnesses. However, as we will see in the chapter on schizophrenia, it has been hard to define any biologic deficits that explain the social deficit.

Autism Spectrum

Kanner first described autism in 1943 at Johns Hopkins University. We now envision autism as anchoring the more extreme end of a spectrum of disorders characterized by the following:

- Severe social dysfunctions
- Early communication failure
- Presence of repetitive, rigid, and stereotypic behaviors

Asperger's disorder and childhood disintegrative disorder are other conditions in the autism spectrum, which are believed to share common biologic foundations. These conditions are now considered a less severe form of the underlying disorder.

Eye Aversion

The social dysfunctions constitute the core deficits of the disorders. The inability to understand other people's feelings and a failure to establish reciprocal relationships emerge early in those with autism. Robert Schultz et al. at Yale have developed techniques to study this aspect of autism. They used eye-tracking technology to study spontaneous viewing patterns while watching video clips of complex social situations. They showed clips from the 1967 movie *Who's Afraid of Virginia Woolf?* to subjects with autism and age- and IQ-matched normal controls.

Figure 17.14 shows a drawing of one scene from the movie. In the foreground, two adults lean toward each other in a flirtatious interchange. The woman's husband is in the background, silent, but irritated by his wife's behavior. The eye movements from a control (brown) and an autistic subject (black) are collapsed onto this one scene. Note how the healthy control subject focuses on the eyes of the actors. Additionally, the control's focus moves from face to face, literally outlining the charged social triangle.

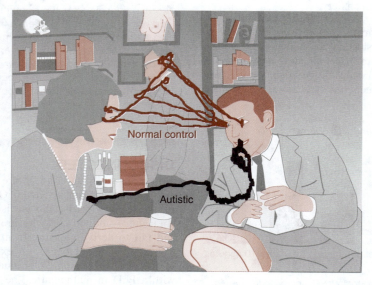

FIGURE 17.14 A drawing of a scene from *Who's Afraid of Virginia Woolf?* shows the different aspects of the movie that subjects with autism (*black*) and normal controls (*brown*) track with their eyes. (Adapted from Klin A, Jones W, Schultz R, et al. Defining and quantifying the social phenotype in autism. *Am J Psychiatry*. 2002;159[6]:895–908. Reprinted with permission from the *American Journal of Psychiatry* [Copyright © 2002]. American Psychiatric Association. All Rights Reserved.)

The autistic subject, on the other hand, attends to less relevant aspects of the scene. This subject displays the following three findings commonly seen in subjects with autism:

- Avoidance of the eyes
- Focus on the mouth
- Preferential attention to objects rather than people

Clearly, this method of observation fails to gather the subtle social cues that are essential to understand the thoughts and feelings of other people. A quantitative assessment of 15 subjects with autism and 15 controls demonstrated significant and substantial differences in time spent observing eyes and mouths from similar film clips. A 2017 study with toddlers with autism found that when appropriately cued, they would look at the eyes on a video and did not look away any faster than the control groups. This suggests that eye aversion, at least at the time of initial diagnosis, is not due to anxiety or some unpleasantness, but rather due to indifference. That is, the child with autism might not appreciate the social significance of the eyes.

Brain Enlargement

The underlying neuroanatomic abnormalities of autism remain unknown, but appear in part to be widespread neural connectivity disruption that develops in the first years of life. Some parents have reported that their children were developing normally for the first year and a half of life, but then showed a regression in social and/or communication skills. In a clever use of technology, Werner and Dawson had blinded observers review home video tapes of autistic children who were reported to have regressed. Indeed, they noted normal social attention and word babble at 12 months of age, but developed significant impairment by 24 months.

Enlarged brain volume has been the most consistent finding in the neuroscience of autism. In a meta-analysis, Redcay and Courchesne collected studies measuring head circumference and brain size with MRI. The authors noted that for autism the brain size is initially reduced, dramatically increases within the first year of life, but then returns to the normal range by adulthood. In a recent prospective study MRI scans were conducted on 106 infants at high risk for autism (had an older sibling with autism). They discovered an overgrowth (or what they call a hyperexpansion) of the cortical surface area between 6 and 12 months that precedes the brain volume overgrowth observed between 12 and 24 months (Figure 17.15). The authors calculated that autism, diagnosed clinically at 24 months, could be predicted with 80% accuracy based on two brain scans—6 and 12 months. If this can be repeated and verified, we may have a test to diagnose autism months before the clinical symptoms develop—a first in neuroscience.

The above studies show a critical period of subtle aberrant development in those with autism. What goes wrong? One theory is insufficient pruning of synaptic spines. In another remarkable study, a group out of Columbia University Medical Center analyzed postmortem brains of 10 children with autism and 10 healthy controls. With painstaking detailed analysis, they literally counted spines on pyramidal neurons from the temporal lobes and found increased density of spines for those with autism (Figure 17.16). Furthermore, in a follow-up study they gave mice rapamycin, a medication that "restores" normal pruning and the rapamycin reduced autisticlike behavior in mice—an exciting discovery. However, we must be cautious—this is the *mouse model* of autism—not real autism and not in humans.

Mirror Neurons

Mirror neurons were discovered in one of those beautiful serendipitous scientific moments. Researchers in Italy placed an electrode in a neuron in a monkey's motor cortex and noted that it was active when he grabbed an object. Much to their amazement it also became active when the monkey watched someone else grabbing the same object. They called these neurons *mirror neurons* and found that they are not uncommon in the brain. Figure 17.17 shows an example of a mirror neuron.

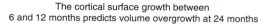

The cortical surface growth between 6 and 12 months predicts volume overgrowth at 24 months

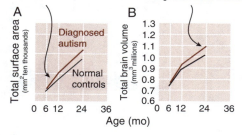

FIGURE 17.15 A: Toddlers who develop autism showed an accelerated expansion of brain *surface* area between 6 and 12 months. **B:** Toddlers with autism have greater total brain *volume* at 24 months. (Adapted with permission from Macmillan Publishers Ltd. Hazlett HC, et al. Early brain development in infants at high risk for autism spectrum disorder. *Nature.* 2017;542:348–351. Copyright 2017.)

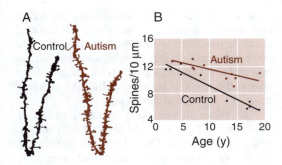

FIGURE 17.16 A: Neurons from people with autism have more spines (less pruning) than found on neurons from normal controls. **B:** Spine density is greater in subjects with autism compared with normal controls. (Adapted from Tang G, et al. Loss of mTOR-dependent macroautophagy causes autistic-like synaptic pruning deficits. *Neuron.* 2014;83:1131–1143. Copyright 2014 with permission from Elsevier.)

Note that the neuron is active both when a human (A) grasps the object and when the monkey (B) grasps the same object. However, the mirroring does not translate to all actions. If the object is grasped with pliers, the neuron does not become active.

Functional imaging studies on humans have also demonstrated mirroring. For example, a person moving a finger or observing a finger move will show similar activity in the same region of the motor cortex. Another study looked for mirroring with facial expressions. In this study, subjects were shown pictures of people displaying emotional expressions (such as happy, sad, angry, etc.). The subjects were instructed to either imitate the expression or just observe the picture. They found similar activity in the premotor region of the cortex,

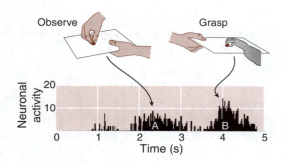

FIGURE 17.17 A neuron in the premotor cortex of a monkey is active when it observes a food morsel grasped by a human **(A)**. The same neuron is active when the monkey grasps the morsel **(B)**. (Adapted with permission from Macmillan Publishers Ltd. Rizzolatti G, Fogassi L, Gallese V. Neurophysiological mechanisms underlying the understanding and imitation of action. *Nat Rev Neurosci.* 2001;2[9]:661–670. Copyright 2001.)

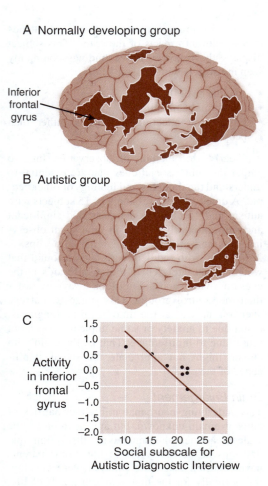

FIGURE 17.18 Functional magnetic resonance imaging studies for normally developing preteens compared with high-functioning age/IQ-matched subjects with autism while imitating emotional facial expressions. The subjects with autism show less activity of the mirror neuronal network, particularly in the frontal cortex. (Adapted with permission from Macmillan Publishers Ltd. Dapretto M, Davies MS, Pfeifer JH, et al. Understanding emotions in others: mirror neuron dysfunction in children with autism spectrum disorders. *Nat Neurosci.* 2006;9[1]:28–30. Copyright 2006.)

regardless of whether the subject was imitating the expression or simply observing.

Additional research by this same group has identified a network of neurons connecting the frontal, parietal, and temporal lobes. Furthermore, they found that imitating emotional facial expressions not only activated this network but also activated the emotional centers of the brain, such as the insula and amygdala. The capacity to reflect another person's emotions may be the neuronal mechanism facilitating empathy. It may be this system that is impaired in disconnected individuals.

Dysfunction of the mirror neuronal network may underlie the lack of empathy in patients with autism. To test this hypothesis, researchers conducted similar facial imitation and observation studies with high-functioning autistic children and normally developing children matched for age and IQ. Their results showed a marked decrease in activation of the mirror neuronal network in the children with autism, particularly in the frontal cortex (Figure 17.18A and B). Additional analysis showed that activity in the frontal cortex during the study correlated with the score on the social subscale of the Autistic Diagnostic Interview (Figure 17.18C).

Treatment

Medical treatments have failed to provide any consistent benefit for the core features of autism. This is likely true because medical interventions fail to correct the synaptic dysregulation that is believed to be the underlying problem of the disorder. However, intensive behavior modification has been shown to be partially effective. One study with children aged 18 to 30 months old found that 2 years of 20 hours a week therapist-led treatment (plus homework with the parents on the weekends) resulted in an increase in IQ of almost 18 points compared with 7 for the control group. Additionally, almost 30% in the treatment group were reclassified to a less severe form of autism after 2 years, while only 5% in the control group received a similar upgrade. These results are consistent with a basic tenet of this book —that environmental interactions (in this case behavior modification) can change the brain, possibly "rewire" some of the synaptic errors, especially when the changes are introduced early in life when the brain is more plastic and developing.

QUESTIONS

1. Which combination of hormones is believed to trigger maternal behavior in rats just prior to delivery?
   a. Rising progesterone and rising estradiol.
   b. Rising progesterone and falling estradiol.
   c. Falling progesterone and rising estradiol.
   d. Falling progesterone and falling estradiol.

2. Oxytocin receptors are found in all of the following except
   a. Uterus.
   b. Paraventricular nucleus.
   c. Preoptic area.
   d. Optic chiasm.

3. Pups born to mothers who are high lickers and groomers show
   a. Increased reluctance to explore a novel environment.
   b. Increased GRs in the hippocampus.
   c. Increased CRH during stress.
   d. Increased corticosterone when restrained.

4. Lightly methylated DNA
   a. Allows greater access to transcription factors.
   b. Results in greater glucocorticoid response to stress.
   c. Decreases gene expression.
   d. Is induced by mothers with low licking and grooming behavior.

5. Romantic love has a strong correlation with activity in the
   a. Ventral tegmental area.
   b. Caudate nucleus.
   c. Nucleus accumbens.
   d. Amygdala.

6. All of the following are false except
   a. Vasopressin promotes pair bonding in male voles.
   b. Meadow voles have more vasopressin.
   c. Transplanting oxytocin receptors induces monogamous behavior in male voles.
   d. Tend-and-befriend behavior modulates dips in oxytocin.

7. Eye tracking studies have shown that autistic subjects
   a. Focus on the eyes.
   b. Avoid looking at objects.
   c. Attend to the subtle social cues.
   d. Prefer to look at the lower face.

8. All of the following are true about mirror neurons except
   a. They play a role in empathy.
   b. They are impaired in autism.
   c. The frontosubcortical network is the most active.
   d. Frontal mirror neurons inactivity correlates with social impairment in autism.

See Answers section at the end of this book.

CHAPTER 18

Memory

The next three chapters will review important aspects of cognition. *Cognition* is loosely defined as the ability to do the following:

- Attend to external or internal stimuli.
- Identify the significance of the stimuli.
- Respond appropriately.

This complex processing takes place in the cortices of the brain. It occurs between the arrival of sensory input and the behavioral reaction. In the following two chapters we will discuss intelligence and attention. Here we will start with memory.

The ability to store information and access it at some future point is one of the most fascinating aspects of the brain. Indeed, some of the first experiments in psychology deal with learning and memory which continues to be hotly studied in modern neuroscience. *Learning* is defined as new information acquired by the nervous system and observed through behavioral changes. *Memory* describes encoding, storage, and retrieval of learned information.

TYPES OF MEMORY

Experts in memory have identified different types and subtypes of memory. Many of these subtle distinctions are not relevant for our purposes. One important distinction is separating memory of details from learning procedures. The facts we learn in school or from historic events of our lives are called *declarative memory* (also called *explicit memory*). This is usually what people are referring to when they speak of memory.

Procedural memory is *nondeclarative memory* (also called *implicit memory* or *somatic memory*). It describes the process of learning a skill or making associations. Examples include learning to ride a bike or playing a musical instrument. This type of memory is outside the conscious thought and actually can deteriorate if one concentrates too hard. Another example includes the exaggerated startle response seen with posttraumatic stress disorder. This reaction is immediate and takes place before the subject is consciously aware of the stimulus.

The importance of separating declarative from nondeclarative memory is that these two types of memory are encoded through different mechanisms in the brain. Likewise, they are disrupted by different central nervous system lesions or disorders—more on this later.

Immediate, Short, and Long
Memories begin to decay as soon as they are formed. The temporal stages of retention are divided into immediate, short term, and long term (Figure 18.1). These are the stages we test in a comprehensive mental status examination. *Immediate memory* (also called *working memory*) describes the ability to hold a few new facts in mind for a matter of seconds. Looking up a new phone number and successfully dialing the number within seconds is an example of this. We test this function when we ask a person to repeat three objects immediately or repeat a series of numbers. Immediate memory must be stored in some temporary state (such as short-term synaptic plasticity) that can be passed along or dissolved and be reused.

Short-term memory describes those memories that exist from seconds to minutes. An example of this process is searching the house for a lost item and remembering where you have looked. We test this process when we ask a patient to repeat three objects in 5 minutes. Both immediate and short-term memories are vulnerable to disruption.

Long-term memories are enduring representations that last for days, months, and years: the historic events and facts of our lives. This requires the development of a more permanent form of

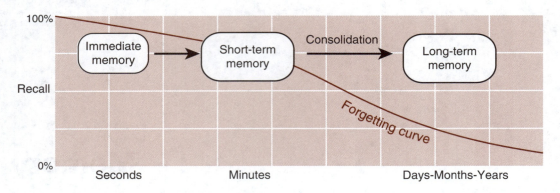

FIGURE 18.1 The temporal stages of memory superimposed on a hypothetical curve of memory retention.

storage. The process of moving information from immediate and short-term memories into long-term memory is called *consolidation*. The physical representation of memories and the areas of the brain dedicated to this function are the focus of this chapter—what do memories look like in the brain, how are they stored, and how do they fade?

ALCOHOLIC BLACKOUTS

Alcoholic blackouts occur when someone has consumed too much alcohol and awakens without memories of what happened the night before. It is believed that the high blood level of alcohol disrupts the consolidation of short-term memories into long-term memories. The drinker failed to preserve lasting images of the party because long-term memories were never formed. This can happen with short-acting hypnotics and benzodiazepines as well.

Amazingly, memories formed before drinking are actually enhanced by alcohol. That is, drinking after learning improves recall compared with not drinking. It is possible that memories already consolidated remain in a more pristine state because there is less interference from new memories that are never fully formed during the drinking.

CELLULAR MECHANISMS

The Canadian psychologist Donald O. Hebb proposed in 1949 that some changes must take place between two neurons for memories to develop. He wrote as follows:

When an axon of cell A is near enough to excite a cell B and repeatedly or persistently takes part in firing it, some growth process or metabolic change takes place in one or both cells such that A's efficacy, as one of the cells firing B, is increased.

This has come to be called *Hebb's postulate* and can be more easily stated as we said in Chapter 1, Introduction, *neurons that fire together, wire together*. Almost 60 years of research has affirmed that the brain changes with learning and experience.

Long-Term Potentiation

In Chapter 5, Receptors and Signaling the Nucleus, we have discussed long-term potentiation (LTP), a laboratory procedure with slices of brain tissue that serves as a model for memory formation. In summary:

- A series of rapid signals between two neurons results in a greater stimulus in the postsynaptic neuron when normal activity resumes (see Figure 5.6).
- Increased activity between two glutamate neurons will open the *N*-methyl-D-aspartate (NMDA) receptor, which results in molecular signals to the nucleus that induce gene expression (see Figure 5.7).
- Gene expression results in structural changes on the neuron such as spine formation on the dendrites (see Figure 5.8).

Protein Synthesis

Real memories in mammals, such as LTP, require gene expression and protein synthesis for consolidation. For example, a rat can be taught to quickly find a submerged platform in a tub of water—called a *water maze* (see Figure 18.2A and B). However, if one group of rats is given intraventricular injections of the protein synthesis inhibitor *anisomycin* 20 minutes before each test, they cannot remember the location of the submerged platform from one session to the next. These rats spend about the same amount of time each day trying to find the submerged platform (Figure 18.2C). Anisomycin inhibits the production of proteins that are needed to consolidate short-term memories into long-term memories.

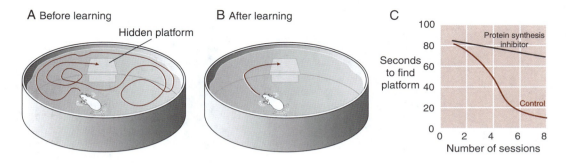

FIGURE 18.2 A rat will learn the location of a hidden platform after several sessions in a pool of water. However, rats given a protein synthesis inhibitor fail to learn **(C)**. (Adapted from Bear MF, Connors BW, Paradiso MA, eds. *Neuroscience: Exploring the Brain*. 4th ed. Baltimore: Lippincott Williams & Wilkins; 2015; Meiri N, Rosenblum K. Lateral ventricle injection of the protein synthesis inhibitor anisomycin impairs long-term memory in a spatial memory task. *Brain Res.* 1998;789[1]:48–55.)

Epigenetics

A new line of research suggests that epigenetic mechanisms may play a role in memory formation. As we discussed in Chapter 6, Genetics and Epigenetics, acetylation of the histones can open up access to the DNA and allow greater gene expression; and we know gene expression is required for protein synthesis. Several laboratories have shown that fear memory, for example, is associated with acetylation of histone H3 in the hippocampus. Likewise, inhibition of the deacetylase enzymes elevated histone acetylation and enhanced long-term memory formation.

In 2009 a group at Massachusetts Institute of Technology (MIT) established a link between histone acetylase inhibition, memory formation, and synaptic plasticity. They were able to show with mice that overexpression of the inhibitor (so there was less acetylation, more tightly closed DNA, and less gene expression) resulted in decreased dendritic spine density, synapse number, synaptic plasticity, and memory formation. Conversely, deficiencies of the acetylase inhibitor (more acetylation—more gene expression) resulted in increased synapse number and memory facilitation. These studies establish an epigenetic mechanism for the formation of long-term memories and suggest possible future sites for intervention for those with memory impairment.

Extinction

Extinction is the gradual reduction in the response to a feared stimulus when the stimulus is repeatedly encountered without an adverse experience. For example, a person who is afraid of bridges will have a reduction in fear if they repeatedly cross the bridge without falling off or the bridge collapsing. Extinction is the bedrock of behavioral therapy and one of the most effective treatments for anxiety disorders.

Several lines of evidence suggest that extinction is accomplished through the development of

new memories rather than erasing the old memories. Studies have established this by looking at the effect of anisomycin on extinction. Rats given intraventricular injections of anisomycin before repeated exposure to a stimulus (without the negative consequences) fail to show extinction the following day. In other words, the new *learning* did not *erase* the old memories.

Faster Extinction?

Wouldn't it be ideal if we could give patients a medication that would enhance learning and speed up the process of extinction? In previous editions we have discussed the use of exposure therapy in conjunction with D-cycloserine, an antibiotic used to treat tuberculosis, which is also a partial agonist at the NMDA receptor. D-Cycloserine will open the NMDA receptor and intensify the signal the postsynaptic nucleus receives. With this in mind researchers at Emory gave height-sensitive patients D-cycloserine or placebo before just two sessions in a virtual elevator. They found a 50% reduction in fear for those on the active medication. This was an exciting preliminary finding.

Unfortunately, subsequent research has not been as impressive. A recent meta-analysis of D-cycloserine and exposure-based treatment reported "a small, nonsignificant benefit of D-cycloserine augmentation compared to placebo." This is disappointing with regard to D-cycloserine, but the concept of a "psychotherapy enhancer" remains viable. At this time the best examples are the psychedelic agents, but more on this in another chapter.

Structural Plasticity

Some memories last an entire lifetime. These long-term memories persist despite surgical anesthesia, epileptic seizures, and drug abuse. Protein

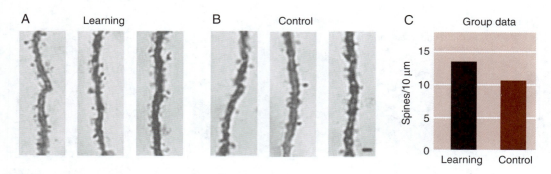

FIGURE 18.3 Rats taught to blink when a sound preceded a puff of air to their eyes showed greater spine density 24 hours later. (Adapted with permission of Society for Neuroscience, from Leuner B, Falduto J, Shors TJ. Associative memory formation increases the observation of dendritic spines in the hippocampus. *J Neurosci*. 2003;23[2]:659–665.)

molecules are not stable enough to survive these insults. Therefore, long-term memories must be the result of more stable formations such as structural changes (as seen with LTP) or they might be continuously rebuilt throughout one's life. In a previous chapter we discussed several examples of cortical strengthening secondary to learning and practicing, for example, monkeys spinning a wheel and humans playing a musical instrument. These studies establish that the cortex changes with learning.

Synaptogenesis

One mechanism that could explain learning-associated changes in the cortical structure is some type of synaptic growth. Indeed, there is considerable evidence showing that learning increases branching and synapse formation. We have already discussed that rats living in an enriched environment show greater branching and spine formation on their hippocampal neurons.

Spines are the small protrusions on the shaft of the dendrite. They are believed to represent the formation of new synapses thereby increasing communication between neighboring neurons. It has long been suggested that new spines are involved in memory formation. Leuner et al. tested this theory by teaching rats to blink in anticipation of a puff of air to the eye. After 24 hours, they found that the conditioned rats showed a 27% increase in spine formation on the pyramidal cells from the hippocampus. The reader can perceive the structural difference in the examples shown in Figure 18.3. Additionally, these changes were blocked with an NMDA antagonist. Therefore, new memories correlate with new spines.

Neurogenesis

Another mechanism that could explain the development of stable memories which can last a human life span is the formation of new neurons. We now know

that new neurons are regularly developed throughout adulthood. We have seen that rats exposed to an enriched environment, for example, also showed greater neurogenesis. Are the new neurons produced to hold memories of the enriched environment?

Leuner et al. by again teaching rats to anticipate a puff of air, looked at learning and neurogenesis. They found that those animals that showed a better performance with the task also had more new neurons surviving several days after the instruction. In other words, the greater the mastery of the skill, the greater the number of newly developing neurons that survived.

Perhaps the most compelling data regarding learning and neurogenesis come from Nottemohm and his work with songbirds. We hope the readers have stored in their long-term memory from Chapter 16, Sex and the Brain, that Nottemohm established that male canaries have a sexually dimorphic brain region called the *high vocal center* (HVC), which is directly involved in song production. Further, the HVC fluctuates in size during the year with seasonal changes in the reproductive hormones.

The relevance of the HVC for this chapter has to do with learning new songs and the changes in the HVC. The male canary changes his song repertoire over the course of 12 months by adding new notes and discarding others. Additionally, the number of new neurons added to the HVC fluctuates throughout the year. Of particular interest, the addition of new song notes and new neurons correlate (Figure 18.4). Although not definitive, it appears that the memory of the songs come and go with the development and loss of neurons in the HVC.

More recently a group in Toronto has shown an inverse relationship between neurogenesis in the hippocampus and memory persistence. First, they established that infant mice have more neurogenesis in the dentate gyrus than do adult mice and also display increased forgetting—what they call *infantile*

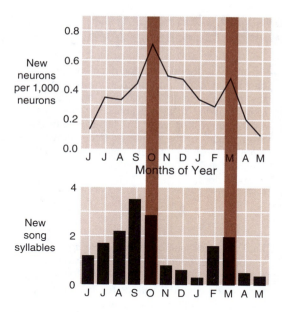

FIGURE 18.4 The development of new neurons correlates with the development of new song syllables. (Adapted from Kirn J, O'Loughlin B, Kasparian S, et al. Cell death and neuronal recruitment in the high vocal center of adult male canaries are temporally related to changes in song. *Proc Natl Acad Sci U S A*. 1994;91[17]:7844–7848. Copyright [1994] National Academy of Sciences, U.S.A.)

amnesia. Then they established that increasing neurogenesis in adult mice promotes forgetting. Last they showed that reducing neurogenesis in infant mice increases memory persistence. They conclude that the hippocampus encodes experiences, but because we cannot remember all experiences, neurogenesis must be one "process that promotes degradation of hippocampus-dependent memories, most likely by reconfiguring dentate gyrus-CA3 circuits." In other words, more neurogenesis means more forgetting.

STRESS AND MEMORY

Singularly traumatic experiences are known to produce long-lasting, intense (but not necessarily accurate) memories. Chronic stress, on the other hand, corrupts the memory-storage process. Humans who were given stress levels of cortisol demonstrate impaired declarative memory within days. As we discussed in Chapter 7, Hormones and the Brain, the likely mechanism is excess glucocorticoids causing atrophy of hippocampal dendrites, shrinking the hippocampus, and decreasing hippocampal neurogenesis.

Reconsolidation

Until recently, the prevailing belief about memories was that once consolidated they were resistant to change. That is, convulsions, protein synthesis inhibitors, or head trauma cannot erase long-term memories. However, Nader et al.'s study suggested that long-term memories can return to a labile state, vulnerable to disruption, before being consolidated again. This phenomenon is called *reconsolidation*. The essential feature of reconsolidation is that the memory must be reactivated for this process to occur.

To understand reconsolidation it is important to understand the details of the study. First, rats are taught to associate a sound with an adverse stimulation, such as a foot shock. When the rats hear the sound again, they "freeze"—a sign of fear in rodents. The researchers can quantify the percent of time the animals spend "frozen." Then the rats are exposed to the sound without the foot shock, but this time they receive the protein synthesis inhibitor anisomycin injected directly into their amygdala. Amazingly, when tested again, they do not "freeze." In other words, they show no fear. They appear to have forgotten what they learned. By analogy it is as though the long-term memory was ice, which melts to water when reactivated and then freezes again in the reconsolidation process—but now in a different shape.

What about with humans? A recent study out of the Netherlands with patients receiving electroconvulsive therapy (ECT) suggests the mechanism is the same. In the study, patients were told two emotionally laden stories. One story was reviewed just prior to anesthesia and ECT. A day later patients were quizzed about both stories. The memory of the story recalled prior to ECT was no better than chance and was significantly worse than the recall of the story that was *not* reviewed before ECT. It appears that the memory of the story reviewed prior to ECT went back to a "liquid" state and failed to "freeze" (reconsolidate) due to the amnesia of ECT.

Although there is still much to be learned about reconsolidation, it provides a possible explanation for some of the healing power of psychotherapy. Do patients reactivate their memories in the course of telling their stories? But then, because the patient is in a safe setting, the memory can be reconsolidated without as much negative affect. Hopefully, this is true and can be better used in the future as a way to improve the effectiveness of psychotherapy. Or perhaps we could use ECT or other forms of brain stimulation to help with the pain of traumatic memories.

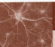

FAULTY EYEWITNESS IDENTIFICATION AND RECONSOLIDATION

DNA technology has opened a window on some major errors in the criminal justice system. Hundreds of inmates have been released from jails and prisons when the DNA evidence shows that they could not have committed the crime. Eyewitness identification errors account for the largest single cause of wrongful incarcerations. Even more amazing, some eyewitnesses refuse to accept the DNA evidence. They persist in believing their identification.

Although there are many reasons a memory can be wrong, reconsolidation may explain the persistence in maintaining an inaccurate identification. It is possible that the victim, when confronted with the lineup, reactivates the memory of the crime. At that moment the memory returned to a labile state, which is then reconsolidated, but now with the face of the wrong culprit.

ORGANIZATION OF DECLARATIVE MEMORY

One of the great mysteries of neuroscience involves finding the location of long-term declarative memories. Where are they stored in the brain? How are they formed and why do they decay? Unfortunately, there are only basic explanations for these intriguing questions.

Hippocampus

The hippocampus is crucial for consolidation of long-term memories. The importance of the hippocampus became painfully obvious with the famous case of H.M. H.M. had struggled with minor seizures since the age of 10 and major seizures since the age of 16. Despite aggressive anticonvulsant medications, the seizures increased in frequency and ultimately the patient was unable to work. In 1953, at the age of 27, H.M. underwent a large bilateral resection of the medial temporal lobes in an effort to remove the nidus of the seizures. Figure 18.5 shows the areas of the brain removed.

The surgery successfully quieted the seizures, but unfortunately left H.M. with profound anterograde amnesia. Although his personality remained the same and his IQ even improved a bit from 104 to 112, he displayed severe and pervasive memory impairments. Specifically, he showed normal immediate memory, but could not consolidate those memories into enduring traces. For example, when a person exited and reentered his room within a few minutes, H.M. was unaware of that person's earlier visit. However, his remote memories remained intact. In fact, he would frequently speak of events before the surgery, in part because he was not developing new memories. To use a computer metaphor, it is as though H.M. has a "read only"

hard drive for memory storage. He could retrieve old memories but could not write new ones.

This unfortunate outcome for H.M. highlighted the essential role of the medial temporal lobe in forming long-term memories. Subsequent studies with animals and humans have established the hippocampus and the parahippocampal gyrus as crucial for encoding and consolidating memories of events and objects in time and space. For example, numerous studies have shown that lesions of a rat's hippocampus impair its ability to remember the location of the hidden platform in a water maze.

Further studies with H.M. established that the amnesia was not as widespread as initially perceived. For example, H.M. was asked to participate in a mirror-tracing task. While viewing his hand in a mirror, H.M. was asked to trace a star while keeping the pencil between the lines. H.M. improved at this task in 10 trials on the first day (Figure 18.6). He did even better on the second and third days. Remarkably, when asked about the task, he stated he had never seen the test before. This highlights what we addressed at the beginning of the chapter: there are different types of memory. H.M.'s explicit memory is disrupted, but his implicit memory remains intact. Consequently, this type of memory must be stored through different mechanisms—ones that are independent of the hippocampus.

H.M. died in December 2008. Studies shortly before his death showed that his declarative memory deficit was not as absolute as dense thought. For example, he was able to draw a reasonably accurate floor plan of his house although he had moved there 5 years after his operation. Likewise, when he looks in a mirror he is not startled by his appearance. This suggests that some declarative memories were being stored.

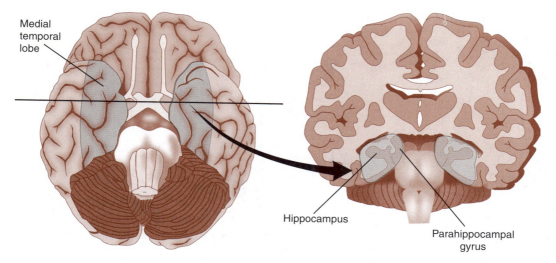

FIGURE 18.5 Two views of H.M.'s brain identifying the areas that were removed in surgery, which left him with anterograde amnesia. (Adapted from Bear MF, Connors BW, Paradiso MA, eds. *Neuroscience: Exploring the Brain*. 4th ed. Baltimore: Lippincott Williams & Wilkins; 2015.)

In 2014 a postmortem examination of H.M.'s brain was published that included his real name (Henry Molaison) and provided more precise details about the extent of the ablative brain surgery—which was primarily the anterior hippocampus and entorhinal cortex. More of the posterior hippocampus was spared than had been anticipated. However, the entorhinal cortex functions as the conduit for cortical sensory information moving into the hippocampus. Therefore there was less hippocampal damage than expected but almost complete severing of the means of getting information into the hippocampus. Finally, the amygdalae were almost entirely absent, which may explain his dampened emotions and lack of initiative.

MEMORY AND PLEASURE

We discussed in Chapter 12, Pleasure, that memories associated with getting high could induce cravings in drug addicts. Conversely, it is well documented that pleasure enhances learning. Indeed, dopamine neurons from the ventral tegmental area directly innervate the medial temporal lobe. Recent brain imaging studies have shown simultaneous activation of the ventral tegmental area and medial temporal lobe when subjects are remembering rewarding experiences.

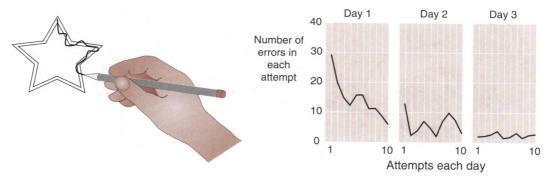

FIGURE 18.6 The mirror-tracing task asks subjects to trace between two stars while watching their hand in a mirror. The patient H.M. showed improvement at this task although he had no recollection of having taken the test before. (Adapted from Blakemore C. *Mechanics of the Mind*. Cambridge, UK: Cambridge University Press; 1978.)

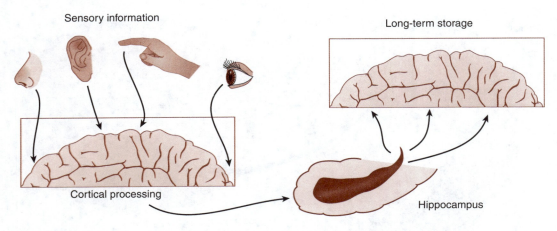

FIGURE 18.7 Experiences enter the brain through the senses and are initially processed in the cortex. This information then goes to the hippocampus before being stored in the cortex.

Neocortex

Sensory information comes into the brain and is processed in specific regions of the neocortex. Efferent projections from these cortical areas are passed along to the *entorhinal cortex* that serves as the major hub between the cortex and the hippocampus. The hippocampus has efferent projections back to cortical regions, which appear to serve as storage sites for long-term memories. Figure 18.7 is a schematic representation of this process.

Damage to the hippocampus impairs the formation of new memories, but what affects remote memories? Bayley et al. examined eight patients with damage to their medial temporal lobes. All patients had problems storing new memories, but largely retained the ability to recall remote autobiographic memories. Only the three patients who also had significant additional damage to the neocortex showed impairment with remote memories. However, the exact location of long-term memories remains a mystery. It appears that remote memories are stored throughout the cortex rather than in one specific location. Anatomic studies with monkeys have established hippocampal projections to the cortical regions shown in Figure 18.8. These studies suggest that declarative memories are stored in the dorsolateral prefrontal cortex, cingulate gyrus, parietal lobe, and temporal lobe.

System Consolidation

When your computer saves a file to the hard drive, that data is placed in a specific location where it

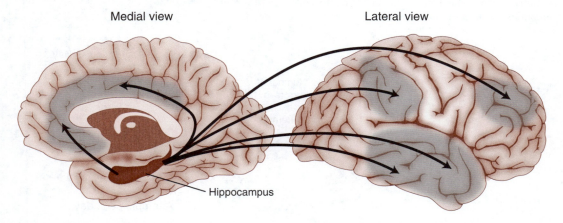

FIGURE 18.8 Efferent projections from the hippocampus go to the cortical areas shaded in *gray*. It is thought that long-term declarative memories are physically contained within these regions. The exact mechanism remains a mystery. (Adapted with permission from Van Hoesen GW. The parahippocampal gyrus: new observations regarding its cortical connections in the monkey. *Trends Neurosci*. 1982;5:345–350. Copyright 1982 with permission from Elsevier.)

remains unchanged until it is modified. When we put items in our closets, they stay in the same location until we return for them. Storage in the brain, on the other hand, is more dynamic. There is evidence that memories undergo continuing remodeling even weeks and months after they are formed. This process is called *system consolidation*.

Looking at which part of the brain is activated during retrieval of recent and remote memories provides a good understanding of system consolidation. Researchers in France taught mice to navigate a maze. Placing the mice back in the maze at either 5 days or 25 days reactivated those memories. Cerebral metabolic activity was then measured in a mouse functional scanner (we're not kidding). At 5 days the mice had greater activity in their hippocampus. Those tested after 25 days had less activity in the hippocampus and greater activity in the cortical regions such as the cingulate gyrus and frontal cortex. This shows that memories are initially dependent on hippocampus. Then, by some process of consolidation that occurs over days, the memories become independent of the hippocampus and reside in a distributed pattern in the cortex.

The same researchers also looked at the remodeling of memories within layers of the cortex. As before, they taught the mice to negotiate a maze and then retested their memory at either 1 day or 30 days. This time they sacrificed the mice and measured Fos (a marker of gene activation) in the parietal cortex. They found that total Fos activity was the same at days 1 and 30. However, the location of activity within the layers of the parietal cortex changed from days 1 to 30. Figure 18.9 shows the change in Fos activity by layer. Note how the recent memory activates neurons in layers V and VI. Memory after 30 days, in comparison, shows greater activity in layers II and III.

These studies show that memories in the brain are not simply created and stored in a fixed and static receptacle awaiting recall. Memories appear to undergo remodeling as they become independent of the hippocampus and possibly as they are relocated in the layers of the cortex. And all this is done "off-line," without conscious recall of the memory, possibly during sleep.

Recently, a group at University of California, Riverside, postulated that episodic memories acquired during the day are temporarily stored in the hippocampus and relayed up to the cortex during the night for long-term storage. They found evidence (which requires way too much math to comprehend) that alternating electrical activity between the hippocampus and cortical neurons during deep sleep strengthens synaptic connections that are believed to be the physical manifestation of memory storage. This may be one explanation for what the brain is doing during sleep to strengthen memories.

FORGETTING

From the standpoint of a mental health practitioner, problems with forgetting may be more relevant in day-to-day clinical practice than problems with forming new memories. Sometimes patients forget too much, as with Alzheimer's disease, or, at the other extreme, cannot forget horrific traumatic memories they wish would disappear. Although the cellular and molecular mechanisms of learning and memory are becoming clearer, the mechanisms of forgetting remain poorly understood.

The importance of forgetting can be understood from a standpoint of storage. Our brains are simply not large enough to retain all the details of our lives. To further minimize what is retained it is likely the brain only stores broad outlines of the information. An example of this can be shown with Figure 18.10. Although the reader has seen pennies thousands of times over the past years, it is still hard to correctly identify the accurate drawing of the penny. This example highlights one reason we fail to remember: detailed memories were never stored in the first place. Likewise, any interference at the time of consolidation will impair future recall. However, this is different from forgetting what was once learned.

Numerous experiments have documented a continuous decline for remote memories with the passage of time. The "forgetting curve" in Figure 18.1 shows a hypothetical drop in the ability to

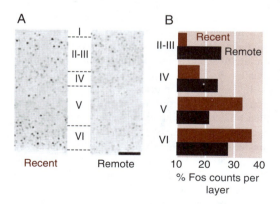

FIGURE 18.9 A: Micrographs from parietal lobes of mice tested at day 1 (recent) and day 30 (remote). **B:** Percentage of Fos counts per layer. (Micrograph from Maviel T, Durkin TP, Menzaghi F, et al. Sites of neocortical reorganization critical for remote spatial memory. *Science.* 2004;305[5680]:96–99. Reprinted with permission from AAAS.)

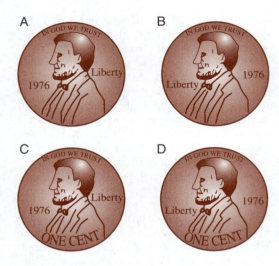

A **B**

C **D**

FIGURE 18.10 Because the brain retains so few details about objects, it is hard to identify which penny is an actual representation of the 1-cent coin. Few viewers will recognize that none of the drawings are a good match because Lincoln is facing the wrong direction.

recall unrehearsed information with the passage of time. Memories simply grow weaker as we age. How this occurs is poorly understood.

One possible mechanism assumes a passive decay over time. If the connections holding the memory are not used, they become weaker with time. Alternatively, the memory could be overwritten with new information and distorted or lost. Figuratively, it is as though an unused path through the woods is lost as the forest grows over it.

Actively forgetting is another possible mechanism that the brain could use. In this case it would be more like going through one's closet and throwing away items not being used. Recent research suggests that active forgetting does occur in the brain.

In Chapter 5, Receptors and Signaling the Nucleus, we discussed how protein kinases phosphorylate transcription factors such as cyclic adenosine monophosphate responsive element–binding protein (CREB) to promote gene expression. As is typical in the Yin and Yang mechanisms of the body, different proteins *dephosphorylate* CREB and turn off gene expression. The proteins that dephosphorylate are called *protein phosphatases*, and one of them, called *protein phosphatase 1* (PP1), has been implicated in forgetting. But first researchers established that inhibiting PP1 enhanced learning efficacy.

In a second experiment in a water maze, the researchers tested memory for the location of the hidden platform. Mice with PP1 inhibition remembered equally well at 8 weeks as they did on day 1. However, the control mice showed a decay in memory of the platform location as early as 2 weeks and seemed to have completely forgotten by 8 weeks. These results suggest that forgetting is an active function perpetrated by the brain to clean out old memories—possibly to make room for new information.

Electroconvulsive Therapy

One of the great controversies in psychiatry involves ECT and memory loss. There is no question about failure to remember experiences around the time of the procedure. The electrically induced seizure disrupts formation of new memories, so patients never recall details of the treatment or shortly afterward. However, some patient groups have vigorously complained that ECT also erases long-term memories (retrograde amnesia). This was a difficult issue to tease out until the development of autobiographical interviews, which could be individualized to each patient and then administered before and after the ECT.

Harold Sackeim and his group prospectively studied the cognitive effects of ECT on 347 patients at seven hospitals in New York City. At the 6-month follow-up examination, scores on the Mini-Mental Status Examination (as a comparison) had improved from baseline for almost all patients. However, some patients showed persistent deficits for autobiographical memories compared with the pretreatment baseline. Further analysis showed that retrograde amnesia correlated with electrode placement (Figure 18.11). Patients who received bilateral ECT forgot some of their past history while patients receiving unilateral ECT improved their autobiographical recall.

If long-term memories are a stronger connection between neurons (as we discussed above), then bilateral ECT must in some way disrupt the connections in the cortex. How this happens is a mystery. Some have postulated that the electricity and convulsion induce an outpouring of biochemical molecules such as glutamate and glucocorticoids, which possibly are toxic to the cortical connections. Fortunately, the benefits found with unilateral ECT suggest the problem is not an essential feature of successful treatment. Furthermore, newer developments with shorter pulse widths (ultrabrief right unilateral ECT) have reduced the memory problems even further.

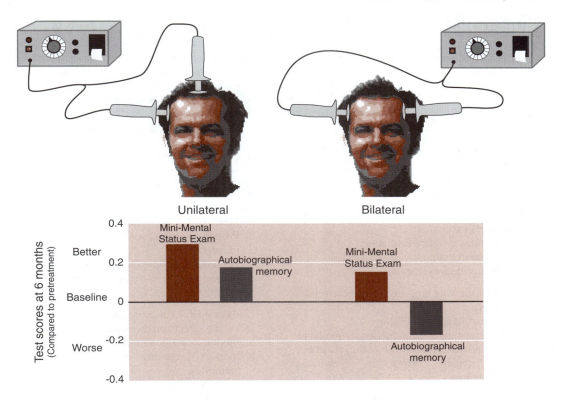

FIGURE 18.11 Long-term autobiographical memories deteriorated after electroconvulsive therapy (ECT) for patients who received bilateral ECT, but not for patients receiving unilateral ECT. (Data from Sackiem HA, et al. The cognitive effects of electroconvulsive therapy in community settings. *Neuropsychopharmacology*. 2007;32:244–254.)

MIND OF A MNEMONIST

Some people have extraordinary memories. One such person was studied at length in Russia for over 30 years during the time of Stalin. This man, called S. by the psychologist Alexander Luria, had an unbelievable capacity to accurately recall long lists of words, syllables, or numbers. For example, when shown the nonsense formula in the figure below, S. studied it briefly and then after a few minutes reproduced it without error. Even more remarkable, when spontaneously and without warning asked to recall the formula 15 years later, he did so flawlessly.

$$N \cdot \sqrt{d^2 \times \frac{85}{vx}} \cdot \sqrt[3]{\frac{276^2 \cdot 86x}{n^2v \cdot \pi 264}} \ \ n^2b{=}sv \ \frac{1624}{32^2} \cdot r^2s$$

A nonsense mathematical formula created to test S.'s memory. (Adapted from *The Mind of a Mnemonist: A Little Book About a Vast Memory* by A. R. Luria, translated from the Russian by Lynn Solotaroff. Cambridge, Mass.: Harvard University Press, Copyright © 1968 by Michael Cole.)

S. had an unusual ability to generate vivid enduring images in his mind. When asked to recall the items, he simply recalled the images and read them as one would read symbols on a page. Although the stable quality of these images allowed S. to earn a living as a performing mnemonist, it also cluttered his mind. He had trouble forgetting. S. was actually encumbered by past visual images that were activated by similar topics in conversation and reading. The associated images led to mental wanderings taking his mind far from the task in front of him. His gift for details interfered with his grasp of the "big picture."

Was there something different about S.'s brain? Unfortunately, S. lived before the time of brain imaging technology, so any differences in his brain's size or functions that might explain his extraordinary memory remain unknown. He also lived before the revolution in genetics. Might he have had an unusual variant of a protein synthesis gene that allowed for better immediate memory formation?

QUESTIONS

1. Learning to tie shoes is what kind of memory?
   a. Declarative.
   b. Implicit.
   c. Explicit.
   d. Antegrade.

2. Which answer does not fit?
   a. Short-term memory.
   b. DNA $\Rightarrow$ RNA.
   c. Gene expression.
   d. Protein synthesis.

3. Anisomycin
   a. Enhances extinction.
   b. Accelerates memory formation.
   c. Limits neurogenesis.
   d. Inhibits protein synthesis.

4. All of the following are true about reconsolidation except
   a. It was an unexpected finding.
   b. It suggests long-term memories are mailable.
   c. Is demonstrated with the use of D-cycloserine.
   d. Helps explain errors in eyewitness identification.

5. The patient H.M. is impaired with the following?
   a. Ability to build new long-term memories.
   b. Retrieve long-term memories.
   c. Develop new procedural memories.
   d. Understand explicit instructions.

6. Evidence of system consolidation includes?
   a. More mature memories are more dependent on the hippocampus.
   b. Mature memories are more prevalent in the prefrontal cortex.
   c. Cortical layers II and III have less remote memories.
   d. Older memories are more active in the neocortex.

7. All of the following are true about forgetting long-term memories except
   a. Memories decay with time.
   b. Protein phosphatases have been implicated in forgetting.
   c. Forgetting can be enhanced with anisomycin.
   d. Interference during consolidation increases forgetting.

8. Unilateral ECT for depression has all of the following effects on memory except
   a. Inhibits consolidation.
   b. Induces forgetting of remote long-term memories.
   c. Improves cognition.
   d. Some memories are completely lost.

See Answers section at the end of this book.

CHAPTER 19

Intelligence

INTELLIGENCE

The topic of intelligence can generate strong feelings. Specifically, the idea that there is one monolithic kind of intelligence that is reflected by a single number plotted on a bell-shaped curve is hard to accept. Can one number determine a person's life? Other variables such as interpersonal skill, emotional resilience, creativity, and motivation are factors independent of intelligence, which are critical for success in a career or in life. Likewise, a person can show great aptitude in one area, yet struggle in another. Having said that, it is important to acknowledge there is considerable evidence of a general mental ability called *intelligence*, which has a predictive value.

It has been shown that all credible tests of mental ability rank individuals in about the same way; that is, people who do well on one type of test tend to do well on the others and *vice versa*. Such tests (e.g., the Wechsler Intelligence Scale, which gives an IQ score) are believed to measure some global element of intellectual ability. This global element is called "*g*" or fluid intelligence. *g* is conceptualized as reasoning and novel problem-solving ability. Others have described it as the ability to deal with complexity. There is no pure measure of *g*. An IQ score is an approximation of *g*.

Some argue that *g* is only useful to predict academic success or success in situations that resemble school. Arguing against this, others point to data showing the predictive correlates between IQ and employment, marriage, incarceration, and income. From our standpoint, we are interested in the associations between *g* and the neural substrate of the brain.

Genetics

Before we delve into the neuroscience of intelligence, it is worth discussing some compelling studies on the heritability of cognitive skills. The Colorado Adoption Project that started in 1975 followed up 200 adopted children from childhood through adolescence. They compared the cognitive ability of the children with their adoptive parents and their biologic parents. A control group of children raised by their biologic parents was included for comparison.

Figure 19.1 shows the correlations for verbal and spatial abilities over time between the children and the parents. Note how the adopted children have almost zero correlation between them and their adopted parents. Their cognitive skills more closely match their biologic parents. Another finding of interest is that the correlations improve with age. We become more like our biologic parents as we age—at least with regard to intelligence.

Beijing Genomics Institute (BGI) in Shenzhen, China, has embarked on a quest to find the genetics of intelligence. BGI is the largest gene-sequencing facility in the world. They have gathered DNA and IQ results from thousands of very bright subjects and are sifting through the code looking for biologic clues to intelligence—a daunting and somewhat disturbing plan.

Brain Size

A consistent finding in neuroscience has been the association between brain size and intelligence; that is, all other things being equal, bigger brains really are better. Nottebohm in his work with songbirds found a noteworthy example. The reader will remember that male songbirds have an enlarged high vocal center (HVC) that plays an essential role in his song production. Nottebohm meticulously recorded the diversity of song syllables that

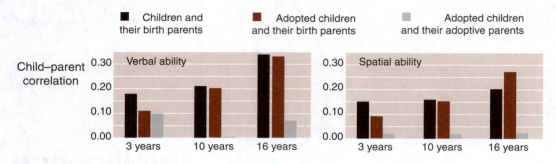

FIGURE 19.1 The correlation between children and their biologic parents increases with age for verbal and spatial abilities. The shared environment between adopted children and their parents had little effect on verbal or spatial intelligence scores. (Adapted from Plomin R, DeFries JC. The genetics of cognitive abilities and disabilities. *Sci Am*. 1998;278[5]:62–69. Reproduced with permission. Copyright © 1998 *Scientific American*, a division of Nature America, Inc. All rights reserved.)

each bird produced and then compared this with the size of his HVC. The results are plotted in Figure 19.2 and show a good correlation.

An extensive song repertoire is not the same as reasoning and problem solving. It is probably closer to having a large fund of knowledge (sometimes called *crystalline intelligence*). However, for our purposes it shows an association between brain size and a learned task.

With humans, there is a long history of studies comparing brain size and intelligence. In the early days they would simply compare head circumference (hat size) with rough estimates of intelligence. However, there is more to intelligence than just brain size, otherwise whales and elephants would have ruled the world. The important

variable is the relative size of the brain to the size of the body.

The Smartest Animal

Why are humans so smart? Or, to put this another way, what features of the human brain distinguish it from the brains of other mammals? If we are so much smarter, one would think it would be easy to spot the differences between our brains and that of our closest animal relatives. Unfortunately, it is hard to find anatomic correlates that explain the significant leap in intelligence we see in humans.

There are several variables that have been suggested such as brain size, relative brain weight, or number of cortical neurons, but for almost every variable there is some species that exceeds or is at least equal to humans. A cat has more cortical neurons relative to brain weight than do humans, and dolphins have almost the same relative brain weight compared with body weight as humans do. Cats and dolphins are smart animals but they cannot design a house, write a play, or solve algebra problems.

There is no single variable that marks the superior human intelligence. The explanation appears to be a combination of relative size and speed and connectedness of communication.

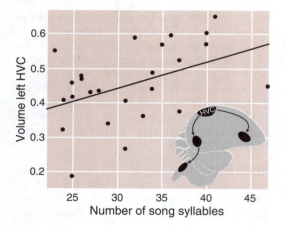

- Relatively large brain compared to body weight
- Large number of cortical neurons
- Numerous synaptic connections
- Thick, fast axons that transmit signals quickly
- Short distance between neurons

In other words, humans have more cortical neurons with faster conduction velocities that make more connections than do elephants, dolphins, or the other great apes.

Our superior intelligence is often attributed to our large prefrontal cortex (PFC)—the home of

FIGURE 19.2 Adult male canaries with a large repertoire of song syllables also tend to have a large high vocal center (HVC) while those with small repertoire have a small HVC. (Adapted from Nottebohm F. [2004.] The road we travelled: discovery, choreography, and significance of brain replaceable neurons. *Ann N Y Acad Sci*. 1016:628–658.)

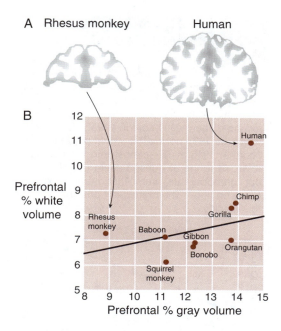

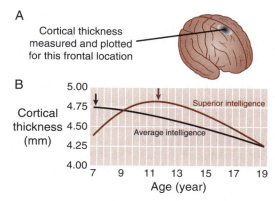

FIGURE 19.4 Measurements at the indicated point of the right superior frontal gyrus **(A)**. Comparison of the cortical thickness at the point in **A** through adolescence for those with superior intelligence compared with those with average intelligence **(B)**. (Adapted by permission from Macmillan Publishers Ltd. Shaw P, Greenstein D, Lerch J, et al. Intellectual ability and cortical development in children and adolescents. *Nature*. 2006;440[7084]:676–679. Copyright 2006.)

FIGURE 19.3 Gray matter and white matter comparisons in the prefrontal cortex (PFC) for rhesus monkeys and humans **(A)**. The proportion of white matter in the PFC (compared with total white matter) is larger for humans than other primates **(B)**. (Adapted by permission from Macmillan Publishers Ltd. Schoenemann PT, Sheehan MJ, Glotzer LD. Prefrontal white matter volume is disproportionately larger in humans than in other primates. *Nat Neurosci*. 2005;8[2]:242–252. Copyright 2005.)

executive function. However, comparative studies have found the proportional human PFC to be inline with that of the great apes and may be smaller than that in elephants and whales. A better explanation may be the proportion of white matter to gray matter in the frontal cortex. Recent magnetic resonance imaging (MRI) studies on humans and other primates compared the relative volumes of white and gray matter in the PFC. The largest difference was found with the PFC white matter (Figure 19.3). The authors suggested that this difference might be a measure of "connectional elaboration." They postulate that the superior cognitive skills in humans could be a result of more and faster connections, not just more neurons.

The Smartest Humans

Shortly after his death, Einstein's brain was removed by a pathologist at the Princeton Hospital who assumed the world *had* to examine the brain of such a genius. Almost certainly this was not Einstein's last wish. The journey of his brain since 1955 is an entertaining story, but not great science. Most remarkable is the *unremarkable* appearance of the brain of the man who first voiced the theory of relativity. Einstein's brain is just one example of the difficulty of finding neuroanatomical correlates for intelligence.

Modern imaging studies allow the in vivo measurement of brain volume in multiple subjects. McDaniel conducted a meta-analysis of imaging studies comparing brain volume and intelligence. He identified 37 high-quality studies with a total of 1,530 people. The correlation between brain volume and intelligence across the studies was 0.33. In other words, differences in brain volume may explain some of the differences in IQ, but there is much more that remains unexplained.

Measurements of intelligence remain relatively stable over a person's life span. Yet, we know that the brain is a dynamic organ with more remodeling capability than we could have imagined just a decade ago. Likewise, there is a shrinking of the gray matter starting in adolescence. It is unclear how these fluctuations relate to intelligence.

Giedd et al. at National Institute of Mental Health (NIMH) completed a longitudinal study of cortical thickness and intellectual ability from childhood through adolescence for more than 300 children. The most significant finding was that it was not the absolute thickness of the gray matter that correlated best with intelligence, but rather the rate of change. This was most prominent in the PFC. Figure 19.4 shows the cortical thickness for one location on the right superior frontal gyrus for subjects with superior intelligence and average intelligence. Note how those with superior intelligence have less gray matter when very young, which peaks later, and then shows a more rapid thinning compared with the average children.

These findings are not what were expected. Smart children do not simply have more gray matter. Rather, it is the dynamic properties (perhaps even efficient pruning of unneeded connections) of the cortical maturation that are somehow superior in intelligent children. The significance of this finding remains unclear, but suggests that refinement, not size, is the hallmark of intelligence.

Parents and their teenage children provide an alternative way to examine the topic of intelligence. We would expect parents and children to have similar intellectual abilities. Yet we would seek out the parents if we wanted advice and counsel—not the "know-it-all" teens. However, with almost every anatomical measure of the brain, the teen brain is superior: thickness of gray matter, number of neurons, and number of synaptic connections, for example. It does not make sense—the teens have more brain matter but the adults have more wisdom. The only brain structure that seems to correlate with adult wisdom is frontal lobe white matter, which peaks around 39 years of age (see Figure 8.8). This is further evidence that connectivity may be the secret to intelligence.

Smart people postulate that higher intelligence is the result of network efficiency. That is, faster and more accurate transfer of information around the brain makes a person smarter. Research supports this belief. In one study of brain-damaged patients, there was a correlation between lower intelligence and damage to the long white matter tracts (arcuate and superior longitudinal fasciculus) that connect the frontal and parietal lobe. Numerous diffusion tensor imaging studies have shown correlations between intelligence and the integrity of the white matter tracts—implying that more efficient white matter tracts transmit information faster which enhances intelligence. Finally, functional imaging studies (functional MRI (fMRI)) have examined what is called *functional connectivity*—meaning the capacity of distant brain regions to work together. For example, a number of studies suggest connectivity between the parietal and frontal lobes is critically involved in intelligence.

In summary, the essence of intelligence in the brain remains a mystery. The studies mentioned above suggest that numerous neurons, densely packed, with rapid connections between the frontal cortex and other regions of the brain facilitate cognitive performance. More neurons, talking faster to each other, likely make for a smarter brain.

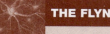

THE FLYNN EFFECT

James Flynn has shown that if IQ scores were not renormalized every generation, the average scores would significantly increase. This suggests we are getting smarter. For example, the mean score in 1995 was 100 and using the 1995 norms this would put the mean score in 1918 at 75—almost into the mentally retarded range. It doesn't seem possible that our grandparents were that stupid. What's going on here? The brain can't possibly evolve this quickly.

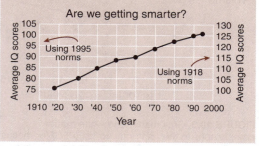

Are we getting smarter?

Brilliance and Mental Illness

There is a popular belief in an association between "genius" and "madness"—a "fine line" is often stated. Numerous books have been written on the topic, but these case studies are more anecdote than science. Prospective research is needed. A recent study out of Sweden sheds some much-needed light on the issue.

Sweden's social policies and national registries allow for the comparison of academic achievement with later psychiatric hospitalization. All students in Sweden are required to attend school until the summer in which they turn 16. Grades from the final year of compulsory education are normalized based on a national distribution, and an average is calculated for each student. These scores were compared with psychiatric diagnoses for subsequent hospitalization. The results are shown in Figure 19.5.

It appears that exceptional academic achievement is a risk factor for bipolar disorder. For males with excellent grades, there was a fourfold increase in risk of developing bipolar disorder compared with students with average grades. Students with the lowest grades had a modest (twofold) increased risk compared with average students. Schizophrenia, on the other hand, is uniformly associated with poor school performance, and high grades are in fact protective.

The results lend some credence to the book entitled "Brilliant Madness" which was coauthored

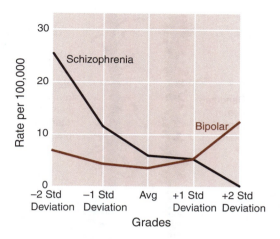

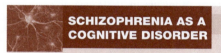

FIGURE 19.5 Students whose average grades at the age of 16 years were two standard deviations above the norm were more likely to develop bipolar disorder and less likely to develop schizophrenia. (Adapted from MacCabe JH, Lambe MP, Cnattingius S, et al. Excellent school performance at age 16 and risk of adult bipolar disorder: national cohort study. *Br J Psychiatry*. 2010;196:109–115.)

by Patty Duke about her struggle with bipolar disorder. It certainly seems that activated bipolar patients are thinking too fast—racing thoughts is the clinical term. Are some racing thoughts advantageous? Is a little bit helpful for academic performance, but too much is called mental illness?

SCHIZOPHRENIA AS A COGNITIVE DISORDER

Kahn and Keefe have proposed that schizophrenia be viewed as a cognitive disorder. They posit that intellectual underperformance is a risk factor for schizophrenia, cognitive decline precedes the onset of psychosis, cognitive impairment is related to outcome and is not improved with antipsychotic treatment. "Putting the focus back on cognition may facilitate finding treatments for the illness before psychosis ever emerges."

Performance Enhancement

There is considerable interest in medications or brain stimulation devices that could enhance cognitive performance. Interventions to increase problem-solving skills would be valuable tools in the treatment of disorders such as traumatic brain injury, Alzheimer's disease, and schizophrenia. However, there would be a large demand from people without disorders seeking to enhance their cognitive performance. The prospect of "lifestyle" medications for intelligence is worrisome, especially in a meritocracy such as ours where profession and income are largely dependent on school performance and intelligence.

Although a blockbuster intelligence boosting treatment is more the realm of science fiction, there are several products currently used by people looking for an advantage. The best-known agents are the stimulants such as the amphetamines and methylphenidate. Surveys of college students have reported the abuse and misuse of the stimulant medications. Although the estimates vary widely, the practice appears to be common in US colleges. In general, students at more competitive universities, members of fraternities, and those with lower grades are at greater risk for misuse of the stimulants. But misuse is not limited to college students. An informal online survey by *Nature* readers found that 20% of the almost 1,500 respondents reported using performance enhancing medications, most commonly methylphenidate (62%).

DISORDER

ATTENTION DEFICIT HYPERACTIVITY DISORDER

It is not uncommon in clinical practice for a parent to try out their child's stimulant and experience a favorable response. The parent will conclude that they also have attention deficit hyperactivity disorder (ADHD). Often such parents will present with a request for a prescription for themselves. However, improved productivity while taking methylphenidate or amphetamine is a normal response and does not constitute the presence of a disorder.

Other pharmacologic agents are also believed to enhance cognitive skills. Modafinil marketed for narcolepsy and excessive fatigue has been shown to improve cognitive performance in healthy subjects, as have caffeine and nicotine. In general, any agent that increases energy appears to improve cognitive performance—or at least the perception of enhanced performance.

Fortunately, someone has finally studied the cognitive effects of stimulants in healthy young adults. A group at the University of Pennsylvania administered a battery of cognitive tests including episodic memory, working memory, inhibitory control, creativity, and general intelligence, as well as verbal and math SAT's on young adult subjects without ADHD. Thirteen tests were conducted over several days when the subjects were blindly taking 20 mg of Adderall or placebo..., and, remarkably, there was no difference in the scores. However, when asked, the participants *believed* they performed better when taking amphetamine. Therefore, it's possible people feel smarter, but do not actually perform any better. However, even if amphetamines do not make us smarter on tests, they still may enhance productivity regardless of diagnosis.

DEFICITS

It is beyond the scope of this text to review all known cognitive deficits. However, mental retardation (MR) and dyslexia, in particular, shed light on the neuroscience of cognitive impairment. Both have distinct abnormalities that give us greater understanding of the brain.

Mental Retardation
Dendritic Pathology

MR is a nonprogressive developmental disorder affecting global cognitive function. By definition, MR is characterized by an IQ of 70 or below (two standard deviations below the norm of 100). In the United States, this comprises approximately 1% to 2% of the population. There are numerous causes of MR, including genetic aberrations, toxin exposure in utero, and malnutrition.

Severe forms of MR often have readily apparent structural abnormalities, for example, microcephaly. However, most subjects with MR show little, if any, obvious changes in brain anatomy. Their brains appear normal when examined with MRI. In the 1970s, researchers began postmortem examination of the brains of retarded children and discovered extensive dendritic spine abnormalities (Figure 19.6). Subsequent studies established aberrant spine morphology and/or reduced dendritic branching as a consistent finding in MR in a variety of syndromes.

The importance of spine architecture for learning and memory has been discussed in several chapters in this book (e.g., see Figures 8.13, 12.13, 16.6, and 18.3). It is reasonable to assert that deficits in spine morphology impair the network connectivity essential for information processing. Likewise, it is only a short step to imagine that problems with information processing play a large role in the cognitive deficits of MR.

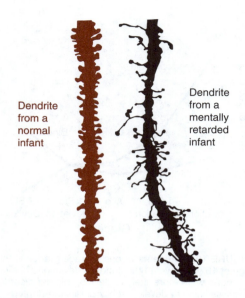

Dendrite from a normal infant

Dendrite from a mentally retarded infant

FIGURE 19.6 Dendrites from a healthy child and one with mental retardation (MR), highlighting the abnormal spine morphology in the child with MR. (Adapted from Purpura DP. Dendritic spine "dysgenesis" and mental retardation. *Science*. 1974;186[4169]:1126–1128. Reprinted with permission from AAAS.)

Environmental and Nurturing Deprivation

Deprivation in early infancy is a well-known cause of cognitive impairment. Draconian studies on animals have established the lasting impact of early environmental impoverishment. The fall of the totalitarian government ruled by Nicolae Ceausescu in Romania in 1989 gave the world a group of unfortunate children who could be systematically studied to document the long-term effects of early deprivation.

During the Ceausescu regime, orphaned children were raised in institutions under conditions of severe deprivation. When Romania was opened to the world by the new government, the shocking condition of these children was revealed. Most were severely malnourished, with significant developmental delays. European and American families responded by adopting many of these children.

It is assumed that most of these children were put into the institutions as very young babies. Consequently, the age at which they were adopted approximates the length of time they were raised in a deprived environment. Likewise, it is assumed that these children moved into enriched environments after adoption.

The cognitive skills of 131 of these adoptees have been studied and compared with 50 UK adoptees who were adopted before 6 months of age. IQ tests have been administered to all these children

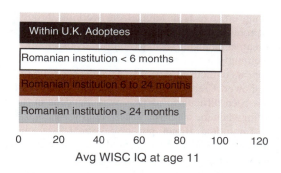

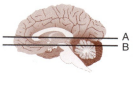

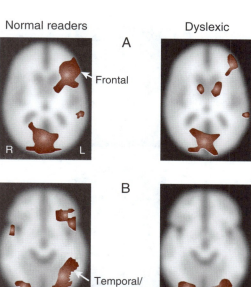

FIGURE 19.7 A dose–response effect is shown for different amounts of institutional deprivation on IQ at 11 years of age. WISC, Wechsler Intelligence Scale for Children. (Adapted from Beckett C, Maughan B, Rutter M, et al. [2006.] Do the effects of early severe deprivation on cognition persist into early adolescence? Findings from the English and Romanian adoptees study. *Child Dev.* 77[3]: 696–711.)

throughout their childhood. Significant improvements were seen at the assessments of 4-year-old and 6-year-old Romanian children. Many children displayed an encouraging "catch-up" with the UK adoptees. The examination results of the 11-year-old Romanian adoptees were reported and are shown in Figure 19.7.

The figure highlights the profound and lasting effects of early institutional deprivation. Of particular interest is the dose–response relationship between IQ and the number of years spent in an impoverished environment. Children removed from deprivation before 6 months of age had almost no lasting impairment. However, those children who stayed in the institutions for more than 6 months had 20-point reductions compared with the UK adoptees. These results substantiate the work by Hubel and Wiesel (Chapter 8, Plasticity and Adult Development) regarding critical periods of brain development.

Dyslexia

Unlike MR, dyslexia is a localized impairment. Classified as a learning disorder, dyslexia presents as an unexpected difficulty in reading in a person with otherwise normal intelligence and motivation. Dyslexia may be the most common neurobehavioral disorder in children. Estimates of the prevalence range from 5% to 17.5%.

Although speech develops naturally, reading is an acquired skill. Children must learn that letters on a page represent the sounds of spoken language. Children with dyslexia have trouble decoding the letters into the sounds of words. Comprehension can be normal once the word is recognized, but sounding out the word is laborious. Reading is

FIGURE 19.8 Children with dyslexia and healthy readers were scanned while reading. Normal readers showed greater activation of the frontal region as well as the temporal/occipital region. (Adapted with permission from Shaywitz SE, Shaywitz BA. Dyslexia (specific reading disability). *Biol Psychiatry.* 2005;57[11]:1301–1309. Copyright 2005 with permission from Elsevier.)

effortful and slow for such children. Additionally, the impairment does not spontaneously remit.

The Shaywitzs at Yale have been studying dyslexia for over 30 years. In a large study, they examined 144 children (70 with dyslexia) in an fMRI. The children read real words and pseudowords while being scanned. Figure 19.8 shows the difference in activity in the brains of the normal readers compared with those with dyslexia. Note the increased activity for normal readers at two regions in the left hemisphere: a frontal region and a temporal/occipital region. These regions are thought to be critical for analyzing written words.

In a remarkable application of their findings, Shaywitz et al. conducted a treatment study to see if the dormant regions in the dyslexic children could be awakened. Thirty-seven children, who were second or third graders, with dyslexia received 50 minutes of daily tutoring in their schools for 1 year—a hearty intervention. They focused on phonics: associating letters and combinations

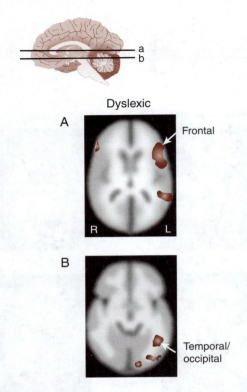

Dyslexic

A — Frontal

R   L

B — Temporal/occipital

FIGURE 19.9 Dyslexic children who received a phonics-based reading intervention over one school year showed increased activation in the regions of the brain associated with fluent reading. (Adapted with permission from Shaywitz SE, Shaywitz BA. Dyslexia (specific reading disability). *Biol Psychiatry*. 2005;57[11]:1301–1309. Copyright 2005 with permission from Elsevier.)

of letters with sounds. Children in the treatment group showed improved reading accuracy, fluency, and comprehension after 1 year.

Of particular interest were the results of the repeated fMRIs 1 year after the study ended (2 years after the start of the study). The baseline scans subtracted from the follow-up scans revealed regions activated in the intervening years. The newly activated regions (Figure 19.9) correspond to the same regions active in fluent readers: frontal and temporal/occipital. This study is further evidence that cognitive exercises can change the brain.

CREATIVITY

Creativity is conceptualized as the capacity to generate novel approaches to a problem. However, any fool can make a mess and call it art. The talent comes in producing something new as well as meaningful and even useful. Furthermore,

being creative is different from working through a problem and testing all the available solutions. Creative moments seem to come to us in a flash—seemingly out of nowhere—often when the mind appears unfocused, e.g., driving in the car or taking a shower. Creative moments feel different, but it has been difficult to identify what happens in the brain when the creative "juices are flowing."

Limb and Braun put professional jazz pianists in an fMRI and measured their brain activity when playing an overlearned musical sequence (scales) or improvising. They reported that improvisation required suppression of the dorsolateral PFC—the part of the brain they feel is responsible for self-monitoring and volitional control. Limb believes the emergence of the creative spirit requires turning off self-criticism.

It is a popular belief that creativity is localized to the right brain. Daniel Pink's "A Whole New Mind: Why Right-Brainers Will Rule the Future," a book that was on the New York Times bestseller list for 101 weeks and has been translated into 24 languages, is a good example of this sort of belief. Pink argues that the future belongs to people who can use their right brain—storytellers, inventors, designers—in general, people who are more creative. Pink and others purport that the right brain is the locus for art and creativity while the left brain is more mathematical and logical. Is this true or just an urban legend? What does the science show?

Review of the Literature

Dietrich and Kanso in 2010 reviewed the literature on studies designed to identify the neural underpinnings of creative behavior and found 72 studies reported in 63 articles. They divided the studies into three categories (divergent thinking, artistic creativity, and insight) and looked for patterns in the neuroimaging and neuroelectric findings. Their conclusion is straightforward and unequivocal—it's a mess!

With the possible exception of diffuse prefrontal activation during the creative moment, creativity is not localized to *any* area of the brain. Specifically, they noted that creativity is "not particularly associated with the right brain or any part of the right brain." They concluded that a variety of areas of the brain have been identified in one study or another, but then fail to replicate in numerous other studies. In short, the best we can say at this time is that the creative spirit uses the PFC—not a particularly enlightening insight. The problem may be the failure of subdividing creativity into appropriate categories or the limitations of our current imaging equipment or that creativity arises out of the connection between many areas and is not localizable to any one brain region.

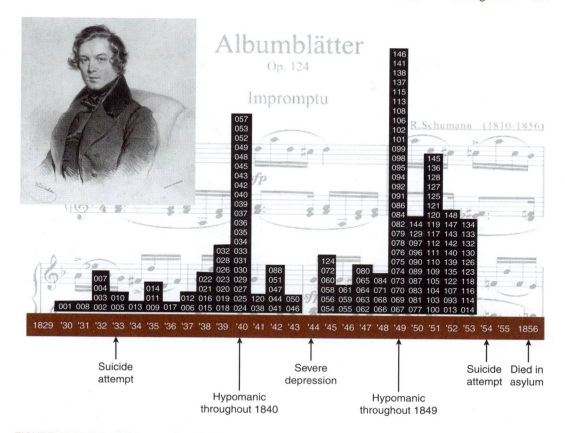

FIGURE 19.10 Robert Schumann's works graphed by opus number and year of completion provide a visual display of the creative potential of hypomania and the devastating effects of depression. Robert Schumann, Wien 1839, lithography by Joseph Kriehuber. (Data from Slater E, Meyer A, 1959.)

Creativity and Mental Illness

Another interesting aspect of creativity is the association with mental illness. Individuals such as artist Vincent van Gogh, writer Ernest Hemingway, and Nobel laureate John Nash are good case examples of highly imaginative people who also struggled with mental illness. The composer Robert Schumann provides one of the most compelling examples of mental illness and the creation of art (Figure 19.10). Schumann attempted suicide twice and eventually died in an asylum. He had two particularly productive periods of his life during which he also had symptoms of hypomania. Graphing his musical works by the years he created them shows a remarkable fluctuation in productivity with mood.

A larger study supports a correlation between creativity and mental illness. Combining results from two older studies, from a time when people were more likely to have taken the Minnesota Multiphasic Personality Inventory, the authors found that scores for writers and highly creative writers fell between normal controls and patients with psychosis (Figure 19.11). It is important to note that the highly creative writers were not necessarily mentally ill, just sharing some of the traits of the seriously mentally ill.

A recent analysis out of Sweden—searching databases that the Swedes are so prone to collect examined the likelihood of having received in-patient psychiatric treatment and employment in a creative occupation (such as author, visual artist, university professor, etc.). They found that individuals with bipolar disorder and the healthy siblings of people with bipolar disorder or schizophrenia were "overrepresented in creative professions." However, patients with schizophrenia or unipolar depression did not differ from controls in the creative professions.

The similarity between creativity and mental illness may be related to decreased filtering of thoughts and sensations. A good example of

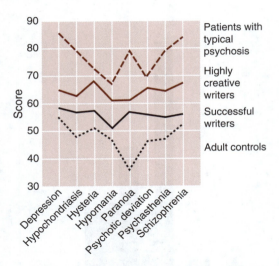

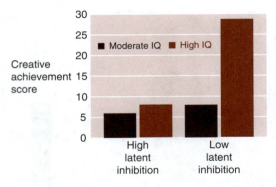

FIGURE 19.12 Undergraduate students with high IQ and low latent inhibition (the ability to filter out irrelevant stimuli) showed greater creative achievement. (Adapted from Carson SH, Peterson JB, Higgins DM. [2003.] Decreased latent inhibition is associated with increased creative achievement in high-functioning individuals. *J Pers Soc Psychol*. 85[3]:499–506. http://dx.doi.org/10.1037/0022-3514.85.3.499.)

FIGURE 19.11 The Minnesota Multiphasic Personality Inventory allows the plotting of symptom severity across a spectrum—the upper graph being more severe symptoms. Highly creative writers and successful writers fall between typical psychotic patients and healthy controls. (Adapted from Simonton DK. Are genius and madness related? Contemporary answers to an ancient question. *Psychiatric Times*. 2005;22[7]:21–23. Copyright Dean K Simonton.)

unfiltered thoughts occurs when we dream during sleep. In this uninhibited state we experience a wild variety of thoughts that are—if nothing else—unique and creative. Some think dreaming is similar to psychosis. The important point is that when the inhibitions are off (as with sleep), the mind is open to new associations. Yet, few of the new ideas are useful.

Latent inhibition describes one cognitive mechanism known to filter extraneous sensations during the awake state. *Latent inhibition* is defined as an animal's unconscious capacity to screen out and ignore stimuli that are irrelevant. Specific tests can measure an individual's capacity to ignore irrelevant stimuli. The significance to this discussion is that individuals with less ability to screen out extraneous stimuli have been shown to be more creative. Additionally, this same trait is associated with increased propensity toward psychosis. In other words, a little less inhibition may promote more creative thinking, but too much may be problematic.

A study with Harvard undergraduate students found an intriguing association between latent inhibition, IQ, and creativity. The authors categorized the students by IQ and capacity for latent inhibition. They also determined each student's creative achievement. Students scored high on creative achievement if they had published a

book, recorded a musical composition, patented an invention, or won a prize for a scientific discovery. The results of this analysis are shown in Figure 19.12.

The figure reflects that smart people who tend to filter less are more creatively productive. The authors concluded such individuals have access to more information, but also have the brainpower to handle the additional information and are consequently more likely to make original connections. However, the authors agreed with the proposition that too much unfiltered sensory information in lower IQ individuals may be a feature of psychotic thinking.

Loosening the Frontal Lobes

Artistic expression may be enhanced with loosening of frontal lobe control. Three examples suggest this to be true. The first is of an artist with evolving frontotemporal dementia whose creative expression blossomed as her illness progressed. The patient was a high school art teacher who had been painting since she was a child. In 1986, at the age of 43 years, she began developing cognitive problems. The demands of running a class became too much, and in 1995 she took early retirement. An MRI showed moderate bifrontal atrophy along with mild left temporal atrophy. However, while she was losing cognitive skills, she was also becoming increasingly expressive in her artistic work. Her paintings, which had been previously traditional, were now impressionistic, abstract, and emotional. Apparently, the inhibitions within the PFC were removed as the disease progressed and the patient became less constrained as an artist. However, when the dementia progressed too far, her painting ceased entirely.

James C. Harris who used to write a monthly commentary about artwork on the cover of Archives of General Psychiatry, and is also the director of the Johns Hopkins Developmental Neuropsychiatry Clinic, recently wrote about the remarkable drawings discovered in the Chauvet Cave. Dated to approximately 31,000 years ago, the animal drawings have a realistic perspective that seems impossible for Cro-Magnon man (Figure 19.13). How could these "primitive" people produce such expressive work? Dr Harris speculates that there is reciprocal relationship between artistic representation and frontal lobe development.

The final example is a longitudinal study of a girl described as an autistic savant whose graphic skills enabled her to draw with amazing perspective as early as 4 years old even though she virtually had no language skills. However, as she matured and her intellectual ability improved, she lost her artistic touch. These three examples highlight a conflicting relationship in the frontal lobes between artistic creativity and

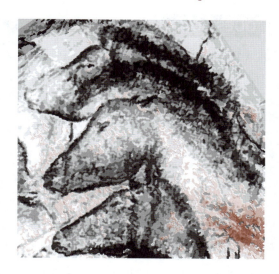

FIGURE 19.13 Drawings in the Chauvet Cave made 31,000 years ago. Did the primitive Paleolithic frontal cortex allow for greater artistic expression?

cognitive skills. There is some functional connection within the frontal lobes in which "more" improves cognitive skills but "less" frees-up artistic expression.

QUESTIONS

1. All of the following apply to *g* except
   a. Fund of knowledge.
   b. Novel problem solving.
   c. Fluid intelligence.
   d. Ability to handle complexity.

2. All of the following are true about the male canary's HVC except
   a. The size is influenced by testosterone.
   b. Greater volume equals greater repertoire of songs.
   c. The size is an indirect measure of *g*.
   d. The size fluctuates with the seasons.

3. Indications that the PFC is a major site of intelligence include all of the following except
   a. Active during problem solving.
   b. Lesions produce problem-solving deficits.
   c. Larger relative size in more intelligent animals.
   d. Larger proportion of gray matter in humans compared with other primates.

4. Impaired spine formation on dendrites is seen with all of the following except
   a. Opioid abuse.
   b. Memory formation.
   c. Mental retardation.
   d. Impoverished environment.

5. All of the following are true about dyslexia except
   a. Impaired ability to decode words.
   b. Right hemisphere problem.
   c. Inactive temporal/occipital region during reading.
   d. Increased frontal activity with proper treatment.

6. Most creative individuals in the sciences have the following except
   a. Active PFC.
   b. Low latent inhibition.
   c. Mental illness.
   d. Above average IQ.

See Answers section at the end of this book.

CHAPTER 20

Attention

INTRODUCTION

The last aspect of cognition that we will review is the ability to attend to external or internal stimuli. Like memory, attention is one of the oldest and most studied areas of cognitive science. One hundred years ago researchers used stopwatches and psychological tests to measure attention. In the latter half of the 20th century, the placement of microelectrodes into the brains of monkeys opened the door to investigating the capacity of individual neurons to attend. Now with brain imaging studies we can observe, in real time, the shifting focus of an awake human solving a puzzle—with or without medication. One hundred years of research have given us a better understanding of the power of the brain to focus on relevant stimuli, although many aspects of the neurobiology of attention remain elusive.

Attention in a broad sense describes the mechanism that weighs the importance of various stimuli and selects the one that will receive the brain's focus. The brain has limited capacity for attention. Numerous psychological tests have demonstrated the brain's finite capacity to attend as more and more stimuli are added. A relevant example from modern life involves driving while talking on a cell phone. A phone conversation detracts from developments on the road—contrary to what the driver thinks. A recent study found that drivers using a cell phone had a fourfold increase in the chance of a serious accident—hands-free phones were equally problematic.

The capacity to concentrate and maintain one's attention is inversely related to the ability to ignore other stimuli. Responding to other stimuli—whether internal or external—changes the brain's focus. The brain cannot attend if it is wandering from one thought to another. The border collie in Figure 20.1 shows an example of highly selective attention. The dog is not only focused on the Frisbee, but is also actively ignoring other objects of potential interest around him. In this state he will ignore female dogs, squirrels, children, even food. He will not sniff the scent of other dogs or leave his own mark on the shrubbery. He tunes out diversions to focus solely on the flying sphere.

Athletes provide another example of the intimate relationship between attending and ignoring. The quarterback who has dropped into the pocket

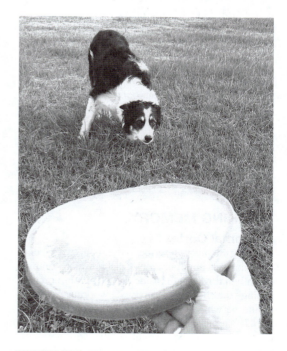

FIGURE 20.1 A border collie ignores everything else around him while focusing on the Frisbee.

and is able to ignore all the noise and violence around him while he searches for an open receiver is an extraordinary example of attending and ignoring. Likewise, when the artist or the absent-minded professor gets lost in work, they are ignoring most sensory inputs coming into their brain. Improving attention and concentration is accomplished by both reducing distractions and enhancing focus.

Measuring Attention

Continuous performance tests (CPTs) give an objective estimate of an individual's attention and impulsivity. Subjects watch a computer screen and hit a button or click a mouse whenever a specified sequence of symbols or letters appears (Figure 20.2A). Such tests reflect the subject's capacity to attend as well as the ability to restrain impulsive answers. Results are compared with normative data for individuals in one's age group.

Attention changes across the life span. Figure 20.2B shows the percent errors on one CPT (Test of Variables of Attention) for 1,590 individuals from the ages of 4 to 80+ years. Note how attention improves with age until the senior years. These findings appear to roughly correlate with the myelination of the white matter in the frontal lobes (see Figure 8.8).

ATTENTION DEFICIT HYPERACTIVITY DISORDER AND ADULTHOOD

Attention deficit hyperactivity disorder (ADHD) was once considered a childhood disorder. More recently, it has become popular for adults to get treatment for this condition. However, a meta-analysis of follow-up studies found that most children with ADHD fail to meet the full criteria for the disorder as adults—only 10% to 15%.

WORKING MEMORY

Prefrontal Cortex

Working memory describes what is actively being considered at any moment. If the conscious brain is actually a tiny person inside a control room orchestrating the body's responses, working memory would be what he sees on the monitors in front of him. It is temporary, limited in capacity, and must be continually refreshed. Traditionally, working memory has been associated with the prefrontal cortex (PFC). It most certainly resides there but may also include connections with the parietal lobes.

Trauma to the PFC impairs working memory. Phineas Gage is the most famous case that shows the effects of frontal brain damage on working memory. He was the young railroad worker mentioned in Chapter 14, Anger and Aggression, who had a tamping iron explode through his frontal cortex. He went from being responsible and organized to impulsive and inattentive. His inability to sustain a thought in his working memory could be considered the root cause of his wandering attention.

Researchers developed a way to test working memory in monkeys, called the *delayed-response task*. In this task, a monkey is shown a piece of fruit being placed in one of the two randomly chosen receptacles (Figure 20.3). This is called the *cue*. Someone pulls down a screen obscuring the monkey's field of vision, and lids are placed over both receptacles. When the screen is lifted, the monkey gets one chance to remove the correct lid and receive his reward. The significance of this test is that the monkey must hold the visual image of the location of the fruit in his working memory during the delay period. Healthy monkeys learn this task quickly. Monkeys with frontal lobe lesions perform poorly.

In the 1970s, researchers began putting microelectrodes into individual neurons in the PFC of monkeys while they participated in the delayed-response task (Figure 20.4A). They found that neurons reacted differently during the task. Some neurons were active only during the cue and response periods, whereas other neurons became active during the delay period (Figure 20.4B).

The delay neurons start firing with the presentation of the cue and stop with the response. These neurons seem to hold the memory of the task—literally the neural equivalent of working memory (although it is more likely a network of neurons). When the monkeys incorrectly responded, the delay neurons were usually inactive. If the monkeys were distracted during the delay period, the delay neurons usually have settled and the monkeys make incorrect responses or do not respond at all.

After the studies, the researchers sacrificed the monkeys and identified the location of the microelectrodes. The locations in the right PFC from several monkeys are shown in Figure 20.4C. The cue neurons and delay neurons are shown in different colors. Note how the delay neurons are more common than the cue neurons, showing the importance of holding a thought in working memory. Also, it appears that the delay neurons cluster together in what we imagine is part of the network of working memory.

A

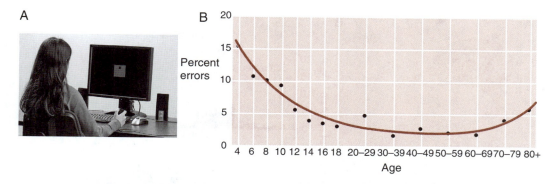

FIGURE 20.2 **A:** Subject taking the Visual T.O.V.A. test, © 2017 The TOVA Company. **B:** Percent errors as measured by the Test of Variables of Attention (TOVA) are age dependent. (Data from Greenberg LM, Crosby RD. *A Summary of Developmental Normative Data on the T.O.V.A. Ages 4 to 80+.* Unpublished manuscript available through the TOVA Company; 1992.)

Catecholamines

Working memory is modulated by the catecholamines: dopamine (DA) and norepinephrine (NE). Pharmacologic interventions that increase DA and NE in the PFC enhance working memory and improve attention. Alternatively, agents that block DA receptors, such as haloperidol, have been shown to degrade performance on delayed-response tasks.

Phillips et al. examined the relationship between accuracy on a delayed-response task and DA release in the PFC. They placed microdialysis probes in the PFC of rats (see Figure 12.4A), which allowed continual analysis of extracellular DA concentrations while the rat performed the task. The rats were tested using an eight-arm radial maze (Figure 20.5A). In the *training* phase, rats were given 5 minutes to explore a radial arm maze that had four randomly chosen arms baited with food. During the *delay*, the rats were confined at the center of the maze in the dark from 30 minutes to 6 hours. In the *test* phase, food was placed on the opposite arms from the training phase and the

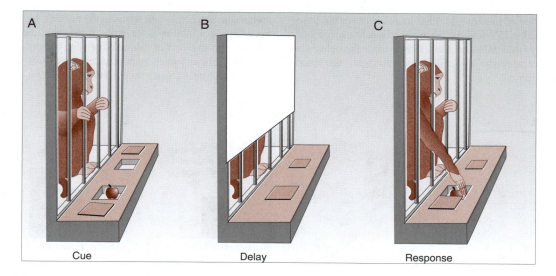

FIGURE 20.3 The delayed-response task. **A:** The screen is raised and the monkey observes a piece of fruit placed in one of the wells. **B:** The screen is lowered and the wells are covered. **C:** After a specific period of time the screen is raised and the monkey has one chance to remember the correct location of the fruit. (Adapted from Purves D, Augustine GJ, Fitzpatrick D, et al. *Neuroscience.* 3rd ed. Sunderland, MA: Sinauer; 2004, by permission of Oxford University Press, USA.)

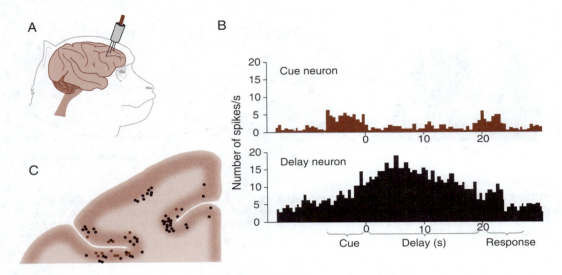

FIGURE 20.4 A: Microelectrodes placed into individual neurons in the prefrontal cortex (PFC) and monitored during the delayed-response task. **B:** Neuronal activity in cue neurons (*brown*) and delay neurons (*black*) during the delayed-response task. **C:** The location of the cue and delay neurons in the right PFC. (Adapted from Fuster JM. Unit activity in prefrontal cortex during delayed-response performance: neuronal correlates of transient memory. *J Neurophysiol*. 1973;36[1]:61–78.)

rats were given 5 minutes to locate the rewards. Errors were scored as entries into unbaited arms. Extracellular DA was analyzed at baseline and during the testing phase.

The results show an inverse correlation between extracellular DA in the PFC during the testing phase and errors (Figure 20.5B). Less DA, more errors. When the delay was only 30 minutes, the efflux of DA into the PFC increased over the baseline by 75% and the rat made only a few error journeys into unbaited arms. However, as the delay was increased the DA efflux decreased and the errors mounted.

There is another interesting development regarding attention and the other catecholamine: NE. Stimulating the vagus nerve causes activation of the locus coeruleus and an immediate release of NE throughout the cortex. By pairing vagus nerve stimulation (VNS) with a behavior, one can help the brain "pay attention" to that behavior and cause the brain to change. VNS can be done either through implanted wires in the neck or, more recently, in a noninvasive way, through surface stimulation over either the neck or vagus fibers in the ear. This approach is now in clinical trials in tinnitus and poststroke rehabilitation.

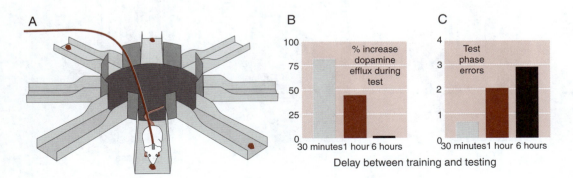

FIGURE 20.5 A: Radial arm maze with four arms baited. **B:** Percent increase in extracellular dopamine at the testing phase. **C:** Errors at the testing phase. (Data from Phillips AG, Ahn S, Floresco SB. Magnitude of dopamine release in medial prefrontal cortex predicts accuracy of memory on a delayed response task. *J Neurosci*. 2004;24[2]:547–553.)

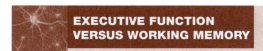

EXECUTIVE FUNCTION VERSUS WORKING MEMORY

The terms executive function and working memory are often used synonymously in the literature. Some researchers prefer one term while others prefer the other, but they are not synonymous. Executive function includes working memory as well as other higher-level cognitive skills such as organizing priorities and planning initiation strategies. Although executive function and working memory describe different functions in the brain, they share the same underlying mechanisms. Both reside in the PFC, are impaired with frontal lobe damage, and fluctuate with catecholamine modulation.

Biofeedback

Neurofeedback (also called *electro EEG biofeedback*) is a treatment option that allows patients to exercise their brain to improve attention and concentration. As we have discussed, the EEG frequencies are divided into four groups (see Figure 15.3). Beta waves are the frequency pattern produced when a person is alert and concentrating. The goal of neurofeedback is for the patient to generate more beta rhythm and less alpha and theta rhythms.

Neurofeedback uses a computer that interprets the EEG frequencies generated by the user and provides them with feedback through a symbol on the computer screen. For example, the symbol will move up with beta rhythm and down with all other EEG frequencies. The user learns to move the image up the screen by producing beta rhythms, which in turn strengthens the neurons that focus attention. It is the mental equivalent of lifting weights.

Although there have not been large, randomized controlled trials, results in the literature are about 75% positive. A group in Montreal completed a small controlled trial with functional imaging before and after biofeedback treatment in children with ADHD. Treatment consisted of 40 sessions of neurofeedback, each lasting an hour, over 15 weeks. The neurofeedback group not only improved their scores on measures of attention, but also increased the activation of the anterior cingulate cortex (Figure 20.6). Once again we see that the brain is not a static organ and responds to exercise and training. More recently a group in the Netherlands assigned 112 children with ADHD to neurofeedback, methylphenidate, or physical exercise. All interventions improved working memory; neurofeedback and methylphenidate reduced theta

activity, but the stimulant showed superior effects on tests of attention and inhibitory control.

The inverse is also true. That is, not exercising the brain—or worse, watching "mindless" television— seems to make the brain lazy. Longitudinal studies have linked childhood television viewing with subsequent attentional problems in adolescence—more TV results in poorer focus. A recent study examined the immediate effects on 4-year-old children of watching a segment of Sponge Bob. Children who watched 9 minutes of the cartoon, as compared with those who spent 9 minutes drawing, showed impairments in executive function (such as self-regulation, delay of gratification, and working memory) when tested immediately after the intervention. The fast-paced nature of some television fails to train the brain to focus and attend. Is this one reason we are seeing a surge in the diagnosis of attentional disorders?

REWARD AND IMPULSE CONTROL

Controlling the impulse to take an immediate, smaller reward rather than waiting for the larger, delayed reward is essential for completing any project. People who cannot control these impulses perpetually fall behind. The famous marshmallow studies at Stanford almost 50 years ago showed the profound effect that good impulse control has on later accomplishments.

In the study, 4-year-old children were sequestered in a room with an assistant who placed a marshmallow on a table. The children were told that the assistant had to run an errand and would be stepping out of the room. They were also told they could eat the one marshmallow, but if they could *wait* until the assistant returned, they could have *two* marshmallows. The assistant left the room for approximately 15 minutes and the children's response was monitored. Some children ate the marshmallow as soon as the assistant exited the room, whereas the rest showed varying degrees of self-restraint.

The social and academic performance of these children was reassessed in their adolescence. The children who were better at inhibiting the impulse to immediately eat the one marshmallow were more resilient, confident, and dependable as adolescents. Additionally, they were more successful students and even scored higher on the SAT. The SAT scores for the more impulsive children were approximately 100 points less than those who were able to wait.

Clearly, the ability to suppress the desire to grab the immediate reward is associated with behaviors that have a profound impact on one's life. People

A Neuropsychological testing

Test	Before	After
Digit Span	9.8	11.6*
Continuous Performance Test	77.5	85**
Conners Parent Rating Scale Inattention	71.6	58.9***
Conners Parent Rating Scale Hyperactivity	79.4	64.3*

*$P < .05$ **$P < .005$ ***$P < .001$

B Imaging study

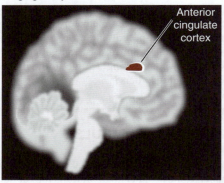

Anterior cingulate cortex

FIGURE 20.6 A: Neuropsychological testing improved after 40 sessions of neurofeedback. **B:** The anterior cingulate cortex showed greater activity after the neurofeedback treatment. (Adapted with permission from Levesque J, Beauregard M, Mensour B. Effect of neurofeedback training on the neural substrates of selective attention in children with attention-deficit/hyperactivity disorder: a functional magnetic resonance imaging study. *Neurosci Lett.* 2006;394[3]:216–221. Copyright 2006 with permission from Elsevier.)

	Impulsive Eaters	Patient Waiters
Verbal	524	610
Math	528	652

who can delay gratification and control their impulses appear to achieve more in the long run.

Nucleus Accumbens and Dopamine

Attention and impulsivity are opposite sides of the same coin. Both are controlled, in part, by DA activity in the nucleus accumbens (NAc). Pleasurable activities increase the release of DA in the NAc (see Figure 12.6). People are less likely to respond to other stimuli if they are pursuing activities they enjoy. Stimulant medications also increase the DA released at the NAc and improve impulse control.

Patients report that stimulants enable them to block out irrelevant stimuli with greater ease.

Clearly, other areas of the brain influence the NAc. For example, the orbitofrontal cortex, the hippocampus, and the amygdala are three regions with important projections to the NAc (see Figure 12.3). However, the NAc is uniquely wired to focus attention on the more favorable rewards.

Other evidence of the role of the NAc in impulsive behavior comes from lesion studies on rats. Rats can learn to choose a larger, delayed reward over a smaller, immediate reward, but they need an intact NAc. The rats with damaged NAc become more impulsive and choose the immediate reward more frequently.

Impulsivity and Youth

Why are adolescents so impulsive and prone to taking risks? One possible explanation is that the frontal cortex has not yet matured—an issue discussed in Chapter 14, Anger and Aggression, in the context of explaining impulsive aggression. Another explanation points to the NAc and dopaminergic tone.

BOREDOM

It is no great revelation to say that people have a hard time staying focused on boring tasks. The stimulant medications may improve attention (at least in part) by increasing the level of interest perceived by the brain. Volkow et al. gave methylphenidate or placebo to normal young men and imaged their brains while they solved math problems. When taking methylphenidate, the men found math less boring and more exciting.

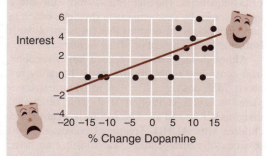

Changes in extracellular DA at the striatum correlated with interest in normal adults solving math problems. (Adapted from Volkow ND, Wang GJ, Fowler JS, et al. Evidence that methylphenidate enhances the saliency of a mathematical task by increasing dopamine in the human brain. *Am J Psychiatry.* 2004;161[7]:1173–1180. Reprinted with permission from the *American Journal of Psychiatry* [Copyright © 2004]. American Psychiatric Association. All Rights Reserved.)

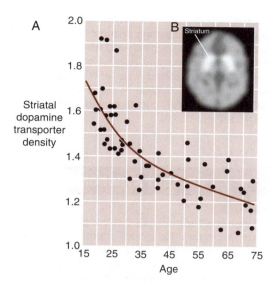

FIGURE 20.7 **A:** The density of the dopamine (DA) transporter at the striatum as a function of age. **B:** Distribution of DA transporter in the human brain. (Adapted with permission from Mozley PD, Acton PD, Barraclough ED, et al. Effects of age on dopamine transporters in healthy humans. *J Nucl Med.* 1999;40[11]:1812–1817, © by the Society of Nuclear Medicine and Molecular Imaging, Inc.)

The DA reuptake pump (called the *DA transporter*) has been used as a measure of dopaminergic tone. New technology allows the imaging of the DA transporter density. Studies have examined the DA transporter density at the striatum (the region that contains the NAc) and show a decline with age (Figure 20.7). Note the more precipitous drop in early adulthood.

Other researchers have shown that drug-naïve patients with ADHD have, on average, a slightly higher density in DA transporter at equivalent ages. For example, a 30-year-old patient with ADHD has the DA transporter density of a normal 22-year-old. Therefore, it appears that high DA transporter density (seen with younger individuals and patients with ADHD) correlates with more impulsive behavior, whereas lower density correlates with matured impulse control.

Drug Addiction

The cravings that drug addicts experience for their drug of choice might be the most extreme example of seeking immediate gratification. When a drug addict gets this kind of urge, there are few concerns about long-term consequences. Every clinician knows horror stories of addicts who have squandered the family savings just to get high. What is the role of the NAc in addictive behavior?

We know that chronic cocaine use down-regulates the DA receptors at the NAc (see Figure 12.11). Likewise, we have shown that amphetamines and opioids alter the morphology of dendritic spine on neurons in the NAc (see Figure 12.13). These results and the behavior of the addicts suggest that drug abuse damages the NAc. Such an effect might be the pharmacologic equivalent of lesioning the NAc—an effect that enhances impulsive behavior.

ATTENTION DEFICIT HYPERACTIVITY DISORDER

Genetics

ADHD travels in families. It is one of the most heritable psychiatric disorders we know. Pooled analyses of twin studies suggest the heritable rate may be as high as 76%, but the search to identify the specific genes has been disappointing. Pharmacologic and neuroimaging studies suggest a dopaminergic hypothesis for ADHD. Indeed the genes for the DA transporter and the D4 DA receptor have been implicated in a number studies. However, not all findings are replicated and meta-analysis shows only small effects of individual genes—the usual genetic finding in mental illness.

Several genome-wide association studies have been conducted in an unbiased search for candidate genes. A 2015 review of the topic reported that a number of genes have been implicated in a number of studies. Unfortunately, the authors concluded, "the number of associated variants (and their effect size) is small and when considered together they explain a small proportion of the variation in ADHD. Moreover it appears that each of these risk variants is neither necessary nor sufficient to cause ADHD." Probably not a bad description about the genetics of all psychiatric disorders, as we currently understand them.

Brain Size

As discussed earlier, working memory and impulse control are important features of attention and are usually impaired in patients with ADHD. As would be expected, dysfunctions in the PFC and striatum are the most common abnormal brain findings reported for ADHD.

However, the most comprehensive neuroscientific studies on children with ADHD come from Judith Rapoport's laboratory at the National Institute of Mental Health (NIMH). They have conducted several large prospective case–control magnetic resonance imaging (MRI) studies of the brains of children with ADHD. One study produced multiple

MRI scans of 150 children with ADHD and 139 age- and sex-matched controls. Sixty percent of the participants had at least two scans.

The most interesting finding was that children with ADHD had smaller total brain volumes by approximately 5% compared with controls. The difference held true for all four cerebral lobes (including white matter and gray matter), as well as the cerebellum. The trajectory of the total brain volumes did not change as the children aged, nor was it affected by the use of stimulant medication.

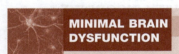

MINIMAL BRAIN DYSFUNCTION

In the past, ADHD was called *minimal brain dysfunction*, a term now considered derogatory. The findings from Rapoport's laboratory suggest that those older clinicians, without the benefits of modern imaging studies, had a subtle but accurate understanding of the pathophysiology of ADHD.

Gray Matter Thickness

In a follow-up study, Rapoport's group examined another 300 subjects, half of whom had ADHD. This time, with better technology, they measured regional gray matter thickness. The most unique feature of this second study was that they followed up the clinical outcome as well as the structural changes in the brain of the children over time. They were able to compare the children who grew out of the disorder with those who did not.

The results showed that children with ADHD had global thinning of all the gray matter compared with the controls, although it was most prominent in the PFC. Additionally, both groups showed the usual pruning of the total gray matter as they grew through adolescence (Figure 20.8). However, two regions were unique when correlated with clinical outcome.

1. Children who remained impaired at follow-up had thinner gray matter in the medial PFC at the beginning of the study.
2. Children who grew out of the disorder showed a normalization of the gray matter thickness in the right parietal cortex.

These results imply that the normalization of the parietal cortex may be a compensatory activation of the posterior attentional network. Indeed,

research suggests that the parietal cortex may play a greater role in attention than previously considered. Imaging studies conducted while the subjects attempted to detect and respond to the presence of an infrequent stimulus (a variation on a CPT) showed greater activation of the bilateral parietal lobes in the controls compared with patients with ADHD (Figure 20.9).

NEGLECT SYNDROME

There is other evidence that the parietal lobes are important for good attention. Parietal lesions can cause a neglect syndrome in which patients ignore objects, people, and even parts of their body to one side of the center of gaze. The very existence of parts of the body on the ignored side can be denied (usually the left body). The figure shows an example of a patient after a right parietal stroke attempting to copy some drawings. Note how he fails to copy details from the left side of the drawings. It has been proposed that the parietal cortex is involved in attending to objects at different positions in extracellular space.

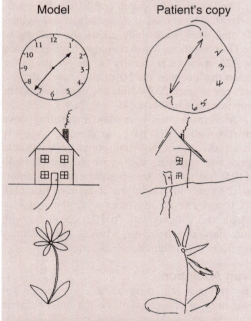

A patient after a right parietal stroke attempts to copy the drawings on the left and neglects aspects of the drawings that are in his left visual field. (From Springer SP, Deutsch G. *Left Brain, Right Brain*. 5th ed. New York: Worth Publishers; 1998.)

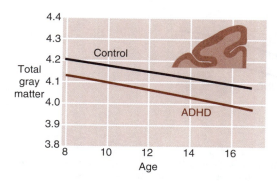

FIGURE 20.8 Total gray matter thickness for children with attention deficit hyperactivity disorder (ADHD) compared with controls. (Data from Shaw P, Lerch J, Greenstein D, et al. Longitudinal mapping of cortical thickness and clinical outcome in children and adolescents with attention-deficit/hyperactivity disorder. *Arch Gen Psychiatry*. 2006;63[5]:540–549.)

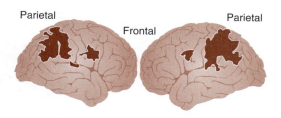

FIGURE 20.9 Regions of significantly greater activation in healthy subjects relative to the attention deficit hyperactivity disorder (ADHD) group during a target detection task. (Adapted from Tamm L, Menon V, Reiss AL. Parietal attentional system aberrations during target detection in adolescents with attention-deficit/hyperactivity disorder: event-related fMRI evidence. *Am J Psychiatry*. 2006;163[6]:1033–1043. Reprinted with permission from the *American Journal of Psychiatry* [Copyright © 2006]. American Psychiatric Association. All Rights Reserved.)

Timing and Cerebellum

Some researchers suggest that deficits in time perception are an integral feature of ADHD. Children with ADHD are known to have problems with temporal information processing and the timing of motor tasks. Clinical tests such as estimates of time duration or the reproduction of timed sequences are frequently impaired in children with ADHD. The finger tapping studies by Ben-Pazi provide a specific example of this problem. Children were asked to replicate the same frequency of the presented stimuli by tapping the space bar on a computer. Children with ADHD were less capable of replicating the stimuli and tended to tap faster than the stimulus presentation—getting ahead of themselves. The authors speculate that the rhythmic tapping problems reflect an abnormal oscillatory mechanism for those with ADHD.

These rhythmic motor abnormalities may represent a larger timing problem for patients with ADHD. In other words, the problem is greater than just replicating the tapping of a metronome. The problems with timing may contribute to the impairments seen with higher cognitive skills required to plan and complete a project. Inconsistencies in performance, responding too fast or too slow, and procrastination are behaviors that may be impaired due to temporal processing deficits. For example, patients with ADHD typically overestimate the time left to finish a project. In short, patients with ADHD may have trouble with project planning and completion due to problems getting into a good rhythm and maintaining a consistent pace.

The cerebellum, traditionally conceptualized as controlling motor coordination, has been identified as a possible culprit in the etiology of ADHD.

Studies such as those from Rapoport's laboratory have documented smaller cerebellum volumes in patients with ADHD (Figure 20.10). Likewise, stimulant medications are known to activate the cerebellum. Finally, the cerebellum is believed to play an important role in timing responses.

In summary, it is clear that the PFC and striatum play large roles in the pathophysiology of ADHD. More recent studies suggest that the parietal cortex and cerebellum may also contribute to the problems that ADHD patients experience.

Long-Term Effects of Stimulants

There are two kinds of stimulants widely used in our society. The first kind, cocaine and methamphetamine, is primarily obtained illegally on the street. The second, methylphenidate and amphetamine, is available with a prescription. Both classes of medication produce an outpouring of DA. One of the ironies of psychiatry is that the first group is studied by substance abuse clinicians, whereas the second group of stimulants is studied by clinicians treating ADHD. To a large extent, the two groups are focusing on alternative features of the effects of DA stimulation.

A multicriteria decision analysis of drug harm in the UK compared harm to the user for 20 drugs of abuse. The top three harmful drugs were crack cocaine, heroin, and methamphetamine. The next three were alcohol, cocaine, and amphetamine. Four of the top six harmful drugs are CNS stimulants. On the other side of the academic isle is the research showing that stimulant medication may actually "normalize" some structural abnormalities in the brain. So, on the one hand, abusing stimulants damages the brain (see Figure 12.11), while on the other hand, stimulant medications seem to normalize the brain. How can this be?

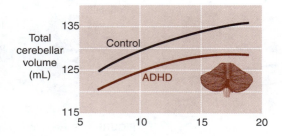

FIGURE 20.10 Children with attention deficit hyperactivity disorder (ADHD) have smaller total cerebellar volume compared with unaffected controls. (Adapted by permission from Macmillan Publishers Ltd. Castellanos FX, Tannock R. Neuroscience of attention-deficit/hyperactivity disorder: the search for endophenotypes. *Nat Rev Neurosci.* 2002;3[8]:617–628. Copyright 2002.)

The difference may be the timing of the subject analysis. The substance abusers are evaluated once they are *off* their drugs. The stimulant users—typically patients with ADHD—are usually assessed *on* the medication. Almost no studies in the ADHD literature compare the effects on the brain of subjects who stay on the medication with those who stop it.

Cortical thickness in children and adolescents, although not adults, can be "normalized" by regular stimulant use as shown in Figure 20.11. However, those patients who stopped the medication between the ages of 12.5 and 16.4 years experienced a more rapid thinning of their cortical thickness in the left frontal lobe—an area of importance in ADHD. Clearly the "normalization" is the result of gene expression activated by the stimulant medication. When the stimulants are stopped, the genes too shut down and the

cortex thins. The relevant question is this: what effect have the medications had on the brain in the long term?

This is an important question because more people are taking more stimulant medications for a longer period of time, and what will their brains look like when the medications are discontinued? Will the brain resume the structure it would have had without any exposure to medication—or will it be worse—or will it be better? The importance of this question is highlighted by recent studies finding increased incidence of Parkinson's disease in addicts abusing methamphetamine. And, more troubling is a large, but as yet unpublished analysis looking at the use of diet pills in the sixties and seventies and later problems in the nineties. Patients who had taken Benzedrine and/or Dexedrine to lose weight were 60% more likely to develop Parkinson's

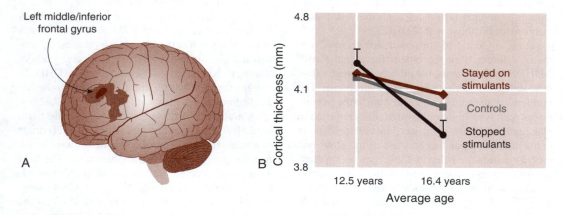

FIGURE 20.11 Prospective study of cortical thickness at the left middle/inferior frontal gyrus for 43 youths with attention deficit hyperactivity disorder (ADHD). (Adapted from Shaw PS, Sharp WS, Morrison M, et al. Psychostimulant treatment and developing cortex in ADHD. *Am J Psychiatry.* 2009;166[1]:58–63. Reprinted with permission from the *American Journal of Psychiatry* [Copyright © 2009]. American Psychiatric Association. All Rights Reserved.)

A

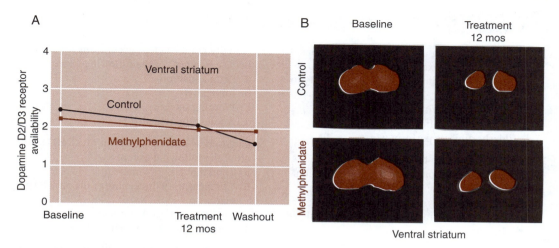

FIGURE 20.12 Dopamine D2/D3 receptor availability measure in the ventral striatum. **A:** Average changes. **B:** PET scans of D2/D3 receptors before and after the study. (Adapted by permission from Macmillan Publishers Ltd. Gill KE, et al. Chronic treatment with extended release methylphenidate does not alter dopamine systems or increase vulnerability for cocaine self-administration: a study in nonhuman primates. *Neuropsychopharmacology*. 2012;37:2555–2565. Copyright 2012.)

disease as adults. More long-term studies are needed.

The encouraging news, since our last edition, is the findings of several controlled trials that included brain imaging. Two of these are long-term placebo–controlled treatment studies with peri-adolescent/adolescent male monkeys. The monkeys were tested at baseline, after 12 to 18 months of therapeutic level doses of oral stimulant medication, and after 3 to 6 months washout. Although the studies were a bit different, neither found problems with physical growth, vulnerability to cocaine abuse, cognitive measures, or DA markers in the brain. Figure 20.12A shows the average dopamine D2/D3 receptor availability in the ventral striatum for all monkeys and B shows representative PET scans from an animal in the control group and one in the methylphenidate group. Note how all animals showed reduced D2/D3 availability over the course of the study. Lastly, a large placebo controlled trial

of methylphenidate in Germany with adults with ADHD found no cerebral volume loss in those patients taking the stimulant compared with placebo, although there was a trend toward cerebral gray matter increase in those on the medication.

Before we get too complacent, we should say a word about long-term benefits with stimulant treatment. Although short-term studies demonstrate improvements, studies lasting over a year have been disappointing. James Swanson, one of the lead investigators in the large NIMH Multimodal Treatment Study of Children with ADHD (MTA), said in a recent *Nature* interview, "I don't know of any evidence that's consistent that shows that there's any long-term benefit of taking the medication." It is not clear why long-term studies are so equivocal, but this is a common finding in a wide range of mental health interventions and may be a product of the difficult nature of changing the brain.

QUESTIONS

1. All of the following are true about continuous performance tests except
   a. They give an estimate of a subject's ability to attend.
   b. Scores change with age.
   c. Treatment will affect the scores.
   d. Elderly subjects perform worst.

2. A delayed-response task measures
   a. The subject's capacity to delay gratification.
   b. Impulsivity.
   c. Working memory.
   d. Relative dopamine activity at the nucleus accumbens.

3. The goal of neurofeedback is for the subjects to improve their attention by spending more time in which rhythm?
   a. Alpha.
   b. Beta.
   c. Theta.
   d. Delta.

4. Stimulant medications improve attention and concentration through the following mechanisms except
   a. Increase norepinephrine efflux in the striatum.
   b. Increase norepinephrine efflux in the PFC.
   c. Increase activity in the cerebellum.
   d. Increase interest in new activities.

5. Activity at the nucleus accumbens (or striatum) helps explain all of the following except
   a. Drug addiction.
   b. Impulsivity
   c. Working memory.
   d. Adolescent behavior.

6. Children who fail to grow out of ADHD show all of the following except
   a. Total thinner gray matter.
   b. Compensatory thickening of the parietal gray matter.
   c. Smaller total cerebellum volume.
   d. Less prefrontal gray matter.

7. Which structure is associated with which finding in ADHD?
   1. Prefrontal cortex.
   2. Cerebellum.
   3. Nucleus accumbens.
   4. Parietal cortex.

   A. Compensatory gray matter thickening.
   B. Temporal processing.
   C. Working memory.
   D. Delay of gratification.

See Answers section at the end of this book.

Disorders

CHAPTER 21

Depression

INTRODUCTION

We will wrap up this review of neuroscience by looking closer at the pathophysiology of four common psychiatric disorders. The first will be the depressive disorders. Although we will often use the term *depression*, the reader should keep in mind that there are probably a multitude of discrete diseases that all end up with the syndrome we now call depression. For example, psychotic depression, atypical depression, bipolar depression, and pathologic grief may be variants of the same phenomenon or they could be different conditions with different mechanisms of action. We have no objective measures to distinguish between the depressive disorders at this time. In the 1920s, we would have talked about pneumonia as one disease, as they all produced coughs and fever, although we now know that there are many different causes of pneumonia (e.g., tuberculosis, pneumococcus, Black Death, etc.).

Depression is a common condition recognized by Hippocrates (melancholia). Yet in spite of all the technologic advances since the time of the ancient Greeks, we know surprisingly little more about the pathophysiology of the disorder. We know even less about bipolar disorder.

Monoamine Hypothesis

The accidental discovery in the 1950s that the tricyclic and monoamine oxidase inhibitor medications could relieve depression symptoms transformed the treatment of the disorder. Numerous spin-off medications have been developed since the 1950s. Most are safer and better tolerated than the earlier medications, but none are more effective. In addition, they all work through the same mechanism: the monoamines. This has driven the common conceptualization of depression as a disorder of serotonin or norepinephrine (NE) or both.

Again, we see that treatment response generates theories about the pathophysiology. Clinicians call this the *monoamine hypothesis*, and the lay public calls it a *chemical imbalance*. Unfortunately, neither is an accurate description of the biologic mechanisms of depression. At least three factors argue against the monoamine hypothesis as being the only cause of depression:

1. Medications take 6 to 10 weeks to reach full effectiveness, although the neurotransmitter activity at the synapse is altered within a few doses.
2. Studies of neurotransmitter levels in the plasma, cerebrospinal fluid, and brain tissue have failed to find consistent deficiencies in patients who are depressed compared with healthy controls.
3. Although significantly heritable, genome-wide association studies have failed to identify monoamine genes as culprits in patients with depression.

Clearly, the depressions are more complex than the simple replacement of an insufficient neurotransmitter.

The Depressed Brain

If you were going to biopsy the brain of a patient with depression, where you would stick the needle? What you would look for? Structural imaging, functional imaging, and postmortem studies have established five regions that are consistently dysfunctional in most patients with depression. The five regions are shown in Figure 21.1. Note the extensive prefrontal involvement.

It is tempting to match depressive symptoms from the *Diagnostic and Statistical Manual of Mental Disorders* (*DSM*) criteria with specific regions in the brain. For example, anhedonia can be attributed to dysfunction of the nucleus accumbens (NAc) or cognitive deficits to the anterior cingulate or dorsolateral

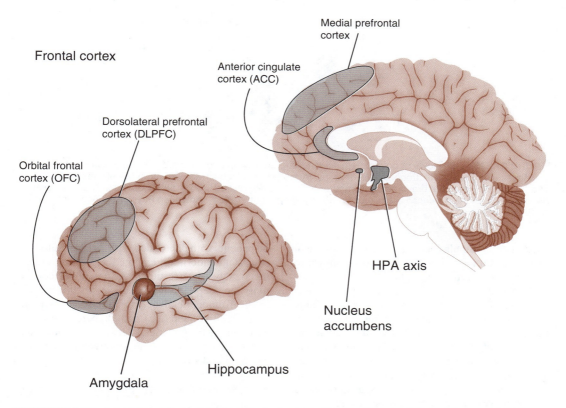

FIGURE 21.1 The five major regions of dysfunction in depressed brains. HPA, hypothalamic–pituitary–adrenal.

prefrontal cortex (PFC). However, although a few symptoms seem to match up with a brain region, most do not. Most symptoms are likely the product of simultaneous dysfunction in several regions.

Alternatively, it is possible to envision depression as the result of underactivity in some regions (e.g., the frontal lobes) and overactivity in others (e.g., the amygdala and hypothalamic–pituitary–adrenal [HPA] axis). This is smugly appealing as we can imagine the symptoms of depression matching to brain regions. For example, the underactive PFC produces low motivation, lack of hope, and low appetite, whereas the overactive amygdala produces insomnia, anxiety, and suicidal thoughts. But evidence for this symptom matching to specific regions has been inconsistent.

Over the past 20 years, numerous imaging studies have been administered to patients with depression in an effort to identify the characteristic dysfunction of the depressed brain. Studies have been conducted with positron emission tomography (PET) and functional magnetic resonance imaging (fMRI) when the brain is idle or performing tasks—both cognitive tasks and emotional responses. Results have been inconsistent.

A 2017 meta-analysis of functional neuroimaging studies compared depressed patients with healthy controls while they were all being challenged with cognitive tasks or emotional provocations. They found inconsistencies across the studies and a failure to replicate results. Nothing jumped out as a consistent marker of depression. The authors speculated this might be due to differences in the tasks performed, the heterogeneity of depressive disorders, differences in investigated populations, and publishing biases. Regardless, it is all discouraging.

Frontal Cortex

Response to treatment further clouds the water. Examining just the resting brain (what we call the idling brain—using PET or single photon emission computed tomography [SPECT] scans), we find remarkably differing responses in the PFC to successful treatment. For example, Figure 21.2 shows the effect that electroconvulsive therapy (ECT) has on the brain. Note how a successful course of ECT turns *down* the frontal cortex. A study using cognitive-behavioral therapy showed a similar response. However, paradoxically antidepressants,

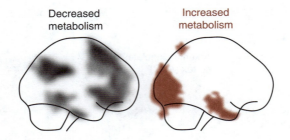

Decreased
metabolism

Increased
metabolism

FIGURE 21.2 Sagittal views of positron emission tomography scans on an average group of patients after a successful course of electroconvulsive therapy. (Adapted from Nobler MS, Oquendo MA, Kegeles LS, et al. Decreased regional brain metabolism after ECT. *Am J Psychiatry*. 2001;158[2]:305–308. Reprinted with permission from the *American Journal of Psychiatry* [Copyright © 2001]. American Psychiatric Association. All Rights Reserved.)

vagus nerve stimulation (VNS), and transcranial magnetic stimulation (TMS) have been shown to *increase* the activity of the PFC.

How can these successful treatments have such disparate effects on the frontal cortex? We think one explanation is that depression results from dysfunctional communication between the frontal cortex and subcortical regions. Successful treatment restores harmony between the regions. A frontal cortex that is organized and more appropriately responsive (whether more active or less active compared with pretreatment) may be less depressed. It may not be the idling rate of activity in the region that is pathologic in depression but rather the relationship between the PFC and the associated other regions in the depression or mood-regulating network.

This brings us to *functional connectivity*—an imaging technique designed to look for synchronicity of different brain regions—which is believed to be an assessment of the integrity of brain networks. Technically, functional connectivity is a mathematical calculation estimating correlations between different regions of the brain. Using fMRI images of the brain taken every 2 seconds over 10 minutes, the computer calculates areas that correlate between different brain regions in activity (or lack of activity). The most famous network identified in this manner is the *default mode network* or just the *default network*. This is the network that becomes active when someone (with their head in a scanner) closes their eyes and relaxes—or daydreams—lets the mind wander (see Figure 21.3). This replicated network is thought to be independent of and different from task-based networks such as the attention or emotional networks.

Study of functional connectivity is a hot topic, particularly in diseased states that are believed to have aberrant connections. The hope is that the strength (or lack of strength) of a network will be a biologic marker of an illness or facilitate treatment choices. A number of studies have been conducted

on patients with depression with mixed results—no consistent pattern has emerged. However, a recent meta-analysis of resting-state functional connectivity in depression found "hypoconnectivity" in the frontoparietal network (believed to represent cognitive clouding) and "hyperconnectivity" between the frontoparietal network and the default network (suggestive of the negative rumination so common in depression).

THE HYPOTHALAMIC–PITUITARY–ADRENAL AXIS

Since the 1950s it has been recognized that depressed patients have excessive activity of the HPA axis. Figure 21.4 shows the increased plasma cortisol levels over 24 hours in patients with depression compared with controls. The hypercortisolemia is stimulated by increased expression

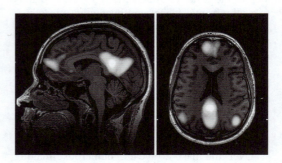

FIGURE 21.3 Resting-state functional magnetic resonance imaging showing the default mode network—when subjects are "resting" rather than involved in goal-oriented or attention-demanding tasks. (From Graner J, Oakes TR, French LM, Riedy G. Functional MRI in the investigation of blast-related traumatic brain injury. *Front Neurol*. 2013. Copyright © 2013 Graner, Oakes, French, and Riedy. https://doi.org/10.3389/fneur.2013.00016.)

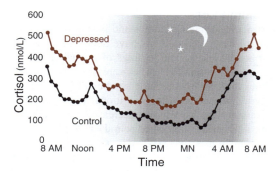

FIGURE 21.4 Diurnal mean plasma cortisol in depressed patients and healthy controls. (Adapted from Deuschle M, Schweiger U, Weber B, et al. Diurnal activity and pulsatility of the hypothalamic-pituitary-adrenal system in male depressed patients and healthy controls. *J Clin Endocrinol Metab.* 1997;82[1]:234–238, by permission of Oxford University Press.)

of corticotropin-releasing hormone (CRH) and reduced feedback inhibition of the HPA axis. As discussed in Chapter 7, Hormones and the Brain, one theory of depression postulates that chronic, unremitting stress leads to the inability of the brain to turn down the HPA axis.

Postmortem studies of depressed patients have shown an increased number of neurons in the paraventricular nucleus of the hypothalamus that are believed to drive the increased activity in the HPA axis. It is unclear why these patients have more neurons in the hypothalamus—probably genetic or a reaction to chronic stress—but we always say that.

Some patients with excess cortisol—either taken orally or generated internally—have reduced hippocampal volume. A meta-analysis of MRI studies has confirmed that hippocampal volume is reduced in patients with depression. Possibly the excess cortisol produced by depressed patients is toxic to the hippocampus and causes the volume loss, or they could be born with smaller hippocampus—a finding we will see when we discuss posttraumatic stress disorder (PTSD).

Effective treatments for depression (such as antidepressants, ECT, and lithium) are known to restore normal HPA function in most patients. It is postulated that this effect is due to increased glucocorticoid receptor production stimulated by the treatments, which has the effect of making the hypothalamus more receptive to negative feedback from cortisol. Finally, effective treatment of depression is believed to preserve and possibly restore hippocampal function (more on this later). A healthy hippocampus provides more inhibitory feedback on the HPA axis, as shown in Figure 7.9.

In summary, depression appears to result in the breakdown of the normal relationship between the hippocampus and the HPA axis. Increased cortisol from the adrenal gland causes hippocampal damage, which results in decreased inhibitory feedback on the HPA axis—which in turn causes increased cortisol release, etc.

Restoring normal functioning of the HPA axis as a treatment focus has generated considerable interest. Several groups have tested CRH receptor blockers as novel treatments for depression. Although the early small studies were favorable, the results were

DEPRESSION LABORATORY TEST

The overactivation of the HPA axis is so consistent in depression that there were early efforts to use it as a laboratory test to diagnose depression. Unfortunately, the sensitivity and specificity of increased adrenocorticotropic hormone (ACTH) for depression are not to the level where it is clinically useful. Other medical conditions also result in elevations of ACTH, and there is even a subset of depressed patients who have low ACTH!

The dexamethasone suppression test was piloted in the early 1980s in an alternative attempt to develop a laboratory test for depression. Patients are given dexamethasone at 11 PM, and cortisol levels are drawn the next morning. Dexamethasone binds to the glucocorticoid receptors, which in turn inhibits the secretion of ACTH and subsequently cortisol. Healthy

subjects will suppress the release of cortisol. Depressed patients will fail to suppress the cortisol and show a bump in their cortisol level the next morning. Unfortunately, the test has not been sensitive or specific enough—only 25% to 40%. It fails to detect many patients who are truly depressed, and some general medical conditions (such as Cushing's disease or even general stress of a chronic medical illness) also cause the HPA axis to fail to suppress cortisol.

Subsequently, with the availability of CRH, a new test has been developed using both dexamethasone and CRH (dex/CRH). Although the dex/CRH test is more accurate (the sensitivity increases to 80%), the clinical utility of this cumbersome test as a diagnostic tool remains doubtful.

not consistent and were associated with a risk of hepatotoxicity. Research in this area has stalled.

REWARD DYSFUNCTION

As discussed in Chapter 12, Pleasure, the drive for rewards (such as food, sex, revenge, reading this book, etc.) is mediated through the NAc with its dopaminergic projects from the ventral tegmental area. One theory of depression proposes that depressed patients, particularly those with anhedonia, suffer from impairment of the reward system. Various research studies support this as a possible mechanism of depression:

- Depressed patients show reduced reward responsiveness as measured by computer games that reward for correct answers.
- Depressed patients show a weaker response to rewards in the NAc compared with healthy controls—and even less for those with recurrent depression.
- Stimulants (dopamine agonists) are occasionally used to augment antidepressant treatment.
- Deep brain stimulation (DBS) of the NAc in treatment-resistant depression has been beneficial for some patients.

However, as noted in Chapter 12, other evidence (e.g., sweet taste test) suggests that depressed patients can feel the joy but lack energy and motivation to pursue it. The NAc may play a role in some depressions, in our opinion, but this is not the salient feature of major depression.

Finally, there is speculation about the role of the opioid system in mood regulation, although actual neuroscience markers are hard to find. The primary evidence comes from studies showing improved mood with opioid medications, as we discussed in Chapter 11, Pain. When one's world is gray, opioids relieve emotional as well as physical pain—although at great risk. This may be one of the reasons it is so difficult to get some people off opioids.

NEUROGENESIS AND BRAIN-DERIVED NEUROTROPHIC FACTOR

As discussed in Chapter 8, Plasticity and Adult Development, the brain is more dynamic than previously thought. The brain contains undeveloped stem cells that can migrate and mature into neurons or glial cells. There is compelling evidence that this process is disrupted in depression and gets corrected with successful treatment.

Volume Loss

Structural imaging studies and postmortem analysis of depressed patients have documented subtle volumetric loss. The findings of a smaller hippocampus (mentioned earlier) are the best known, but other findings include smaller PFC, cingulate gyrus, and cerebellum. Additionally, microscopic examinations have shown decreased cortical thickness as well as diminished neural size. One possible explanation is that HPA axis activation is neurotoxic to the brain. Another possibility involves a disruption of normal nerve growth.

The prospect that depression is related to problems with nerve growth factors opens a new way to conceptualize the pathophysiology of the disorder. A failure of neurogenesis and growth factor proteins, such as brain-derived neurotrophic factor (BDNF), may cause subtle shrinkage of the brain in depression.

BDNF is one of a family of neurotrophins that regulates the differentiation and survival of neurons (see Figure 8.10). Most likely there are a multitude of growth factor proteins maintaining and stimulating nerve growth, but BDNF is the most widely studied at this point. Figure 21.5 shows a dramatic example of the effects of BDNF on serotonergic neurons in the rat cortex. Saline or BDNF was infused directly into the rat frontal cortex for 21 days. Then the animals were sacrificed, and the cortex at the site of the infusion was stained for 5-hydroxytryptamine (5-HT) neurons. Note the remarkable arborization of the 5-HT axons in the cortex of the rat exposed to BDNF.

Growth factor proteins such as BDNF provide ongoing maintenance of neurons in the brain. Disruption of these nerve growth factors results in the reduction in the size of neurons, as well as some cell loss. Such reductions and loss may produce psychiatric symptoms.

It is difficult to assess the quantity and quality of BDNF in living humans, so the evidence connecting BDNF and depression is indirect. A postmortem analysis of suicide subjects found a marked decrease in BDNF in their PFC and hippocampus compared with controls (see Figure 21.6).

Psychiatric Treatment and Brain-Derived Neurotrophic Factor

Of particular interest are the increases in BDNF and neurogenesis seen with treatments that relieve depression. In rats, the following interventions have been shown to increase BDNF:

1. Antidepressants
2. Lithium
3. Stimulation treatments: ECT, TMS, and VNS
4. Estrogen
5. Exercise

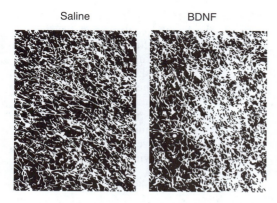

Saline   BDNF

FIGURE 21.5 Brain-derived neurotrophic factor (BDNF) infused directly into the rat frontal cortex results in a supranormal branching of 5-hydroxytryptamine axons. (Adapted with permission of Society for Neuroscience, from Mamounas LA, Blue ME, Siuciak JA, et al. Brain-derived neurotrophic factor promotes the survival and sprouting of serotonergic axons in rat brain. *J Neurosci*. 1995;15[12]:7929–7939.)

This is a remarkable discovery. It is the first time that one mechanism of action has been found that could explain how all these disparate modes of treatments relieve depression. (Presumably, psychotherapy would also increase BDNF, but no one has yet developed a credible animal model that can be tested.)

With humans, there are less data on studies following depression treatment and BDNF levels. A recent study from the University of California, San Francisco (UCSF) examined serum BDNF levels in depressed patients before and after the initiation of antidepressant treatment. The results were compared with those of healthy control subjects. Although serum BDNF levels are not as accurate as direct central measurements, the results are still impressive (see Figure 21.7). The BDNF levels in the depressed patients before treatment were significantly less than the levels in the healthy subjects. After 8 weeks of antidepressant treatment, the serum BDNF levels increased significantly and no longer differed from those of the controls.

Neurogenesis

Numerous studies have shown that increased BDNF leads to increased neurogenesis. Therefore, interventions that increase BDNF might also increase the development of new nerve cells. A unique study with rats has demonstrated that fluoxetine stimulates neurogenesis in about the same amount of time as it takes for humans to respond to the treatment. The rats given fluoxetine did not generate new neurons at a rate any different from placebo after 5 days but did separate from placebo by 28 days (see Figure 21.8). It also took 28 days for the rats to change their behavior—demonstrate a greater willingness to move into open, bright areas to eat (depressed rats stay more in the shadows).

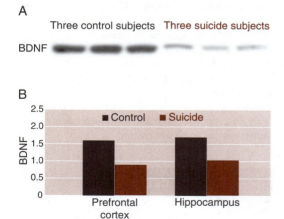

FIGURE 21.6 A: Western blots showing the immunolabeling of brain-derived neurotrophic factor (BDNF) in the prefrontal cortex in three control subjects and three suicide subjects. **B:** Averaged BDNF in the prefrontal cortex and hippocampus for both groups. (Data from Dwivedi Y, Rizavi HS, Conley RR, et al. Altered gene expression of brain-derived neurotrophic factor and receptor tyrosine kinase B in postmortem brain of suicide subjects. *Arch Gen Psychiatry*. 2003;60[8]:804–815.)

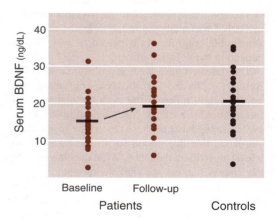

FIGURE 21.7 Serum brain-derived neurotrophic factor (BDNF) levels in depressed patients before and 8 weeks after escitalopram or sertraline treatment compared with healthy controls. (Adapted with permission from Wolkowitz OM, Wolf J, Shelly W, et al. Serum BDNF levels before treatment predict SSRI response in depression. *Prog Neuropsychopharmacol Biol Psychiatry*. 2011;35:1623–1630. Copyright 2011 with permission from Elsevier.)

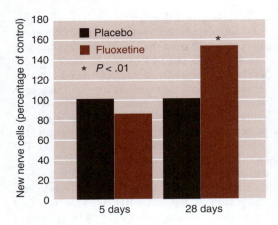

FIGURE 21.8 New neurons (neurogenesis) at 5 and 28 days in rats given placebo and fluoxetine. (Adapted from Santarelli L, Saxe M, Gross C, et al. Requirement of hippocampal neurogenesis for the behavioral effects of antidepressants. *Science*. 2003;301[5634]:805–809. Reprinted with permission from AAAS.)

Scarring the DNA

Nestler et al. at the University of Texas Southwestern Medical Center have taken these ideas one step further. They have looked at the effect of animal models of depression on the DNA that codes for BDNF. First, they stressed mice by placing them in the presence of a different aggressor mouse for 10 consecutive days. The exposed mice—called *defeated mice*—were later socially avoidant with unfamiliar mice. Such a reaction is similar to that of humans with depression and PTSD. The messenger RNA (mRNA) that encodes for BDNF was analyzed in the defeated mice and comparable controls. As expected, it was greatly reduced in the defeated mice.

The defeated mice were given imipramine, fluoxetine, or placebo for 30 days. The antidepressants not only reversed the avoidant behavior but also returned the BDNF mRNA to almost normal levels. On the basis of these results the researchers speculated that depression (or in this case, social defeat) must affect the DNA. What they have found may change the way we view depression.

We discussed in Chapter 6, Genetics and Epigenetics, how DNA must unravel for the mRNA to be transcribed (see Figure 6.6). Likewise, we discussed in Chapter 17, Social Attachment, the profound effect that a mother rat's behavior has on gene expression (see Figure 17.7). The results from Nestler's laboratory suggest that depression too may be a disorder of gene expression—or what they call *gene silencing*.

The region of the DNA that codes for BDNF was examined in the defeated mice as well

as healthy controls. Figure 21.9 presents the findings. The healthy controls had few methyl groups attached to the histones that package the DNA. In the defeated mice, the methyl groups were greatly increased, which had the effect of limiting access to the DNA. The antidepressant-treated group had the addition of many acetyl groups to the histones, although there was no change in the number of methyl groups. The acetyl groups have the effect of opening up the DNA and allowing BDNF mRNA to be transcribed.

Human studies examining methylation of the DNA in depressed patients have not been conducted. Although we would never biopsy the brain of a living depressed person, it would be interesting to compare methylation of the DNA in postmortem studies of depressed patients and nondepressed controls.

In summary, these studies suggest a mechanism for depression. Stress in conjunction with a genetic vulnerability decreases growth factor proteins (such as BDNF) because of "clogging" of the DNA. This leads to thinning of the neuronal structures, which results in depressive symptoms (see Figure 21.10). These structural changes make the prefrontal limbic governing system vulnerable to disruption and dysregulation. Stress, loss, or other processes cause the system to lose self-regulation. Furthermore, it appears that effective treatments such as antidepressants, lithium, ECT, and exercise (and presumably psychotherapy and good social support) will reverse the process. Presumably the treatment increases the production of growth factor proteins, such as BDNF, which results in renewed neuronal growth, more resilient self-regulating circuits, and a return to healthy mood.

Clearly, this is a simplistic description of what is a very complex and heterogenous process. Much more remains to be discovered.

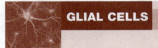

GLIAL CELLS

An unexpected finding in postmortem studies of depressed patients has been the reduced number and density of glial cells in the PFC. Subsequent studies have shown that electroconvulsive seizures in rats will increase proliferation of new glial cells but not new neurons in the PFC. Glial cells may play a larger role in depression and its treatment than traditionally believed.

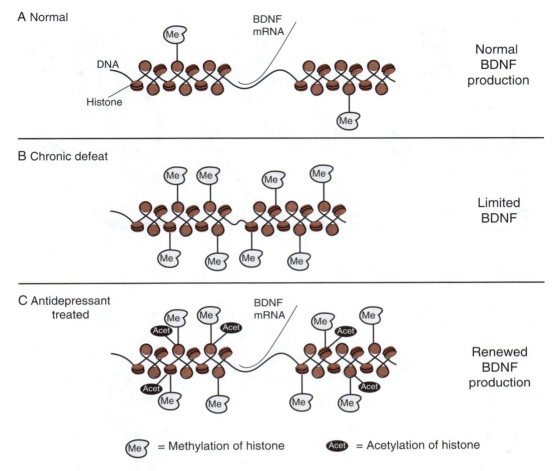

Me⟩ = Methylation of histone   Acet = Acetylation of histone

FIGURE 21.9 **A:** DNA must unravel to transcribe messenger RNA (mRNA) needed for protein translation such as brain-derived neurotrophic factor (BDNF). **B:** Chronic defeat (and possibly depression) caused excessive methylation of the histones, which blocks access to the DNA. **C:** Antidepressant treatment renews access to the DNA by adding acetyl groups to the histones. (Data from Tsankova NM, Berton O, Renthal W, et al. Sustained hippocampal chromatin regulation in a mouse model of depression and antidepressant action. *Nat Neurosci.* 2006;9[4]:519–525.)

Ketamine

One of the most interesting recent findings in psychiatry is the rapid antidepressant response to the old anesthetic, ketamine—an *N*-methyl-D-aspartate (NMDA) blocker (see Figure 5.2). Not only does this offer a unique approach to the treatment of depression—tweaking the glutamate neurons—but also a single IV administration can have a robust response in less than 2 hours in upward of 75% of the subjects—lasting several days to 2 weeks. There are few interventions with such a hearty response—sleep deprivation, intrathecal thyrotropin-releasing hormone, or winning the lottery—all with limited duration.

Ketamine infusion is not FDA approved for the treatment of depression, nor covered by insurance. Regardless, infusion clinics have popped up around the country in response to the demand. However, ketamine is not without problems. Dissociation, hallucination, and addiction are the big issues, and we do not know the long-term effects from frequent infusions. Also we believe some of the effectiveness of ketamine is due to its effect on the opioid receptors—and we know all the problems that receptor causes.

Searching for the mechanism of action—how ketamine induces a rapid lifting of mood—has generated a lot of research. The general consensus is that gene expression turns on protein synthesis and downstream phosphorylation modulates synaptic plasticity. Research at Yale demonstrated that ketamine could reverse anhedonia and induce synaptogenesis in the PFC in the animal model of depression (chronic stress). Other studies have

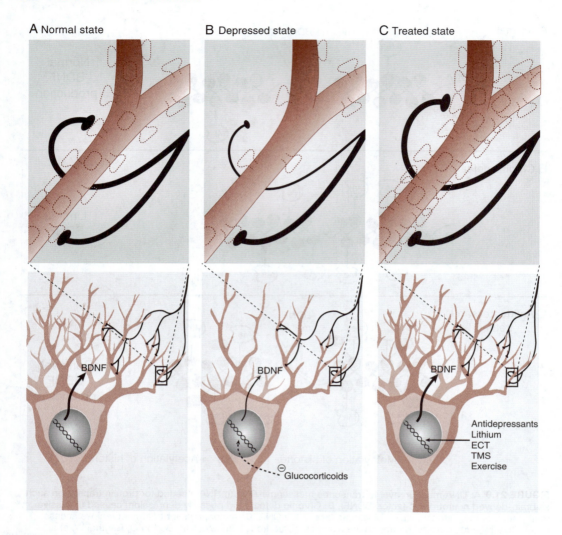

A Normal state

B Depressed state

C Treated state

BDNF

BDNF

BDNF

Antidepressants
Lithium
ECT
TMS
Exercise

⊖ Glucocorticoids

FIGURE 21.10 Stress and genetics cause deviation from normal state **(A)** to result in decreased growth factor protein production, which reduces neural substrate **(B)**. Effective treatment reverses this process **(C)**. BDNF, brain-derived neurotrophic factor; ECT, electroconvulsive therapy; TMS, transcranial magnetic stimulation. (Adapted by permission from Macmillan Publishers Ltd. Berton O, Nestler EJ. New approaches to antidepressant drug discovery: beyond monoamines. *Nat Rev Neurosci.* 2006;7[2]:137–151. Copyright 2006.)

shown that ketamine increases the production of BDNF in the hippocampi and that BDNF-knockout mice fail to show the usual clinical response to an infusion.

How does ketamine induce synaptogenesis (if this is the antidepressant mechanism)? It is hard to imagine that blocking the NMDA receptor—a widespread receptor associated with learning and memory—can have such a dramatic effect on mood. Research recently published out of the University of Maryland suggests it is a metabolite of ketamine (hydroxynorketamine) that is essential for the anti-depressant effects. In a variety of experiments, they blocked seemingly everything else and established

it is the metabolite working through the α-amino-3-hydroxy-5-methyl-4-isoxazole propionate receptor (see Figure 5.2) that improves mood. Furthermore, they showed that the metabolite does not induce dissociation in mice (*how is that tested?*) and appears to have no abuse/addiction liability. If shown to be effective and safe in humans, the authors believe they will have discovered a novel mechanism for the treatment of depression.

Deep Brain Stimulation

DBS is like a cardiac pacemaker for the brain—there are a pulse generator implanted under the skin, thin wires that transmit the pulse, and

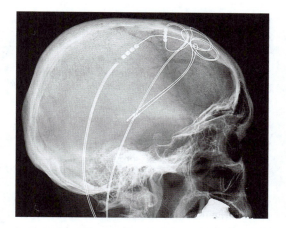

FIGURE 21.11 X-ray of electrodes placed in the brain for deep brain stimulation for Parkinson's disease. (Courtesy of Hellerhoff.)

electrodes at the end that emit an electrical charge (see Figure 21.11). DBS is an effective treatment option for Parkinson's disease but is still experimental for treating depression. We hear remarkable stories of patients with treatment-resistant depression reporting dramatic improvements in mood on the operating table when the electrodes are turned on. Unfortunately, controlled trials have not been so impressive. In two recent trials, DBS for treatment-resistant depression was terminated early because of lack of benefit.

When electrodes are inserted for cardiac arrhythmias or Parkinson's disease, the location for the electrodes is based on knowledge of the pathology—for example, the sinoatrial node of the heart or the subthalamic nucleus for Parkinson's disease. But we do not know the pathology of depression so we do not know where to point the electrode, although a number of locations have been tried, e.g., subcallosal cingulate gyrus, NAc, medial forebrain bundle, and ventral capsule are the most common. Perhaps whatever causes, depression is widespread throughout the brain and reversing this is difficult with simple focal stimulation.

GENES AND ENVIRONMENT

Some people encounter a stressful life event and bounce back with astounding resilience. Others, faced with the same life experience, lapse into depression. The general consensus is that depression (and most mental illness for that matter) results from the interaction of dubious genes and difficult environmental events. In 2003, Avshalom Caspi published a remarkable paper in Science that purported to identify a gene that could explain why people respond differently to life's challenges.

There are two versions for the gene that produces the serotonin transporter (the reuptake pump in the synapse): a short one that is less effective and a long one. Caspi and his colleagues collected

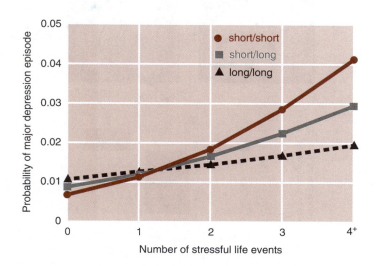

FIGURE 21.12 Individuals with the long allele for the serotonin transporter are less likely to develop depression when dealing with life's stresses in this landmark study. Unfortunately, subsequent studies failed to replicate these impressive findings. (Adapted from Caspi A, Sugden K, Moffitt TE, et al. Influence of life stress on depression: moderation by a polymorphism in the 5-HTT gene. *Science.* 2003;301:386–389. Reprinted with permission from AAAS.)

information from 26-year-old subjects—stressful life events in the past 5 years and presence of major depression in the past year—and correlated these data with the genes for the serotonin transporter. The results are graphed in Figure 21.12. Individuals with copies of the short allele *and* stressful events were predisposed to develop major depression.

This was one of the most famous studies in psychiatry in the previous decade. A copy seemed to appear in every PowerPoint presentation on depression. Unfortunately, a meta-analysis 6 years later demonstrated that combining the results from 14 studies "yielded no evidence that the serotonin transporter genotype alone or in interaction with stressful life events is associated with elevated risk of depression." These disappointing results are probably a product of focusing on one gene (when depression is more likely the result of numerous genes) and the illusion of pattern effects in small studies. Most of us believe depression results from the interaction of genes and environment, but research remains hampered by our inability to identify the important genes.

BIPOLAR DISORDER

Bipolar disorder is a prevalent illness with strong genetic links and unique clinical features. Unfortunately, there is little to report about the neuroscience of bipolar disorder. This may be due to the difficultly in distinguishing the subtle differences in bipolar patients' brains from those with unipolar depression as well as healthy controls. Furthermore, bipolar disorder also has similarities

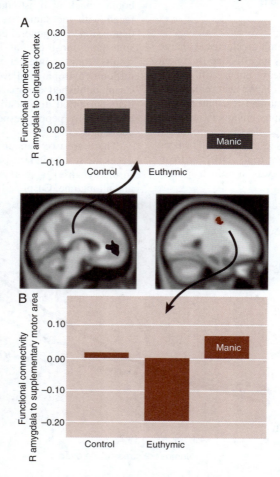

FIGURE 21.13 A: Manic patients display reduced connectivity between the amygdala and anterior cingulate gyrus compared with euthymic bipolar patients and healthy controls. **B:** Manic patients show increased connectivity between amygdala and supplementary motor area. (Adapted with permission from Brady RO, et al. State dependent cortico-amygdala circuit dysfunction in bipolar disorder. *J Affect Disord*. 2016;201:79–87. Copyright 2016 with permission from Elsevier.)

to schizophrenia. The essential feature of bipolar disorder—episodes of mania—is clinically very distinctive but has no obvious structural, functional, or molecular markers yet identified in the brain.

Global Activation

One would think that manic episodes would be easy to differentiate in functional imaging studies— if the subjects could remain still long enough in the scanner. In a manic episode the patient's brain appears to be revved up—going way too fast. One would imagine that the manic brain would "light up" in a functional imaging study, but that has not been the case. Studies following patients in and out of manic episodes with multiple functional scans have failed to find changes in brain metabolism.

More recently the focus has shifted to functional connectivity. A group out of McLean Hospital has compared bipolar patients in manic states with euthymic bipolar patients and healthy controls. Using an fMRI to measure functional connectivity, they found disrupted functional connectivity in manic patients compared with the other groups. Specifically they found *decreased* connectivity between the amygdala and anterior cingulate cortex and *increased* connectivity between the amygdala and the supplemental motor area (see Figure 21.13). In a longitudinal study the authors followed 10 bipolar patients and scanned them in both mood states. This "within"-subject study replicated their earlier findings.

It is unclear if these findings give us more insight into the manic state, and it remains to be seen if they can be replicated (a problem with connectivity studies), but it is exciting to find alterations in the brain for a condition that is clinically so obvious.

Lithium and Gray Matter

Some imaging studies have found decreased size and activity in the PFC of patients with bipolar disorder—similar to that found in patients with unipolar depression. We mentioned earlier that lithium has been shown to stimulate BDNF synthesis. A group at Wayne State University conducted a clever study matching these two concepts. They examined the gray matter volume changes in bipolar patients after initiating lithium treatment. MRI scans were conducted at baseline and after 4 weeks of lithium. A computer outlined and measured the gray matter volume in each scan (see Figure 21.14). Of the 10 patients, 8 showed significant increases in total gray matter volume—averaging 3%.

Subsequent studies by other groups have replicated these data. Of interest, valproic acid has not been shown to have the same effect.

Bipolar Summary

Although these studies are interesting, they fail to provide the neuroscientific basis for bipolar disorder that we would like to see. Haldane and Frangou reviewed the literature on imaging studies

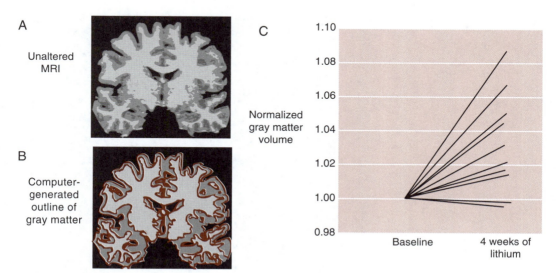

FIGURE 21.14 Gray matter in magnetic resonance imaging (MRI) **(A)** is outlined and quantified in the computer **(B)**. The change in gray matter volume is shown after 4 weeks of lithium treatment **(C)**. (Adapted from Moore GJ, Bebchuk JM, Wilds IB, et al. Lithium-induced increase in human brain grey matter. *Lancet.* 2000;356[9237]:1241–1242. Copyright 2000 with permission from Elsevier.)

on patients with bipolar disorder. They suggest that bipolar patients share some features with unipolar depression (reduced activity in the PFC). Yet other areas such as the amygdala are larger and more active in the bipolar patients. The authors suggest that bipolar disorder may be the result of abnormal interactions between the PFC and subcortical regions such as the amygdala—an abnormality they claim is not seen with unipolar depression. Clearly, more research is needed on this interesting topic.

BDNF UTOPIA?

One can get the impression that nerve growth factors such as BDNF are the solution to all problems. Although future psychiatric treatments may provide better ways to restore nerve growth factor deficiencies in mentally ill patients, it will not be as simple as just finding ways to get more BDNF into the brain. Too much BDNF in some regions of the brain may be detrimental. For example, Nestler et al. using the same "defeated mouse" protocol found that the defeated mice had increased BDNF in the NAc. The researchers speculate that the development of the social phobia seen with the defeated mice may be related to too much BDNF in the brain's reward system. Additionally, "too much growth, in an uncontrolled manner," is another way to describe cancer.

QUESTIONS

1. All the following are true about the mono-amine hypothesis except
   a. It is often called a chemical imbalance.
   b. It explains the delay in response seen with depression treatments.
   c. It proposes deficiencies in 5-HT and NE in depressed patients.
   d. It suffers from a lack of supporting findings.

2. Postmortem studies in depressed patients have found all of the following except
   a. Reduced neurons in the hypothalamus.
   b. Thinning of the gray matter in certain regions.
   c. Diminished neuronal size.
   d. Reduced glial cells.

3. Antidepressants may decrease depressive symptoms and improve neural survival through which of the following effects?
   a. Increase glucocorticoids and increase BDNF.
   b. Increase glucocorticoids and decrease BDNF.
   c. Decrease glucocorticoids and increase BDNF.
   d. Decrease glucocorticoids and decrease BDNF.

4. Goals for effective treatment of depression include all of the following except
   a. Decrease HPA activity.
   b. Protect the hippocampus.
   c. Restore normal sleep architecture.
   d. Awaken the PFC.

5. Which intervention has not been shown to increase BDNF in animal models?
   a. Cognitive-behavioral therapy.
   b. Exercise.
   c. Transcranial magnetic stimulation.
   d. Estrogen.

6. Possible culprits in the etiology of depression include all of the following except
   a. Cytotoxic effects of cortisol.
   b. Insufficient limbic activity.
   c. Genetic predisposition for sufficient nerve growth factors.
   d. Disorganized prefrontal activity.

7. One plausible explanation for antidepressant effectiveness is
   a. Removing methyl groups from scarred DNA.
   b. Restoring 5-HT and NE to their normal levels.
   c. Restoring access to the DNA.
   d. Neuroprotective effects on mRNA.

8. The pathologic mechanism of bipolar disorder is best described as
   a. Excessive prefrontal activity in manic episodes and decreased activity during depression.
   b. Too much BDNF in subcortical structures.
   c. Cortisol activation of excessive electrical activity.
   d. None of the above.

See Answers section at the end of this book.

CHAPTER 22

Anxiety

INTRODUCTION

Anxiety is part of a mechanism developed in higher animals to handle adverse situations. The anxiety response can be conceptualized as part of the brain's alarm system firing during times of perceived danger. The characteristic responses including avoidance, hypervigilance, and increased arousal have evolved to evade the wolf lurking in the woods. Unfortunately, in many individuals, the mechanism is overactive. The alarm fires too frequently. Such people cannot seem to turn down their internal alarm even when the feared animal is on the endangered species list.

Diagnostic and Statistical Manual

The Diagnostic and Statistical Manual (DSM) system categorizes anxiety into a multitude of different disorders (such as generalized anxiety disorder [GAD], obsessive–compulsive disorder [OCD], posttraumatic stress disorder [PTSD], etc.). Although each disorder has unique clinical features, it is not clear whether they actually describe different pathologic states. The disorders have the following similar characteristics:

1. Most patients with an anxiety disorder will have features of other anxiety disorders as well as depression—comorbidity is the norm.
2. Many of the disorders respond to similar treatment interventions: selective serotonin reuptake inhibitors (SSRIs), benzodiazepines, exposure therapy, and so on.
3. There is little evidence to show that different disorders stem from different regions of the brain.

Work out of Peter Lang's anxiety clinic at the University of Florida has demonstrated a dimensional model of anxiety consistent with the RDoC initiative. In an analysis of over 400 patients, they found a wide range of distress within DSM disorders. Using a general measure of anxiety, they showed that patients with more disorders are more distressed—or what they call anxious misery (see Figure 22.1A). For example, patients with panic and agoraphobia are more anxious than patients with just panic. Or patients with PTSD and multiple traumas are more anxious than most patients with PTSD from a single trauma. Likewise, the addition of depression to anxiety increased the anxious misery. Of more importance, those with more anxious misery were more impaired and least responsive to treatment.

Lang et al. also looked at physiologic reactivity. Patients were asked to listen to threatening stories that were interrupted with a "brief acoustic probe" (that's what they call a sudden 95-dB noise), at which time patients blink as a defensive reaction. So, they measured the startle reaction (blinking) and change in heart rate to the "acoustic probe." Paradoxically, the patients with the most anxious misery were also the *least* reactive to the noise (see Figure 22.1B).

It is important to not presume the hyporeactors as less distressed, but rather that they are less reactive to specific threats when they are already on edge. Lang and his colleagues believe that the more anxious patients have become disorganized and perceive threats *everywhere*. They have overgeneralized their fears and fail to distinguish between real and benign threats. The key point for us is that this may be a better way to diagnosis anxiety—on a dimensional scale, combining self-report with physiologic biomarkers. We believe that the reaction to perceived threat is mediated in similar pathways in the brain in patients with various DSM anxiety disorders. The one potential exception is OCD, which has unique mechanisms in the brain and will be reviewed separately.

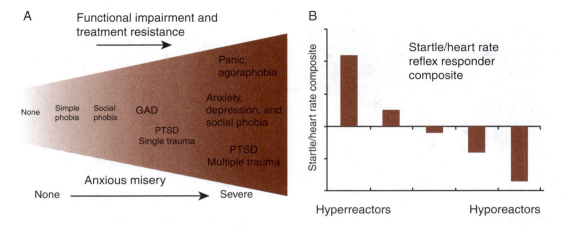

FIGURE 22.1 **A:** Anxiety is best seen as a spectrum of anxious misery rather than discrete disorders. **B:** Paradoxically, the most anxious people are less startled in laboratory conditions. (Adapted from Lang PJ, et al. [2016.] RDoC, DSM, and the reflex physiology of fear: a biodimensional analysis of the anxiety disorders spectrum. *Psychophysiology*. 53:336–347.)

Acute Stress

The body's reaction to an acutely stressful situation is well known to all of us. The characteristic rapid heart rate, dry mouth, and sweaty palms are the body's response to increased sympathetic activity generated by a stressful situation (see Figure 2.10). Less readily apparent are the endocrine responses to acute stress.

In the late 1970s, Ursin et al. studied the endocrinologic responses of young Norwegian military recruits during parachute training. During the exercise, the recruits repeatedly jumped off a 12-m tower and slid down a long sloping wire to learn the basic skills of parachuting. The training was designed to give the jumper a realistic sensation of the initial free fall. Measures of anxiety and performance skill as well as serum hormone levels were captured at baseline and after each jump.

Initially, anxiety was high and performance was poor. As the days and number of jumps progressed, anxiety subsided and the skills improved. The endocrinologic measures, shown in Figure 22.2, followed a similar pattern. Presumably, the anxiety induces changes in the releasing hormones, which alter the pituitary hormones and ultimately the peripheral hormones. Note how testosterone levels drop with the stress of the jumping, whereas the other measures increase. Sapolsky would likely point out that maintenance of sexual characteristics becomes a low priority in an emergency.

Although the average individual shows a peak in the endocrine response at the start of a difficult task, which usually subsides as the person gains mastery, this is not true for everyone. Some people have more exaggerated and persistent endocrine reactions. Kirschbaum et al. looked at salivary cortisol levels

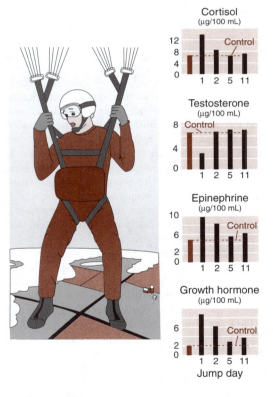

FIGURE 22.2 The stress of learning to parachute, on young recruits, results in changes in hormones, which return to baseline as the anxiety decreases. (Adapted from Rosenzweig MR, Breedlove SM, Watson NV. *Biological Psychology*. 4th ed. Sunderland, MA: Sinauer; 2005, by permission of Oxford University Press, USA. Graphs adapted from Ursin H, Baade E, Levine S. *Psychobiology of Stress: A Study of Coping Men*. New York: Academic Press; 1978.)

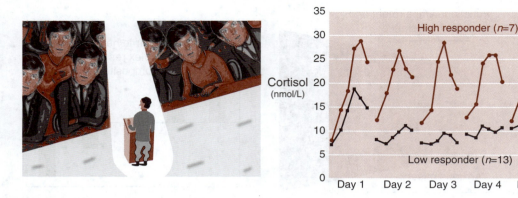

FIGURE 22.3 Men stressed by public speaking over five consecutive days showed different patterns of adrenocortical response. (Graph adapted from Kirschbaum C, Prussner JC, Stone AA, et al. Persistent high cortisol responses to repeated psychological stress in a subpopulation of healthy men. *Psychosom Med.* 1995;57[5]:468–474. Illustration adapted from Images.com.)

in 20 men exposed to five consecutive days of public speaking. For the total group, the average cortisol levels jumped on the first day and then gradually declined over the following days. However, the men could be divided into two groups: high responders and low responders. Figure 22.3 shows the cortisol levels for these two groups.

Note how the cortisol in the low responders peaked the first day but then quickly returned to baseline levels on the following days. These individuals appear to adjust rapidly to the stress of public speaking. The high responders, on the other hand, showed higher, more persistent peaks of cortisol. Such people appear to have a harder time turning off the stress response. Presumably, they have a stronger alarm response in the brain, which is driving this endocrine reaction. Alternatively, they have a weak or faulty regulatory system that fails to extinguish the response.

Cortisol has been implicated as a culprit in the development of anxiety after trauma, although not everyone agrees if it is too much or too little. Some researchers believe that the consolidation of emotional memories and development of PTSD are exacerbated by *insufficient* cortisol. They cite studies showing lower levels of cortisol in PTSD patients and anecdotal studies that found that patients who received hydrocortisone in the ICU for septic shock were less likely to develop PTSD. Several small placebo-controlled trials conducted in emergency departments within hours of the trauma showed that patients who received hydrocortisone went on to have fewer PTSD symptoms. Wow! Wouldn't it be wonderful if we could mitigate the emotional effects of trauma and reduce the risk of developing PTSD.

Other researchers cite studies showing increased levels of cortisol with PTSD. This group believes that *excess* cortisol sensitizes the amygdala. They want to block the glucocorticoid receptors after the development of PTSD. Early studies have been positive, so the Veterans Administration is conducting a randomized trial of mifepristone (RU-486, the "abortion pill") to block the glucocorticoid receptors after the development of PTSD. The take-home message is that hypothalamic–pituitary–adrenal (HPA) axis is somewhat influential in PTSD, although the details are fuzzy. Hopefully we'll know more by the next edition of this book.

NEURONAL CIRCUITRY

A plethora of research points to the prefrontal cortex (PFC), amygdala, hippocampus, and HPA axis as the regions involved with anxiety (Figure 22.4). However, if there is one organ that represents an alarm system in the brain, it is the amygdala.

Amygdala

In their classic studies with rhesus monkeys in the 1930s, Heinrich Klüver and Paul Bucy identified the amygdala as a structure that is essential for the expression of numerous emotions. They removed large segments of the temporal lobes from wild monkeys and transformed the monkey's temperament. Aggressive and easily frightened monkeys were changed into docile, calm creatures.

The monkeys virtually became tame. They did not react fearfully to strange humans or even a snake. Of particular interest, the monkeys failed to learn from negative experience. One monkey, bitten by a snake, later approached a snake again as if

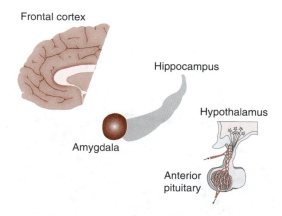

FIGURE 22.4 The important regions of the brain affecting anxiety.

nothing had happened—a clear example of the survival value of anxiety. The entire constellation of symptoms is called the *Klüver–Bucy syndrome* and includes a host of other bizarre features, such as hypersexuality and a tendency to transfer objects to the mouth.

In the intervening years, it has been demonstrated that the emotional changes of the Klüver–Bucy syndrome can be elicited with the removal of just the amygdala. Other evidence points to the amygdala as an important region in the recognition and management of fear:

1. Electric stimulation of the amygdala in animals elicits fearful behavior, for example, freezing and tachycardia.
2. Humans with damaged amygdala exhibit impaired fear conditioning.
3. Functional imaging studies of humans show activation of the amygdala during fear learning.

Recognizing Danger

Sensory information enters the brain by way of the thalamus. All neurons carrying auditory and visual information synapse first in the thalamus before being relayed to the appropriate cortical region for analysis. Information about danger is particularly important and needs to be recognized quickly. Work by Joseph LeDoux et al. at New York University has shown that the amygdala quickly receives some preliminary information about possible threats even before it is processed in the cortex.

Figure 22.5 shows an example of a person coming upon a rattlesnake. This life-threatening visual information proceeds from the eyes to the thalamus. However, the thalamus sends fast but rudimentary signals to the amygdala at the same

time that the full information is passed back to the visual cortex. The amygdala in turn sends responding signals to the muscles, sympathetic nervous system, and hypothalamus. The person jumps even before being consciously aware of what has been seen. LeDoux has shown with rats that the fear response is preserved even if the neural connections between the thalamus and cortex are cut. In essence, the animal startles without knowing why.

We have all had the experience of being frightened when seeing something, only to realize that it was just a rope or shadow—not a real threat. It is the fast track from the thalamus directly to the amygdala that causes the false alarm. This is considered to be "unconscious" or preconscious. We jump before we are aware. Patients with anxiety disorders can have exaggerated startle responses. They are burdened with an exaggerated, unconscious reaction to what are actually harmless events.

Anticipatory Anxiety

Some people dread personal interactions in which they will be the focus of attention. Typically, they fear they will embarrass themselves. The anticipatory anxiety can restrict what they do and impede their social life and career path trajectory.

An imaging study looked at the activity in the brain of such patients who were asked to anticipate making a public speech. By subtracting the activity during anticipation from that at rest, they identified the areas of activity. Patients showed greater activity in their amygdala as well as hippocampus and insula. Figure 22.6A shows the functional magnetic resonance imaging (fMRI) slice at the level of the amygdala.

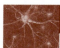

TREATMENT

AMYGDALA ACTIVITY

A small study in Sweden looked at the effects of cognitive–behavioral therapy (CBT) and the antidepressant citalopram on brain activity in patients with social phobia. Both treatments were equally effective, and both reduced the amygdala activation after 9 weeks of treatment. The degree of amygdala attenuation was associated with clinical improvement 1 year later.

Anticipatory anxiety is not all bad. Figure 22.6B shows the hypothetical upside-down U-curve that many think represents the benefits and problems with anticipatory anxiety. Some anxiety is beneficial and actually improves performance; however,

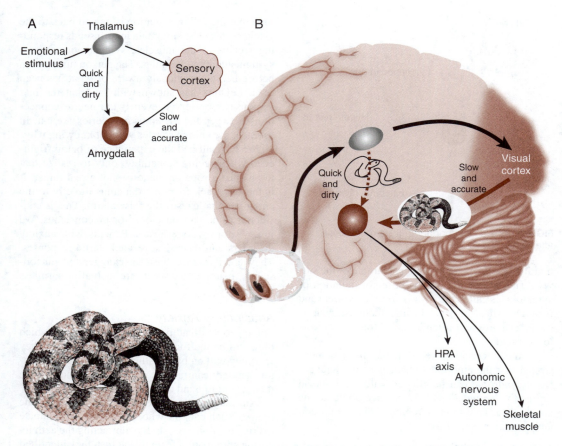

FIGURE 22.5 Two representations, **(A)** and **(B)**, showing the quick and slow tracks that emotionally stimulating sensory information takes to the amygdala after entering the brain through the thalamus. HPA, hypothalamic–pituitary–adrenal. (Adapted from LeDoux JE. Emotion, memory and the brain. *Sci Am*. 1994;270[6]:50–57. Illustration by Roberto Osti.)

too much of it is overwhelming and results in a poorer outcome.

Amygdala Memories

There is evidence that primitive emotionally relevant memories are stored in the amygdala. For example, in rodents:

1. Long-term potentiation (LTP) can be induced in the amygdala.
2. Protein synthesis inhibitors injected directly into the amygdala will prevent the formation of fear conditioning.
3. Chronic stress will induce increased dendritic branching in the amygdala.

These results suggest that the typical structural changes that are observed with memory formation occur in the amygdala in reaction to fearful circumstances. This may be one reason why traumatic events are so persistent. Fearful experiences form quickly, and enduring

memories then reside in both the neocortex as well as the amygdala.

Prefrontal Cortex

One of the central components of anxiety is the feeling that one is not in control. Patients will complain of increased anxiety when they lose control, for example, when the door closes on an airplane or when their social support drives off—anytime they feel trapped. Feeling in control, on the other hand, calms anxiety. The ability to reappraise a difficult situation into more favorable terms is a function of executive control. Rational reappraisal is a central feature of CBT.

The ability to cognitively master difficult circumstances and gain control likely resides in the PFC. Clearly, the PFC plays an important role in managing anxiety. However, the exact prefrontal regions involved (such as medial, lateral, or orbital) are ill-defined, although the medial prefrontal cortex (mPFC) gets the most attention. The mPFC,

A

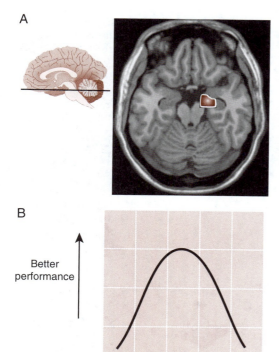

B

Better performance

Increasing anxiety

FIGURE 22.6 A: Increased activity at the level of the amygdala when patients with anxiety anticipate making a public speech. **B:** Hypothetical upside-down U-curve showing benefits and problems of anticipatory anxiety. (fMRI from Lorberbaum JP, Kose S, Johnson MR, et al. Neural correlates of speech anticipatory anxiety in generalized social phobia. *Neuroreport.* 2004;15[18]:2701–2705.)

which includes the anterior cingulate gyrus, is well connected to the amygdala.

In a simple conceptualization, we can imagine that the mPFC applies the brakes to the amygdala. Several lines of evidence highlight the role of the mPFC in anxiety.

1. Lesions of the mPFC in rats reduce the ability to extinguish fears.
2. Stimulation of the mPFC inhibits a learned fear response; that is, the rat does not show anxiety.
3. The mPFC lights up in functional imaging studies when fear is evoked in healthy subjects.
4. Subjects with anxiety disorders have reduced activity in the mPFC.

Taken together, these findings suggest that anxiety in part results from the reciprocal relation between PFC and amygdala (Figure 22.7). This has been shown clearly in a clever study with traumatized combat veterans and firefighters. The subjects were shown pictures of faces expressing various

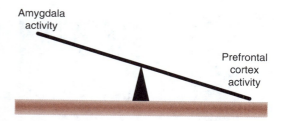

FIGURE 22.7 In simple terms, anxiety disorders may be the result of too much activity in the amygdala and not enough activity in the prefrontal cortex.

emotions during fMRI scanning (Figure 22.8A). The activity in the brain when the subjects were viewing the happy face was subtracted from the brain activity when viewing the fearful face. The subjects with PTSD were compared with healthy controls.

Figure 22.8 B and C shows the results of the brain scans. Note how subjects with PTSD, under the circumstances of the study, show *increased* activity in their amygdala and *decreased* activity in their PFC. In essence, in these traumatized subjects their PFC is insufficiently powered and unable to turn down the "alarm" in the amygdala.

Hippocampus

The hippocampus, an area involved with explicit memory acquisition, appears to interact with the amygdala during encoding of emotional memories. Although the exact role of the hippocampus in anxiety disorders remains unclear, it is an area frequently active in imaging studies during fearful situations.

A number of studies have documented smaller hippocampi in anxious patients. It was proposed that an activated HPA axis produced too much cortisol, which presumably shrank the hippocampus. However, a unique study with twins turned this theory upside down.

Gilbertson et al. recruited 40 pairs of twins, in which one of each pair was exposed to combat in Vietnam and the other had stayed home. (Who knew such a study was possible?) With an MRI the researchers measured the hippocampal volume of each twin. Additionally, the presence and severity of PTSD in the combat-exposed twin was assessed. As with previous reports, the twins who were diagnosed with PTSD had smaller hippocampal volumes (Figure 22.9A). However, the most remarkable finding was that the PTSD score from the combat-exposed twin had a similar correlation with the hippocampal volume of the twin who had *stayed at home* (Figure 22.9B). To put it simply, the best prediction of the size of a combat veteran's hippocampus is not his exposure to trauma but rather the size of his twin's hippocampus.

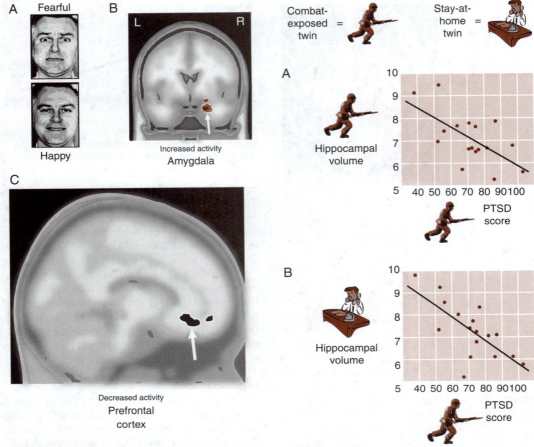

FIGURE 22.8 A: Traumatized subjects and controls were shown pictures of fearful faces and happy faces while in a functional magnetic resonance imaging (fMRI). The patients displayed increased activity in the amygdala **(B)** and decreased activity in the prefrontal cortex (PFC) **(C)** compared with the controls. Activity in the PFC and amygdala had an inverse correlation for the traumatized patients. (**A:** Adapted with permission of Macmillan Publishers Ltd. From Calder AJ, Lawrence AD, Young AW. Neuropsychology of fear and loathing. *Nat Rev Neurosci.* 2001;2[5]:352–363. **B, C:** Data from Shin LM, Wright CI, Cannistraro PA, et al. A functional magnetic resonance imaging study of amygdala and medial prefrontal cortex responses to overtly presented fearful faces in posttraumatic stress disorder. *Arch Gen Psychiatry.* 2005;62[3]:273–281.)

FIGURE 22.9 **A:** The correlation between hippocampal volume and posttraumatic stress disorder (PTSD) score for the combat-exposed twin. **B:** The correlation between the stay-at-home twin's hippocampal volume and the PTSD score of his combat-exposed twin brother. (Adapted by permission from Macmillan Publishers Ltd. Gilbertson MW, Shenton ME, Ciszewski A, et al. Smaller hippocampal volume predicts pathologic vulnerability to psychological trauma. *Nat Neurosci.* 2002;5[11]:1242–1247. Copyright 2002.)

This finding brings to light one of the great discoveries in neuroscience. It is the interaction between nature and nurture that results in mental illness (Figure 22.10). In other words, those at increased risk for developing PTSD are those individuals with a small hippocampus and exposure to trauma. Neither alone is sufficient.

Taken together, these findings suggest an important role for the hippocampus in the

development of anxiety. These early preliminary data suggest that there is something neuroprotective about a large hippocampus that mitigates the development of PTSD, even when someone is exposed to unimaginable trauma. Hypothetically, a larger hippocampus is better able to limit the acquisition of haunting memories or more efficient at extinguishing them once they develop.

Two recent twin studies published in 2012 corroborated the Gilbertson findings. In one study with women, a smaller hippocampus correlated with a diagnosis of GAD. In a large study with male twins, hippocampal volume correlated with self-esteem.

ALCOHOLISM AND ANXIETY

There is controversy about the relation between alcoholism and anxiety. Acute alcohol intoxication reduces anxiety. Many clinicians believe that substance abusers are self-medicating their anxiety with alcohol and other γ-aminobutyric acid (GABA) agonists. Longitudinal and genetic studies support this perception for some patients.

However, there is compelling evidence that chronic alcohol exposure induces long-term central nervous system adaptations that cause anxiety. For example, the following have been observed.

1. Withdrawal from alcohol increases anxiety temporarily, which then decreases as abstinence persists.
2. Studies on twins have shown that anxiety disorders are common in the alcoholic twin but not in the sober twin.
3. Rats exposed to chronic alcohol show alterations in GABA receptors.

4. Abstaining alcoholics showed a decreased benzodiazepine receptor distribution in the frontal cortex and cerebellum compared with controls (see figure).

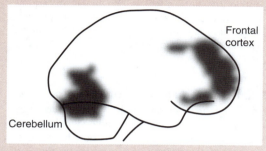

(Data from Abi-Dargham A, Krystal JH, Anjilvel S, et al. Alterations of benzodiazepine receptors in type II alcoholic subjects measured with SPECT and [123I]iomazenil. *Am J Psychiatry.* 1998;155[11]:1550–1555.)

NEUROTRANSMITTERS AND CELL BIOLOGY

γ-Aminobutyric Acid

GABA is the major inhibitory neurotransmitter in the brain. Activating GABA neurons calms down the brain. Too much GABA activation causes sluggishness and even coma. The GABA receptor has several sites that bind with other substances, which has the effect of enhancing the inhibitory activity of the GABA neurons. Figure 5.3 shows that ethanol, barbiturates, and benzodiazepines are known to bind with the GABA receptor. It is no wonder that people use and abuse these substances to calm down and reduce anxiety.

Abnormalities in the benzodiazepine GABA receptor have been implicated as a possible cause of anxiety disorders. Results of the original imaging studies and more recent genetic studies suggest that alterations in the structure or concentration of the benzodiazepine GABA receptor may predispose individuals to anxiety. However, the hypotheses have not been consistently or conclusively established.

Norepinephrine

The norepinephrine (NE) neurons with cell bodies in the locus coeruleus (shown in Figure 4.5) are believed to be part of the stress response system and play an important role in anxiety. The following evidence supports this belief.

1. NE neurons project to the amygdala.
2. Stressed rats show increases in NE release.
3. NE stimulates the release of corticotropin-releasing hormone, which in turn activates the HPA axis.
4. Peripheral NE (the sympathetic branch of the autonomic nervous system) produces somatic symptoms of anxiety: racing heart, sweating, dry mouth, and so on.

With this in mind, blocking NE with the β blocker propranolol has been proposed as a treatment to prevent the development of PTSD, that is, giving a β blocker in the acute aftermath of trauma (such as in the emergency department, on the battle field, etc.) to inhibit the NE stimulation and limit the development of haunting memories. Early small studies reported mild to moderate effects. Subsequent larger, controlled trials have been disappointing.

THE PARADOX OF ANTIDEPRESSANTS AND ANXIETY

If the NE system is part of the anxiety response, why does blocking NE reuptake, and consequently increasing NE at the synapse, relieve anxiety? How can more be less? For example, antidepressants such as the highly noradrenergic imipramine and the NE reuptake inhibitor reboxetine are known to reduce panic attacks. This does not make sense.

This paradox highlights that our understanding of anxiety and how the antidepressants calm the nervous system are in need of further study. Most likely, the antidepressants reduce anxiety by growth or increased strengthening of inhibitory networks.

Brain-Derived Neurotrophic Factor

This brings us back to a topic we first addressed in Chapter 5, Receptors and Signaling the Nucleus,—LTP. Figures 5.5–5.8 show how excessive stimulation alters the signals to the cell nucleus, which affects gene expression and ultimately changes the structure of the neurons. LTP is an analogy for trauma-induced anxiety (PTSD). With anxiety, we see heightened activity in the amygdala and reduced activity in the PFC and hippocampus. Clearly, something changes in the traumatized anxious brain. The missing ingredient may be growth factor proteins (such as brain-derived neurotrophic factor [BDNF]) that can alter the structure and function of the neural networks.

Animal studies have shown that BDNF is essential for the acquisition and extinction of anxiety.

1. BDNF transcription is increased in the amygdala after fear conditioning.

2. When BDNF is selectively deleted from the hippocampus in mice, they show impaired ability to extinguish conditioned fear.
3. BDNF in the lateral part of the dorsolateral prefrontal cortex (DLPFC) appears to control fear memory formation, whereas BDNF in the medial DLPFC is necessary for fear extinction.

In summary, this research implies that the development of anxiety and the failure to extinguish it, likely, occur through the production of growth factor proteins in specific regions of the brain. These conflicting roles for BDNF show how difficult it would be to develop an effective antianxiety treatment involving BDNF that would go to the whole brain. BDNF has different roles in various brain regions; any treatment would need to be only focally targeted or delivered.

EARLY ADVERSITY

Early adverse experiences have a significant impact on the later development of anxiety. Harry Harlow established with monkeys the profound negative impact of being raised without a mother or peer relationship. He replaced the mother of infant rhesus monkeys with an inanimate surrogate object during the first months of life. The infant monkeys displayed long-term deficits in social adaptation as well as increased anxiety-related behaviors.

We have discussed examples in which early experience changes neural structures. For example, the following have been observed:

1. Rats raised in standard wire cages have less dendritic branching than those raised in an enriched environment.
2. Licking and grooming by the rat mother affects the pup's response to stress (see Figure 17.5).

3. Children raised in Romanian orphanages have lower IQs (see Figure 19.7).

A recent study looked at the effect of breast-feeding on anxiety in humans. Children whose parents separated or divorced when the children were between the ages of 5 and 10 years were assessed for anxiety when they turned 10. The children who were breast-fed had less anxiety and more resilience in response to the difficult circumstances. Although we know very little about the effects of breast-feeding on the human brain, the results of this study seem strikingly similar to what Michael Meaney found with his high lick and groom mother rats. Extra attention at an early stage of life may be neuroprotective.

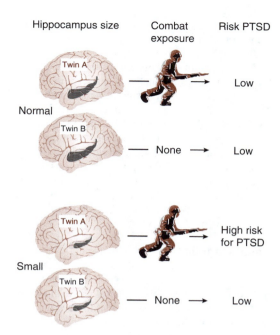

Hippocampus size Combat exposure Risk PTSD

FIGURE 22.10 The risk for developing posttraumatic stress disorder (PTSD) is highest among individuals with a small hippocampus and exposure to trauma.

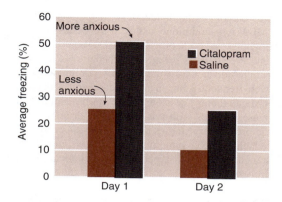

FIGURE 22.11 Rats treated with an antidepressant had a more difficult time extinguishing fear as measured by time spent "frozen" when hearing a tone previously associated with a foot shock. (Adapted with permission from Burghardt NS, et al. Chronic antidepressant treatment impairs the acquisition of fear extinction. *Bio Psychiatry*. 2013;73:1078–1086. Copyright 2013 with permission from Elsevier.)

AUGMENTING PSYCHOTHERAPY

Medications or psychotherapy diminish anxiety through different but equally effective mechanisms. Combining the two treatment modalities is generally believed to be more efficacious than either of them alone, although this has not been established. As a matter of fact, some research suggests that psychotherapeutic medications limit the learning that is essential for effective psychotherapy. How can this be true?

A recent study out of Columbia University looked at fear extinction after 22 days of citalopram or placebo in rodents. Fear extinction, which we discussed in Chapter 18, Memory, is the technique of reducing anxiety by repeated exposure to the feared stimulus. In the study, the feared stimulus was an auditory tone that had been followed by a shock. In the extinction phase, when all medications had been stopped, the rats only heard the tone—no shock (Whew!). The extinction testing measured how much time the rats stood "frozen" after hearing the tone and was conducted over 2 days. (Freezing is a defensive reaction in rats. Figure 14.3 shows a rat "frozen" in fear.) Figure 22.11 displays the

results. Note that the rats treated with the SSRI fared worse.

In a follow-up review, Burghardt, the lead author in the aforementioned study, examined numerous rodent studies that investigated SSRI treatment and fear learning. She concluded that SSRIs decrease fear *acquisition*, meaning the rats are less likely to develop new fears while on medication, which may explain the anxiolytic effect of SSRIs. However, the SSRIs also impair fear *extinction*, which may be "problematic therapeutically...when SSRI treatment is combined with exposure-based CBT." Therefore it is possible that SSRIs reduce anxious feelings but also impede therapy-initiated recovery. Burghardt believes that this occurs because SSRIs reduced plasticity in the amygdala and hippocampus, which may be necessary to develop new memories.

It is difficult to conduct studies like this with humans, but there are a few older studies that compared CBT with or without medication and then followed the patients after the medications were stopped. The medications used were imipramine, alprazolam, or sertraline in three different studies for anxiety disorders. After the medications were stopped, patients treated with medication and CBT fared *worse* than the subjects who received CBT alone. As with the rat studies, the human results suggest that some medications obstruct learning.

The psychedelics offer a potential shining light in these otherwise discouraging efforts to find a medication that can augment psychotherapy. The best studies have combined two or three sessions of 3,4-methylenedioxymethamphetamine (MDMA)—commonly known as ecstasy—with ongoing psychotherapy for PTSD. What is different here (besides using a psychedelic) is that the patients do not take the MDMA continuously or even frequently but just before several separated in-depth therapy sessions. The FDA has authorized phase III trials with this Schedule I drug because the preliminary studies have been so successful in reducing PTSD symptoms. Finally, we may have something that will expedite the psychotherapeutic process.

OBSESSIVE–COMPULSIVE DISORDER

OCD is classified as an anxiety disorder in the DSM nomenclature. However, some clinicians conceptualize OCD as an entirely different kind of disorder. They see OCD as one extreme of a spectrum of repetitive behavioral problems: body dysmorphic disorder, certain eating disorders, gambling, and even autism. These conditions are frequently called *OC spectrum disorders*. Others conceptualize OCD as a movement disorder, where

the obsessions are likely repetitive tics or movements. OCD not uncommonly co-occurs with tics or Tourette's syndrome.

Regardless of the nomenclature controversy, OCD is unique among the anxiety disorders because it is driven by different neural networks. The first indication occurred in the 1930s after the von Economo's encephalitis pandemic from 1917 to 1926. Patients who had recovered from the original infection often subsequently developed OCD or parkinsonism—which implicated the basal ganglia. Symptoms of OCD are also seen with other disorders that affect the basal ganglia: Tourette's syndrome, Parkinson's disease, Sydenham's chorea, and so on.

Basal Ganglia

The basal ganglia are subcortical structures that are usually associated with movement and motor control. Disruption of the basal ganglia leads to disorders such as Huntington's disease, Parkinson's disease, and hemiballismus. However, the exact function of the basal ganglia in OCD remains unclear.

The basal ganglia are made up of interconnected nuclei—the caudate, putamen, and globus pallidus (Figure 22.12). The caudate and putamen

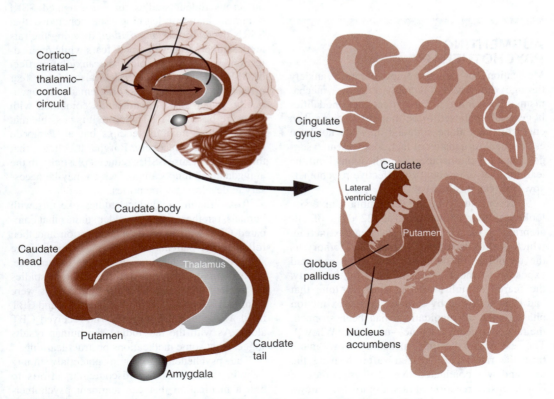

FIGURE 22.12 The structures of the basal ganglia and how they reside within the brain.

together are called the *striatum* and also contain the nucleus accumbens (NAc). Many areas of the cerebral cortex send signals to the basal ganglia, which are relayed to the thalamus, which in turn sends an impulse back to the cortex. This loop is called the cortico–striatal–thalamic–cortical circuit.

Functional imaging studies of obsessing OCD patients have repeatedly shown increased activity in the orbitofrontal cortex, anterior cingulate gyrus, and basal ganglia. It is presumed that these areas light up because of looping signals within the cortico–striatal–thalamic–cortical circuit. Treatment interventions, whether with psychotherapy or medications, show decreased activity in the basal ganglia for those who respond. However, the particular circuit may depend on the particular ritual: washing, checking, or hoarding seem to activate slightly different regions.

Psychosurgery

There is a long and troubling history of attempts to treat mental illness with neurosurgical interventions. Understandably, many are reluctant to even consider neurosurgery as a treatment option for psychiatric diseases. However, there is good evidence that some limited procedures with treatment-resistant patients can diminish OCD symptoms.

Different techniques are preferred in various regions of the world. In the United States, the popular technique is anterior cingulotomy, which is based on the concept of interrupting the circuit between the anterior cingulate gyrus and basal ganglia. Figure 22.13 shows the location of the lesions in postsurgical MRI scans.

Follow-up studies found that approximately 30% of the anterior cingulotomy patients have a 35% or greater reduction on the Yale–Brown Obsessive–Compulsive Scale. Complications include urinary incontinence and seizures but appear to be infrequent. A different technique used more regularly in Europe is anterior capsulotomy. Although this procedure appears to be more effective, it is also associated with more complications, for example, cognitive and affective dysfunction.

More recently, deep brain stimulation (DBS) has been studied as a way to treat severe and intractable OCD in a manner that is reversible and more flexible. The FDA has issued a humanitarian device exemption to allow psychiatrists to treat treatment-resistant OCD patients with DBS. The bilateral leads are implanted with the intention to interrupt this cortico–subcortical circuit (similar to Figure 21.11).

The results from a multicenter double-blind placebo-controlled trial with DBS for severe and treatment-resistant OCD have recently been announced and are not as encouraging as we had hoped. They had a heck-of-a-time finding enough patients—only 27—and that required extending the study for several years beyond initial projections. In the end, the active treatment was not superior to placebo treatment (electrodes implanted but not active) in reducing obsessive–compulsive symptoms. However, the active treatment group did report superior functional improvement (e.g., more likely to venture outside the home), which may be a more important result. Ultimately, this suggests that there is more to treating OCD than simply interrupting an aberrant cortico–striatal circuit.

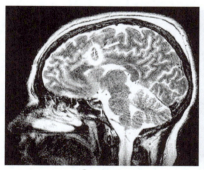

Sagittal

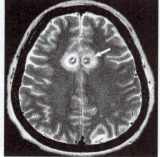
Axial

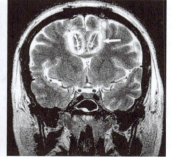
Coronal

FIGURE 22.13 Three views of anterior cingulotomy for treatment-resistant obsessive–compulsive disorder (OCD). The *white arrows* show the location of the lesions. The *white rings* around the lesions are secondary edema from the procedure. (Redrawn from Richter EO, Davis KD, Hamani C, et al. Cingulotomy for psychiatric disease: microelectrode guidance, a callosal reference system for documenting lesion location, and clinical results. *Neurosurgery.* 2004;54[3]:622–628; discussion 8–30, by permission of Oxford University Press.)

There are promising new data with transcranial magnetic stimulation (TMS) for OCD. The focal point of the stimulation is the supplementary motor area (SMA)—and area of the cortex just in front of the motor cortex—that contributes to control of movement in ways that are still not understood. A multisite trial found that inhibiting the SMA followed by exposure therapy reduced OCD symptoms more than did sham TMS and exposure therapy. These data are now in front of the FDA for potential approval of this approach.

BENZODIAZEPINES AND ALZHEIMER'S DISEASE

An observational study by French and Canadian researchers has reported a dose–effect relationship between benzodiazepine use and risk of Alzheimer's disease. Longer use and medications with longer half-life had a stronger association. A pathophysiologic mechanism is not readily evident, although benzodiazepines are associated with memory impairment. However, correlation is not causation. Early symptoms of Alzheimer's disease could have caused anxiety which led to increased benzodiazepine use.

QUESTIONS

1. Which hormone initially drops because of the stress of parachute jumping?
   a. Glucocorticoids.
   b. Gonadotropins.
   c. Growth hormone.
   d. Mineralocorticoids.

2. All of the following are true about the Klüver–Bucy syndrome except
   a. Made aggressive monkeys tame.
   b. Induced hypersexuality.
   c. Identified the hippocampus as important for anxiety.
   d. Was elicited through removal of most of the temporal lobe.

3. Evidence that the amygdala is important to experiencing fear?
   a. Ischemic damage increases fear response.
   b. Electrical stimulation reduces freezing and heart rate.
   c. Emotional trauma has no effect on the amygdala.
   d. Treatment reduces activity in the amygdala.

4. The recognition of a threatening object includes all of the following except
   a. The brain reacts once all the signals are analyzed.
   b. Signals from the amygdala stimulate heart rate.
   c. Auditory and visual information proceed to the thalamus.
   d. Memories modulate the amygdaloid response.

5. Stimulation of the mPFC has what effect on a rat's fear response?
   a. Inhibits the expression of anxiety.
   b. Impairs extinction.
   c. Increases the activity in the amygdala.
   d. Decreases activity in the anterior cingulate gyrus.

6. The best estimate of the volume of a combat veteran hippocampus is
   a. The total duration of trauma he experienced.
   b. The intensity of combat trauma he experienced.
   c. The level of glucocorticoids in the morning at rest.
   d. The size of his twin's hippocampus.

7. Medications decrease anxiety in all the following ways except
   a. Increase the GABA inhibitory signal.
   b. Increase BDNF production at the NAc.
   c. Modulation of the NE neurons.
   d. Quieting the amygdala.

8. Imaging studies show increased activity in all the following regions in OCD patients except
   a. Orbitofrontal cortex.
   b. Anterior cingulate gyrus.
   c. Amygdala.
   d. Basal ganglia.

See Answers section at the end of this book.

CHAPTER 23

Schizophrenia

HISTORIC PERSPECTIVE

Over 100 years ago, Emil Kraepelin, a German psychiatrist, described the syndrome now called *schizophrenia*. Bleuler actually coined the term *schizophrenia*. Kraepelin called it *dementia praecox*. Kraepelin's major contribution to psychiatry was recognizing that schizophrenia and manic depression are likely different disorders. The mental function of the patient with schizophrenia has a persistent deteriorating course, whereas the patient with manic depression will experience periods of remission. Figure 23.1 shows a modern interpretation of the clinical course of schizophrenia.

Kraepelin was convinced that schizophrenia was an organic disease of the brain and spent considerable time and energy conducting postmortem studies on the brains of patients with schizophrenia. They had a good track record of finding the pathology, as one of his colleagues was the neuropathologist Alois Alzheimer. Unfortunately, Kraepelin was never able to discover a specific abnormality in the brains of schizophrenic patients. This pattern was to continue for a long time.

Numerous postmortem studies were conducted over the next 70 years comparing the brains of schizophrenic patients with healthy controls. Still no distinguishing pathology was isolated. The absence of gliosis in the tissue was of particular interest. Gliosis, sometimes called the *glial scar*, is considered the hallmark of neurodegenerative disorders and is found with such conditions as Huntington's and Alzheimer's diseases, as well as with trauma and ischemia.

The absence of any significant neuropathology along with the burgeoning interest in psychoanalytic theory led to psychosocial explanations for schizophrenia. Terms such as the *refrigerator mother* or the *double-bind* were developed to explain the psychological turmoil that presumably caused schizophrenia.

Some clinicians even speculated that patients voluntarily chose to be psychotic to avoid conflict in their lives. Seriously, *smart* people actually said that.

Although the development of chlorpromazine (Thorazine) in the early 1950s dramatically changed the treatment of schizophrenia, the identification of biologic abnormalities remained elusive. In 1972, Plum summarized the frustration when he called schizophrenia the *graveyard of neuropathologists*. Schizophrenia was actually dropped from the preeminent neuropathology textbook (Greenfield's Neuropathology) for the next two editions and only added back in 1997. It was the emergence of significant findings on brain imaging studies that finally ended the debate about whether there are quantifiable (measurable) changes in the brain (more on this in the next section).

Although we follow convention and use the term "schizophrenia," many researchers are struck by the variations between patients. For example, some patients have no hallucinations and mostly struggle with negative symptoms, whereas other patients have chronic hallucinations and few negative symptoms. To remind readers of this heterogeneity, some use the term "the schizophrenias." In this book we will use the standard term, schizophrenia.

MODERN EPIDEMIC?

E. Fuller Torrey calls schizophrenia an invisible plague. He believes that schizophrenia is a modern illness that has increased so gradually that the change is not perceptible during any single person's lifetime. Additionally, the changes in diagnostic criteria that occur over the decades make comparisons between generations difficult. In spite of these difficulties, there is evidence to support Dr Torrey's belief.

The ancient Greeks and Romans were astute observers of human behavior. Reviews of the

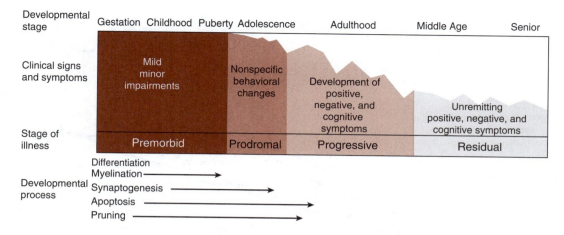

FIGURE 23.1 The typical clinical course of schizophrenia includes a relatively normal childhood interrupted in late adolescence or early adulthood by a dramatic deterioration from which few remit. (Adapted with permission from Lewis DA, Lieberman JA. Catching up on schizophrenia: natural history and neurobiology. *Neuron.* 2000;28[2]:325–334. Copyright 2000 with permission from Elsevier.)

writings from ancient times provide the following descriptions of conditions that we easily recognize:

1. Epilepsy
2. Migraine headache
3. Melancholia
4. Anxiety
5. Chronic alcoholism
6. Delirium

The ancient writers described psychotic symptoms including hallucinations and delusions. However, in almost every case the psychosis cleared. There are no reports that describe an initial psychotic break in late adolescence or early adulthood with a chronic unremitting course. The absence of a condition that looks like schizophrenia stands in contrast to the good clinical descriptions of other neuropsychiatric syndromes. This softly suggests that the illness was not present in ancient Greece or Rome.

The 19th and 20th centuries saw an explosion in the institutionalization of patients with chronic mental illness. Many of these patients had schizophrenia. Figure 23.2 shows the growth in institutionalized patients as a percentage of the total population in four countries. There are many reasons for confining the seriously mentally ill: industrial revolution, changes

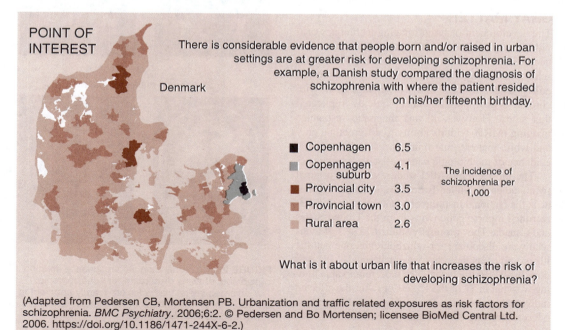

POINT OF INTEREST

There is considerable evidence that people born and/or raised in urban settings are at greater risk for developing schizophrenia. For example, a Danish study compared the diagnosis of schizophrenia with where the patient resided on his/her fifteenth birthday.

Denmark

■ Copenhagen	6.5	
■ Copenhagen suburb	4.1	The incidence of schizophrenia per 1,000
■ Provincial city	3.5	
■ Provincial town	3.0	
■ Rural area	2.6	

What is it about urban life that increases the risk of developing schizophrenia?

(Adapted from Pedersen CB, Mortensen PB. Urbanization and traffic related exposures as risk factors for schizophrenia. *BMC Psychiatry.* 2006;6:2. © Pedersen and Bo Mortensen; licensee BioMed Central Ltd. 2006. https://doi.org/10.1186/1471-244X-6-2.)

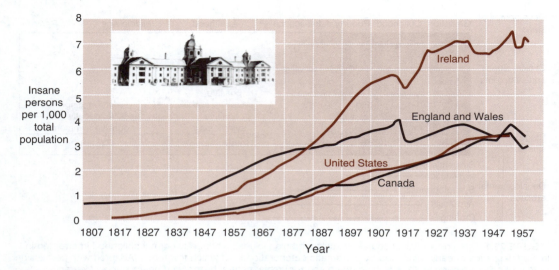

FIGURE 23.2 The epidemic of mental illness in the last two centuries. (Adapted from Liberman RP, Musgrave JG, Langlois J. Taunton State Hospital, Massachusetts. *Am J Psychiatry.* 2003;160[12]:2098. Reprinted with permission from the *American Journal of Psychiatry* [Copyright © 2003]. American Psychiatric Association. All Rights Reserved.)

in social norms, lack of effective treatments, and so on. An additional explanation is the emergence of a psychiatric epidemic.

Although we may never know for sure whether schizophrenia is a modern epidemic or has been around for ages, the topic raises the issue of etiology. What causes schizophrenia? We will start with what is known about the brains of patients with schizophrenia.

GRAY MATTER

The development of brain imaging techniques provided a way to examine schizophrenic brains in live people. The first computed tomography scans in schizophrenia were published in 1976 and showed enlarged lateral ventricles in a group of patients with chronic schizophrenia. Others quickly replicated this study. However, it was magnetic resonance imaging (MRI), with its ability to differentiate gray and white matters, that finally provided irrefutable evidence of the biologic nature of schizophrenia.

The most famous MRI studies were the original twin studies. E. Fuller Torrey, Daniel Weinberger et al. at the National Institute of Mental Health (NIMH) recruited monozygotic twins from the United States and Canada. They originally studied 15 sets of twins who were discordant for schizophrenia: one had the illness, whereas the other was unaffected. MRI was done in all 30 participants. The most remarkable finding was that in 12 of the 15 sets of twins the affected individual was easily identified by visual inspection of corresponding coronal scans (Figure 23.3).

35-year-old female identical twins

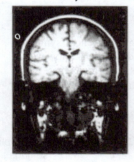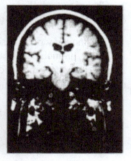

28-year-old male identical twins

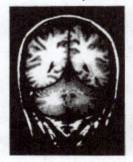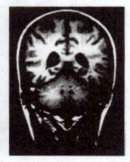

FIGURE 23.3 Coronal magnetic resonance imaging of two sets of twins discordant for schizophrenia. The enlarged lateral ventricles are readily apparent in the subjects on the right. (Courtesy of Drs E. Fuller Torrey and Daniel Weinberger.)

A

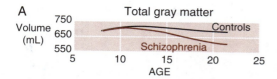

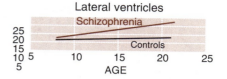

B

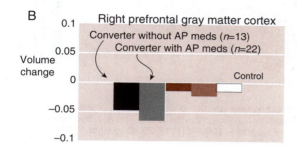

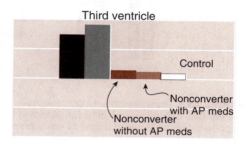

FIGURE 23.4 A: Children with schizophrenia have greater loss of brain gray matter as well as enlargement of the ventricles during adolescence. **B:** Youth at high risk for psychosis show similar brain changes unaffected by antipsychotic (AP) medication. (**A:** Adapted from Sporn AL, et al. Progressive brain volume loss during adolescence in childhood-onset schizophrenia. *Am J Psychiatry.* 2003;160:2181–2189. Reprinted with permission from the *American Journal of Psychiatry* [Copyright © 2003]. American Psychiatric Association. All Rights Reserved. **B:** Adapted with permission from Cannon TD, Chung Y, He G, et al. Progressive reduction in cortical thickness as psychosis develops: a multisite longitudinal neuroimaging study of youth at elevated clinical risk. *Biol Psychiatry.* 2015;77:147–157. Copyright 2015 with permission from Elsevier.)

The results of the twin study have been replicated and extended. The most common finding remains enlarged ventricles, but better technology has allowed more detailed analysis. Patients with schizophrenia show consistent but subtle decreases in total brain volume and total gray matter volume. These results provide an explanation for the increased ventricle size; that is, the ventricles expand to fill the void left by the loss of gray matter.

Judith Rapoport's laboratory performed sequential MRI scans on children with childhood-onset schizophrenia and compared the findings with age-matched controls in an effort to follow up the changes in the brain that occur during adolescence. They found that the rate of change was greater for those children with schizophrenia. Figure 23.4A shows that the children with schizophrenia had striking loss of gray matter and expanded ventricles.

A more recent study followed children at high risk for developing schizophrenia (e.g., they had a parent with schizophrenia.) Everyone received an MRI scan, which was repeated again at 12 months. They followed 274 cases along with 135 healthy controls—everyone was in their late teenage years or early 20s. During the study, 35 individuals developed psychosis—which they called converting. This study is unique because they also separated individuals who were taking antipsychotic medication from those who did not. The results are shown in Figure 23.4B. As with

other studies, the people who developed psychosis showed more gray matter loss in the frontal lobes and increased ventricle size. The good news is that antipsychotic medications do not appear to worsen the brain tissue loss, although the study is small.

Adolescence is a time of remodeling the connections in the brain to create a more efficient organ. Processes such as pruning, apoptosis, and synaptogenesis are accepted features of the maturing brain (see Figures 8.8, 19.4, and 20.8). Studies such as the one described here suggest that schizophrenia may be the result of overly aggressive remodeling of the gray matter.

The process of gray matter reduction occurs in the same time frame as the usual onset of schizophrenic symptoms. Besides this correlation, some genetic studies suggest that aberrant expression of genes that control synaptic plasticity contributes to the development of schizophrenia.

Reduced Neuropil Hypothesis

As stated before, traditional microscopic examination of the gray matter of schizophrenics will not identify anything unusual. Therefore it has been difficult to explain the gray matter loss. Investigators at Yale used labor-intensive three-dimensional analytic tools to estimate cellular densities. They compared neuronal density in three regions of the brain from patients with schizophrenia and from healthy controls. The regions were Brodmann's areas 9 and

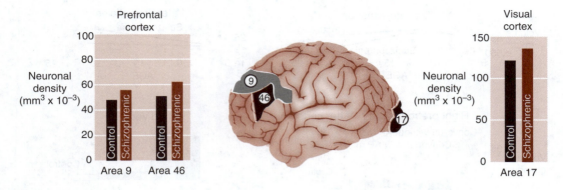

FIGURE 23.5 Patients with schizophrenia have increased neuronal density in all three areas of the brain tested. Glial density was no different. (Adapted from Selemon LD, Goldman-Rakic PS. The reduced neuropil hypothesis: a circuit based model of schizophrenia. *Biol Psychiatry*. 1999;45[1]:17–25. Copyright 1999 with permission from Elsevier.)

46 in the prefrontal cortex (PFC) and area 17 in the visual cortex. They found increased density of neurons but not glial cells in the gray matter of schizophrenic patients (Figure 23.5).

It appears that schizophrenic patients have the same number of neurons as do healthy controls, but they are packed together in less space, called the *reduced neuropil hypothesis*. The tighter packaging of the schizophrenic neurons results from reduced cell size, less branching, and decreased spine formation. Figure 23.6A shows a drawing of this process. Figure 23.6B and C shows examples of actual spine formation from schizophrenic patients and controls, as well as average spine densities. The key point is that it is not neuronal loss, but rather the loss of the richness of the dendritic connections that causes the reduced gray matter in schizophrenia. Presumably, this is one of the causes of the faulty information processing in patients with schizophrenia.

What causes the shrinking (increase density) of the gray matter? We discussed one theory in Chapter 9, Immunity and Inflammation,—a finding *so exciting*; we felt compelled to present it early in this book. The new finding suggests that pruning is a natural process modulated through the immune system by mechanisms such as the C4 protein, which means immune system markers are used to identify which synapses are to be removed. Unfortunately, this is done to excess in schizophrenics. A study, even more recent than that one, suggests it is the smallest spines that are lost while larger spines are retained.

One further point worth mentioning is that these studies highlight the extensive whole-brain involvement of schizophrenia. That is, it is not a focal disorder of just one region of the brain. Rather, schizophrenia seems to affect almost the entire cortex, as well as other parts of the brain as we shall see. Furthermore, we do not know if this thinning of the brain is an on-going process continually occurring over the life span or a one-time hit from which individuals rarely recover.

Functional Brain Imaging

Traditionally, the hallmark of schizophrenia has been the hallucinations and delusions. In actuality, the symptoms of schizophrenia are made up of many symptoms organized into the following three categories.

1. Positive symptoms: hallucinations and delusions
2. Negative symptoms: lack of motivation, apathy, and so on
3. Cognitive impairment

The cognitive dysfunction, which includes problems with attention, memory, and executive function, may be the most detrimental aspect of the illness and has a greater negative impact on the individual than the positive symptoms. Likewise, cognitive functioning is the best predictor of long-term outcome from the disorder. We discussed in Chapter 19, Intelligence, that some insightful clinicians believe schizophrenia might be better categorized as a cognitive disorder rather than as a psychotic disorder because cognitive impairments are a more clinically significant feature of the illness. We would do well to remember Kraepelin's term—*Dementia* praecox.

The pattern of cognitive impairment in schizophrenia implicates the frontal cortex. *Hypofrontality* is a term sometimes used to describe this problem. However, functional imaging studies of the resting brain have given inconsistent results. Weinberger et al. recognized that the best measure of frontal

A
Healthy control gray matter

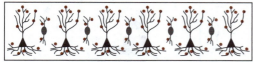

Schizophrenic gray matter

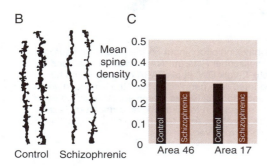

B   C

Control   Schizophrenic

Mean spine density

0.5
0.4
0.3
0.2
0.1
0

Area 46   Area 17

Control   Schizophrenic   Control   Schizophrenic

FIGURE 23.6 A: Schematic representation of the increased density but decreased size of schizophrenic gray matter. **B:** Drawings of actual dendrites and spines from pyramidal neurons in the dorsolateral prefrontal cortex of controls and schizophrenic patients. **C:** Mean spine density in frontal cortex and visual cortex from controls and schizophrenic patients. (**A:** Data from Selemon LD. Increased cortical neuronal density in schizophrenia. *Am J Psychiatry*. 2004;161[9]:1564. **B and C:** Data from Glantz LA, Lewis DA. Decreased dendritic spine density on prefrontal cortical pyramidal neurons in schizophrenia. *Arch Gen Psychiatry*. 2000;57[1]:65–73.)

lobe function requires engaging the individual in a cognitive challenge while performing the scan.

To test this theory, patients and healthy controls underwent xenon, XE 133, inhalation procedure for regional cerebral blood flow measurements (a positron emission tomography scan) while they were performing the Wisconsin Card Sort test (Figure 23.7). The control subjects showed increased activation of their frontal lobes while performing the test, but the schizophrenic patients did not. Furthermore, there was a good correlation between the change in blood flow in the frontal cortex and percent errors on the test. It is presumed that atrophic, disconnected neuronal cells cause the PFC dysfunction and consequently the cognitive impairment.

Inhibitory Neurons

The activity of the large pyramidal neurons in the gray matter is modulated by smaller local interneurons (see Figure 2.3). Most of the interneurons are

A

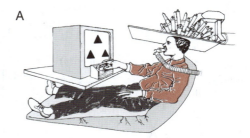

B   Normal   Schizophrenic   More activity / Less activity

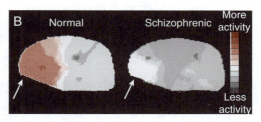

C

% Change in PFC activity

20
15
10
5
0
−5
−10
−15

0   10   20   30   40   50   60   70
% Error

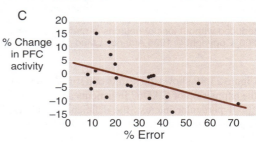

FIGURE 23.7 A: Subjects were scanned while performing the Wisconsin Card Sort task. **B:** Healthy subjects displayed increased blood flow to the prefrontal cortex (PFC), whereas those with schizophrenia did not. **C:** Percent errors on the task correlated with change in PFC blood flow. (Adapted with permission from Weinberger DR, Berman KF, Zec RF. Physiologic dysfunction of dorsolateral prefrontal cortex in schizophrenia. I. Regional cerebral blood flow evidence. *Arch Gen Psychiatry*. 1986;43[2]:114–124. Copyright © 1986 American Medical Association. All rights reserved.)

γ-aminobutyric acid (GABA) neurons and hence inhibitory. There are several types of GABA neurons. Figure 23.8A shows two of them: the parvalbumin in brown and the calretinin in black. The location of their inhibitory input seems to have different effects on the pyramidal neuron.

The GABA interneurons are important in the discussion of schizophrenia because there is evidence that the parvalbumin neurons are impaired in patients with the disorder. GABA is synthesized from a number of enzymes, one of which is called *glutamic acid decarboxylase* (GAD). One form of messenger RNA (mRNA) that encodes for GAD (GAD67) has been shown repeatedly to be decreased in patients with schizophrenia. It is one of the most consistent findings in postmortem studies.

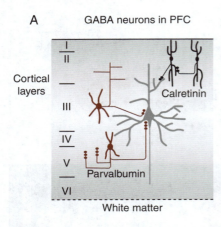

A   GABA neurons in PFC

Cortical layers

Calretinin

Parvalbumin

White matter

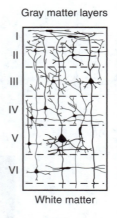

Gray matter layers

White matter

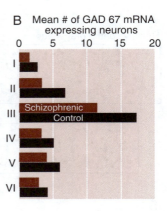

B   Mean # of GAD 67 mRNA expressing neurons

Schizophrenic
Control

FIGURE 23.8 A: γ-Aminobutyric acid (GABA) interneurons have inhibitory input on the pyramidal neurons in the prefrontal cortex (PFC). **B:** Mean number of GAD67 messenger RNA (mRNA) expression neurons by gray matter layer. (**A:** Adapted from Tamminga C, Hashimoto T, Volk DW, et al. GABA neurons in the human prefrontal cortex. *Am J Psychiatry.* 2004;161[10]:1764. Reprinted with permission from the *American Journal of Psychiatry* [Copyright © 2004]. American Psychiatric Association. All Rights Reserved. **B:** Adapted with permission from Akbarian S, Kim JJ, Potkin SG, et al. Gene expression for glutamic acid decarboxylase is reduced without loss of neurons in prefrontal cortex of schizophrenics. *Arch Gen Psychiatry.* 1995;52[4]:258–266. Copyright © 1995 American Medical Association. All rights reserved.)

Figure 23.8B shows the results of a study comparing the expression of GAD67 in patients and controls.

Of particular interest, the deficiency in GAD67 expressing interneurons seems to be limited only to the parvalbumin neurons and is not found in other GABA neurons. Furthermore, the number of parvalbumin neurons is not reduced in patients with schizophrenia. Therefore the GABA neurons that are implicated in schizophrenia are not deficient in total number but have decreased expression of important genes that might impair the function of the cortex.

More recent research conducted with frontal lobe specimens from the University of Pittsburgh brain bank looked at the excitatory synaptic density on the inhibitory neurons. They found an 18% reduction in excitatory input on the parvalbumin neurons for patients with schizophrenia compared with healthy controls. No difference was found for the calretinin neurons. The authors speculate the reduced excitatory input on the parvalbumin neurons reduces their activity, which in turn reduces the inhibition of the pyramidal neurons.

Working memory depends on the coordinated firing of pyramidal neurons in the PFC. The inhibitory interneurons are essential for synchronizing the output from the pyramidal neurons, where the real decisions are made. Tasks such as the delayed response task (see Figure 20.3) require inhibitory control to bridge the time between stimulus presentation and behavioral response. The cognitive impairment in patients with schizophrenia may be due to a failure to properly coordinate the pyramidal neurons.

WHITE MATTER

The white matter tracts that interconnect different regions of the cortex, as well as connecting the cortex with the deeper brain structures, may also play an important role in the disruption of communication in the brain. White matter is composed of the myelinated axons that transport the signals generated by the neurons. Figure 23.9 shows a drawing of some of the long and short white matter tracts. Disruption of the integrity of the white matter tracts leads to degradation of the neuronal signal.

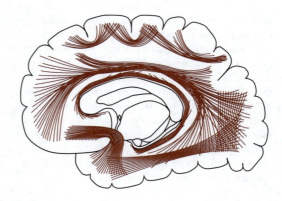

FIGURE 23.9 A drawing of the white matter tracts connecting various regions in the brain. (Adapted from Gray H. *Anatomy of the Human Body*; 1918.)

Imaging

MRI studies on patients and controls have found a small but nonsignificant trend toward reduced white matter in schizophrenia. Other studies using the more recently developed DTI technology (see Figure 3.13) have found abnormalities in patients with schizophrenia compared with healthy controls. Some insight into the significance of these findings can be gleaned from comparing the result of DTI studies in other demyelinating diseases. For example, multiple sclerosis and human immunodeficiency virus (both known to induce cognitive impairment and hallucinations with some patients) also produce changes in the DTI analysis. These results suggest that all three diseases may share some similar white matter degradation—with subsequent disruption in neural signaling.

A recent study from the University of Toronto performed DTI imaging studies on patients with schizophrenia and healthy controls. They graded the schizophrenic patients on a negative symptom scale and found those patients with more negative symptoms (impaired emotional expression and social function) also had more white matter tract disruption. This suggests what we all believe but so far have not been able to prove that different clinical presentations of schizophrenia involve different neural deficits.

Myelin

Oligodendrocytes

Oligodendrocytes are one of the glial cells that support the neurons. Specifically, the oligodendrocytes grow layers of myelin that insulate the axons and enhance the speed of transmission of neural impulses (see Figure 3.10). Diseases that affect the integrity of the myelin sheath impair the function of the brain and can cause psychotic symptoms in some cases. One particular disease—metachromatic leukodystrophy—usually begins with demyelination of the frontal lobes.

The rare late-onset form of metachromatic leukodystrophy occurs in about the same time frame as schizophrenia—from adolescence to young adulthood. Reviews of such cases have noted that over half the individuals had psychotic symptoms including auditory hallucinations and bizarre delusions.

Others have looked at the oligodendrocyte population in patients with schizophrenia. Hof et al. counted the number of oligodendrocytes in the white matter of Brodmann's area 9. They found that there was a 27% decrease in the number of oligodendrocytes in the patients with schizophrenia compared with the controls (see Figure 23.10).

The application of microarray analysis (see Figure 1.10) has further implicated the involvement

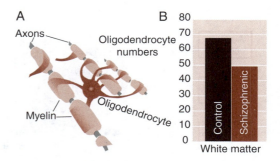

FIGURE 23.10 A: One oligodendrocyte can provide the myelin covering over many axons. **B:** Patients with schizophrenia have fewer oligodendrocytes in their white matter. (**B:** Graph adapted with permission from Hof PR, Haroutunian V, Friedrich Jr VL, et al. Loss and altered spatial distribution of oligodendrocytes in the superior frontal gyrus in schizophrenia. *Biol Psychiatry*. 2003;53[12]:1075–1085. Copyright 2003 with permission from Elsevier.)

of myelin in schizophrenia. Hakak et al. applied postmortem tissue from patients with schizophrenia and controls to microarray chips to identify gene expression. In other words, they wanted to see which genes were active in which subjects.

More than 6,000 genes were compared between the schizophrenia and control subjects. Only 17 genes were significantly downregulated in the schizophrenia patients. Of these, six were myelin related. The other 11 showed no particular pattern. The authors concluded that deficient oligodendrocytes and myelination are likely involved in schizophrenia.

AUDITORY HALLUCINATIONS

In 1863, Broca described lesions of the left frontal cortex in patients with language expression deficits (see Figure 1.6). Roughly 10 years later, Wernicke described a different language deficit associated with lesions of the superior temporal lobe. The region Wernicke described was a part of what is now called the *auditory cortex*. The perception of sound starts in the ear, then proceeds through the brain stem and thalamus before reaching the auditory cortex on the superior aspect of the temporal lobe (see Figure 23.11). White matter tracts called the *arcuate fasciculus* connect the auditory cortex with the frontal cortex.

Wernicke and later Kraepelin both postulated that auditory hallucinations were due to temporal lobe abnormalities. Indeed, an auditory aura preceding a seizure suggests the temporal lobe as the nidus of the electric activity. Likewise, hallucinations can result from strokes that involve the temporal lobes.

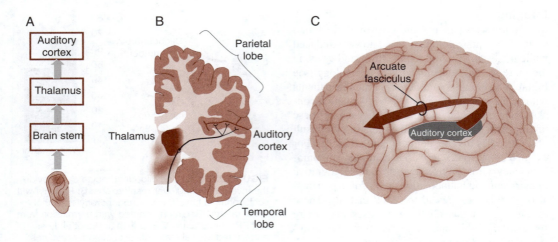

FIGURE 23.11 A: Pathways from the ear to the cortex. **B:** Auditory signals synapse in the thalamus before reaching the auditory cortex. **C:** The arcuate fasciculus is composed of white matter tracts that connect the auditory cortex with the frontal cortex.

Therefore neurologic causes of auditory hallucinations point to the temporal lobe. Until recently, it was just speculation about the neuronal correlates of auditory hallucinations with schizophrenia.

A group in Switzerland has done extensive imaging studies of schizophrenic patients when they were hallucinating. In the past, the time it took to scan a person was so long that it obscured the difference between the hallucinating state and the nonhallucinating state. Now with rapid fMRI scans the differences can be detected. Patients were asked to press a button with the onset of hallucinations and keep it pressed for as long as they lasted. Images during hallucinations were compared with images when the voices were silent. Figure 23.12A shows the activity in the gray matter of the auditory cortex during hallucinations for one patient.

significantly more alterations of the white matter tracts of the arcuate fasciculus (Figure 23.12B).

Taken together, these studies suggest that auditory hallucinations are derived from abnormalities in the regions that register external sounds. The patient with auditory hallucinations may misidentify inner speech as coming from an external source due to lack of integrity of the system. It is reminiscent of a phone or television picking up other signals and playing more than one sound track at a time.

These studies highlight the complexity of schizophrenia (or the schizophrenias). For just one symptom, abnormalities have been identified in both the gray matter and white matter for patients with schizophrenia. Clearly, schizophrenia is a confusing disorder with diverse and numerous effects on multiple areas of the brain.

POINT OF INTEREST

Numerous researchers have documented a correlation between auditory hallucinations and the size of the temporal lobe; that is, a smaller temporal lobe predicts more hallucinations. This seems counterintuitive. Why does less brain tissue produce positive symptoms?

This same research group used DTI imaging to look at white matter tracts in schizophrenic patients with hallucinations compared with patients without hallucinations and healthy controls. Remarkably, they found that patients with hallucinations have

ETIOLOGY

We have tried to establish that schizophrenia appears to be a disorder of impaired communication. It is not as though the wires are completely severed—more like the signals are noisy and full of inaccuracies. There is no specific brain region affected, rather a dysfunction of circuits and cells within and between regions. Additionally, the onset of the full disorder suggests a neurodevelopmental disruption. It is plausible to envision that schizophrenia results from the abnormal expression of genes that govern maturational processes. However, what goes wrong and how does this happen?

A
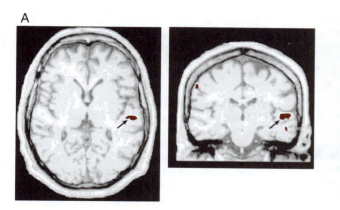

B
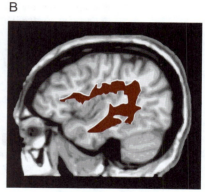

FIGURE 23.12 **A:** Functional magnetic resonance imaging showing the gray matter regions activated when they are experiencing auditory hallucinations. **B:** Diffusion tensor imaging showing the areas of altered white matter tracts for patients who hear auditory hallucinations compared with healthy controls. (**A:** Data from Dierks T, Linden DE, Jandl M, et al. Activation of Heschl's gyrus during auditory hallucinations. *Neuron.* 1999;22[3]:615–621. Copyright 1999 with permission from Elsevier. **B:** Data from Hubl D, Koenig T, Strik W, et al. Pathways that make voices: white matter changes in auditory hallucinations. *Arch Gen Psychiatry.* 2004;61[7]:658–668.)

Genetics

One of the most consistent findings in schizophrenia research is the heritable nature of the illness and related illnesses. Figure 1.1 shows the striking power of the genes with this disorder. The closer one is related to someone with schizophrenia, the more likely that person is to get the illness. However, even the monozygotic twin of a person with schizophrenia only has approximately a 50% chance of getting the illness. Furthermore, patients with schizophrenia are less likely to procreate. If this is a genetic disorder with Mendelian properties, we would expect it to decline in frequency over many generations. Clearly, there is more involved than just genes in the traditional sense.

Environment

Prenatal Complications

Adverse environmental events are known to be potential triggers for developing schizophrenia. We mentioned at the beginning of this chapter the increased risk for those born in urban settings versus rural areas. Maternal infection is another well-known risk factor for schizophrenia. Obstetric complications are also associated with schizophrenia. A large prospective study that followed up children from birth through adulthood found that the odds of schizophrenia increased linearly with increasing number of hypoxia-associated obstetric complications.

Famine

Two large epidemiologic surveys of in utero exposure to maternal starvation have shown an increased risk of schizophrenia among the offspring. The first was the Nazi blockade of western Netherlands from October 1944 to May 1945 (called the *Dutch Hunger Winter*) in which daily food rations fell to less than 500 calories per person per day. The second instance was the famine caused by the so-called *Great Leap Forward* in China from 1960 to 1961. In both situations children in utero during the famine doubled their chances of developing schizophrenia in early adulthood. The results from China are shown in Figure 23.13. Some speculate that the lack of folate in the diet had a detrimental effect on the developing fetal brain. Folate is needed for DNA synthesis and repair. Its absence can lead to chromosomal instability. (Is this why the Irish, with their persistent famines, experienced a greater epidemic of mental illness? see Figure 23.2.)

Finnish Adoption Study

We have a highly heritable disorder that is affected by environmental factors. There are many other environmental factors than we have mentioned

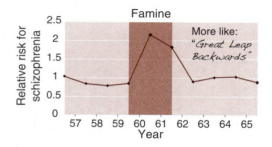

FIGURE 23.13 The relative rate of developing schizophrenia doubled for those born during the famine during 1960 to 1961 in one region of China.

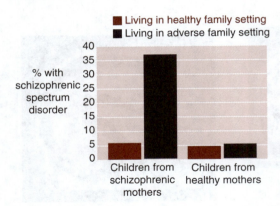

FIGURE 23.14 Children born to schizophrenic mothers and raised in more dysfunctional family environments were at increased risk of developing schizophrenic spectrum disorders.

here, but the big question is: how do environment and genetics conspire to induce schizophrenia? The Finnish Adoption Study provides some interesting data to help us understand this interaction. Researchers collected the names of all women who were hospitalized in Finland from 1960 to 1979 and diagnosed with schizophrenia. Then they identified the children from these women who were adopted away. They collected a similar number of adopted children as matched controls.

Detailed and blinded assessments were made of the adoptive families by experienced psychiatrists. Using specific scales, they divided families into those that were healthy and those that were dysfunctional. Additionally, each child was assessed for a schizophrenia spectrum disorder based on *Diagnostic and Statistical Manual of Mental Disorders, Third Edition, Revised* (DSM-III-R) criteria, for example, schizophrenia, delusional disorder, depressive disorder with psychotic features, schizotypal personality disorder, and so on.

The remarkable results of this study are shown in Figure 23.14. Only the children born to mothers with schizophrenia *and* raised in an adverse family

household showed an increased risk of developing schizophrenic spectrum disorders. This is a good example of a genetic–environment interaction. Children at genetic risk for schizophrenia appear to be more sensitive to problems in the environment.

Where Are the Genes?

In Chapter 9, Immunity and Inflammation, we showed the Manhattan plot (sometimes called the "skyline" graph) of the largest genomic search for genetic causes of schizophrenia. The Psychiatric Genomic Consortium combined all accessible genetic data (37,000 cases and 113,000 controls) and, with some massive number crunching, found 108 inherited variations in the genetic code associated with schizophrenia. Figure 23.15 shows the recent study (also available in Figure 9.6A—where you can actually read the numbers) compared with the 2011 analysis that found only five significant sites—quite a jump in just a few years. The difference was the result of the larger sample size. The experts tell us, unfortunately, this still only accounts for 3.5% of the risk for schizophrenia. Therefore the vast majority of heritability remains hidden. (Where's the other 96.5%?)

The genetic variations that have been identified converge around pathways involved in communication, cellular ion channels, memory and learning, and—the largest signal—the immune system. In spite of these discoveries, the mechanism or mechanisms that cause schizophrenia remain a mystery. Much to everyone's amazement, virtually all the genetic loci are in the noncoding regions of the DNA—what used to be called "junk DNA." This means that genetic errors do not result in changes to the amino acid sequence nor affect the structure of proteins. Therefore, unlike sickle cell anemia, where one change in an amino acid results in a slightly altered protein, which in turn does not fold properly, with schizophrenia, errors produce unknown results. Furthermore, each variation in Figure 23.15 increases the chances of getting schizophrenia by about 10%, or at most 20%—a very small effect. Consequently, schizophrenia is not

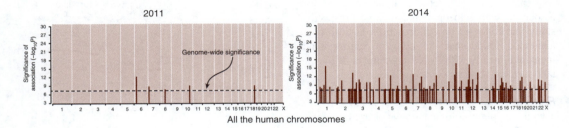

FIGURE 23.15 Comparison of genome-wide association studies in 2011 and 2014. (Adapted from NIMH press release. Schizophrenia's genetic "skyline" rising. July 22, 2014.)

one big genetic change that causes the disease, nor even several smaller errors that add up to the illness. It is much more confusing than that. How do we make sense of this?

Gene Expression

In several chapters of this book we have discussed the enduring effects that life events can have on the DNA. Environmental events change the genes— a cardinal feature of the neuroscience model (see Figure 6.12). Enhancing or silencing specific genes through epigenetic changes can alter behavior. This enables animals to adapt their behavior to their particular environment. However, some events seem to silence important genes and have devastating effects on behavior. Schizophrenia may be such a condition.

Researchers are starting to look at changes in gene expression in patients with schizophrenia as a way to better understand the disorder. To proceed with such an examination, an important protein must be first identified and then the DNA that encodes for that protein must be analyzed. One protein that has been identified is reelin, a protein expressed by GABA interneurons. Reelin is recognized as crucial for neuronal migration, axonal branching, and synaptogenesis throughout brain development. Additionally, reelin and its mRNA are reduced in postmortem brains of schizophrenic patients.

We have previously discussed that adding methyl groups to DNA limits gene expression—the methyl groups prevent the transcription factors from "zipping" off some mRNA. Tsuang et al. at the University of California in San Diego looked at the methylation of the reelin DNA from gray matter from postmortem brains of patients with schizophrenia. Not surprisingly, they found a distinct methylated signal in 73% of the schizophrenic samples but only in 24% of the control samples. To put it in another way, the reelin DNA of the schizophrenic patients was three times more likely to be methylated.

Not only does this give a possible mechanism to explain the failure of gene expression in patients with schizophrenia but also fits with known environmental events that increase the risk of developing the disorder. For example, transient ischemia is known to increase DNA methylation. Likewise, folate is necessary for normal DNA methylation. This may explain why fetal hypoxia and maternal famine predispose some individuals to develop schizophrenia. Furthermore, epigenetic mechanisms, which do not show up on genome-wide studies, may be one mechanism that explains the missing heritability.

The take-home message is this: There are likely to be multiple genetic vulnerabilities to schizophrenia, which are rarely expressed but not uncommon. Insults from the environment, such as diet,

infection, ischemia, etc., have detrimental and lasting effects on the DNA, which likely affects how genes are expressed. Those individuals having both genetic vulnerability and environmental insult are the ones who develop schizophrenia.

OLDER FATHERS

Older fathers are more likely to have increased de novo germline mutations, and schizophrenia is associated with increased paternal age. An analysis of genome-wide DNA sequencing from 78 Icelandic families (219 individuals) found that it is the age of the father that determines the number of de novo mutations in the child. As the father's age at conception of the child increases, the number of single nucleotide polymorphisms increases. A 20-year-old father passes along on average 25 mutations, whereas a 40-year-old father passes on about 65.

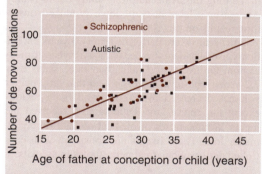

(Adapted by permission from Macmillan Publishers Ltd. Kong A, et al. Rate of de novo mutations and the importance of father's age to disease risk. *Nature*. 2012;488:471–475. Copyright 2012.)

Dopamine Hypothesis

It does not seem proper to write an entire chapter on schizophrenia without mentioning dopamine (DA). The DA hypothesis is an old and enduring theory purporting that overactivity of the DA system is part of the pathogenesis of schizophrenia. It was first proposed in 1966 on the basis of pharmacologic studies. DA blocking agents provided the first effective treatment for the positive symptoms of schizophrenia. Furthermore, amphetamines, which increase DA at the synaptic cleft, can induce psychosis.

Although popularity of the DA blocking agents is at an all time high, the belief that DA over activity causes schizophrenia has dwindled. Modulation of DA activity may be effective in diminishing psychotic symptoms, but there is minimal evidence to implicate the DA neurons in the pathogenesis of the disorder. Howes and Kapur put it nicely in their review of the DA hypothesis when they proposed that DA dysregulation is the final common pathway of psychosis, which is manipulated by "upstream factors." Most likely it is the disconnections among the glutamate and GABA neurons that are the etiopathogenesis of schizophrenia.

ANTIPSYCHOTICS AND THE SHRINKING BRAIN

One of the foremost concerns in the treatment of psychosis is the long-term effect of antipsychotic medications. Medications change gene expression, which can, in some instances, propagate irreversible adverse outcomes, e.g., tardive dyskinesia. Although medications can be beneficial in the short run, we do not know the effects on the brain in the long run. A decade-long study out of Nancy Andreasen's laboratory in Iowa produced unsettling results on this issue.

MRI scans were performed every 3 years on 211 first-episode patients treated with antipsychotic medication. On average, patients had three scans over 7.2 years. The investigators found that gray matter volumes decreased over time in all brain regions except the cerebellum. Patients who received the higher lifetime doses of medication had more gray matter loss. These results are consistent with controlled antipsychotic treatment studies in animals.

Two more recent studies continue this disturbing trend. The first study followed cortical thickness in patients who were medicated compared with those unmedicated after their first episode of schizophrenia. The group on antipsychotic medication had greater cortical thinning of the PFC and temporal regions compared with the unmedicated group. However, the medicated group showed more activation of the dorsolateral PFC and better performance when tested in an fMRI, compared with the unmedicated group.

The second important study was an extended follow-up of a randomized trial of early medication reduction/discontinuation. In the original study, patients presenting with first-episode psychosis were randomly assigned to medication reduction/discontinuation or maintenance treatment, after 6 months of remission. Eighteen months after randomization, the reduction/discontinuation group was twice as likely to relapse. However, when followed up 5 years after the end of the first study (total of 7 years), the reduction/discontinuation group was doing better than the maintenance group. They were twice as likely to have recovered (40% vs 18%) and achieve functional remission (46% vs 20%). And, there was no significant difference in symptom remission (69% vs 67%).

We are caught in a bind. The mediations that can have such a profound beneficial effect with schizophrenia, additionally, may actually slightly damage the brain over time. The potential neurotoxicity of antipsychotic medications reminds us to avoid unnecessary treatment and to use the lowest dose possible whenever we can.

QUESTIONS

1. Neurodevelopmental causes that could explain schizophrenia include excessive amounts of all of the following except
   a. Pruning.
   b. Synaptogenesis.
   c. Apoptosis.
   d. Myelination

2. Evidence that schizophrenic is a biologic disorder includes all of the following except
   a. The difference in lateral ventricles in the twin study.
   b. Gliosis in the PFC.
   c. Gray matter reduction in childhood onset schizophrenia.
   d. Hypofrontality.

3. All of the following support the reduced neuropil hypothesis except
   a. Oligodendrocyte dysfunction.
   b. Reduced neural cell size.
   c. Limited spine formation on the dendrites.
   d. Increased density of gray matter.

4. Evidence that GABA interneurons are impaired in schizophrenia.
   a. Increased methylation of calretinin DNA.
   b. Reduced parvalbumin neurons.
   c. Reduced GAD67.
   d. Increased reelin.

5. All of the following suggest white matter impairment in schizophrenia except
   a. Microarray analysis.
   b. Diffusion tensor imaging.
   c. Oligodendrocyte cell counts.
   d. Significantly reduced white matter volume.

6. Auditory hallucinations have been shown to activate which region on fMRI?
   a. Superior temporal lobe.
   b. Broca's area.
   c. Wernicke's area.
   d. Arcuate fasciculus.

7. All are plausible theories on the etiology of schizophrenia, except
   a. Methylation of DNA.
   b. Spontaneous mutations.
   c. DA hypothesis.
   d. Genetic–environment interactions.

8. Match up the following:
   1. Bleuler   A. Psychoanalytic theory
   2. E. Fuller Torrey B. Distinguished schizo-
   3. Kraepelin   phrenia from bipolar
   4. Plum   disorder
   5. Refrigerator   C. Hypofrontality
      mother   D. Invisible epidemic
   6. Wisconsin Card   E. Coined the term
      Sort   schizophrenia
                        F. Graveyard of
                           neuropathologists

See Answers section at the end of this book.

CHAPTER 24

Alzheimer's Disease

HISTORIC PERSPECTIVE

Human Longevity

Although historic records indicate that older people have always existed in human societies, old age was once rare. Before the 20th century, few people lived beyond 50 years. Now, 95% of the children born in developed countries live past that age (Figure 24.1). Changes in health care, sanitation, and nutrition (to name a few) have had a profound impact on life expectancy. The ultimate result is that more and more people are living to ripe old ages. With more people living into their geriatric years, the aging-related central nervous system (CNS) disorders are becoming common.

All nerve cells are affected by aging. Sensory and motor skills decline with age. Neurodegenerative disorders such as Parkinson's disease, amyotrophic lateral sclerosis, and Huntington's disease become more prevalent as people get older. Cellular and molecular changes that accumulate over time render neurons

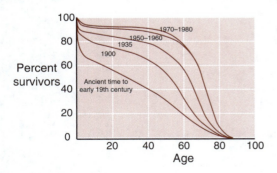

FIGURE 24.1 The percentage of people living beyond the age of 60 has increased dramatically in the past two centuries. (Adapted with permission from Springer, from Thorbecke G, ed. *Biology of Aging and Development*. New York: Springer; 1975.)

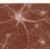

POINT OF INTEREST

The maximum human life span is approximately 125 years and has not changed in over 100,000 years. Cell culture studies suggest that each species has a biologic clock that influences its life span. For example, fibroblasts will only divide a limited number of times before dying. The number of divisions is related to that species' life span (see table).

Life Span and Cell Division of Different Species

Species	Maximum Life Span (y)	Maximum Fibroblast Doubling
Galapagos tortoise	175	125
Man	125	60
Mouse	4	28

The important point is that life span and age-related illnesses such as dementia are likely to be controlled by different mechanisms.

vulnerable to damage. Most likely, the damage results from a combination of genetic vulnerability and environmental hits, but we say that about everything.

Dementia, the progressive deterioration of cognitive skills, is perhaps the most worrisome development for all of us. There are numerous causes of dementia, including cerebral vascular accidents, alcoholism, and infections. Alzheimer's disease (AD) is the most common cause of dementia. The surge in dementia cases as the baby boomers age is expected to overwhelm the health care system unless some intervention is discovered.

Alois Alzheimer

The disease we now call Alzheimer's was first discussed when Alois Alzheimer presented a case in 1906 of a woman with the early onset of dementia. Her symptoms started in middle age with a change in personality and mild memory impairment. She was institutionalized when she became paranoid and unmanageable. Alzheimer repeatedly examined the woman as he followed her deteriorating clinical course. Four and a half years after her initial symptoms, she was bedridden in a fetal position until she died.

The autopsy revealed gross atrophy of the cortex without localized foci. With the application of the new staining methods (see Figure 1.8), Alzheimer found sclerotic plaques scattered throughout the cortex, especially in the upper layers. Additionally, he noted that many of the cortical neurons were reduced to dense bundles of neurofibrils. Alzheimer thought that his description of plaques and neurofibrillary tangles in a patient with "presenile dementia" was a new and unique condition.

In fact, Alzheimer's finding was cognitive loss associated with the following:

1. Cortical atrophy
2. Plaques outside the neurons
3. Tangles inside the neurons

These findings have become the description of the dementia that bears his name. Figure 24.2 shows a schematic representation of what Alzheimer might have seen when he looked through his microscope.

ALZHEIMER'S DISEASE

Surprisingly, what Alzheimer saw roughly a 100 years ago remains the focus of current research. However, the application of modern technology has greatly advanced the understanding of the pathophysiology of atrophy, plaques, and tangles.

Cortical Atrophy

The most striking feature of the Alzheimer's brain is the dramatic shrinkage of the cortical tissue secondary to neuronal cell death. AD is a bit like losing hair. It starts years before it is actually noticed and progresses slowly. In some people it starts sooner and proceeds faster. Furthermore, almost everyone experiences some hair loss with aging.

Brain volume loss is also a "normal" feature of aging. Brain volume peaks in adolescence and then declines as much as 0.2% to 0.5% per year. Patients with AD experience accelerated neural loss. Likewise, some people are genetically predisposed to early-onset AD.

Examination of the AD brain at autopsy shows extensive atrophy. Figure 24.3 compares two views of normal brains with AD brains. The enlargement of the ventricles and sulci in combination with the decreased tissue are easily recognized—and a bit unsettling for those of us in middle age.

Brain imaging, although not yet diagnostic for early AD, can document the volume loss and contrast the changes for those with and without AD.

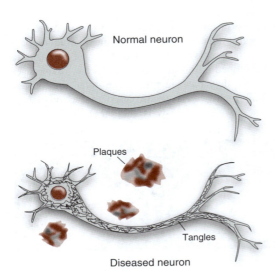

FIGURE 24.2 Alzheimer's disease includes the constellation of neuronal shrinkage, plaques, and neurofibrillary tangles.

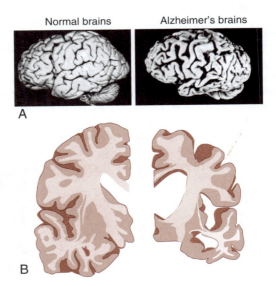

FIGURE 24.3 Gross examination (**A**) and coronal slices (**B**) show the extensive shrinkage of the brain from Alzheimer's disease. (**A:** Courtesy of George Grossberg and the St. Louis University Alzheimer's Brain Bank.)

Figure 24.4 shows the results of sequential magnetic resonance imaging (MRI) on one patient destined to develop familial AD. Note how his brain atrophy proceeds faster than a healthy elderly control. It is also of interest that the symptoms of AD did not appear until significant brain tissue was lost.

The decrease in energy metabolism secondary to the extensive neuronal damage can be seen in functional imaging studies such as positron emission tomography (PET). Figure 24.5 shows the marked reduction in glucose metabolism in a patient with AD compared with a healthy control. The difference is so prominent that some have suggested that PET could be used to differentiate patients with AD from those aging normally. A large European study including more than 500 subjects found 93% sensitivity and specificity for separating mild to moderate AD from normal controls. Unfortunately, they were not as effective at separating AD from other forms of dementia, and PET is even less helpful in diagnosing patients with mild cognitive impairment and determining whether they will go on to develop AD.

Amyloid Plaques

The extracellular deposits that Alzheimer saw are called *amyloid plaques*, which is a bit of a misnomer. They are actually aggregates of fibrous protein and not amyloid at all. It was not until 1984 that the primary component of the plaques was found to be a small protein called *amyloid-β* or *A-β*. (To add to the confusion, the most common term used in the literature is beta-amyloid or β-amyloid.) Specifically, it is a long 42-amino acid chain called A-β-42 that seems to be the real culprit, although there may be others that are more noxious.

A-β is cleaved from a larger molecule called *amyloid-β precursor protein* (APP). APP is a large protein protruding through the cell wall (Figure 24.6). It is found in cells throughout the body but is prominent in neurons. The functions of APP are not fully understood but may include regulating neuronal survival, neural neurite outgrowth, and synaptic plasticity.

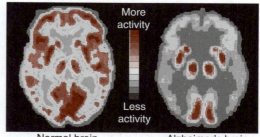

FIGURE 24.5 Positron emission tomography images showing glucose metabolism in a normal brain compared with an Alzheimer's disease (AD) brain. Note the reduced activity in the frontal and temporal regions of the AD brain. (Adapted by permission from Macmillan Publishers Ltd. Mattson MP. Pathways toward and away from Alzheimer's disease. *Nature.* 2004;430[7000]:631–640. Copyright 2004. https://doi.org/10.1038/nature02621.)

APP is cleaved into smaller portions by at least two enzymes called β- and γ-*secretases*. The final cleavage results in the generation of A-β-42 (and others) that coalesces into long filaments. It is the clumping of the filaments that form the "amyloid" plaques. Pharmacologic inhibition of the activity of the secretase enzymes has been of interest to those seeking ways to slow down the development of plaques, although a recent large Phase 3 trial by Merck was halted because there was "virtually" no chance of a beneficial outcome.

Amyloid Hypothesis

Many believe that amyloid plaques are the source of the problem with AD. Two lines of reasoning suggest this is true. First, some people carry a genetic predisposition for early-onset AD usually developed before the age of 65 years. In all cases where they have identified the gene, the genetic abnormality causes an increased production of A-β. The toxicity of A-β is the other evidence that

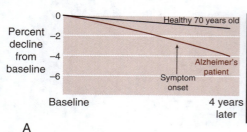

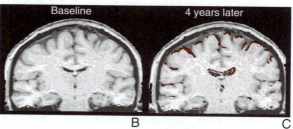

FIGURE 24.4 A: Sequential magnetic resonance imaging (MRI) scans show the aggressive brain atrophy in a patient with Alzheimer's disease (AD) compared with healthy geriatric controls. **B:** MRI in a patient with AD at baseline and **(C)** 4 years later. Brown overlay represents tissue loss compared with baseline. (Adapted from Fox NC, Schott JM. Imaging cerebral atrophy: normal ageing to Alzheimer's disease. *Lancet.* 2004;363[9406]:392–394. Copyright 2004 with permission from Elsevier.)

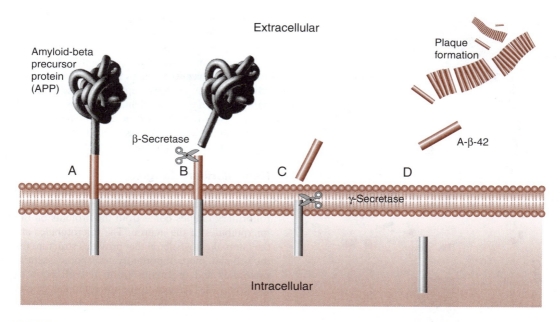

FIGURE 24.6 Amyloid plaques are formed from the cleavage of amyloid precursor protein into smaller proteins that clump together.

supports the amyloid hypothesis. A-β is toxic to neurons grown in petri dishes. Furthermore, A-β can impair the development of long-term potentiation as well as memory for a maze in rodents.

Investigators in England have reported the results of a long-term study with marmoset monkeys. The monkeys received cerebral injections of A-β or other brain tissue that did not contain β-amyloid. When the monkeys died, their brains were analyzed for amyloid plaques (Figure 24.7). Monkeys that were injected with A-β were much more likely to have cerebral amyloidosis at autopsy. These results not only confirm the toxic effects of A-β but also imply that the presence of A-β seeds the progression.

The exact mechanisms of the toxicity of A-β remain murky. Some research studies suggest that it is the soluble form of the protein that causes the damage, called A-β oligomers. Other research studies suggest that it is not the A-β-42 protein, but different A-β proteins as yet unidentified. Furthermore, it is not clear why the plaques coalesce in the first place. Some evidence hints that the genetic forms of AD result from an overproduction of APP, whereas the more common sporadic cases result from the failure to clear the excess A-β. Clearly, efforts to treat the disorder would benefit from better understanding of these concerns.

Imaging Amyloid

The first step in any treatment approach is an accurate diagnosis of the condition. Historically, the gold standard for the diagnosis of AD has been at autopsy—a bit late to start treatment. As noted earlier, imaging studies are poor at differentiating AD from other forms of dementia. More recently, researchers have been looking at ways to detect the presence of amyloid deposits in subjects even before symptoms appear. In 2012, the FDA approved florbetapir F18 (Amyvid) for PET imaging of the brain in cognitively impaired adults. Florbetapir binds to amyloid in the brain and gives an estimate of the density of the plaques. Figure 24.8 shows the results of a scan comparing a healthy control with a patient with AD. With this scan, unlike

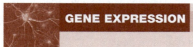

GENE EXPRESSION

In the previous chapters we have discussed how the addition of methyl groups to the DNA can silence gene expression, which, in turn, can produce psychiatric symptoms. The opposite may be happening with Alzheimer's disease, that is, the awakening of improper gene expression through *demethylation*. There is some indirect evidence that demethylation of the DNA sequence coding for β-secretase results in increased production of that enzyme. This could result in greater production of A-β and a faster progression of the disease.

A

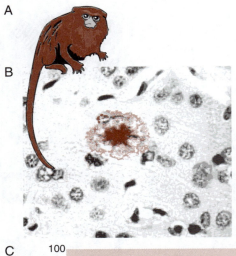

B

C

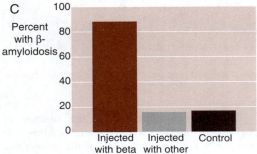

Percent with β-amyloidosis

100
80
60
40
20
0

Injected with beta amyloid | Injected with other brain tissue | Control

FIGURE 24.7 Marmoset monkeys **(A)** can develop cerebral amyloid plaques **(B)**. Monkeys injected with A-β were much more likely to develop amyloidosis in the next 3 to 4 years. (Adapted by Ridley RM, Baker HF, Windle CP, et al. Very long-term studies of the seeding of beta-amyloidosis in primates. *J Neural Transm.* 2006;113:1243–1251. With permission of Springer.)

Alzheimer's disease   Healthy control

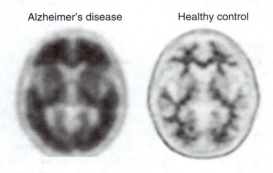

FIGURE 24.8 A positive scan on the left shows high uptake of florbetapir F18 in the cortical gray matter indicating the presence of amyloid plaques. A negative scan (on the right) is paradoxically a healthier brain. (Images courtesy of Avid Radiopharmaceuticals, a wholly owned subsidiary of Eli Lilly and Company.)

the PET scan in Figure 24.5, the subject with the disease lights up when the florbetapir attaches to the amyloid deposits.

The current utility of a florbetapir PET scan is to identify reversible causes of cognitive decline, other than AD, such as depression. The ultimate utility of such a scan—identifying early stages of the disease so that treatment can be started prior to substantial neural cell loss—awaits the development of effective treatments.

Neurofibrillary Tangles

The other major pathologic finding with AD is the intracellular neurofibrillary tangles. The neurofibrillary tangles come from the proteins on the microtubules of the neuron. The microtubules are the internal cytoskeleton that provides structure for the cell and, more importantly, transports essential molecules and organelles from the cell body to the synapses. Damage to the microtubules causes the peripheral aspects of the neuron to effectively starve.

The tau proteins bind to the microtubules and provide stability. The problem seems to start with the hyperphosphorylation of the tau proteins (Figure 24.9). Too many phosphates attached to the tau proteins cause them to detach from the microtubules. It is these detached proteins that clump together and form the neurofibrillary tangles, which in turn clog the neuron's axons and dendrites and cause the cell to die. What causes the hyperphosphorylation remains unclear but seems to be initiated by β-amyloid—possibly soluble A-β that diffuses across the cell wall.

 CEREBRAL SPINAL FLUID

Tau protein is increased in the cerebral spinal fluid (CSF) of patients with AD. The diagnostic accuracy of the disease may be enhanced from measurements of specific proteins in the CSF, as well as better imaging studies—in patients with signs of cognitive decline.

Alzheimer's Disease Progression

AD is a relentlessly progressive disorder. There are no remissions. The first signs are marked by subtle decline in memory. As the disease advances, changes in personality and language skills develop. Eventually even motor functions are impaired. Understanding the spread of the pathology of AD gives a greater appreciation of the changing clinical picture.

The progression of the disease can be staged by the development and progression of neurofibrillary tangles. In a landmark analysis of more than 2,500 brains in Germany over 10 years, Braak documented the insidious evolution of AD as shown in Figure 24.10. The initial stages start in the entorhinal cortex of the hippocampus. From there the disease spreads into the temporal and frontal cortices. The final stages involve the entire brain, with the greatest deposits remaining in the regions where it all started.

TREATMENT

If nothing is done to prevent or treat AD, the number of cases is expected to quadruple in the next 40 years. Current treatments can temporarily improve cognition in those afflicted but do nothing to alter the underlying pathophysiology or delay the unrelenting progression. Perhaps even more discouraging is that we do not even know which pathology of AD is most detrimental: amyloid plaques, neurofibrillary tangles, or some upstream event that precedes the development of plaques and tangles.

Most research studies have focused on amyloid, but anti-tau medications are under investigation as well. Regardless of the focus, recent studies have been disappointing. Despite encouraging results in animal studies or small studies with humans, no medication has been found to prevent or reverse AD. Two large Phase 3 trials, the kind of studies the US pharmaceutical industry is famous for, reported negative results in the same issue of The New England Journal of Medicine in 2014. Both agents, solanezumab (Lilly) and bapineuzumab (Janssen), are anti-amyloid-β monoclonal antibodies but showed no significant improvement compared with placebo. This is not good. Those of us on the other

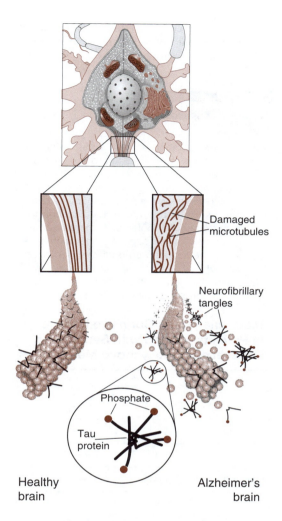

FIGURE 24.9 Hyperphosphorylation of the tau proteins produces neurofibrillary tangles that damage the microtubules. The result is impaired axonal transport and ultimately cell death.

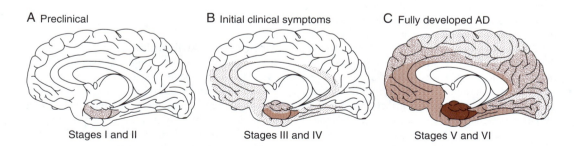

FIGURE 24.10 The spread of neurofibrillary tangles in Alzheimer's disease (AD). (Adapted from Braak H, Braak E. Frequency of stages of Alzheimer-related lesions in different age categories. *Neurobiol Aging*. 1997;18[4]:351–357. Copyright 1997 with permission from Elsevier.)

side of our life curve hope the scientific community does something quick to reverse this discouraging trend. Here are a few of the favorable prospects.

Vaccine

Immunizations against childhood diseases have transformed the risks of growing up. The possibility of using vaccines to treat and/or prevent AD is an exciting application of this old intervention, which could likewise revolutionize growing old. The trick is to get the immune system to attack the amyloid plaques without irritating other parts of the brain or inciting an inflammatory response in the CNS.

The vaccine was initially tested in mice genetically engineered to overexpress APP (APP mice). Such mice will develop amyloid plaques and memory loss by the age of 12 months. They have become the accepted animal model of AD. Immunotherapy with APP mice has produced extraordinary results (Figure 24.11). Clearing of amyloid plaques and preservation of cognitive functions have been repeatedly documented in animal studies.

In 2001, clinical trials of a synthetic version of the β-amyloid protein for use as a vaccine were started in humans. Preliminary safety studies were completed without a hitch. Unfortunately, the larger Phase 2 study had to be stopped after several months when 6% of the participants developed an excessive inflammatory response (meningoencephalitis). Further analysis has suggested that T-cell activation may have been the problem.

Follow-up studies on the 372 subjects who were immunized have found some encouraging results. Those individuals who did mount an antibody response to A-β showed subtle signs of improved memory and cognitive skills. Furthermore, postmortem studies of a few patients have documented clearing of the amyloid plaques in some regions of their brains.

In 2012, a group in Sweden published what appears to be the next step in the vaccine story. This vaccine, called CAD106, is designed to mount an antibody response against a small portion of the A-β molecule without activating the T cells (humeral response but not cellular). A small double-blind Phase 1 study of 58 patients with mild to moderate AD was conducted to establish safety and tolerability. Although almost every patient developed minor side effects (such as sore throat, headache, fatigue, etc.), none developed meningoencephalitis. (Whew!) In 2017, the results of a larger Phase 2b study (121 patients) were published with similar results. CAD106 elicited a specific immune response to A-β with an acceptable safety profile but no advantage in clinical efficacy. The authors want to keep moving forward and

advocated for larger Phase 3 studies. Therefore this exciting treatment option continues to progress, although without robust benefits.

ANTIPSYCHOTICS

Alzheimer's original patient was ultimately admitted to his ward because of her uncontrollable psychotic symptoms. Currently most clinicians would quickly place such a patient on a new generation antipsychotic medication. Yet, the use of antipsychotic medications for AD is not without problems. A meta-analysis looked at the effect of second-generation antipsychotic medications on cognitive decline in patients with AD. They found that the medications actually worsened the cognitive decline when compared with placebo (see table).

Meta-analysis of Cognitive Decline in Patients Treated with Second Generation Antipsychotic Medications

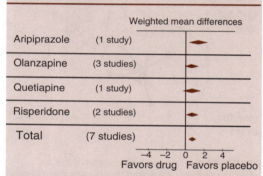

		Weighted mean differences
Aripiprazole	(1 study)	
Olanzapine	(3 studies)	
Quetiapine	(1 study)	
Risperidone	(2 studies)	
Total	(7 studies)	
		−4 −2 0 2 4
		Favors drug Favors placebo

(Adapted from Schneider LS, et al. Efficacy and adverse effects of atypical antipsychotics for dementia: meta-analysis of randomized, placebo-controlled trials. *Am J Ger Psych.* 2006;14[3]:191–210. Copyright 2006 with permission from Elsevier.)

Monoclonal Antibodies

An alternative to activating a person's immune system with a vaccine is to give them antibodies already formed poised to attack the offending agent (passive immunity). Called monoclonal antibodies, we already mentioned two such agents that were colossal failures—maybe that's a little harsh. Another monoclonal antibody, aducanumab, has shown remarkable encouraging results—although in small studies. One hundred and sixty five patients with prodromal or mild AD, as well as positive on an A-β PET scan, were randomized

Hippocampus from APP genetically engineered mice

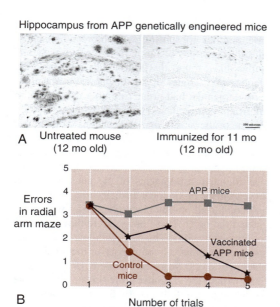

A   Untreated mouse   Immunized for 11 mo
     (12 mo old)   (12 mo old)

B   Number of trials

FIGURE 24.11 A: Slices of amyloid precursor protein (APP) mice hippocampi show the accumulation of amyloid plaques without and with the A-β vaccination. **B:** Vaccinated mice display memory similar to control mice and superior to the APP mice. (**A:** From Lemere CA, Maier M, Jiang L, et al. Amyloid-beta immunotherapy for the prevention and treatment of Alzheimer disease: lessons from mice, monkeys, and humans. *Rejuvenation Res.* 2006;9[1]:77–84, courtesy of Cynthia A. Lemere. Published by Mary Ann Liebert, Inc., New Rochelle, NY. **B:** Adapted by permission from Macmillan Publishers Ltd. Morgan D, Diamond DM, Gottschall PE, et al. A beta peptide vaccination prevents memory loss in an animal model of Alzheimer's disease. *Nature.* 2000;408[6815]:982–985. Copyright 2000.)

to monthly infusions of placebo or four increasing doses of aducanumab.

The results are astounding. PET scans at baseline and 1 year later show remarkable clearing of amyloid (Figure 24.12A). At the end of the study the amyloid was reduced in a dose-dependent manner (Figure 24.12B). But most pleasing, the medication slowed the cognitive decline in a similar dose-dependent fashion (Figure 24.12C). Now this is what we've been looking for!

It is not clear why this monoclonal antibody is so effective at clearing the plaque. Smarter people than us speculate that aducanumab selectively binds to the harmful soluble A-β oligomers that are harder to measure and more difficult to remove. Or it is possible that this antibody is more effective at recruiting the microglia that does the grunt work to clear the plaques.

The treatment is not without problems. Some patients developed what is called amyloid-related imaging abnormalities (ARIAs), which are seen on MRI as cerebral edema or small hemorrhages. Patients can experience headaches, change in mental status, and/or gait disturbances form ARIA, but no one in the study went to the hospital. Subjects on higher doses of aducanumab were more likely to develop ARIA (Figure 24.12D), so a medium dose may clear the amyloid without undue risk. Phase 3 trials are under way.

Nerve Growth Factor

The neuronal loss from AD might be prevented or at least limited with appropriate stimulation from growth factor proteins. Animal studies suggest

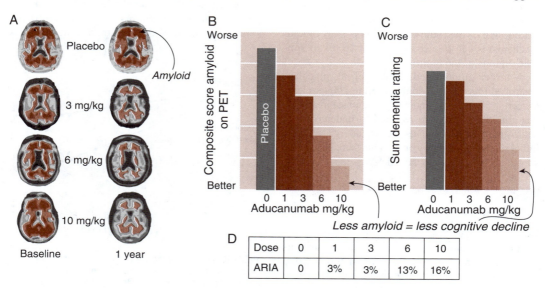

Less amyloid = less cognitive decline

Dose	0	1	3	6	10
ARIA	0	3%	3%	13%	16%

FIGURE 24.12 Sorry for making such a nosey, crowded illustration, but there is SO much good information in this study. Best to see text for details. (Adapted by permission from Macmillan Publishers Ltd. Sevigny J, et al. The antibody aducanumab reduces Aβ plaques in Alzheimer's disease. *Nature.* 2016;537:50–56. Copyright 2016.)

growth factor proteins may be useful for treating neurodegenerative diseases such as AD. Specifically, nerve growth factor (NGF, see Figure 8.9) has been shown to prevent cholinergic degeneration and improve memory in animals. The problem arises in choosing a method to deliver the NGF to the brain. The molecule is too large to cross the blood–brain barrier. Likewise, direct infusion into the ventricles results in excessive stimulation and intolerable side effects, for example, pain and glial cell infiltration.

An alternative method of delivery entails hijacking the DNA in autologous fibroblasts using retroviral vectors. Such fibroblasts can be induced to express NGF. In turn, they can be placed directly into the brain of the subject and deliver NGF within a few millimeters of the nucleus basalis of Meynert, where the cholinergic neuronal degeneration occurs. Because the fibroblasts are autologous, they do not activate an immune response.

Researchers at the University of California in San Diego completed a Phase 1 trial with eight patients with probable AD. Fibroblasts producing NGF were injected into the subjects' cholinergic basal forebrain. Two patients had significant complications from the surgery, but with five of the remaining six, cognition stabilized or improved during the 6 to 18 months after injection. PET scans showed increased activity.

In a recent follow-up, the brains of 10 patients who underwent this NGF gene therapy were examined after death. They all "exhibited a trophic response to NGF in the form of axonal sprouting toward the NGF source." Although this treatment will not halt the development of amyloid plaques or neurofibrillary tangles, it does show that NGFs may play a role in reducing the symptoms of AD. Additionally, the study highlights that unique mechanisms can be used to deliver NGFs to specific regions of the brain.

A larger randomized, double-blind, placebo-controlled Phase 2 trial commenced in 2009 seeking to recruit 50 patients. Patients in the placebo arm of this ambitious study are required to undergo sham neurosurgery. As much as we would not wish to inflict sham neurosurgery on anyone, there is no other way to accurately assess the efficacy of the treatment.

PREVENTION

Brain Reserve

Postmortem studies have found that a substantial proportion of people have the histopathology of AD but not the cognitive failings of dementia. Prospective studies suggest the number may be as high as 40%. Some believe that this is due to *brain reserve*; that is, greater neural substrate

buffers against the clinical expression of the disease (similar to starting with more adipose tissues during times of famine). Indeed, prospective studies have found that individuals who have the plaques and tangles at death, but were not clinically demented, had greater number of neurons in the frontal, parietal, and temporal cortices.

One of the most remarkable studies on this topic was the Nun Study, in which they determined the correlation between early verbal skills and later cognitive impairment. The researchers completed extensive cognitive assessments of the nuns older than 75 years in their retirement. In their early 20s, the nuns had completed an autobiographic essay when they entered the order. These essays were blindly graded for linguistic ability. The nuns with low idea density and low grammatical complexity in the autobiographies written 50 years earlier were 15 times more likely to have low cognitive scores in late life. In other words, cognitive skills in early life serve as a reserve against developing cognitive impairment later on.

A follow-up study has taken this analysis one step further by including postmortem brain examination. This study included 156 individuals in whom the researchers could correlate educational background, level of cognition before death, and amyloid load in the brain at autopsy. The results are shown in Figure 24.13. The individuals with greater years of education had less cognitive impairment even with increasing amyloidosis. The authors concluded that education is associated with factors that somehow reduce the effect of amyloid on cognition. They estimated that the difference between 15 years of education and 22 years is equivalent to approximately 2.6 years of amyloid progression. We hope this information provides some relief for the sort of person reading this book.

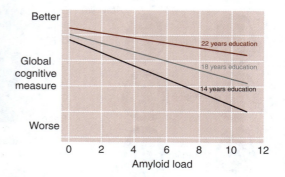

FIGURE 24.13 The cognitive impairment associated with amyloidosis is minimized by increasing years of education. (Adapted from Bennett DA, Schneider JA, Wilson RS, et al. Education modifies the association of amyloid but not tangles with cognitive function. *Neurology.* 2005;65[6]:953–955.)

"Use it or lose it" is one of the mantras resulting from this line of research: The implication being that exercising the brain is neuroprotective against the pathology of AD. Clearly, the research described here shows that smarter, more educated people have greater brain resilience. What we do not know is whether these people were born with a larger reserve of neural substrate or whether a lifetime of cognitive enrichment stimulated neuronal growth that protected their brains from the effects of AD.

Caloric Restriction

Caloric restriction is known to enhance longevity. Dietary restriction may also retard the effects of AD. Studies with animals suggest that low-calorie diets may protect the brain in the following ways:

1. Limiting oxidative stress
2. Reducing DNA damage
3. Increasing brain-derived neurotrophic factor production

A recent study shows the profound effects that calorie restriction can have on amyloid deposits in nonhuman primates. A colony of squirrel monkeys was raised on a diet reduced by 30% and compared with a freely eating control group. As the monkeys died of natural causes, their temporal cortical tissues were measured for β-amyloid, APP, and the secretase enzymes.

The monkeys on dietary restriction showed no change in the amount of APP molecule but a remarkable reduction in A-β. The activity of β- and γ-secretase enzymes (Figure 24.6) was no different between the two groups. However, α-secretase was almost 100% more active in the diet-restricted group. α-Secretase is an enzyme that cuts the APP molecule in a manner that limits the production of β-amyloid. It seems that caloric restriction enhances the activity of an enzyme that prevents the buildup of amyloid plaques.

Although caloric restriction may be effective in altering the buildup of β-amyloid, it seems unlikely to be used by the large number of people at risk for AD. Indeed, the industrial societies that are at most risk for AD are also the ones struggling with the obesity epidemic. However, if treatments that reduce hunger or enhance satiety can be developed, these could be reasonable pharmacologic approaches to forestalling AD.

The Lancet Commission

In 2017, the Lancet Commission published an extensive review on the latest information about Dementia Prevention, Intervention, and Care. It has 62 pages with 665 references. We have not read every word, although it might increase our cognitive reserve if we did. The lay press jumped on the authors' conclusion—"prevention is better than cure." The authors list nine potentially modifiable risk factors for dementia (see Table 24.1). They postulate that one-third of the cases can be prevented with proper intervention. This is the best we can do right now.

One of the delights of writing this new edition is revisiting promising treatments from previous editions. Many treatment interventions, which looked effective, have proven to be no better than placebo in larger studies. Nowhere is that more evident than with the treatment of dementia. However, that all could change in the near future. As Tom Hanks said in *Cast Away*, "who knows what the tide will bring in" tomorrow. We can't wait to see what's in the next edition.

TABLE 24.1

Potential Risk Factors for Dementia That Can Be Prevented

		Relative risk of dementia
Early life (age <18 y)	Less education (none or only primary school)	1.6
Midlife (age 45–65 y)	Hypertension	1.6
	Obesity	1.6
	Hearing loss	1.9
Later life (age >65 y)	Smoking	1.6
	Depression	1.9
	Physical inactivity	1.4
	Social isolation	1.6
	Diabetes	1.5

CABERNET SAUVIGNON

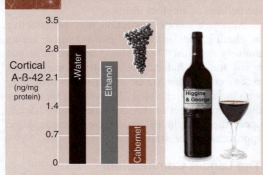

Alzheimer's modeled mice showed significant reductions in cortical β-amyloid with daily Cabernet Sauvignon. (Adapted from Wang J, Ho L, Zhao Z, et al. Moderate consumption of Cabernet Sauvignon attenuates Abeta neuropathology in a mouse model of Alzheimer's disease. *FASEB J.* 2006;20:2313–2320.)

It is with great pleasure that we report the results of a study showing the cerebral benefits of moderate doses of red wine. Mice altered to overexpress APP were given daily supplements of California Cabernet Sauvignon, ethanol, or water. The wine group had not only superior memory function but also less β-amyloid in their cortex (see figure).

We think that anyone who has finished reading every word of this book should celebrate with a little California Cabernet Sauvignon. Heck, it will give a little tweak to the nucleus accumbens, as well as promote β-amyloid clearance—all in moderation of course.

QUESTIONS

1. One hundred and twenty five years?
   a. Life expectancy.
   b. Fibroblast duration.
   c. Maximum cell divisions.
   d. Life span.

2. Alzheimer identified all of the following except
   a. Cortical atrophy.
   b. Amyloid plaques.
   c. β-Amyloid.
   d. Neurofibrillary tangles.

3. All of the following are increased in AD except
   a. Amyloid-β precursor protein.
   b. A-β-42.
   c. Ventricular size.
   d. CSF tau protein.

4. Neurofibrillary tangles are composed of
   a. Damaged microtubules.
   b. Extracellular protein tangles.
   c. Excessively phosphorylated tau.
   d. Untransportable cellular products.

5. The goal of the Alzheimer's vaccine is to increase which of the following?
   a. A-β-42.
   b. T-cell activation.
   c. Memory performance.
   d. Anti-Aβ antibodies.

6. Increases with calorie restriction.
   a. Amyloid-β precursor protein.
   b. α-Secretase.
   c. β-Secretase.
   d. γ-Secretase.

See Answers section at the end of this book.

Bibliography

CHAPTER 1

1. Bailey CH, Chen M. Morphological basis of long-term habituation and sensitization in Aplysia. *Science*. 1983;220:91–93.
2. Bear MF, Connors BW, Paradiso MA, eds. *Neuroscience: Exploring the Brain*. 4th ed. Baltimore, MD: Lippincott Williams & Wilkins; 2015.
3. Bouchard TJ. Twin studies of behavior: new and old findings. In: Schmitt A, Atzwanger K, Grammer K, et al. eds. *New Aspects of Human Ethology* . New York, NY: Plenum Publishing; 1997:121–140.
4. Finger S. *Minds Behind the Brain: A History of the Pioneers and Their Discoveries*. New York, NY: Oxford University Press; 2000.
5. Friend SH, Stoughton RB. The magic of microarrays. *Sci Am*. 2002;286:44–53.
6. Gottesman II. *Schizophrenia Genesis*. New York, NY: WH Freeman; 1991.
7. Insel TR. The NIMH Research Domain Criteria (RDoC) Project: precision medicine for psychiatry. *Am J Psychiatry*. 2014;171:395–397.
8. Ioannidis JPA. Excess significance bias in literature on brain volume abnormalities. *Arch Gen Psychiatry*. 2011;68:773–780.
9. Kandel ER. In: *Search of Memory: The Emergence of a New Science of Mind*. New York, NY: WW Norton & Co.; 2006.
10. Mertens J, Wang QW, Kim Y, et al. Differential responses to lithium in hyperexcitable neurons from patients with bipolar disorder. *Nature*. 2015;527:95–99.
11. Open Science Collaboration. Psychology. Estimating the reproducibility of psychological science. *Science*. 2015;349:aac4716.
12. Rorden C, Karnath HO. Using human brain lesions to infer function: a relic from a past era in the fMRI age? *Nat Rev Neurosci*. 2004;5:813–819.
13. Russell R, Duchaine B, Nakayama K. Super-recognizers: people with extraordinary face recognition ability. *Psychon Bull Rev*. 2009;16:252–257.
14. Shen HH. News feature: better models for brain disease. *Proc Natl Acad Sci U S A*. 2016;113:5461–5464.
15. Tye KM, Deisseroth K. Optogenetic investigation of neural circuits underlying brain disease in animal models. *Nat Rev Neurosci*. 2012;13:251–266.
16. Zimmer C. *Soul Made Flesh: The Discovery of the Brain—And How It Changed the World*. New York, NY: Free Press; 2004.

CHAPTER 2

1. Abbott NJ, Ronnback L, Hansson E. Astrocyte-endothelial interactions at the blood–brain barrier. *Nat Rev Neurosci*. 2006;7(1):41–53.
2. Bear MF, Connors BW, Paradiso MA, eds. *Neuroscience: Exploring the Brain*. 4th ed. Baltimore, MD: Lippincott Williams & Wilkins; 2015.
3. Behrstock S, Ebert A, McHugh J, et al. Human neural progenitors deliver glial cell line-derived neurotrophic factor to parkinsonian rodents and aged primates. *Gene Ther*. 2005;13(5):379–388.
4. Bower JM, Parsons LM. Rethinking the "lesser brain". *Sci Am*. 2003;289(2):50–57.
5. Cowan WM. The development of the brain. *Sci Am*. 1979;241(3):113–133.
6. Fuster JM. *The Prefrontal Cortex*. 5th ed. Cambridge, MA: Academic Press; 2015.
7. Gabathuler R. Blood-brain barrier transport of drugs for the treatment of brain diseases. *CNS Neurol Disord Drug Targets*. 2009;8(3):195–204.
8. Goodkind M, Eickhoff SB, Oathes DJ, et al. Identification of a common neurobiological substrate for mental illness. *JAMA Psychiatry*. 2015;72(4):305–315.
9. Kandel ER, Schwartz JH, Jessell TM, Siegelbaum SA, Hudspeth AJ, eds. *Principles of Neural Science*. 5th ed. New York, NY: McGraw-Hill; 2012.
10. Latvala A, Kuja-Halkola R, Ruck C, et al. Association of resting heart rate and blood pressure in late adolescence with subsequent mental disorders: a longitudinal population study of more than 1 million men in Sweden. *JAMA Psychiatry*. 2016;73:1268–1275.
11. Lewis DA. Structure of the human prefrontal cortex. *Am J Psychiatry*. 2004;161(8):1366.
12. Mashour GA, Walker EE, Martuza RL. Psychosurgery: past, present, and future. *Brain Res Brain Res Rev*. 2005;48(3):409–419.
13. Nestler EJ, Hyman SE, Malenka RC. *Molecular Neuropharmacology: A Foundation for Clinical Neuroscience*. 2nd ed. New York, NY: McGraw-Hill; 2009.
14. Salloway SP, Malloy PF, Duffy JD, eds. *The Frontal Lobes and Neuropsychiatric Illness*. Washington, DC: American Psychiatric Publishing, Inc; 2001.
15. Snell RS. *Clinical Neuroanatomy: A Illustrated Review with Questions and Explanations*. 3rd ed. Philadelphia, PA: Lippincott Williams & Wilkins; 2001.
16. Welch MJ, Meltzer EO, Simons FE. H1-antihistamines and the central nervous system. *Clin Allergy Immunol*. 2002;17:337–388.

CHAPTER 3

1. Bear MF, Connors BW, Paradiso MA, eds. *Neuroscience: Exploring the Brain*. 4th ed. Baltimore, MD: Lippincott Williams & Wilkins; 2015.

2. Breedlove SM, Watson NV. *Biological Psychology*. 7th ed. Sunderland, MA: Sinauer; 2013.
3. Fields RD. The other half of the brain. *Sci Am*. 2004;290(4):54–61.
4. Haydon PG. GLIA: listening and talking to the synapse. *Nat Rev Neurosci*. 2001;2(3):185–193.
5. Insel TR. Faulty circuits. *Sci Am*. 2010;302(4):44–51.
6. Kaufmann WE, Moser HW. Dendritic anomalies in disorders associated with mental retardation. *Cereb Cortex*. 2000;10(10):981–991.
7. Kolb B, Forgie M, Gibb R, et al. Age, experience and the changing brain. *Neurosci Biobehav Rev*. 1998;22(2):143–159.
8. Tian GF, Azmi H, Takano T, et al. An astrocytic basis of epilepsy. *Nat Med*. 2005;11(9):973–981.

CHAPTER 4

1. Bear MF, Connors BW, Paradiso MA, eds. *Neuroscience: Exploring the Brain*. 4th ed. Baltimore, MD: Lippincott Williams & Wilkins; 2015.
2. Breedlove SM, Watson NV. *Biological Psychology*. 7th ed. Sunderland, MA: Sinauer; 2013.
3. Cooper JR, Bloom FE, Roth RH. *The Biochemical Basis of Neuropharmacology*. 8th ed. New York, NY: Oxford University Press; 2003.
4. Goff DC, Coyle JT. The emerging role of glutamate in the pathophysiology and treatment of schizophrenia. *Am J Psychiatry*. 2001;158(9):1367–1377.
5. Holmes A, Heilig M, Rupniak NM, et al. Neuropeptide systems as novel therapeutic targets for depression and anxiety disorders. *Trends Pharmacol Sci*. 2003;24(11):580–588.
6. Iversen L. Cannabis and the brain. *Brain*. 2003;126(pt 6):1252–1270.
7. Lai TW, Zhang S, Wang YT. Excitotoxicity and stroke: identifying novel targets for neuroprotection. *Prog Neurobiol*. 2014;115:157–188.
8. Nestler EJ, Hyman SE, Malenka RC. *Molecular Neuropharmacology: A Foundation for Clinical Neuroscience*. 2nd ed. New York, NY: McGraw-Hill; 2009.
9. Purves D, Augustine GJ, Fitzpatrick D, et al. *Neuroscience*. 6th ed. Sunderland, MA: Sinauer; 2017.
10. Risacher SL, McDondal BC, Tallman EF, et al. Association between anticholinergic medication use and cognition, brain metabolism, and brain atrophy in cognitively normal older adults. *JAMA Neurol*. 2016;73:721–732.
11. Shan L, Dauvillers Y, Siegel JM. Interactions of the histamine and hypocretin systems in CNS disorders. *Nat Rev Neurol*. 2015;11:401–413.
12. Snyder SH, Ferris CD. Novel neurotransmitters and their neuropsychiatric relevance. *Am J Psychiatry*. 2000;157(11):1738–1751.
13. Stahl SM. *Stahl's Essential Psychopharmacology: Neuroscientific Basis of Practical Applications*. 3rd ed. New York, NY: Cambridge University Press; 2008.
14. Strand FL. *Neuropeptides: Regulators of Physiological Processes*. London: MIT Press; 1999.
15. Tsen G, Williams B, Allaire P, et al. Receptors with opposing functions are in postsynaptic microdomains under one presynaptic terminal. *Nat Neurosci*. 2000;3(2):126–132.
16. Vohora D, Bhowmik M. Histamine H3 receptor antagonists/inverse agonists on cognitive and motor processes: relevance to Alzheimer's disease, ADHD, schizophrenia, and drug abuse. *Front Syst Neurosci*. 2012;6:1–10.

CHAPTER 5

1. Bear MF, Connors BW, Paradiso MA, eds. *Neuroscience: Exploring the Brain*. 4th ed. Baltimore, MD: Lippincott Williams & Wilkins; 2015.
2. Breedlove SM, Watson NV. *Biological Psychology*. 7th ed. Sunderland, MA: Sinauer; 2013.
3. Engert F, Bonhoeffer T. Dendritic spine changes associated with hippocampal long-term synaptic plasticity. *Nature*. 1999;399(6731):66–70.
4. Huang YZ, Edwards MJ, Rounis E, et al. Theta burst stimulation of the human motor cortex. *Neuron*. 2005;45:201–206.
5. Kroeze WK, Hufeisen SJ, Popadak BA, et al. H1-histamine receptor affinity predicts short-term weight gain for typical and atypical antipsychotic drugs. *Neuropsychopharmacology*. 2003;28(3):519–526.
6. LeDoux J. *The Synaptic Self. How Our Brains Become Who We Are*. New York, NY: Viking; 2002.
7. Nestler EJ, Hyman SE, Malenka RC. *Molecular Neuropharmacology: A Foundation for Clinical Neuroscience*. 2nd ed. New York, NY: McGraw-Hill; 2009.
8. Purves D, Augustine GJ, Fitzpatrick D, et al. *Neuroscience*. 6th ed. Sunderland, MA: Sinauer; 2017.
9. Ressler KJ, Rothbaum BO, Tannenbaum L, et al. Cognitive enhancers as adjuncts to psychotherapy: use of D-cycloserine in phobic individuals to facilitate extinction of fear. *Arch Gen Psychiatry*. 2004;61(11):1136–1144.
10. Rogawski MA, Loscher W. The neurobiology of antiepileptic drugs. *Nat Rev Neurosci*. 2004;5(7):553–564.
11. Strohle A, Romeo E, di Michele F, et al. Induced panic attacks shift gamma-aminobutyric acid type A receptor modulatory neuroactive steroid composition in patients with panic disorder: preliminary results. *Arch Gen Psychiatry*. 2003;60(2):161–168.
12. Tecott LH, Smart SL. Monoamine neurotransmitters. In: Sadock BJ, Sadock VA, eds. *Kaplan and Sadock's Comprehensive Textbook of Psychiatry*. 8th ed. Philadelphia, PA: Lippincott Williams & Wilkins; 2005:49–60.
13. Victor M, Ropper AH. *Adams and Victor's Principles of Neurology*. 7th ed. New York, NY: McGraw-Hill; 2001.

CHAPTER 6

1. Adriani W, Leo D, Guarino M, et al. Short-term effects of adolescent methylphenidate exposure on brain striatal gene expression and sexual/endrocrine parameters in male rats. *Ann N Y Acad Sci*. 2006;1074:52–73.
2. Cook EH, Scherer SW. Copy-number variations associated with neuropsychiatric conditions. *Nature*. 2008;455:919–923.
3. Cross-Disorder Group of the Psychiatric Genomics Consortium. Identification of risk loci with shared effects on five major psychiatric disorders: a genome-wide analysis. *Lancet*. 2013;381(9875):1371–1379.
4. Dick DM, Riley B, Kendler KS. Nature and nurture in neuropsychiatric genetics: where do we stand? *Dialogues Clin Neurosci*. 2010;12:7–23.
5. Higgins ES. The new genetics of mental illness. *Sci Am Mind*. 2008;19:40–47.
6. Jirtle RL, Skinner MK. Environmental epigenomics and disease susceptibility. *Nat Rev Genet*. 2007;8:253–262.
7. Kaati G, Bygren LO, Pembrey M, Sjostrom M. Transgenerational response to nutrition, early life circumstances and longevity. *Eur J Hum Genetics*. 2007;15:784–790.

8. Kong A, Frigge ML, Masson G, et al. Rate of *de novo* mutations and the importance of father's age to disease risk. *Nature*. 2012;488:471–475.

9. Lincoln T, Joyce GF. Self-sustained replication of an RNA enzyme. *Science*. 2009;323:1229–1232.

10. Kananen L, Surakka I, Pirkola S, et al. Childhood adversities are associated with shorter telomere length at adult age both in individuals with anxiety disorder and controls. *PLoS One*. 2010;5:e10826.

11. Kendler KS, Prescott CA. *Genes, Environment and Psychopathology: Understanding the Causes of Psychiatric and Substance Use Disorders*. New York, NY: Guilford Press; 2006.

12. Maher B. The case of the missing heritability. *Nature*. 2008;456:18–21.

13. Mattick J. Deconstructing the dogma: a new view of evolution and genetic programming of complex organisms. *Ann N Y Acad Sci*. 2009;1178:29–46.

14. Miller BH, Wahlestedt C. MicroRNA dysregulation in psychiatric disease. *Brain Res*. 2010;1338:89–99.

15. Nestler EJ. Epigenetic mechanisms of drug addiction. *Neuropharmacology*. 2014;76:259–268.

16. Pennisi E. Shining a light on the genome's "dark matter". *Science*. 2010;330:1614.

17. Psychiatric GWAS Consortium Coordinating Committee. Genome wide association studies: history, rationale and prospects for psychiatric disorders. *Am J Psychiatry*. 2009;166:540–556.

18. Strachan T, Read A. *Human Molecular Genetics*. 4th ed. New York, NY: Garland Science; 2011.

19. Waterland RA, Jirtle RL. Transposable elements: targets for early nutritional effects on epigenetic gene regulation. *Mol Cell Biol*. 2003;23:5293–5300.

20. Williams NM, Zaharieva I, Martin A, et al. Rare chromosomal deletions and duplications in attention-deficit hyperactivity disorder: a genome-wide analysis. *Lancet*. 2010;376:1401–1408.

CHAPTER 7

1. Azukizawa M, Pekary AE, Hershman JM, et al. Plasma thyrotropin, thyroxine, and triiodothyronine relationships in man. *J Clin Endocrinol Metab*. 1976;43(3):533–542.

2. Bauer M, Heinz A, Whybrow PC. Thyroid hormones, serotonin and mood: of synergy and significance in the adult brain. *Mol Psychiatry*. 2002;7(2):140–156.

3. Bauer M, London ED, Silverman DH, et al. Thyroid, brain and mood modulation in affective disorder: insights from molecular research and functional brain imaging. *Pharmacopsychiatry*. 2003;36(suppl 3):S215–S221.

4. Bauer M, Whybrow PC. Thyroid hormone, neural tissue and mood modulation. *World J Biol Psychiatry*. 2001;2(2):59–69.

5. Bear MF, Connors BW, Paradiso MA, eds. *Neuroscience: Exploring the Brain*. 4th ed. Baltimore, MD: Lippincott Williams & Wilkins; 2015.

6. Bradley RG, Binder EB, Epstein MP, et al. Influence of child abuse on adult depression. *Arch Gen Psychiatry*. 2008;65:190–200.

7. Breedlove SM, Watson NV. *Biological Psychology*. 7th ed. Sunderland, MA: Sinauer; 2013.

8. Constant EL, de Volder AG, Ivanoiu A, et al. Cerebral blood flow and glucose metabolism in hypothyroidism: a positron emission tomography study. *J Clin Endocrinol Metab*. 2001;86(8):3864–3870.

9. Fava M, Labbate LA, Abraham ME, et al. Hypothyroidism and hyperthyroidism in major depression revisited. *J Clin Psychiatry*. 1995;56(5):186–192.

10. Forrest D, Reh TA, Rusch A. Neurodevelopmental control by thyroid hormone receptors. *Curr Opin Neurobiol*. 2002;12(1):49–56.

11. Gordon JT, Kaminski DM, Rozanov CB, et al. Evidence that 3,3,5-triiodothyronine is concentrated in and delivered from the locus coeruleus to its noradrenergic targets via anterograde axonal transport. *Neuroscience*. 1999;93(3):943–954.

12. Guintivano J, Brown T, Newconer A, et al. Identification and replication of a combined epigenetic and genetic biomarker prediction suicide and suicidal behaviors. *JAMA Psychiatry*. 2014;171:1287–1296.

13. Kim JJ, Diamond DM. The stressed hippocampus, synaptic plasticity and lost memories. *Nat Rev Neurosci*. 2002;3(6):453–462.

14. Lupien SJ, de Leon M, de Santi S, et al. Cortisol levels during human aging predict hippocampal atrophy and memory deficits. *Nat Neurosci*. 1998;1(1):69–73.

15. Marangell LB, Ketter TA, George MS, et al. Inverse relationship of peripheral thyrotropin-stimulating hormone levels to brain activity in mood disorders. *Am J Psychiatry*. 1997;154(2):224–230.

16. McEwen BS. Protective and damaging effects of stress mediators. *N Engl J Med*. 1998;338(3):171–179.

17. Nestler EJ, Hyman SE, Malenka RC. *Molecular Neuropharmacology: A Foundation for Clinical Neuroscience*. 2nd ed. New York, NY: McGraw-Hill; 2009.

18. Raison CL, Miller AH. When not enough is too much: the role of insufficient glucocorticoid signaling in the pathophysiology of stress-related disorders. *Am J Psychiatry*. 2003;160(9):1554–1565.

19. Rupprecht R, Holsboer F. Neuroactive steroids: mechanisms of action and neuropsychopharmacological perspectives. *Trends Neurosci*. 1999;22(9):410–460.

20. Sapolsky RM. *Why Zebras Don't Get Ulcers: An Updated Guide to Stress, Stress-Related Diseases, and Coping*. New York, NY: Barns & Noble Books; 1998.

21. Sapolsky RM. Stress and plasticity in the limbic system. *Neurochem Res*. 2003;28(11):1735–1742.

22. Shelton R, Osuntokun O, Heinloth AN, Corya SA. Therapeutic options for treatment-resistant depression. *CNS Drugs*. 2010;24:131–161.

23. Snell RS. *Clinical Neuroanatomy: A Illustrated Review with Questions and Explanations*. Philadelphia, PA: Lippincott Williams & Wilkins; 2001.

24. Starkman MN, Giordani B, Gebarski SS, et al. Decrease in cortisol reverses human hippocampal atrophy following treatment of Cushing's disease. *Biol Psychiatry*. 1999;46(12):1595–1602.

25. Starkman MN, Giordani B, Gebarski SS, et al. Improvement in learning associated with increase in hippocampal formation volume. *Biol Psychiatry*. 2003;53(3):233–238.

26. Vaidya VA, Castro ME, Pei Q, et al. Influence of thyroid hormone on 5-HT(1A) and 5-HT(2A) receptor-mediated regulation of hippocampal BDNF mRNA expression. *Neuropharmacology*. 2001;40(1):48–56.

27. Wolkowitz OM, Rothschild AJ. *Psychoneuroendocrinology: The Scientific Basis of Clinical Practice*. Washington, DC: American Psychiatric Publishing, Inc; 2003.

28. van Zuiden M, Geuze E, Willemen HL, et al. Pre-existing high glucocorticoid receptor number predicting development of posttraumatic stress symptoms after military deployment. *Am J Psychiatry*. 2011;168:89–96.

29. Zorumski CF, Mennerick S. Neurosteroids as therapeutic leads in psychiatry. *JAMA Psychiatry*. 2013;70(7):659–660.

CHAPTER 8

1. Antonini A, Stryker MP. Rapid remodeling of axonal arbors in the visual cortex. *Science*. 1993;260(5115): 1819–1821.
2. Bartzokis G, Lu P, Tinqus K, et al. Lifespan trajectory of myelin integrity and maximum motor speed. *Neurobiol Aging*. 2010;31(9):1554–1562.
3. Bear MF, Connors BW, Paradiso MA, eds. *Neuroscience: Exploring the Brain*. 4th ed. Baltimore, MD: Lippincott Williams & Wilkins; 2015.
4. Bhardway RD, Curtis MA, Spalding KL, et al. Neocortical neurogenesis in humans is restricted to development. *Proc Natl Acad Sci U S A*. 2006;103(33): 12564–12568.
5. Bratt-leal AM, Loring JF. Stem cells for Parkinson's disease. In: Tuszynski MH, ed. *Translational Neuroscience: Fundamental Approaches for Neurological Disorders*. Springer; 2016:187–202.
6. Breedlove SM, Watson NV. *Biological Psychology*. 7th ed. Sunderland, MA: Sinauer; 2013.
7. Brown J, Cooper-Kuhn CM, Kempermann G, et al. Enriched environment and physical activity stimulate hippocampal but not olfactory bulb neurogenesis. *Eur J Neurosci*. 2003;17(10):2042–2046.
8. Elbert T, Candia V, Altenmuller E, et al. Alteration of digital representations in somatosensory cortex in focal hand dystonia. *Neuroreport*. 1998;9(16):3571–3575.
9. Gage FH. Mammalian neural stem cells. *Science*. 2000;287(5457):1433–1438.
10. Gage FH. Brain, repair yourself. *Sci Am*. 2003;289(3): 46–53.
11. Gogtay N, Thompson PM. Mapping gray matter development: implications for typical development and vulnerability to psychopathology. *Brain Cogn*. 2010;72:6–15.
12. Gould E, Reeves AJ, Graziano MS, et al. Neurogenesis in the neocortex of adult primates. *Science*. 1999;286(5439):548–552.
13. Goyal MS, Raichle ME. Gene expression-based modeling of human cortical synaptic density. *PNAS*. 2013;110(16):6571–6576.
14. Heim CM, Mayberg HS, Mletzko T, et al. Decreased cortical representation of genital somatosensory field after childhood sexual abuse. *Am J Psychiatry*. 2013;170: 616–623.
15. Huttenlocher PR, Dabholkar AS. Regional differences in synaptogenesis in human cerebral cortex. *J Comp Neurol*. 1997;387(2):167–178.
16. Johnson JS, Newport EL. Critical period effects in second language learning: the influence of maturational state on the acquisition of English as a second language. *Cognit Psychol*. 1989;21(1):60–99.
17. Kell CA, von Kriegstein K, Rosler A, et al. The sensory cortical representation of the human penis: revisiting somatotopy in the male homunculus. *J Neurosci*. 2005;25:5984–5987.
18. Levi-Montalcini R. The nerve growth factor. *Ann N Y Acad Sci*. 1964;118:149–170.
19. Merzenich MM, Nelson RJ, Stryker MP, et al. Somatosensory cortical map changes following digit amputation in adult monkeys. *J Comp Neurol*. 1984;224(4):591–605.
20. Mirescu C, Peters JD, Gould E. Early life experience alters response of adult neurogenesis to stress. *Nat Neurosci*. 2004;7(8):841–846.
21. Munte TF, Altenmuller E, Jancke L. The musician's brain as a model of neuroplasticity. *Nat Rev Neurosci*. 2002;3(6):473–478.
22. Nestler EJ, Hyman SE, Malenka RC. *Molecular Neuropharmacology: A Foundation for Clinical Neuroscience*. 2nd ed. New York, NY: McGraw-Hill; 2009.
23. Pantev C, Engelien A, Candia V, et al. Representational cortex in musicians. Plastic alterations in response to musical practice. *Ann N Y Acad Sci*. 2001;930: 300–314.
24. Purves D, Augustine GJ, Fitzpatrick D, et al. *Neuroscience*. 6th ed. Sunderland, MA: Sinauer; 2017.
25. Silver J, Miller JH. Regeneration beyond the glial scar. *Nat Rev Neurosci*. 2004;5(2):146–156.
26. Tabakow P, Raisman G, Fortuna W, et al. Functional regeneration of supraspinal connections in a patient with transected spinal cord following transplantation of bulbar olfactory ensheathing cells with peripheral nerve bridging. *Cell Transplant*. 2014;23:1631–1655.
27. Takagi Y, Takahashi J, Saiki H, et al. Dopaminergic neurons generated from monkey embryonic stem cells function in a Parkinson primate model. *J Clin Invest*. 2005;115(1):102–109.
28. Taub E, Uswatte G. Constraint-induced movement therapy: bridging from the primate laboratory to the stroke rehabilitation laboratory. *J Rehabil Med*. 2003;(suppl 41):34–40.
29. Talahashi T, Shirane R, Sato S, Yoshimoto T. Developmental changes of cerebral blood flow and oxygen metabolism in children. *AJNR Am J Neuroradiol*. 1999;20:917–922.
30. Wiesel TN. Postnatal development of the visual cortex and the influence of environment. *Nature*. 1982;299(5884):583–591.

CHAPTER 9

1. Bauer S, Kerr BJ, Patterson PH. The neuropoietic cytokine family in development, plasticity, disease and injury. *Nat Rev Neurosci*. 2007;8:221–232.
2. Cahalan S. *Brain on Fire: My Month of Madness*. 2013. Simon & Schuster.
3. Clarke MC, Tanskanen A, Huttunen M, Whittaker JC, Cannon M. Evidence for an interaction between familial liability and exposure to infection in the causation of schizophrenia. *Am J Psychiatry*. 2009;166:1025–1030.
4. Coico R, Sunshine G. *Immunology: A Short Course*. 6th ed. Hoboken, NJ: Wiley-Blackwell; 2009.
5. Compston A, Coles A. Multiple sclerosis. *Lancet*. 2008;372:1502–1517.
6. Faulkner JR, Herrmann JE, Woo MJ, Tansey KE, Doan NB, Sofroniew MV. Reactive astrocytes protect tissue and preserve function after spinal cord injury. *J Neurosci*. 2004;24:2143–2155.
7. Glaser R, Kiecolt-Glazer JK. Stress-induced immune dysfunction: implications for health. *Nat Rev Immunol*. 2005;5:243–251.
8. Graeber MB, Streit WJ. Microglia: biology and pathology. *Acta Neuropathol*. 2005;119:89–105.
9. Hoofnagle JH, Seeff LB. Peginterferon and ribavirin for chronic hepatitis C. *N Engl J Med*. 2006;355:2444–2451.
10. Kadhim HJ, Duchateau J, Sebire G. Cytokines and brain injury: invited review. *J Intensive Care Med*. 2008;23:236–249.
11. LaFond RE, Lukehart SA. Biological basis for syphilis. *Clin Microbiol Rev*. 2006;19:29–49.
12. Lucas SM, Rothwell NJ, Gibson RM. The role of inflammation in CNS injury and disease. *Br J Pharmacol*. 2006;147:S232–S240.

13. Maes M, Yirmyia R, Noraberg J, et al. The inflammatory & neurodegenerative hypothesis of depression: leads for future research and new drug developments in depression. *Metab Brain Dis.* 2009;24:27–53.

14. Martinez D, Trifilieff P. Cocaine vaccine: research review. *Am Soc Add Med Mag.* Fall 2013.

15. McClure M, Wessely S. Chronic fatigue syndrome and human retrovirus XMRV. Three studies now refute the original study reporting the link. *BMJ.* 2010;340:489–490.

16. Miller AH, Raison CL. The role of inflammation in depression: from evolutionary imperative to modern treatment target. *Nat Rev Immunol.* 2016;16:22–34.

17. Owen N, Poulton T, Hay FC, Mohamed-Ali V, Steptoe A. Socioeconomic status, C-reactive protein, immune factors, and responses to acute mental stress. *Brain Behav Immun.* 2003;17:286–295.

18. Panagiotakos DB, Dimakopoulou K, Katsouyanni K, et al. Mediterranean diet and inflammatory response in myocardial infarction survivors. *Int J Epidemiol.* 2009;38:856–866.

19. Padgett DA, Marucha PT, Sheridan JF. Restraint stress slows cutaneous wound healing in mice. *Brain Behav Immun.* 1998;12:64–73.

20. Potvin S, Stip E, Sepehry AA, Gendron A, Bah R, Kouassi E. Inflammatory cytokine alterations in schizophrenia: a systematic quantitative review. *Biol Psychiatry.* 2008;63:801–808.

21. Raison CL, Rutherford RE, Woolwine BJ, et al. A randomized controlled trial of the tumor necrosis factor antagonist infliximab for treatment-resistant depression. *JAMA Psychiatry.* 2013;70(1):31–41.

22. Reichert WM. *Indwelling Neural Implants: Strategies for Contending with the In Vivo Environment.* Boca Raton, FL: CRC Press, Taylor & Francis Group; 2008.

23. Sanchez-Vellegas A, Delgado-Rodriquez M, Alonso A, et al. Association of the Mediterranean diet pattern with the incidence of depression. *Arch Gen Psychiatry.* 2009;66:1090–1098.

24. Sekar A, Bialas AR, de Rivera H, et al. Schizophrenia risk from complex variation of complement component 4. *Nature.* 2016;530:177–183.

25. Silver J, Miller JH. Regeneration beyond the glial scar. *Nat Rev Neurosci.* 2004;5:146–156.

26. Sompayrac L. *How the Immune System Works.* 3rd ed. Malden, MA: Blackwell Publishing; 2008.

27. Sternberg EM. Neural regulation of innate immunity: a coordinated nonspecific host response to pathogens. *Nat Rev Immunol.* 2006;6:318–328.

28. Tyring S, Gottlieb A, Papp K, et al. Etanercept and clinical outcomes, fatigue, and depression in psoriasis: double-blind placebo-controlled randomised phase III trial. *Lancet.* 2006;367:29–35.

29. van Rossum CT, Shipley MJ, van de Mheen H, Grobbee DE, Marmot MG. Employment grade differences in cause specific mortality. A 25 year follow up of civil servants from the first Whitehall study. *J Epidemiol Community Health.* 2000;54:178–184.

CHAPTER 10

1. Breedlove SM, Watson NV. *Biological Psychology.* 7th ed. Sunderland, MA: Sinauer; 2013.

2. Chahine M, Chatelier A, Babich O, Grupp JJ. Voltage-gated sodium channels in neurological disorders. *CNS Neurol Disord Drug Targets.* 2008;7(2):144–158.

3. Datta A, Bansal V, Diaz J, et al. Gyri-precise head model of transcranial direct current stimulation: improved spatial focality using a ring electrode versus conventional rectangular pad. *Brain Stimul.* 2009;2:201–207.

4. Flöel A, Meinzer M, Kirstein R, et al. Short-term anomia training and electrical brain stimulation. *Stroke.* 2011;42:2065–2067.

5. Higgins ES, George MS. *Brain Stimulation Therapies for Clinicians.* Washington, DC: American Psychiatric Press; 2008.

6. Hodgkin AL, Huxley AF. Action potentials recorded from inside a nerve fibre. *Nature.* 1939;144:710–711.

7. Koch C. A theory of consciousness. *Sci Am Mind.* 2009;20(4):16–19.

8. Parent A. Giovanni Aldini: from animal electricity to human brain stimulation. *Can J Neurol Sci.* 2004;31(4):576–584.

9. Penfield W, Boldrey E. Somatic motor and sensory representation in the cerebral cortex of man as studied by electrical stimulation. *Brain.* 1937;60:389–443.

10. Penfield W. Engrams in the human brain. Mechanisms of memory. *Proc R Soc Med.* 1968;61(8):831–840.

11. Purves D, Augustine GJ, Fitzpatrick D, et al. *Neuroscience.* 6th ed. Sunderland, MA: Sinauer; 2017.

CHAPTER 11

1. Antonini A, Stryker MP. Rapid remodeling of axonal arbors in the visual cortex. *Science.* 1993;260(5115):1819–1821.

2. Apkarian AV, Sosa Y, Sonty S, et al. Chronic back pain is associated with decreased prefrontal and thalamic gray matter density. *J Neurosci.* 2004;24(46):10410–10415.

3. Bear MF, Connors BW, Paradiso MA, eds. *Neuroscience: Exploring the Brain.* 4th ed. Baltimore, MD: Lippincott Williams & Wilkins; 2015.

4. Beecher HK. Pain in men wounded in battle. *Ann Surg.* 1946;123(1):96–195.

5. Borckardt JJ, Weinstein M, Reeves ST, et al. Postoperative left prefrontal repetitive transcranial magnetic stimulation reduces patient-controlled analgesia use. *Anesthesiology.* 2006;105(3):557–562.

6. Boucher TJ, Okuse K, Bennett DL, et al. Potent analgesic effects of GDNF in neuropathic pain states. *Science.* 2000;290(5489):124–127.

7. Cho ZH, Chung SC, Lee HP, et al. Retraction. *Proc Natl Acad Sci.* 2006;103(27):10527.

8. Coghill RC, McHaffie JG, Yen YF. Neural correlates of interindividual differences in the subjective experience of pain. *Proc Natl Acad Sci U S A.* 2003;100(14):8538–8542.

9. Coghill RC, Sang CN, Maisog JM, et al. Pain intensity processing within the human brain: a bilateral, distributed mechanism. *J Neurophysiol.* 1999;82(4):1934–1943.

10. Colloca L, Beneditti F. Placebos and painkillers: is mind as real as matter? *Nat Rev Neurosci.* 2005;6:545–552.

11. Diatchenko L, Slade GD, Nackley AG, et al. Genetic basis for individual variations in pain perception and the development of a chronic pain condition. *Hum Mol Genet.* 2005;14(1):135–143.

12. Fava M, Memisoglu A, Thase ME, et al. Opioid modulation with buprenorphine/samidorphan as adjenctive treatment for inadequate response to antidepressants: a randomized double-blind placebo-controlled trial. *Am J Psychiatry.* 2016;173:499–508.

13. Franklin GM. Opioids for chronic noncancer pain: a position paper of the American Academy of Neurology. *Neurology.* 2014;83:1277–1284.

14. Grace PM, Strand KA, Galer EL, et al. Morphine paradoxically prolongs neuropathic pain in rats by amplifying spinal NLRP3 inflammasome activation. *Proc Natl Acad Sci.* 2016;113(24):E3411–E3450.

15. Gwilym S, Filippini N, Douaud G, Carr AJ, Tracey I. Thalamic atrophy associated with painful osteoarthritis of the hip is reversed after arthroplasty. *Arthritis Rheum.* 2010;62:2930–2940.

16. Harden RN. Chronic neuropathic pain. Mechanisms, diagnosis, and treatment. *Neurologist.* 2005;11(2):111–122.

17. Hocking B. Epidemiological aspects of "repetition strain injury" in telecom Australia. *Med J Aust.* 1987;147(5):218–222.

18. Hohmann AG, Suplita RL, Bolton NM, et al. An endocannabinoid mechanism for stress-induced analgesia. *Nature.* 2005;435(7045):1108–1112.

19. Hooley JM, Delgado ML. Pain insensitivity in the relatives of schizophrenia patients. *Schizophr Res.* 2001;47(2–3):265–273.

20. Hunt SP, Mantyh PW. The molecular dynamics of pain control. *Nat Rev Neurosci.* 2001;2(2):83–91.

21. Jaffee JH, Strain EC. Opioid-related disorders. In: Sadock BJ, Sadock VA, eds. *Kaplan & Sadock's Comprehensive Textbook of Psychiatry.* 8th ed. Philadelphia, PA: Lippincott Williams & Wilkins; 2005:1265–1290.

22. Kandel ER, Schwartz JH, Jessell TM, Siegelbaum SA, Hudspeth AJ, eds. *Principles of Neural Science* . 5th ed. New York, NY: McGraw-Hill; 2012.

23. Knijnik LM, Dussan-Sarria JA, Rozisky JR, et al. Repetitive transcranial magnetic stimulation for fibromyalgia: systematic review and meta-analysis. *Pain Pract.* 2016;16:294–304.

24. Lutz PE, Kieffer BL. Opioid receptors: distinct roles in mood disorders. *Trends Neurosci.* 2013;36:195–206.

25. Manglik A, Lin H, Aryal DK, et al. Structure-based discovery of opioid analgesics with reduced side effects. *Nature.* 2016;537:185–190.

26. Mardy S, Miura Y, Endo F, et al. Congenital insensitivity to pain with anhidrosis (CIPA): effect of TRKA (NTRK1) missense mutations on autophosphorylation of the receptor tyrosine kinase for nerve growth factor. *Hum Mol Genet.* 2001;10(3):179–188.

27. McMahon SB, Cafferty WB, Marchand F, et al. Immune and glial cell factors as pain mediators and modulators. *Exp Neurol.* 2005;192(2):444–462.

28. Melzack R, Coderre TJ, Katz J, et al. Central neuroplasticity and pathological pain. *Ann N Y Acad Sci.* 2001;933:157–174.

29. Nagasako EM, Oaklander AL, Dworkin RH, et al. Congenital insensitivity to pain: an update. *Pain.* 2003;101(3):213–219.

30. Pariente J, White P, Frackowiak RS, et al. Expectancy and belief modulate the neuronal substrates of pain treated by acupuncture. *Neuroimage.* 2005;25(4):1161–1167.

31. Petrovic P, Kalso E, Petersson KM, et al. Placebo and opioid analgesia—imaging a shared neuronal network. *Science.* 2002;295(5560):1737–1740.

32. Premkumar L. Targeting TRPV1 as an alternative approach to narcotic analgesics to treat chronic pain conditions. *AAPS J.* 2010;12:361–370.

33. Price DD. Psychological and neural mechanisms of the affective dimension of pain. *Science.* 2000;288(5472):1769–1772.

34. Purves D, Augustine GJ, Fitzpatrick D, et al. *Neuroscience.* 6th ed. Sunderland, MA: Sinauer; 2017.

35. Reynolds DV. Surgery in the rat during electrical analgesia induced by focal brain stimulation. *Science.* 1969;164(878):444–445.

36. Rodriguex-Raecke R, Niemeier A, Ihle K, et al. Structural brain changes in chronic pain reflect probably neither damage nor atrophy. *PLoS One.* 2013;8(2):E54475.

37. Schrader H, Obelieniene D, Bovim G, et al. Natural evolution of late whiplash syndrome outside the medicolegal context. *Lancet.* 1996;347(9010):1207–1211.

38. Staiger TO, Gaster B, Sullivan MD, et al. Systematic review of antidepressants in the treatment of chronic low back pain. *Spine.* 2003;28(22):2540–2545.

39. Taylor P, Pezzullo L, Grant S, Bensoussan A. Cost-effectiveness of acupuncture for chronic nonspecific low back pain. *Pain Pract.* 2014;14:599–606.

40. Tenore PL. Psychotherapeutic benefits of opioid agonist therapy. *J Addict Dis.* 2008;27(3):49–65.

41. Tesarz J, Schuster AK, Margmann M, et al. Pain perception in athletes compared to normally active controls: a systematic review with meta-analysis. *Pain.* 2012;153:1253–1262.

42. Volkow ND, McLellan AT. Opioid abuse in chronic pain – misconceptions and mitigation strategies. *NEJM.* 2016;374:1253–1263.

43. Wager TD, Rilling JK, Smith EE, et al. Placebo-induced changes in FMRI in the anticipation and experience of pain. *Science.* 2004;303(5661):1162–1167.

CHAPTER 12

1. Adinoff B. Neurobiologic processes in drug reward and addiction. *Harv Rev Psychiatry.* 2004;12(6):305–320.

2. Adriani W, Spijker S, Deroche-Gamonet V, et al. Evidence for enhanced neurobehavioral vulnerability to nicotine during periadolescence in rats. *J Neurosci.* 2003;23(11):4712–4716.

3. Barbano MF, Cador M. Opioids for hedonic experience and dopamine to get ready for it. *Psychopharmacology (Berl).* 2007;191(3):497–506.

4. Berridge KC, Kringelbach ML. Pleasure systems in the brain. *Neuron.* 2015;86:646–664.

5. Bimpisidis Z, De Luca MA, Pisanu A, Di Chiara G. Lesion of medial prefrontal dopamine terminals abolishes habituation of accumbens shell dopamine responsiveness to taste stimuli. *Eur J Neurosci.* 2013;37:613–622.

6. Bolanos CA, Barrot M, Berton O, et al. Methylphenidate treatment during pre- and periadolescence alters behavioral responses to emotional stimuli at adulthood. *Biol Psychiatry.* 2003;54(12):1317–1329.

7. Buhusi CV, Meck WH. Differential effects of methamphetamine and haloperidol on the control of an internal clock. *Behav Neurosci.* 2002;116(2):291–297.

8. Carlezon Jr WA, Mague SD, Andersen SL. Enduring behavioral effects of early exposure to methylphenidate in rats. *Biol Psychiatry.* 2003;54(12):1330–1337.

9. Clark AE, Diener E, Georgellis Y, Lucas RE. Lags and leads in life satisfaction: a test of the baseline hypothesis. *Econ J.* 2008;118:F222–F243.

10. Curtin K, Fleckenstein AE, Robison RJ, et al. Methamphetamine/amphetamine abuse and risk of Parkinson's disease in Utah: a population-based assessment. *Drug Alcohol Dep.* 2015;146:30–38.

11. Ernst M, Nelson EE, Jazbec S, et al. Amygdala and nucleus accumbens in responses to receipt and omission of gains in adults and adolescents. *Neuroimage.* 2005;25(4):1279–1291.

12. Fone KC, Nutt DJ. Stimulants: use and abuse in the treatment of attention deficit hyperactivity disorder. *Curr Opin Pharmacol*. 2005;5(1):87–93.

13. Garavan H, Pankiewicz J, Bloom A, et al. Cue-induced cocaine craving: neuroanatomical specificity for drug users and drug stimuli. *Am J Psychiatry*. 2000;157(11):1789–1798.

14. Glass JM, Buu A, Adams KM, et al. Effects of alcoholism severity and smoking on executive neurocognitive function. *Addiction*. 2009;104(1):38–48.

15. Goldman D, Barr CS. Restoring the addicted brain. *N Engl J Med*. 2002;347(11):843–845.

16. Higgins ES. Do ADHD drugs take a toll on the brain? *Sci Am Mind*. 2009;20:38–43.

17. Hnasko TS, Sotak BN, Palmiter RD. *Nature*. 2005; 438:854–857.

18. Kalivas PW, Volkow N, Seamans J. Unmanageable motivation in addiction: a pathology in prefrontal-accumbens glutamate transmission. *Neuron*. 2005;45(5):647–650.

19. Kolb B, Gorny G, Li Y, et al. Amphetamine or cocaine limits the ability of later experience to promote structural plasticity in the neocortex and nucleus accumbens. *Proc Natl Acad Sci U S A*. 2003;100(18):10523–10528.

20. Kringelback ML, Berridge KC. Toward a functional neuroanatomy of pleasure and happiness. *Trends Cogn Sci*. 2009;13:479–487.

21. Le AD, Harding S, Juzytsch W, et al. The role of corticotrophin-releasing factor in stress-induced relapse to alcohol-seeking behavior in rats. *Psychopharmacology (Berl)*. 2000;150(3):317–324.

22. Leknes S, Tracey I. A common neurobiology for pain and pleasure. *Nat Rev Neurosci*. 2008;9:314–320.

23. Morgan D, Grant KA, Gage HD, et al. Social dominance in monkeys: dopamine D2 receptors and cocaine self-administration. *Nat Neurosci*. 2002;5(2):169–174.

24. Nestler EJ. Molecular basis of long-term plasticity underlying addiction. *Nat Rev Neurosci*. 2001;2(2):119–128.

25. Nestler EJ, Hyman SE, Malenka RC. *Molecular Neuropharmacology: A Foundation for Clinical Neuroscience*. 2nd ed. New York, NY: McGraw-Hill; 2009.

26. Nestler EJ, Malenka RC. The addicted brain. *Sci Am*. 2004;290(3):78–85.

27. O'Connor MF, Wellisch DK, Stanton AL, Eisenberger NI, Irwin MR, Lieberman MD. Craving love? Enduring grief activates brain's reward center. *Neuroimage*. 2008;42:969–972.

28. Olds J. Pleasure centers in the brain. *Sci Am*. 1956;195:105–112.

29. Pettit HO, Justice Jr JB. Effect of dose on cocaine self-administration behavior and dopamine levels in the nucleus accumbens. *Brain Res*. 1991;539(1):94–102.

30. Robbins TW, Everitt BJ. Drug addiction: bad habits add up. *Nature*. 1999;398(6728):567–570.

31. Robinson TE, Gorny G, Savage VR, et al. Widespread but regionally specific effects of experimenter- versus self-administered morphine on dendritic spines in the nucleus accumbens, hippocampus, and neocortex of adult rats. *Synapse*. 2002;46(4):271–279.

32. Robinson TE, Kolb B. Persistent structural modifications in nucleus accumbens and prefrontal cortex neurons produced by previous experience with amphetamine. *J Neurosci*. 1997;17(21):8491–8497.

33. Robinson TE, Kolb B. Structural plasticity associated with exposure to drugs of abuse. *Neuropharmacology*. 2004;47(suppl 1):33–46.

34. Rosenbloom M, Sullivan EV, Pfefferbaum A. Using magnetic resonance imaging and diffusion tensor imaging to assess brain damage in alcoholics. *Alcohol Res Health*. 2003;27(2):146–152.

35. Schultz W. Multiple reward signals in the brain. *Nat Rev Neurosci*. 2000;1(3):199–207.

36. See RE, Fuchs RA, Ledford CC, et al. Drug addiction, relapse, and the amygdala. *Ann N Y Acad Sci*. 2003;985:294–307.

37. Tenenbaum YS, Weizman A, Rehavi M. *J Mol Neurosci*. 2015;57:231–242.

38. Tremblay L, Schultz W. Relative reward preference in primate orbitofrontal cortex. *Nature*. 1999;398(6729):704–708.

39. Urban KR, Waterhouse BD, Gao WJ. Distinct age-dependent effects of methylphenidate on developing and adult prefrontal neurons. *Bio Psychiatry*. 2012;72:880–888.

40. Volkow ND, Fowler JS. Addiction, a disease of compulsion and drive: involvement of the orbitofrontal cortex. *Cereb Cortex*. 2000;10(3):318–325.

41. Volkow ND, Fowler JS, Wang GJ, et al. Role of dopamine in the therapeutic and reinforcing effects of methylphenidate in humans: results from imaging studies. *Eur Neuropsychopharmacol*. 2002;12(6):557–566.

42. Volkow ND, Li TK. Drug addiction: the neurobiology of behaviour gone awry. *Nat Rev Neurosci*. 2004;5(12):963–970.

43. Wilens TE, Faraone SV, Biederman J, et al. Does stimulant therapy of attention-deficit/hyperactivity disorder beget later substance abuse? A meta-analytic review of the literature. *Pediatrics*. 2003;111(1):179–185.

44. Wilson SJ, Sayette MA, Fiez JA. Prefrontal responses to drug cues: a neurocognitive analysis. *Nat Neurosci*. 2004;7(3):211–214.

45. Zhang X, Newport GD, Callicott R, et al. MicroPET/CT assessment of FDG uptake in brain after long-term methylphenidate treatment in nonhuman primates. *Neurotoxicol Teratol*. 2016;56:68–74.

CHAPTER 13

1. Arch JR. Central regulation of energy balance: inputs, outputs and leptin resistance. *Proc Nutr Soc*. 2005;64(1):39–46.

2. Ayyad C, Andersen T. Long-term efficacy of dietary treatment of obesity: a systematic review of studies published between 1931 and 1999. *Obes Rev*. 2000;1(2):113–119.

3. Bear MF, Connors BW, Paradiso MA, eds. *Neuroscience: Exploring the Brain*. 4th ed. Baltimore, MD: Lippincott Williams & Wilkins; 2015.

4. Berthoud HR. Mind versus metabolism in the control of food intake and energy balance. *Physiol Behav*. 2004;81(5):781–793.

5. Bhatti JA, Nathens AB, Thiruchelvam D, et al. Self-harm emergencies after bariatric surgery: a populatin-based cohort study. *JAMA Surg*. 2016;151:226–232.

6. Bray GA. Medical treatment of obesity: the past, the present and the future. *Best Prac Res Clinic Gastro*. 2014;28:665–684.

7. Breedlove SM, Watson NV. *Biological Psychology*. 7th ed. Sunderland, MA: Sinauer; 2013.

8. Carlson NR. *Physiology of Behavior*. Boston, MA: Pearson Education Inc; 2004.

9. Cone RD. Anatomy and regulation of the central melanocortin system. *Nat Neurosci*. 2005;8(5):571–578.

10. Dallman MF, Pecoraro N, Akana SF, et al. Chronic stress and obesity: a new view of "comfort food". *Proc Natl Acad Sci U S A*. 2003;100(20):11696–11701.

11. Fothergill E, Guo J, Howard L, et al. Persistent metabolic adaptation 6 years after "The Biggest Loser" competition. *Obesity*. 2016;24:1612–1619.
12. Freeman MP. Nutrition and psychiatry. *Am J Psychiatry*. 2010;167:244–247.
13. Havel PJ. Peripheral signals conveying metabolic information to the brain: short-term and long-term regulation of food intake and energy homeostasis. *Exp Biol Med*. 2001;226(11):963–977.
14. Kaati G, Bygren LO, Pembrey M, Sjostrom M. Transgenerational response to nutrition, early life circumstances and longevity. *Eur J Hum Genet*. 2007;15:784–790.
15. Kalm LM, Semba RD. They starved so that others be better fed: remembering Ancel Keys and the Minnesota experiment. *J Nutr*. 2005;135(6):1347–1352.
16. Keesey RE, Boyle PC. Effects of quinine adulteration upon body weight of LH-lesioned and intact male rats. *J Comp Physiol Psychol*. 1973;84(1):38–46.
17. Kroeze WK, Hufeisen SJ, Popadak BA, et al. H1-histamine receptor affinity predicts short-term weight gain for typical and atypical antipsychotic drugs. *Neuropsychopharmacology*. 2003;28(3):519–526.
18. Lorello C, Goldfield GS, Doucet E. Methylphenidate hydrochloride increases energy expenditure in health adults. *Obesity*. 2008;16:470–472.
19. Manini TM. Energy expenditure and aging. *Ageing Res Rev*. 2010;9:1–11.
20. Mineur YS, Abizaid A, Roa Y, et al. Nicotine decreases food intake through activation of POMC neurons. *Science*. 2011;332:1330–1332.
21. Muller MJ, Bosy-Westphal A. Adaptive thermogenesis with weight loss in humans. *Obesity*. 2013;21:218–228.
22. Ochner CN, Kwok Y, Conceicao E, et al. Selective reduction in neural responses to high calorie foods following gastric bypass surgery. *Ann Surg*. 2011;253:502–507.
23. Rapoport JL, Buchsbaum MS, Zahn TP, et al. Dextroamphetamine: cognitive and behavioral effects in normal prepubertal boys. *Science*. 1978;199(4328):560–563.
24. Ravussin E, Valencia ME, Esparza J, et al. Effects of a traditional lifestyle on obesity in Pima Indians. *Diabetes Care*. 1994;17(9):1067–1074.
25. Schwartz MW, Woods SC, Porte Jr D, et al. Central nervous system control of food intake. *Nature*. 2000;404(6778):661–671.
26. Seeley RJ, Woods SC. Monitoring of stored and available fuel by the CNS: implications for obesity. *Nat Rev Neurosci*. 2003;4(11):901–909.
27. Shikora AS, Wolfe BM, Apovian CM, et al. Sustained weight loss with vagal nerve blockade but not with sham: 18-month results of the ReCharge trial. *J Obes*. 2015;2015, Article ID: 365604, 8.
28. Strader AD, Woods SC. Gastrointestinal hormones and food intake. *Gastroenterology*. 2005;128(1):175–191.
29. Stunkard AJ, Sorensen TI, Hanis C, et al. An adoption study of human obesity. *N Engl J Med*. 1986;314(4):193–198.
30. Sumithran P, Prendergast LA, Delbridge E, et al. Long-term persistence of hormonal adaptations to weight loss. *NEJM*. 2011;365:1597–1604.
31. Vaisse C, Clement K, Durand E, et al. Melanocortin-4 receptor mutations are a frequent and heterogeneous cause of morbid obesity. *J Clin Invest*. 2000;106(2):253–262.
32. Volkow ND, Wise RA. How can drug addiction help us understand obesity? *Nat Neurosci*. 2005;8(5):555–560.

CHAPTER 14

1. Bear MF, Connors BW, Paradiso MA. *Neuroscience: Exploring the Brain*. 4th ed. Baltimore, MD: Lippincott Williams & Wilkins; 2015.
2. Birbaumer N, Veit R, Lotze M, et al. Deficient fear conditioning in psychopathy: a functional magnetic resonance imaging study. *Arch Gen Psychiatry*. 2005;62(7):799–805.
3. Blair RJ. Neurobiological basis of psychopathy. *Br J Psychiatry*. 2003;182:5–7.
4. Breedlove SM, Watson NV. *Biological Psychology*. 7th ed. Sunderland, MA: Sinauer; 2013.
5. Brower MC, Price BH. Neuropsychiatry of frontal lobe dysfunction in violent and criminal behaviour: a critical review. *J Neurol Neurosurg Psychiatry*. 2001;71:720–726.
6. Caldwell MF, Van Rybroek G. Effective treatment programs for violent adolescents: programmatic challenges and promising features. *Aggression Violent Behav*. 2013;18:571–578.
7. Coccaro EF, Kavoussi RJ. Fluoxetine and impulsive aggressive behavior in personality-disordered subjects. *Arch Gen Psychiatry*. 1997;54:1081–1088.
8. Coccaro EF, Kavoussi RJ, Hauger RL, et al. Cerebrospinal fluid vasopressin levels: correlates with aggression and serotonin function in personality-disordered subjects. *Arch Gen Psychiatry*. 1998;55:708–714.
9. Damasio H, Grabowski T, Frank R, et al. The return of Phineas Gage: clues about the brain from the skull of a famous patient. *Science*. 1994;264:1102–1105.
10. Decety J, Skelly LR, Kiehl KA. Brain response to Empathy-eliciting scenarios involving pain in incarcerated individuals with psychopathy. *JAMA Psychiatry*. 2013;70:638–645.
11. Ehrenkranz J, Bliss E, Sheard MH. Plasma testosterone: correlation with aggressive behavior and social dominance in man. *Psychosom Med*. 1974;36:469–475.
12. Eisenegger C, Haushofer J, Fehr E. The role of testosterone in social interaction. *Trends Cogn Sci*. 2011;15:263–271.
13. Enserink M. Searching for the mark of Cain. *Science*. 2000;289:575–579.
14. van Erp AM, Miczek KA. Aggressive behavior, increased accumbal dopamine, and decreased cortical serotonin in rats. *J Neurosci*. 2000;20:9320–9325.
15. Flynn JP. The neural basis of aggression in cats. In: Glass DC, ed. *Neurophysicology and Emotion*. New York, NY: Rockefeller University Press; 1967:40–60.
16. Grafman J, Schwab K, Warden D, et al. Frontal lobe injuries, violence, and aggression: a report of the Vietnam Head Injury Study. *Neurology*. 1996;46:1231–1238.
17. Gravett N, Bhagwandin A, Sutcliffe R, et al. Inactivity/sleep in two wild free-roaming African elephant matriarchs – does large body size make elephants the shortest mammalian sleepers? *PLoS One*. 2017;12(3):e0171903.
18. Gregg TR, Siegel A. Brain structures and neurotransmitters regulating aggression in cats: implications for human aggression. *Prog Neuropsychopharmacol Biol Psychiatry*. 2001;25:91–140.
19. Hare RD. *Without Conscience: The Disturbing World of the Psychopaths Among Us*. New York, NY: Guilford Press; 1999.
20. Higley JD, Mehlman PT, Higley SB, et al. Excessive mortality in young free-ranging male nonhuman primates with low cerebrospinal fluid 5-hydroxyindoleacetic acid concentrations. *Arch Gen Psychiatry*. 1996;53(6):537–543.

21. Hoppenbrouwers SS, Nazeri A, de Jesus DR, et al. White matter deficits in psychopathic offenders and correlation with factor structure. *PLoS One*. 2013;8(8):e72375.

22. Kiehl KA, Smith AM, Hare RD, et al. Limbic abnormalities in affective processing by criminal psychopaths as revealed by functional magnetic resonance imaging. *Biol Psychiatry*. 2001;50:677–684.

23. Kiehl KA. *The Psychopath Whisperer: The Science of Those Without Conscience*. New York: Crown Publishers; 2014.

24. Lee GP, Bechara A, Adolphs R, et al. Clinical and physiological effects of stereotaxic bilateral amygdalotomy for intractable aggression. *J Neuropsychiatry Clin Neurosci*. 1998;10(4):413–420.

25. Nelson RJ. *The Biology of Aggression*. New York, NY: Oxford University Press; 2006.

26. Ortiz J, Raine A. Heart rate level and antisocial behavior in children and adolescents: a meta-analysis. *J Am Acad Child Adolesc Psychiatry*. 2004;43(2):154–162.

27. Pardini DA, Raine A, Erickson K, Loeber R. Lower amygdala volume in men is associated with childhood aggression, early psychopathic traits, and future violence. *Bio Psychiatry*. 2014;75:73–80.

28. de Quervain DJ, Fischbacher U, Treyer V, et al. The neural basis of altruistic punishment. *Science*. 2004;305(5688):1254–1258.

29. Raine A. Annotation: the role of prefrontal deficits, low autonomic arousal, and early health factors in the development of antisocial and aggressive behavior in children. *J Child Psychol Psychiatry*. 2002;43:417–434.

30. Raine A. *The Anatomy of Violence: The Biological Roots of Crime*. New York: Pantheon Books; 2013.

31. Raine A, Meloy JR, Bihrle S, et al. Reduced prefrontal and increased subcortical brain functioning assessed using positron emission tomography in predatory and affective murderers. *Behav Sci Law*. 1998;16(3):319–332.

32. Sano K, Mayanagi Y. Posteromedial hypothalamotomy in the treatment of violent, aggressive behaviour. *Acta Neurochir Suppl (Wien)*. 1988;44:145–151.

33. Siegel A, Edinger H, Dotto M. Effects of electrical stimulation of the lateral aspect of the prefrontal cortex upon attack behavior in cats. *Brain Res*. 1975;93:473–484.

34. Tiihonen J, Rautiainen M-R, Ollila HM, et al. Genetic background of extreme violent behavior. *Mol Psychiatry*. 2015;20:786–792.

35. Tricker R, Casaburi R, Storer TW, et al. The effects of supraphysiological doses of testosterone on angry behavior in healthy eugonadal men–a clinical research center study. *J Clin Endocrinol Metab*. 1996;81:3754–3758.

36. Wagner GC, Beuving LJ, Hutchinson RR. The effects of gonadal hormone manipulations on aggressive target-biting in mice. *Aggress Behav*. 1980;6:1–7.

37. Yang Y, Raine A, Narr KL, et al. Localization of deformations within the amygdala in individual with psychopathy. *Arch Gen Psychiatry*. 2009;9:986–994.

CHAPTER 15

1. Acsady L, Harris KD. Synaptic scaling in sleep: the structure of synapses change during sleep. *Science*. 2017;355:457.

2. Bear MF, Connors BW, Paradiso MA, eds. *Neuroscience: Exploring the Brain*. 4th ed. Baltimore, MD: Lippincott Williams & Wilkins; 2015.

3. Breedlove SM, Watson NV. *Biological Psychology*. 7th ed. Sunderland, MA: Sinauer; 2013.

4. Buchsbaum MS, Hazlett EA, Wu J, Bunney WE. Positron emission tomography with deoxyglucose-F18 imaging of sleep. *Neuropsychopharmacology*. 2001; 25:S50–S56.

5. De Vivo L, Bellesi M, Marshall W, et al. Ultrastructural evidence for synaptic scaling across the wake/sleep cycle. *Science*. 2017;355:507–510.

6. Everson CA, Laatsch CD, Hogg N. Antioxidant defense responses to sleep loss and sleep recovery. *Am J Physiol Regul Integr Comp Physiol*. 2005;288(2):R374–R383.

7. Fosse R, Stickgold R, Hobson JA. Brain-mind states: reciprocal variation in thoughts and hallucinations. *Psychol Sci*. 2001;12(1):30–36.

8. Frank MG, Issa NP, Stryker MP. Sleep enhances plasticity in the developing visual cortex. *Neuron*. 2001;30(1):275–287.

9. Guzman-Marin R, Suntsova N, Stewart DR, et al. Sleep deprivation reduces proliferation of cells in the dentate gyrus of the hippocampus in rats. *J Physiol*. 2003;549(pt 2):563–571.

10. Henriksen TEG, Skrede S, Fasmer OB, et al. Blue-blocking glasses as additive treatment for mania: a randomized placebo-controlled trial. *Bipolar Disord*. 2016;18:221–232.

11. Hobson JA. *Sleep*. New York, NY: Scientific American Library; 1989.

12. Hobson JA, Pace-Schott EF. The cognitive neuroscience of sleep: neuronal systems, consciousness and learning. *Nat Rev Neurosci*. 2002;3(9):679–693.

13. Krueger JM, Frank MG, Wisor JP, Roy S. *Sleep Med Rev*. 2016;28:42–50.

14. Kryger MH, Roth T, Dement WC. *Principles and Practice of Sleep Medicine*. 4th ed. Philadelphia, PA: Elsevier Saunders; 2005.

15. Mahowald MW, Schenck CH. Insights from studying human sleep disorders. *Nature*. 2005;437(7063):1279–1285.

16. Mansour HA, Monk TH, Nimgaonkar VL. Circadian genes and bipolar disorder. *Ann Med*. 2005;37(3):196–205.

17. Maret S, Faraguna U, Nelson AB, Cirelli C, Tononi G. Sleep and waking modulate spine turnover in the adolescent mouse cortex. *Nat Neurosci*. 2011;14:1418–1420.

18. Marquie JC, Tucker P, Folkard S, et al. Chronic effects of shift work on cognition: findings from the VISAT longitudinal study. *Occup Environ Med*. 2015;72:258–264.

19. Meddis R. *The Sleep Instinct*. London: Routledge & Kegan Paul; 1977.

20. Mujhametov LM. Sleep in marine mammals. In: Borbely AA, ed. 1984.

21. Nedergaad M. Garbage truck of the brain. *Science*. 2013;340:1529–1530.

22. Nofzinger EA, Buysse DJ, Germain A, et al. Functional neuroimaging evidence for hyperarousal in insomnia. *Am J Psychiatry*. 2004;161(11):2126–2128.

23. Ohayon MM, Carskadon MA, Guilleminault C, et al. Meta-analysis of quantitative sleep parameters from childhood to old age in healthy individuals: developing normative sleep values across the human lifespan. *Sleep*. 2004;27(7):1255–1273.

24. Pace-Schott EF, Hobson JA. The neurobiology of sleep: genetics, cellular physiology and subcortical networks. *Nat Rev Neurosci*. 2002;3(8):591–605.

25. Peigneux P, Laureys S, Fuchs S, et al. Are spatial memories strengthened in the human hippocampus during slow wave sleep? *Neuron*. 2004;44(3):535–545.

26. Purves D, Augustine GJ, Fitzpatrick D, et al. *Neuroscience*. 6th ed. Sunderland, MA: Sinauer; 2017.

27. Ralph MR, Lehman MN. Transplantation: a new tool in the analysis of the mammalian hypothalamic circadian pacemaker. *Trends Neurosci*. 1991;14(8):362–366.

28. Reiter RJ. The melatonin rhythm: both a clock and a calendar. *Experientia*. 1993;49(8):654–664.

29. Saper CB, Scammell TE, Lu J. Hypothalamic regulation of sleep and circadian rhythms. *Nature*. 2005;437(7063):1257–1263.

30. Siegel JM. Sleep viewed as a state of adaptive inactivity. *Nat Rev Neurosci*. 2009;10(10):747–753.

31. Sutherland GR, McNaughton B. Memory trace reactivation in hippocampal and neocortical neuronal ensembles. *Curr Opin Neurobiol*. 2000;10(2):180–186.

32. Taheri S, Lin L, Austin D, et al. Short sleep duration is associated with reduced leptin, elevated ghrelin, and increased body mass index. *PLoS Med*. 2004;1(3):e62.

33. Van Dongen HP, Maislin G, Mullington JM, et al. The cumulative cost of additional wakefulness: dose-response effects on neurobehavioral functions and sleep physiology from chronic sleep restriction and total sleep deprivation. *Sleep*. 2003;26(2):117–126.

34. Walch OJ, Cochran A, Forger DB. A global quantification of "normal" sleep schedules using smartphone data. *Sci Adv*. 2016;2:e1501705.

35. Walsh JK, Krystal AD, Amato DA, et al. Nightly treatment of primary insomnia with eszopiclone for six months: effects on sleep, quality of life, and work limitations. *Sleep*. 2007;30(8):959–968.

36. Wehr TA, Duncan Jr WC, Sher L, et al. A circadian signal of change of season in patients with seasonal affective disorder. *Arch Gen Psychiatry*. 2001;58(12):1108–1114.

37. Wehr TA, Turner EH, Shimada JM, et al. Treatment of rapidly cycling bipolar patient by using extended bed rest and darkness to stabilize the timing and duration of sleep. *Biol Psychiatry*. 1998;43(11):822–828.

38. Xie L, Kang H, Xu Q, et al. Sleep drives metabolic clearance from the adult brain. *Science*. 2013;342:373–377.

39. Yetish G, Kaplan H, Gurven M, et al. Natural sleep and its seasonal variations in three pre-industrial societies. *Curr Biol*. 2015;25:2862–2868.

CHAPTER 16

1. Alexander GM, Hines M. Sex differences in response to children's toys in nonhuman primates (*Cercopithecus aethiops sabaeus*). *Evol Hum Behav*. 2002;23:467–479.

2. Allen LS, Hines M, Shryne JE, et al. Two sexually dimorphic cell groups in the human brain. *J Neurosci*. 1989;9(2):497–506.

3. Bear MF, Connors BW, Paradiso MA, eds. *Neuroscience: Exploring the Brain*. 4th ed. Baltimore, MD: Lippincott Williams & Wilkins; 2015.

4. Ben Zion IZ, Tessler R, Cohen L, et al. Polymorphisms in the dopamine D4 receptor gene (DRD4) contribute to individual differences in human sexual behavior: desire, arousal and sexual function. *Mol Psychiatry*. 2006;11(8):782–786.

5. Breedlove SM, Arnold AP. Hormonal control of a developing neuromuscular system. II. Sensitive periods for the androgen-induced masculinization of the rat spinal nucleus of the bulbocavernosus. *J Neurosci*. 1983;3(2):424–432.

6. Breedlove SM, Watson NV. *Biological Psychology*. 7th ed. Sunderland, MA: Sinauer; 2013.

7. Cohen LS, Altshuler LL, Harlow BL, et al. Relapse of major depression during pregnancy in women who maintain or discontinue antidepressant treatment. *JAMA*. 2006;295(5):499–507.

8. Colapinto J. *As Nature Made Him: The Boy Who was Raised As a Girl*. New York, NY: HarperCollins; 2000.

9. Conn J, Gillam L, Conway GS. Revealing the diagnosis of androgen insensitivity syndrome in adulthood. *Br Med J*. 2005;331(7517):628–630.

10. Dunn KM, Cherkas LF, Spector TD. Genetic influences on variation in female orgasmic function: a twin study. *Biol Lett*. 2005;1(3):260–263.

11. Henderson VW. Alzheimer's disease: review of hormone therapy trials and implications for treatment and prevention after menopause. *J Steroid Biochem Mol Bio*. 2014;142:99–106.

12. Hines M. Sex steroids and human behavior: prenatal androgen exposure and sex-typical play behavior in children. *Ann N Y Acad Sci*. 2003;1007:272–282.

13. Hines M, Ahmed SF, Hughes IA. Psychological outcomes and gender-related development in complete androgen insensitivity syndrome. *Arch Sex Behav*. 2003;32(2):93–101.

14. Hoekzema E, Barba-Muller E, Pozzobon C, et al. Pregnancy leads to long-lasting changes in human brain structure. *Nat Neurosci*. 2017;20:287–296.

15. Jaspers L, Frederik F, Bramer WM, et al. Efficacy and safety of flibanserin for the treatment of hypoactive sexual desire disorder in women. A systematic review and meta-analysis. *JAMA Intern Med*. 2016;176:453–462.

16. Jordan R, Hallam TJ, Molinoff P, Spana C. Developing treatments for female sexual dysfunction. *Clin Pharmacol Ther*. 2011;89(1):137–141.

17. Kreukels BPC, Guillamon. Neuroimaging studies in people with gender incongruence. *Int Rev Psych*. 2016;28:120–128.

18. Laumann EO, Paik A, Rosen RC. Sexual dysfunction in the United States: prevalence and predictors. *JAMA*. 1999;281(6):537–544.

19. LeVay S. A difference in hypothalamic structure between heterosexual and homosexual men. *Science*. 1991;253(5023):1034–1037.

20. Mohnke S, Muller S, Amelung T, et al. Brain alterations in paedophilia: a critical review. *Prog Neurobio*. 2014;122:1–23.

21. Nelson RJ. *An Introduction to Behavioral Endocrinology*. 3rd ed. Sunderland, MA: Sinauer; 2005.

22. Nottebohm F. The road we travelled: discovery, choreography, and significance of brain replaceable neurons. *Ann N Y Acad Sci*. 2004;1016:628–658.

23. Pfaus JG, Shadiack A, Van Soest T, et al. Selective facilitation of sexual solicitation in the female rat by a melanocortin receptor agonist. *Proc Natl Acad Sci U S A*. 2004;101(27):10201–10204.

24. Ponseti J, Granert O, Van Eimeren T, et al. Human face processing is tuned to sexual age preferences. *Biol Lett*. 2014;10:0200.

25. Pope Jr HG, Cohane GH, Kanayama G, et al. Testosterone gel supplementation for men with refractory depression: a randomized, placebo-controlled trial. *Am J Psychiatry*. 2003;160(1):105–111.

26. Purves D, Augustine GJ, Fitzpatrick D, et al. *Neuroscience*. 6th ed. Sunderland, MA: Sinauer; 2017.

27. Rapp SR, Espeland MA, Shumaker SA, et al. Effect of estrogen plus progestin on global cognitive function in postmenopausal women: the Women's Health Initiative Memory Study: a randomized controlled trial. *JAMA*. 2003;289(20):2663–2672.

28. Reiner WG, Gearhart JP. Discordant sexual identity in some genetic males with cloacal exstrophy assigned to female sex at birth. *N Engl J Med*. 2004;350(4):333–341.

29. Roselli CE, Larkin K, Resko JA, et al. The volume of a sexually dimorphic nucleus in the ovine medial preoptic area/anterior hypothalamus varies with sexual partner preference. *Endocrinology*. 2004;145(2):478–483.

30. Rust J, Golombok S, Hines M, et al. The role of brothers and sisters in the gender development of preschool children. *J Exp Child Psychol*. 2000;77(4):292–303.

31. Savic I, Gracia-Falgueras A, Swaab DF. Sexual differentiation of the human brain in relation to gender identity and sexual orientation. *Prog Brain Res*. 2010;186:41–62.

32. Soares CN, Almeida OP, Joffe H, et al. Efficacy of estradiol for the treatment of depressive disorders in perimenopausal women: a double-blind, randomized, placebo-controlled trial. *Arch Gen Psychiatry*. 2001;58(6):529–534.

33. Schule C, Eser D, Baghai C, et al. Neuroactive steroids in affective disorders: target for novel antidepressant or anxiolytic drugs? *Neuroscience*. 2011;191:55–77.

34. Stahl SM. *Essential Psychopharmacology: Neuroscientific Basis of Practical Applications*. 2nd ed. New York, NY: Cambridge University Press; 2000.

35. Wallen K. Nature needs nurture: the interaction of hormonal and social influences on the development of behavioral sex differences in rhesus monkeys. *Horm Behav*. 1996;30(4):364–378.

36. Woolley CS, Weiland NG, McEwen BS, et al. Estradiol increases the sensitivity of hippocampal CA1 pyramidal cells to NMDA receptor-mediated synaptic input: correlation with dendritic spine density. *J Neurosci*. 1997;17(5):1848–1859.

37. Wright DW, Yeatts SD, Silbergleit R, et al. Very early administration of progesterone for acute traumatic brain injury. *NEJM*. 2014;371:2457–2466.

38. Yang LY, Verhovshek T, Sengelaub DR. Brain-derived neurotrophic factor and androgen interact in the maintenance of dendritic morphology in a sexually dimorphic rat spinal nucleus. *Endocrinology*. 2004;145(1):161–168.

39. Zandi PP, Carlson MC, Plassman BL, et al. Hormone replacement therapy and incidence of Alzheimer disease in older women: the Cache County Study. *JAMA*. 2002;288(17):2123–2129.

40. Zucker KJ, Bradley SJ, Oliver G, et al. Psychosexual development of women with congenital adrenal hyperplasia. *Horm Behav*. 1996;30(4):300–318.

CHAPTER 17

1. Aron A, Fisher H, Mashek DJ, et al. Reward, motivation, and emotion systems associated with early-stage intense romantic love. *J Neurophysiol*. 2005;94(1):327–337.

2. Becker JB, Breedlove SM, Crews D, et al. *Behavioral Endocrinology*. 2nd ed. Cambridge, MA: MIT Press; 2002.

3. Bosch OJ, Meddle SL, Beiderbeck DI, et al. Brain oxytocin correlates with maternal aggression: link to anxiety. *J Neurosci*. 2005;25(29):6807–6815.

4. Breedlove SM, Watson NV. *Biological Psychology*. 7th ed. Sunderland, MA: Sinauer; 2013.

5. Bridges RS. Endocrine regulation of parental behavior in rodents. In: Krasnegor NA, Bridges RS, eds. *Mammalian Parenting: Biochemical, Neurobiological and Behavioral Determinants*. New York, NY: Oxford University Press; 1990.

6. Buchen L. In their nurture. *Nature*. 2010;467:146–148.

7. Carr L, Iacoboni M, Dubeau MC, et al. Neural mechanisms of empathy in humans: a relay from neural systems for imitation to limbic areas. *Proc Natl Acad Sci U S A*. 2003;100(9):5497–5502.

8. Dapretto M, Davies MS, Pfeifer JH, et al. Understanding emotions in others: mirror neuron dysfunction in children with autism spectrum disorders. *Nat Neurosci*. 2006;9(1):28–30.

9. Dawson G, Rogers S, Munson J, et al. Randomized, controlled trial of an intervention for toddlers with autism: the Early Start Denver Model. *Pediatrics*. 2010;125(1):e17–e23.

10. Emanuele E, Politi P, Bianchi M, et al. Raised plasma nerve growth factor levels associated with early-stage romantic love. *Psychoneuroendocrinology*. 2006;31:288–294.

11. Engh AL, Beehner JC, Bergman TJ, et al. Behavioral and hormonal responses to predation in female chacma baboons (*Papio hamadryas ursinus*). *Proc R Soc Lond B Biol Sci*. 2006;273(1578):707–712.

12. Felsenfeld G, Groudine M. Controlling the double helix. *Nature*. 2003;421(6921):448–453.

13. Francis D, Diorio J, Liu D, et al. Nongenomic transmission across generations of maternal behavior and stress responses in the rat. *Science*. 1999;286(5442):1155–1158.

14. Hazlett HC, Gu H, Munsell BC, et al. Early brain development in infants at high risk for autism spectrum disorder. *Nature*. 2017;542:348–351.

15. Iacoboni M. Neural mechanisms of imitation. *Curr Opin Neurobiol*. 2005;15(6):632–637.

16. Klin A, Jones W, Schultz R, et al. Visual fixation patterns during viewing of naturalistic social situations as predictors of social competence in individuals with autism. *Arch Gen Psychiatry*. 2002;59(9):809–816.

17. Klin A, Jones W, Schultz R, et al. Defining and quantifying the social phenotype in autism. *Am J Psychiatry*. 2002;159(6):895–908.

18. Li M, Davidson P, Budin R, et al. Effects of typical and atypical antipsychotic drugs on maternal behavior in postpartum female rats. *Schizophr Res*. 2004;70(1):69–80.

19. Lim MM, Wang Z, Olazabal DE, et al. Enhanced partner preference in a promiscuous species by manipulating the expression of a single gene. *Nature*. 2004;429:754–757.

20. Liu D, Diorio J, Tannenbaum B, et al. Maternal care, hippocampal glucocorticoid receptors, and hypothalamic-pituitary-adrenal responses to stress. *Science*. 1997;277(5332):1659–1662.

21. McGowan PO, Sasaki A, D'Alessio AC, et al. Epigenetic regulation of the glucocorticoid receptor in human brain associates with childhood abuse. *Nat Neurosci*. 2009;12(3):342–348.

22. Mcgue M, Lykken DT. Genetic influence on risk of divorce. *Psychol Sci*. 1992;3(6):368–373.

23. Meyer-Lindenberg A, Domes G, Kirsch P, Heinrichs M. Oxytocin and vasopressin in the human brain: social neuropeptides for translational medicine. *Nat Rev Neurosci*. 2011;12:524–538.

24. Moriuchi JM, Ami Klin MA, Jones W. Mechanisms of diminished attention to eyes in autism. *Am J Psychiatry*. 2017;174:26–35.

25. Nelson RJ. *An Introduction to Behavioral Endocrinology*. 3rd ed. Sunderland, MA: Sinauer; 2005.

26. Numan M, Sheehan TP. Neuroanatomical circuitry for mammalian maternal behavior. *Ann N Y Acad Sci.* 1997;807:101–125.
27. Purves D, Augustine GJ, Fitzpatrick D, et al. *Neuroscience.* 6th ed. Sunderland, MA: Sinauer; 2017.
28. Redcay E, Courchesne E. When is the brain enlarged in autism? A meta-analysis of all brain size reports. *Biol Psychiatry.* 2005;58(1):1–9.
29. Rizzolatti G, Fogassi L, Gallese V. Neurophysiological mechanisms underlying the understanding and imitation of action. *Nat Rev Neurosci.* 2001;2(9):661–670.
30. Rosenblatt JS, Siegel HI, Mayer AD. Progress in the study of maternal behavior in the rat: hormonal, nonhormonal, sensory, and developmental aspects. *Adv Study Behav.* 1979;10:225–311.
31. Schultz RT, Anderson GM. The neurobiology of autism and the pervasive developmental disorders. In: Charney DS, Nestler EJ, eds. *Neurobiology of Mental Illness.* 2nd ed. Oxford: Oxford University Press; 2004:954–967.
32. Tang G, Gudsnuk K, Kuo SH, et al. Loss of mTOR-dependent macroautophagy causes austic-like synaptic pruning deficits. *Neuron.* 2014;83:1131–1143.
33. Taylor SE, Klein LC, Lewis BP, et al. Biobehavioral responses to stress in females: tend-and-befriend, not fight-or-flight. *Psychol Rev.* 2000;107(3):411–429.
34. Terkel J, Rosenblatt JS. Maternal behavior induced by maternal blood plasma injected into virgin rats. *J Comp Physiol Psychol.* 1968;65(3):479–482.
35. Walem H, Wastberg L, Henningsson S, et al. Genetic variation in the vasopressin receptor 1a gene (AVPR1A) associates with pair-bonding behavior in humans. *Proc Natl Acad Sci U S A.* 2008;105(37):14153–14156.
36. Weaver IC, Cervoni N, Champagne FA, et al. Epigenetic programming by maternal behavior. *Nat Neurosci.* 2004;7(8):847–854.
37. Werner E, Dawson G. Validation of the phenomenon of autistic regression using home videotapes. *Arch Gen Psychiatry.* 2005;62(8):889–895.
38. Wolff JJ, Gu H, Gerig G, et al. Differences in white matter fiber tract development present from 6 to 24 months in infants with autism. *Am J Psychiatry.* 2012;169(6):589–600.
39. Young LJ, Wang Z. The neurobiology of pair bonding. *Nat Neurosci.* 2004;7(10):1048–1054.
40. Zietsch BP, Westberg L, Santtila P, Patrick J. Genetic analysis of human extrapair mating: heritability, between-sex correlation, and receptor genes for vasopressin and oxytocin. *Evol Hum Behav.* 2015;36:130–136.

CHAPTER 18
1. Akers KG, Martinez-Canabal A, Restivo L, et al. Hippocampal neurogenesis regulates forgetting during adulthood and infancy. *Science.* 2014;344:598–602.
2. Annese J, Schenker-Ahmed NM, Bartsch H, et al. Postmortem examination of patient H.M.'s brain based on histological sectioning and digital 3D reconstruction. *Nature Commun.* 2014;5, Article number: 3122. doi:10.1038/ncomms4122.
3. Barad M. Fear extinction in rodents: basic insight to clinical promise. *Curr Opin Neurobiol.* 2005;15(6):710–715.
4. Bayley PJ, Gold JJ, Hopkins RO, et al. The neuroanatomy of remote memory. *Neuron.* 2005;46(5):799–810.
5. Bear MF, Connors BW, Paradiso MA, eds. *Neuroscience: Exploring the Brain.* 4th ed. Baltimore, MD: Lippincott Williams & Wilkins; 2015.

6. Breedlove SM, Watson NV. *Biological Psychology.* 7th ed. Sunderland, MA: Sinauer; 2013.
7. Corkin S. What's new with the amnesic patient H.M.? *Nat Rev Neurosci.* 2002;3(2):153–160.
8. Frankland PW, Bontempi B. The organization of recent and remote memories. *Nat Rev Neurosci.* 2005;6(2):119–130.
9. Genoux D, Haditsch U, Knobloch M, et al. Protein phosphatase 1 is a molecular constraint on learning and memory. *Nature.* 2002;418(6901):970–975.
10. Guan JS, Haggarty SJ, Giacometti, et al. HDAC2 negatively regulates memory formation and synaptic plasticity. *Nature.* 2009;459(7243):55–60.
11. Hebb DO. *The Organization of Behavior.* New York, NY: Wiley; 1949.
12. Hofmann SG, Smits JAJ, Asnaani A, et al. Cognitive enhancers for anxiety disorders. *Pharmacol Biochem Behav.* 2011;99:275–284.
13. Kandel ER, Schwartz JH, Jessell TM, eds. *Principles of Neural Science.* 4th ed. New York, NY: McGraw-Hill; 2000.
14. Kirn J, O'Loughlin B, Kasparian S, et al. Cell death and neuronal recruitment in the high vocal center of adult male canaries are temporally related to changes in song. *Proc Natl Acad Sci U S A.* 1994;91(17):7844–7848.
15. Kroes MCW, Tendolkar I, Van Wingen GA, Van Waarde JA, Strange BA, Fernandez G. An electroconvulsive therapy procedure impairs reconsolidation of episodic memories in humans. *Nat Neurosci.* 2014;17(2):204–206.
16. Lamprecht R, LeDoux J. Structural plasticity and memory. *Nat Rev Neurosci.* 2004;5(1):45–54.
17. Leuner B, Falduto J, Shors TJ. Associative memory formation increases the observation of dendritic spines in the hippocampus. *J Neurosci.* 2003;23(2):659–665.
18. Leuner B, Mendolia-Loffredo S, Kozorovitskiy Y, et al. Learning enhances the survival of new neurons beyond the time when the hippocampus is required for memory. *J Neurosci.* 2004;24(34):7477–7481.
19. Luria AR. *The Mind of a Mnemonist.* New York, NY: Basic Books; 1968.
20. Maviel T, Durkin TP, Menzaghi F, et al. Sites of neocortical reorganization critical for remote spatial memory. *Science.* 2004;305(5680):96–99.
21. McGuire JF, Wu MS, Piacentini J, McCracken T, Storch EA. A meta-analysis of D-cycloserine in exposure-based treatment: moderators of treatment efficacy, response, and diagnostic remission. *J Clin Psych.* 2017;78(2):196–206.
22. Meiri N, Rosenblum K. Lateral ventricle injection of the protein synthesis inhibitor anisomycin impairs long-term memory in a spatial memory task. *Brain Res.* 1998;789(1):48–55.
23. Mikaelsson MA, Miller CA. The path to epigenetic treatment of memory disorders. *Neurobiol Learn Mem.* 2011;96:13–18.
24. Nader K, Schafe GE, Le Doux JE. Fear memories require protein synthesis in the amygdala for reconsolidation after retrieval. *Nature.* 2000;406(6797):722–726.
25. Nobler MS, Sackeim HA. Neurobiological correlates of the cognitive side effects of electroconvulsive therapy. *J ECT.* 2008;24(1):40–45.
26. Purves D, Augustine GJ, Fitzpatrick D, et al. *Neuroscience.* 6th ed. Sunderland, MA: Sinauer; 2017.
27. Ressler KJ, Rothbaum BO, Tannenbaum L, et al. Cognitive enhancers as adjuncts to psychotherapy: use of D-cycloserine in phobic individuals to facilitate extinction of fear. *Arch Gen Psychiatry.* 2004;61(11):1136–1144.

28. Sackeim HA, Prudic J, Ruller R, et al. The cognitive effects of electroconvulsive therapy in community settings. *Neuropsychopharmacology.* 2007;32:244–454.

29. Santini E, Ge H, Ren K, et al. Consolidation of fear extinction requires protein synthesis in the medial prefrontal cortex. *J Neurosci.* 2004;24(25):5704–5710.

30. Van Hoesen GW. The parahippocampal gyrus: new observations regarding its cortical connections in the monkey. *Trends Neurosci.* 1982;5:345–350.

31. Wei Y, Krishnan GP, Bazhenov M. Synaptic mechanisms of memory consolidation during sleep slow oscillations. *J Neurosci.* 2016;36(15):4231–4247.

CHAPTER 19

1. Andreasen NC. *The Creating Brain: The Neuroscience of Genius.* New York, NY: Dana Press; 2005.

2. Beckett C, Maughan B, Rutter M, et al. Do the effects of early severe deprivation on cognition persist into early adolescence? Findings from the English and Romanian adoptees study. *Child Dev.* 2006;77(3):696–711.

3. Breslau N, Lucia VC, Alvarado GF. Intelligence and other predisposing factors in exposure to trauma and posttraumatic stress disorder. *Arch Gen Psychiatry.* 2006;63(11):1238–1245.

4. Carlsson I, Wendt PE, Risberg J. On the neurobiology of creativity. Differences in frontal activity between high and low creative subjects. *Neuropsychologia.* 2000;38(6):873–885.

5. Carson SH, Peterson JB, Higgins DM. Decreased latent inhibition is associated with increased creative achievement in high-functioning individuals. *J Pers Soc Psychol.* 2003;85(3):499–506.

6. Dierssen M, Ramakers GJA. Dendritic pathology in mental retardation: from molecular genetics to neurobiology. *Genes Brain Behav.* 2006;5(suppl 2):48–60.

7. Dietrich A, Kanso R. A review of EEG, ERP, and neuroimaging studies of creativity and insight. *Psychol Bull.* 2010;136(5):822–848.

8. Glascher J, Rudrauf D, Colom R, et al. Distributed neural system for general intelligence revealed by lesion mapping. *Proc Natl Acad Sci U S A.* 2010;107(10):4705–4709.

9. Gottfredson LS. The general intelligence factor. *Sci Am Presents: Exploring Intell.* 1998;9(4):24–29.

10. Gray JR, Thompson PM. Neurobiology of intelligence: science and ethics. *Nat Rev Neurosci.* 2004;5(6):471–482.

11. Haaz J, Westlye ET, Fjaer S, Espeseth T, Lundervold A, Lundervold AJ. General fluid-type intelligence is related to indices of white matter structure in middle-aged and old adults. *Neuroimage.* 2013;83:372–383.

12. Haier RJ. *The Neuroscience of Intelligence.* Cambridge University Press; 2016.

13. Hearne LJ, Mattingley JB, Cocchi L. Functional brain networks related to individual differences in human intelligence at rest. *Sci Rep.* 2016;6:32328. doi:10.1038/srep32328.

14. Harris JC. Chauvet Cave: the panel of horses. *Arch Gen Psychiatry.* 2011;68(9):869–870.

15. Ilieva I, Boland J, Farah MJ. Objective and subjective cognitive enhancing effects of mixed amphetamine salts in healthy people. *Neuropharmacolgy.* 2013;64:496–505.

16. Jamison KR. Manic-depressive illness and creativity. *Sci Am.* 1995;272(2):62–67.

17. Kahn RS, Keefe RSE. Schizophrenia is a cognitive illness – time for a change in focus. *JAMA Psychiatry.* 2013;70(10):1107–1112.

18. Kyaga S, Lichtenstein P, Boman M, Hutman C, Langstrom N, Landen M. *Br J Psychiatry.* 2011;199:373–379.

19. Limb CJ, Braun AR. Neural substrates of spontaneous musical performance: an fMRI study of jazz improvisation. *PLoS One.* 2008:e1679. doi:10.1371/journal.pone.0001679.

20. MacCabe JH, Lambe MP, Cnattingius S, et al. Excellent school performance at age 16 and risk of adult bipolar disorder: national cohort study. *Br J Psychiatry.* 2010;196:109–115.

21. Maher B. Poll results: look who's doping. *Nature.* 2008;452:674–675.

22. McDaniel MA. Big-brained people are smarter: a meta-analysis of the relationship between in vivo brain volume and intelligence. *Intelligence.* 2005;33(4):337–346.

23. Mell JC, Howard SM, Miller BL. Art and the brain: the influence of frontotemporal dementia on an accomplished artist. *Neurology.* 2003;60(10):1707–1710.

24. Nottebohm F. The road we travelled: discovery, choreography, and significance of brain replaceable neurons. *Ann N Y Acad Sci.* 2004;1016:628–658.

25. Plomin R, DeFries JC. The genetics of cognitive abilities and disabilities. *Sci Am.* 1998;278(5):62–69.

26. Purpura DP. Dendritic spine "dysgenesis" and mental retardation. *Science.* 1974;186(4169):1126–1128.

27. Roth G, Dicke U. Evolution of the brain and intelligence. *Trends Cogn Sci.* 2005;9(5):250–257.

28. Schoenemann PT, Sheehan MJ, Glotzer LD. Prefrontal white matter volume is disproportionately larger in humans than in other primates. *Nat Neurosci.* 2005;8(2):242–252.

29. Shaw P, Greenstein D, Lerch J, et al. Intellectual ability and cortical development in children and adolescents. *Nature.* 2006;440(7084):676–679.

30. Shaywitz SE, Shaywitz BA. Dyslexia (specific reading disability). *Biol Psychiatry.* 2005;57(11):1301–1309.

31. Simonton DK. Are genius and madness related? Contemporary answers to an ancient question. *Psychiatry Times.* 2005;22(7):21–23.

32. Smith ME, Farah MJ. Are prescription stimulants "Smart Pills"? The epidemiology and cognitive neuroscience of prescription stimulant use by normal healthy individuals. *Psychol Bull.* 2011;137(5):717–741.

33. Stix G. Turbocharging the brain. *Sci Am.* 2009;301(4):46–55.

CHAPTER 20

1. Banaschewski T, Becker K, Scherag S, Franke B, Coghill D. Molecular genetics of attention-deficit/hyperactivity disorder: an overview. *Eur Child Adolesc Psychiatry.* 2010;19:237–257.

2. Bear MF, Connors BW, Paradiso MA, eds. *Neuroscience: Exploring the Brain.* 4th ed. Baltimore, MD: Lippincott Williams & Wilkins; 2015.

3. Ben-Pazi H, Shalev RS, Gross-Tsur V, et al. Age and medication effects on rhythmic response in ADHD: possible oscillatory mechanisms? *Neuropsychologia.* 2006;44:412–416.

4. Bobb AJ, Castellanos FX, Addington AM, et al. Molecular genetic studies of ADHD: 1991 to 2004. *Am J Med Genet B Neuropsychiatr Genet.* 2005;132(1):109–125.

5. Cardinal RN, Pennicott DR, Sugathapala CL, et al. Impulsive choice induced in rats by lesions of the nucleus accumbens core. *Science.* 2001;292(5526):2499–2501.

6. Cardinal RN, Winstanley CA, Robbins TW, et al. Limbic corticostriatal systems and delayed reinforcement. *Ann N Y Acad Sci.* 2004;1021:33–50.

7. Castellanos FX, Lee PP, Sharp W, et al. Developmental trajectories of brain volume abnormalities in children and adolescents with attention-deficit/hyperactivity disorder. *JAMA*. 2002;288(14):1740–1748.

8. Castellanos FX, Tannock R. Neuroscience of attention-deficit/hyperactivity disorder: the search for endophenotypes. *Nat Rev Neurosci*. 2002;3(8):617–628.

9. Castner SA, Williams GV, Goldman-Rakic PS. Reversal of antipsychotic-induced working memory deficits by short-term dopamine D1 receptor stimulation. *Science*. 2000;287(5460):2020–2022.

10. Faraone SV, Biederman J, Mick E. The age-dependent decline of attention deficit hyperactivity disorder: a meta-analysis of follow-up studies. *Psychol Med*. 2006;36(2):159–165.

11. Franke B, Meale BM, Faraone SV. Genome-wide association studies in ADHD. *Hum Genet*. 2009;126: 13–50.

12. Fuster JM. Unit activity in prefrontal cortex during delayed-response performance: neuronal correlates of transient memory. *J Neurophysiol*. 1973;36(1):61–78.

13. Gelade K, Bink M, Janssen TWP, Van Mourik R, Maras A, Oosterlaan J. An RCT into the effects of neurofeedback on neurocognitive functioning compared to stimulant medication and physical activity in children with ADHD. *Eur Child Adolesc Psychiatry*. 2017;26:457–468.

14. Greenberg LM, Crosby RD. *A Summary of Developmental Normative Data on the T.O.V.A. Ages 4 to 80+*. Unpublished Manuscript Available through The TOVA Company; 1992.

15. Hawi Z, Cummins TDR, Tong J, et al. The molecular genetic architecture of attention deficit hyperactivity disorder. *Mol Psychiatry*. 2015;20:289–297.

16. Landhuis CE, Poulton R, Welch D, Hancox RJ. Does childhood television viewing lead to attention problems in adolescence? Results from a prospective longitudinal study. *Pediatrics*. 2007;120:532–537.

17. Larisch R, Sitte W, Antke C, et al. Striatal dopamine transporter density in drug naive patients with attention-deficit/hyperactivity disorder. *Nucl Med Commun*. 2006;27(3):267–270.

18. Levesque J, Beauregard M, Mensour B. Effect of neurofeedback training on the neural substrates of selective attention in children with attention-deficit/hyperactivity disorder: a functional magnetic resonance imaging study. *Neurosci Lett*. 2006;394(3):216–221.

19. Lillard AS, Peterson J. The immediate impact of different types of television on young children's executive function. *Pediatrics*. 2011;128:644–649.

20. McEvoy SP, Stevenson MR, McCartt AT, et al. Role of mobile phones in motor vehicle crashes resulting in hospital attendance: a case-crossover study. *BMJ*. 2005;331(7514):428.

21. Mozley PD, Acton PD, Barraclough ED, et al. Effects of age on dopamine transporters in healthy humans. *J Nucl Med*. 1999;40(11):1812–1817.

22. Nakao T, Radua J, Rubia K, Mataix-Cols D. Gray matter volume abnormalities in ADHD: voxel-based meta-analysis exploring the effects of age and stimulant medication. *Am J Psychiatry*. 2011;168(11):1154–1163.

23. Nutt DJ, King LA, Phillips LD. Drug harm in the UK: a multicriteria decision analysis. *Lancet*. 2010;376:1558–1565.

24. Phillips AG, Ahn S, Floresco SB. Magnitude of dopamine release in medial prefrontal cortex predicts accuracy of memory on a delayed response task. *J Neurosci*. 2004;24(2):547–553.

25. Purves D, Augustine GJ, Fitzpatrick D, et al. *Neuroscience*. 6th ed. Sunderland, MA: Sinauer; 2017.

26. Shaw P, Lerch J, Greenstein D, et al. Longitudinal mapping of cortical thickness and clinical outcome in children and adolescents with attention-deficit/hyperactivity disorder. *Arch Gen Psychiatry*. 2006;63(5):540–549.

27. Tamm L, Menon V, Reiss AL. Parietal attentional system aberrations during target detection in adolescents with attention deficit hyperactivity disorder: event-related fMRI evidence. *Am J Psychiatry*. 2006;163(6):1033–1043.

28. Van Elst LT, Maier S, Kloppel S, et al. The effect of methylphenidate intake on brain structure in adults with ADHD in a placebo-controlled randomized trial. *J Psychiatry Neruosci*. 2016;41(6):422–430.

29. Toplak ME, Dockstader C, Tannock R. Temporal information processing in ADHD: findings to date and new methods. *J Neurosci Methods*. 2006;151(1):15–29.

30. Volkow ND. Long-term safety of stimulant use for ADHD: findings from nonhuman primates. *Neuropsychopharmacology*. 2012;37:2551–2552.

31. Volkow ND, Wang GJ, Fowler JS, et al. Evidence that methylphenidate enhances the saliency of a mathematical task by increasing dopamine in the human brain. *Am J Psychiatry*. 2004;161(7):1173–1180.

32. Volkow ND, Wang GJ, Fowler JS, et al. Imaging the effects of methylphenidate on brain dopamine: new model on its therapeutic actions for attention-deficit/hyperactivity disorder. *Biol Psychiatry*. 2005;57(11):1410–1415.

CHAPTER 21

1. Autry A, Adachi M, Nosyreva E, et al. NMDA receptor blockade at rest triggers rapid behavioural antidepressant responses. *Nature*. 2011;475:91–95.

2. Berton O, McClung CA, Dileone RJ, et al. Essential role of BDNF in the mesolimbic dopamine pathway in social defeat stress. *Science*. 2006;311(5762):864–868.

3. Berton O, Nestler EJ. New approaches to antidepressant drug discovery: beyond monoamines. *Nat Rev Neurosci*. 2006;7(2):137–151.

4. Brady RO, Margolis A, Masters GA, Keshavan M, Ongur D. Bipolar mood state reflected in cortico-amygdala resting state connectivity: a cohort and longitudinal study. J Affect Disord. 2017;217:205–209.

5. Caspi A, Sugden K, Moffitt TE, et al. Influence of life stress on depression: moderation by a polymorphism in the 5-HTT gene. *Science*. 2003;301:386–389.

6. Deuschle M, Schweiger U, Weber B, et al. Diurnal activity and pulsatility of the hypothalamus-pituitary-adrenal system in male depressed patients and healthy controls. *J Clin Endocrinol Metab*. 1997;82(1):234–238.

7. Dougherty DD, Rezai AR, Carpenter LL, et al. A randomized sham-controlled trial of deep brain stimulation of the ventral capsule/ventral striatum for chronic treatment-resistant depression. *Bio Psychiatry*. 2015;78:240–248.

8. Drevets WC. Neuroimaging and neuropathological studies of depression: implications for the cognitive-emotional features of mood disorders. *Curr Opin Neurobiol*. 2001;11(2):240–249.

9. Duman RS. The neurochemistry of depressive disorders: preclinical studies. In: Charney DS, Nestler EJ, eds. *Neurobiology of Mental Illness*. 2nd ed. New York, NY: Oxford University Press; 2004:421–439.

10. Dwivedi Y, Rizavi HS, Conley RR, et al. Altered gene expression of brain-derived neurotrophic factor and receptor tyrosine kinase B in postmortem brain of suicide subjects. *Arch Gen Psychiatry*. 2003;60(8):804–815.

11. Haldane M, Frangou S. New insights help define the pathophysiology of bipolar affective disorder: neuroimaging and neuropathology findings. *Prog Neuropsychopharmacol Biol Psychiatry*. 2004;28(6):943–960.

12. Haldane M, Frangou S. Functional neuroimaging studies in mood disorders. *Acta Neuropsychiatr*. 2006;18:88–99.

13. Holsboer F. Stress, hypercortisolism and corticosteroid receptors in depression: implications for therapy. *J Affect Disord*. 2001;62(1–2):77–91.

14. Koss S, George MS. Functional magnetic resonance imaging investigations in mood disorders. In: Soares JC, ed. *Brain Imaging in Affective Disorders*. New York, NY: Marcel Dekker Inc; 2003.

15. Li N, Liu RJ, Dwyer JM, et al. Glutamate N-methyl-D-aspartate receptor antagonists rapidly reverse behavioral and synaptic deficits caused by chronic stress exposure. *Bio Psychiatry*. 2011;69:754–761.

16. Mamounas LA, Blue ME, Siuciak JA, et al. Brain-derived neurotrophic factor promotes the survival and sprouting of serotonergic axons in rat brain. *J Neurosci*. 1995;15(12):7929–7939.

17. Manji HK, Quiroz JA, Sporn J, et al. Enhancing neuronal plasticity and cellular resilience to develop novel, improved therapeutics for difficult-to-treat depression. *Biol Psychiatry*. 2003;53(8):707–742.

18. McQuade R, Young AH. Future therapeutic targets in mood disorders: the glucocorticoid receptor. *Br J Psychiatry*. 2000;177:390–395.

19. Moore GJ, Bebchuk JM, Wilds IB, et al. Lithium-induced increase in human brain grey matter. *Lancet*. 2000;356(9237):1241–1242.

20. Muller VI, Cieslik EC, Serbanescu I, Laird AR, Fox PT, Eickhoff SB. Altered brain activity in unipolar depression revisited. Meta-analyses of neuroimaging studies. *JAMA Psychiatry*. 2017;74(1):47-55.

21. Nobler MS, Oquendo MA, Kegeles LS, et al. Decreased regional brain metabolism after ECT. *Am J Psychiatry*. 2001;158(2):305–308.

22. Rajkowska G, Miguel-Hidalgo JJ, Wei J, et al. Morphometric evidence for neuronal and glial prefrontal cell pathology in major depression. *Biol Psychiatry*. 1999;45(9):1085–1098.

23. Risch N, Herrell R, Lehner T, et al. Interaction between the serotonin transporter gene (5-HTTLPR), stressful life events, and risk of depression. *JAMA*. 2009;301(23):2462–2471.

24. Santarelli L, Saxe M, Gross C, et al. Requirement of hippocampal neurogenesis for the behavioral effects of antidepressants. *Science*. 2003;301(5634):805–809.

25. Tsankova NM, Berton O, Renthal W, et al. Sustained hippocampal chromatin regulation in a mouse model of depression and antidepressant action. *Nat Neurosci*. 2006;9(4):519–525.

26. Videbech P, Ravnkilde B. Hippocampal volume and depression: a meta-analysis of MRI studies. *Am J Psychiatry*. 2004;161(11):1957–1966.

27. Whitton AE, Treatway MT, Pizzagalli DA. Reward processing dysfunction in major depression, bipolar disorder and schizophrenia. *Curr Opin Psychiatry*. 2015;28(1):7–12.

28. Wolkowitz OM, Wolf J, Shelly W, et al. Serum BDNF levels before treatment predict SSRI response in depression. *Prog Neuropsychopharmacol Biol Psychiatry*. 2011;35:1623–1630.

29. Wong ML, Licinio J. Research and treatment approaches to depression. *Nat Rev Neurosci*. 2001;2(5):343–351.

30. Zanos P, Moaddel R, Morris P, et al. NMDAR inhibition-independent antidepressant actions of ketamine metabolites. *Nature*. 2016;533:481–486.

31. Zobel AW, Nickel T, Sonntag A, et al. Cortisol response in the combined dexamethasone/CRH test as predictor of relapse in patients with remitted depression. A prospective study. *J Psychiatr Res*. 2001;35(2):83–94.

CHAPTER 22

1. Abi-Dargham A, Krystal JH, Anjilvel S, et al. Alterations of benzodiazepine receptors in type II alcoholic subjects measured with SPECT and [123I] iomazenil. *Am J Psychiatry*. 1998;155(11):1550–1555.

2. Barlow DH, Gorman JM, Shear MK, et al. Cognitive-behavioral therapy, imipramine, or their combination for panic disorder: a randomized controlled trial. *JAMA*. 2000;283(19):2529–2536.

3. Baxter Jr LR, Schwartz JM, Bergman KS, et al. Caudate glucose metabolic rate changes with both drug and behavior therapy for obsessive-compulsive disorder. *Arch Gen Psychiatry*. 1992;49(9):681–689.

4. Berton O, McClung CA, Dileone RJ, et al. Essential role of BDNF in the mesolimbic dopamine pathway in social defeat stress. *Science*. 2006;311(5762):864–868.

5. Breedlove SM, Watson NV. *Biological Psychology*. 7th ed. Sunderland, MA: Sinauer; 2013.

6. Burghardt NS, Sigurdsson T, Gorman JM, McEwen BS, LeDoux JE. Chronic antidepressant treatment impairs the acquisition of fear extinction. *Bio Psychiatry*. 2013;73:1078–1086.

7. Burghardt NS, Bauer EP. Acute and chronic effects of selective serotonin reuptake inhibitor treatment on fear conditioning: implications for underlying fear circuits. *Neurosci*. 2013;247:253–272.

8. Calder AJ, Lawrence AD, Young AW. Neuropsychology of fear and loathing. *Nat Rev Neurosci*. 2001;2(5):352–363.

9. Charney DS. Neuroanatomical circuits modulating fear and anxiety behaviors. *Acta Psychiatr Scand Suppl*. 2003;417:38–50.

10. Furmark T, Tillfors M, Marteinsdottir I, et al. Common changes in cerebral blood flow in patients with social phobia treated with citalopram or cognitive-behavioral therapy. *Arch Gen Psychiatry*. 2002;59(5):425–433.

11. Gilbertson MW, Shenton ME, Ciszewski A, et al. Smaller hippocampal volume predicts pathologic vulnerability to psychological trauma. *Nat Neurosci*. 2002;5(11):1242–1247.

12. Gross C, Hen R. The developmental origins of anxiety. *Nat Rev Neurosci*. 2004;5(7):545–552.

13. Kirschbaum C, Prussner JC, Stone AA, et al. Persistent high cortisol responses to repeated psychological stress in a subpopulation of healthy men. *Psychosom Med*. 1995;57(5):468–474.

14. Kremen WS, Koenen KC, Afari N, Lyons MJ. Twin studies of posttraumatic stress disorder: differentiating vulnerability factors from sequelae. *Neuropharmacology.* 2012;62:647–653.
15. Kushner MG, Abrams K, Borchardt C. The relationship between anxiety disorders and alcohol use disorders: a review of major perspectives and findings. *Clin Psychol Rev.* 2000;20(2):149–171.
16. Lang PJ, McTeague LM, Bradley MM. RDoC, DSM, and the reflex physiology of fear: a biodimensional analysis of the anxiety disorders spectrum. *Psychophysiology.* 2016;53:336–347.
17. LeDoux JE. Emotion, memory and the brain. *Sci Am.* 1994;270(6):50–57.
18. LeDoux JE. *The Synaptic Self: How Our Brains Become Who We Are.* New York, NY: Viking; 2002.
19. LeDoux JE, Pine DS. Using neuroscience to help understand fear and anxiety: a two-system framework. *Am J Psychiatry.* 2016;173:1083–1093.
20. Likhtik E, Pelletier JG, Paz R, et al. Prefrontal control of the amygdala. *J Neurosci.* 2005;25(32):7429–7437.
21. Lorberbaum JP, Kose S, Johnson MR, et al. Neural correlates of speech anticipatory anxiety in generalized social phobia. *Neuroreport.* 2004;15(18):2701–2705.
22. Mahan AL, Ressler KJ. Fear conditioning, synaptic plasticity and the amygdala: implications for posttraumatic stress disorder. *Trends Neurosci.* 2012;35(1):24–35.
23. Maren S, Ferrario CR, Corcoran KA, et al. Protein synthesis in the amygdala, but not the auditory thalamus, is required for consolidation of Pavlovian fear conditioning in rats. *Eur J Neurosci.* 2003;18(11):3080–3088.
24. Maxmen A. A psychedelic compound in ecstasy moves closer to approval to treat PTSD. *Nature.* 2017. doi:10.1038/nature.2017.21917.
25. Mashour GA, Walker EE, Martuza RL. Psychosurgery: past, present, and future. *Brain Res Brain Res Rev.* 2005;48(3):409–419.
26. Montgomery SM, Ehlin A, Sacker A. Breast feeding and resilience against psychosocial stress. *Arch Dis Child.* 2006;91(12):990–994.
27. Ostrowski SA, Delanhanty DL. Prospects for the pharmacological prevention of post-traumatic stress in vulnerable individuals. *CNS Drugs.* 2014;28:195–203.
28. Otto MW, Smits JAJ, Reese HE. Combined psychotherapy and pharmacotherapy for mood and anxiety disorders in adults: review and analysis. *Clin Psychol: Sci Pract.* 2005;12(1):72–86.
29. Purves D, Augustine GJ, Fitzpatrick D, et al. *Neuroscience.* 6th ed. Sunderland, MA: Sinauer; 2017.
30. Richter EO, Davis KD, Hamani C, et al. Cingulotomy for psychiatric disease: microelectrode guidance, a callosal reference system for documenting lesion location, and clinical results. *Neurosurgery.* 2004;54(3):622–628, discussion 8–30.
31. Shin LM, Wright CI, Cannistraro PA, et al. A functional magnetic resonance imaging study of amygdala and medial prefrontal cortex responses to overtly presented fearful faces in posttraumatic stress disorder. *Arch Gen Psychiatry.* 2005;62(3):273–281.
32. Stein DJ. Obsessive-compulsive disorder. *Lancet.* 2002;360(9330):397–405.
33. Ursin H, Baade E, Levine S. *Psychobiology of Stress: A Study of Coping Men.* New York, NY: Academic Press; 1978.
34. Vyas A, Pillai AG, Chattarji S. Recovery after chronic stress fails to reverse amygdaloid neuronal hypertrophy and enhanced anxiety-like behavior. *Neuroscience.* 2004;128(4):667–673.
35. Willyard C. Remembered for forgetting. *Nat Med.* 2012;18:482–484.
36. Yen CP, Kung SS, Su YF, et al. Stereotactic bilateral anterior cingulotomy for intractable pain. *J Clin Neurosci.* 2005;12(8):886–890.
37. Zhong G, Wang Y, Zhang Y, Zhao Y. Association between benzodiazepine use and dementia: a meta-analysis. *PLoS One.* 2015;10:e0127836.

CHAPTER 23

1. Abdolmaleky HM, Cheng KH, Russo A, et al. Hypermethylation of the reelin (RELN) promoter in the brain of schizophrenic patients: a preliminary report. *Am J Med Genet B Neuropsychiatr Genet.* 2005;134(1):60–66.
2. Adityanjee, Aderibigbe YA, Theodoridis D, et al. Dementia praecox to schizophrenia: the first 100 years. *Psychiatry Clin Neurosci.* 1999;53(4):437–448.
3. Akbarian S, Kim JJ, Potkin SG, et al. Gene expression for glutamic acid decarboxylase is reduced without loss of neurons in prefrontal cortex of schizophrenics. *Arch Gen Psychiatry.* 1995;52(4):258–266.
4. Baumeister AA, Francis JL. Historical development of the dopamine hypothesis of schizophrenia. *J Hist Neurosci.* 2002;11(3):265–277.
5. Black DN, Taber KH, Hurley RA. Metachromatic leukodystrophy: a model for the study of psychosis. *J Neuropsychiatry Clin Neurosci.* 2003;15(3):289–293.
6. Cannon TD, Chung Y, He G, et al. Progressive reduction in cortical thickness as psychosis develops: a multisite longitudinal neuroimaging study of youth at elevated clinical risk. *Bio Psychiatry.* 2015;77:147–157.
7. Chung DW, Fish KN, Lewis DA. Pathological basis for deficient excitatory drive in cortical parvalbumin interneurons in schizophrenia. *Am J Psychiatry.* 2016;173:1131–1139.
8. Davis KL, Stewart DG, Friedman JI, et al. White matter changes in schizophrenia: evidence for myelin-related dysfunction. *Arch Gen Psychiatry.* 2003;60(5):443–456.
9. Dierks T, Linden DE, Jandl M, et al. Activation of Heschls gyrus during auditory hallucinations. *Neuron.* 1999;22(3):615–621.
10. Evans K, McGrath J, Milns R. Searching for schizophrenia in ancient Greek and Roman literature: a systematic review. *Acta Psychiatr Scand.* 2003;107(5):323–330.
11. Glantz LA, Gilmore JH, Lieberman JA, et al. Apoptotic mechanisms and the synaptic pathology of schizophrenia. *Schizophr Res.* 2006;81(1):47–63.
12. Glantz LA, Lewis DA. Decreased dendritic spine density on prefrontal cortical pyramidal neurons in schizophrenia. *Arch Gen Psychiatry.* 2000;57(1):65–73.
13. Gogtay N, Sporn A, Rapoport J. Structural brain MRI studies in childhood-onset schizophrenia and childhood atypical psychosis. In: Lawrie S, Johnstone E, Weinberger D, eds. New York, NY: Oxford University Press; 2004.
14. Hakak Y, Walker JR, Li C, et al. Genome-wide expression analysis reveals dysregulation of myelination-related genes in chronic schizophrenia. *Proc Natl Acad Sci U S A.* 2001;98(8):4746–4751.
15. Harrison PJ. Recent genetic finds in schizophrenia and their therapeutic relevance. *J Psychopharm.* 2015;29:85–96.
16. Ho BC, Andreasen NC, Ziebell S, et al. Long-term antipsychotic treatment and brain volumes. *Arch Gen Psychiatry.* 2011;68(2):128–137.

17. Hof PR, Haroutunian V, Friedrich Jr VL, et al. Loss and altered spatial distribution of oligodendrocytes in the superior frontal gyrus in schizophrenia. *Biol Psychiatry*. 2003;53(12):1075–1085.

18. Howes OD, Kapur S. The dopamine hypothesis of schizophrenia: version III—the final common pathway. *Schizophr Bull*. 2009;35(3):549–562.

19. Hubl D, Koenig T, Strik W, et al. Pathways that make voices: white matter changes in auditory hallucinations. *Arch Gen Psychiatry*. 2004;61(7):658–668.

20. Hulshoff Pol HE, Schnack HG, Bertens MG, et al. Volume changes in gray matter in patients with schizophrenia. *Am J Psychiatry*. 2002;159(2):244–250.

21. Kong A, Frigge ML, Masson G, et al. Rate of de novo mutations and the importance of father's age to disease risk. *Nature*. 2012;488:471–475.

22. Lawrie S, Johnstone E, Weinberger D. *Schizophrenia: From Neuroimaging to Neuroscience*. New York, NY: Oxford University Press; 2004.

23. Lesh TA, Tanase C, Geib BR, et al. A multimodal analysis of antipsychotic effects on brain structure and function in first-episode schizophrenia. *JAMA Psychiatry*. 2015;72:226–234.

24. Lewis DA, Hashimoto T, Volk DW. Cortical inhibitory neurons and schizophrenia. *Nat Rev Neurosci*. 2005;6(4):312–324.

25. Lewis DA, Lieberman JA. Catching up on schizophrenia: natural history and neurobiology. *Neuron*. 2000;28(2):325–334.

26. Liberman RP, Musgrave JG, Langlois J. Taunton State Hospital, Massachusetts. *Am J Psychiatry*. 2003;160(12):2098.

27. MacDonald ML, Alhassan J, Newman JT, et al. Selective loss of smaller spines in schizophrenia. *Am J Psychiatry*. 2017;174:586–594.

28. McClellan JM, Susser E, King MC. Maternal famine, de novo mutations, and schizophrenia. *JAMA*. 2006;296(5):582–584.

29. Pedersen CB, Mortensen PB. Urbanization and traffic related exposures as risk factors for schizophrenia. *BMC Psychiatry*. 2006;6:2.

30. Schizophrenia Working Group of the Psychiatric Genomics Consortium. Biological insights from 108 schizophrenia-associated genetic loci. *Nature*. 2014;511:421–427.

31. Selemon LD. Increased cortical neuronal density in schizophrenia. *Am J Psychiatry*. 2004;161(9):1564.

32. Selemon LD, Goldman-Rakic PS. The reduced neuropil hypothesis: a circuit based model of schizophrenia. *Biol Psychiatry*. 1999;45(1):17–25.

33. Sporn AL, Greenstein DK, Gogtay N, et al. Progressive brain volume loss during adolescence in childhood-onset schizophrenia. *Am J Psychiatry*. 2003;160(12):2181–2189.

34. Suddath RL, Christison GW, Torrey EF, et al. Anatomical abnormalities in the brains of monozygotic twins discordant for schizophrenia. *N Engl J Med*. 1990;322(12):789–794.

35. Tamminga C, Hashimoto T, Volk DW, et al. GABA neurons in the human prefrontal cortex. *Am J Psychiatry*. 2004;161(10):1764.

36. Tienari P, Wynne LC, Sorri A, et al. Genotype-environment interaction in schizophrenia-spectrum disorder. Long-term follow-up study of Finnish adoptees. *Br J Psychiatry Suppl*. 2004;184:216–222.

37. Torrey EF, Miller J. *The Invisible Plague: The Rise of Mental Illness from 1750 to the Present*. New Brunswick, NJ: Rutgers University Press; 2001.

38. Voineskos AN, Foussias G, Lerch J, et al. Neuroimaging evidence for the deficit subtype of schizophrenia. *JAMA Psychiatry*. 2013;79:472–480.

39. Walker E, Kestler L, Bollini A, et al. Schizophrenia: etiology and course. *Annu Rev Psychol*. 2004;55:401–430.

40. Weinberger DR, Berman KF, Zec RF. Physiologic dysfunction of dorsolateral prefrontal cortex in schizophrenia. I. Regional cerebral blood flow evidence. *Arch Gen Psychiatry*. 1986;43(2):114–124.

41. Wunderink L, Nieboer RM, Wiersma D, Sytema S, Nienhuis FJ. Recovery in remitted first-episode psychosis at 7 years of follow-up of and early dose reduction/discontinuation or maintenance treatment strategy: long-term follow-up of a 2-year randomized clinical trial. *JAMA Psychiatry*. 2013;70:913–920.

CHAPTER 24

1. Baas PW, Qiang L. Neuronal microtubules: when the MAP is the roadblock. *Trends Cell Biol*. 2005; 15(4):183–187.

2. Bennett DA, Schneider JA, Wilson RS, et al. Education modifies the association of amyloid but not tangles with cognitive function. *Neurology*. 2005;65(6):953–955.

3. Blennow K, de Leon MJ, Zetterberg H. Alzheimer's disease. *Lancet*. 2006;368(9533):387–403.

4. Braak H, Braak E. Frequency of stages of Alzheimer-related lesions in different age categories. *Neurobiol Aging*. 1997;18(4):351–357.

5. Doody RS, Thomas RG, Farlow M, et al. Phase 3 trials of solanezumab for mild-to-moderate Alzheimer's disease. *NEJM*. 2014;370:311–321.

6. Erickson EL, Voss MW, Prakash RS, et al. Exercise training increases size of hippocampus and improves memory. *PNAS*. 2011;108:3017–3022.

7. Finger S. *Origins of Neuroscience: A History of Explorations into Brain Functions*. Oxford: Oxford University Press; 1994.

8. Fox NC, Schott JM. Imaging cerebral atrophy: normal ageing to Alzheimer's disease. *Lancet*. 2004; 363(9406):392–394.

9. Fuso A, Seminara L, Cavallaro RA, et al. S-adenosylmethionine/homocysteine cycle alterations modify DNA methylation status with consequent deregulation of PS1 and BACE and beta-amyloid production. *Mol Cell Neurosci*. 2005;28(1):195–204.

10. Hayflick L. The future of ageing. *Nature*. 2000;408 (6809):267–269.

11. Herholz K, Salmon E, Perani D, et al. Discrimination between Alzheimer dementia and controls by automated analysis of multicenter FDG PET. *Neuroimage*. 2002;17(1):302–316.

12. Kandel ER, Schwartz JH, Jessell TM, eds. *Principles of Neural Science*. 4th ed. New York, NY: McGraw-Hill; 2000.

13. Lemere CA, Maier M, Jiang L, et al. Amyloid-beta immunotherapy for the prevention and treatment of Alzheimer disease: lessons from mice, monkeys, and humans. *Rejuvenation Res*. 2006;9(1):77–84.

14. Livingston G, Sommerlad A, Orgeta V, et al. Dementia prevention, intervention, and care. *Lancet*. Published online July 20, 2017. https://doi.org/10.1016/S0140-6736(17)31363-6.

15. Mattson MP. Pathways towards and away from Alzheimer's disease. *Nature*. 2004;430(7000):631–639.

16. Mattson MP, Magnus T. Ageing and neuronal vulnerability. *Nat Rev Neurosci*. 2006;7(4):278–294.

17. Morgan D, Diamond DM, Gottschall PE, et al. A beta peptide vaccination prevents memory loss in an animal model of Alzheimer's disease. *Nature*. 2000;7(6815):982–985.

18. Mortimer JA. Brain reserve and the clinical expression of Alzheimer's disease. *Geriatrics*. 1997;52(suppl 2):S50–S53.

19. Qin W, Chachich M, Lane M, et al. Calorie restriction attenuates Alzheimer's disease type brain amyloidosis in squirrel monkeys (*Saimiri sciureus*). *J Alzheimers Dis*. 2006;10:417–422.

20. Ridley RM, Baker HF, Windle CP, et al. Very long term studies of the seeding of beta-amyloidosis in primates. *J Neural Transm*. 2006;113:1243–1251.

21. Salloway S, Sperling R, Fox NC, et al. Two phase 3 trials of bapineuzumab in mild-to-moderate Alzheimer's disease. *NEJM*. 2014;370:322–333.

22. Schenk D, Hagen M, Seubert P. Current progress in beta-amyloid immunotherapy. *Curr Opin Immunol*. 2004;16(5):599–606.

23. Sevigny J, Chiao P, Bussiere T, et al. The antibody aducanumab reduces Aβ plaques in Alzheimer's disease. *Nature*. 2016;537:50–56.

24. Snowdon DA, Kemper SJ, Mortimer JA, et al. Linguistic ability in early life and cognitive function and Alzheimer's disease in late life. Findings from the Nun Study. *JAMA*. 1996;275(7):528–532.

25. Tuszynski MH, Thal L, Pay M, et al. A phase 1 clinical trial of nerve growth factor gene therapy for Alzheimer disease. *Nat Med*. 2005;11(5):551–555.

26. Tuszynski MH, Yang JH, Barba D, et al. Nerve growth factor gene therapy: activation of neuronal responses in Alzheimer disease. *JAMA Neurol*. 2015;72:1139–1147.

27. Vandenberghe R, Riviere ME, Caputo A, et al. 2017;3:10–22.

28. Wang J, Ho L, Zhao Z, et al. Moderate consumption of Carernet Sauvignon attenuates AB neuropathology in a mouse model of Alzheimer's disease. *FASEB J*. 2006;20:2313–2320.

29. Winblad B, Andreasen N, Minthon L, et al. Safety, tolerability, and antibody response of active A immunotherapy with CAD106 in patients with Alzheimer's disease: randomized, double-blind, placebo-controlled, first-in-human study. *Lancet Neurol*. 2012;11:597–604.

30. Wolfe MS. Shutting down Alzheimer's. *Sci Am*. 2006;294(5):72–79.

31. Yang L, Rieves D, Ganley C. Brain amyloid imaging—FDA approval of florbetapir F18 injection. *N Engl J Med*. 2012;367(10):885–887.

Answers to End-of-Chapter Questions

CHAPTER 2
1. b
2. c
3. a
4. c
5. d
6. a
7. b
8. d

CHAPTER 3
1. c
2. a
3. b
4. d
5. a
6. b
7. d
8. a

CHAPTER 4
1. c
2. b
3. d
4. a
5. d
6. c
7. a
8. d

CHAPTER 5
1. c
2. b
3. c
4. a
5. d
6. b
7. d
8. d

CHAPTER 6
1. d
2. c
3. a
4. b
5. c
6. d
7. b

CHAPTER 7
1. c
2. d
3. a
4. c
5. b
6. b
7. a

CHAPTER 8
1. d
2. a
3. b
4. c
5. c
6. a
7. d
8. b

CHAPTER 9
1. d
2. c
3. d
4. a
5. c
6. b

CHAPTER 10
1. E
2. C
3. A
4. G
5. H
6. B
7. D
8. F

CHAPTER 11
1. c
2. b
3. a
4. d
5. c
6. d
7. b
8. a

CHAPTER 12
1. c
2. a
3. d
4. b
5. a
6. c
7. d
8. a
9. b

CHAPTER 13
1. d
2. b
3. a
4. c
5. b
6. a
7. d
8. c

CHAPTER 14
1. Who knows?
2. c
3. b
4. d
5. c
6. a
7. b

CHAPTER 15
1. a
2. b
3. d
4. a
5. c
6. c
7. d
8. c

CHAPTER 16
1. d
2. a
3. c
4. b
5. d
6. c
7. a
8. b

CHAPTER 17
1. c
2. d
3. b
4. a
5. b
6. a
7. d
8. c

CHAPTER 18
1. b
2. a
3. d
4. c
5. a
6. d
7. c
8. b

CHAPTER 19
1. a
2. c
3. d
4. b
5. b
6. c

CHAPTER 20
1. d
2. c
3. b
4. a
5. c
6. b
7. 1. C
   2. B
   3. D
   4. A

CHAPTER 21
1. b
2. a
3. c
4. d
5. a
6. b
7. c
8. d

CHAPTER 22
1. b
2. c
3. d
4. a
5. a
6. d
7. b
8. c

CHAPTER 23
1. d
2. b
3. a
4. c
5. d
6. a
7. c
8. 1. E
   2. D
   3. B
   4. F
   5. A
   6. C

CHAPTER 24
1. d
2. c
3. a
4. c
5. d
6. b

Index

Note: Page numbers followed by "f" indicate figures, "t" indicate tables, and "b" indicate boxes.

A

A-β amyloid, 320b, 322, 323b, 325
  hyperphosphorylation, 320
  long-term potentiation development, 319
  production of, 319b
  toxicity, 318
Ablation studies, 11
Ablative brain surgery, 243
A-β oligomers, 319, 323
Absence seizures, 127, 128f
Acetylase inhibitor, 239
Acetylcholine (ACh), 47–48, 48b, 53, 59, 59b
ACTH (adrenocorticotropic hormone), 48, 49t, 80t,
        83f–84f, 86–87, 87b, 88f, 90f, 95, 118, 118f,
        140b, 210, 218, 218f, 224, 277b
Action potentials, electrical signaling, 32, 36, 37f, 43, 43f,
        48b, 53, 56b, 111, 123, 123f, 125, 126f
  axon hillock, 33
  depolarization, 33, 35f
  voltage-gated sodium channels, 36
Acupuncture, 140–142, 142b
Acute alcohol intoxication, 295b
Acute pain, 143–144
  affective-motivational domain, 134–135, 136f–137f
  nociceptors, 133
  pathways, 133, 136t
  peripheral tissue, 133, 135f
  sensory-discriminative domain, 133–134, 136f
  somatosensory cortex, 133, 134f
  spinal cord, 133, 136f
AD. See Alzheimer's disease (AD)
Addiction, 75, 139, 144, 154, 162, 167, 172t, 175, 227,
        281–282
  craving and frontal cortex, 157–158, 158t
  developmental disorder, 159–160, 160f
  dopamine (DA) receptors, 156–157, 157f
  drug, 267
  global impairments, 156, 157f
  mesolimbic pathway, 156, 157f
  molecular changes, 159
  optogenetics, 11
  psychostimulants, 161, 161f
  relapse, 159
  synaptic remodeling, 158–159, 159f
  treatment, 160–161
Addison's disease, 87, 89, 89b, 218
Adenosine diphosphate (ADP), 29
Adenosine triphosphate (ATP), 29, 56, 57f, 60f
ADHD. See Attention deficit hyperactivity disorder
        (ADHD)

ADP (adenosine diphosphate), 29
Adrenergic receptors, 58–59
Adrenocorticotropic hormone (ACTH), 48, 49t, 80t,
        83f–84f, 86–87, 87b, 88f, 90f, 95, 118, 118f,
        140b, 210, 218, 218f, 224
  depression, 277b
Aducanumab, 322–323, 323f
Adult neuroplasticity
  after amputation, 102, 104f
  cellular changes, 106
  cortical expansion, 102, 104f
  genitalia, 104–105, 105f
  maladaptive neuroplasticity, 105, 106f
  musician's Brain, 104
  nerve regeneration, 106
Affective-motivational domain, 133–135, 136t,
        136f–137f, 137
Aging, 75b, 89–90, 166f, 174b, 200, 205, 316–318
  normal sleep, 195, 196f
Agonists, 53–54, 58, 100, 154, 218, 219b, 239, 278, 295
Agouti gene, 73f–74f, 74–75
Agouti-related peptide (AGRP), 168
AGRP (agouti-related peptide), 168
AIS (androgen insensitivity syndrome), 210–211, 212f
  diagnosis, 212b
Alcoholism, 2, 3, 15, 55, 56b, 116b, 128b, 148, 152, 156,
        157f, 159–160, 204b, 205, 218, 238b, 269, 316
  and anxiety, 295b
  blackouts, 269
  memory, 238b
  monozygotic (identical) twins, 3
Alertness, 45, 45f, 47, 89, 192f, 265, 124, 126
Alzheimer's disease (AD), 7, 9, 21, 47– 48, 59, 75b, 98,
        100, 118, 201, 254, 302
  amyloid plaques, 318–320, 319b, 319f–320f
  benzodiazepines, 300b
  cognitive loss, 317
  cortical atrophy, 317–318, 317f–318f
  forgetting, 245
  history, 317
  and hormone therapy, 217
  neurofibrillary tangles, 320–321, 320b, 321f
  neuronal shrinkage, plaques and neurofibrillary
        tangles, 317, 317f
  presenile dementia, 317
  prevention, 324–325, 324f, 325t, 326b
  sclerotic plaques, 317
  treatment for, 321–324, 322b, 323f
α-Amino-3-hydroxy-5-methyl-4-isoxazole propionate
        (AMPA) receptor, 54, 55f, 61, 62f, 282

Amino acid receptors, 53
γ-aminobutyric acid (GABA), 54–55
glutamate, 54, 55f
Amino acids, 26, 46, 48, 79, 125, 166, 312, 318
γ-aminobutyric acid (GABA), 42–43, 42b, 43f
glutamate, 42, 42b
glycine, 42–43
oxytocin, 230, 230f
γ-Aminobutyric acid (GABA), 16, 35b, 41–43, 42b, 43f,
53–55, 55f, 56b, 124, 128b, 154, 156, 157f,
160–161, 205, 307–308, 308f, 313, 314
agonists, 295b
benzodiazepine, 295
hormones, 79, 80f
Ammon's horn, 21, 21f
Amphetamines, 58, 152, 154, 158, 158f–159f, 161, 172t,
175, 175f, 181, 199b, 224, 253b, 253–254, 267,
269, 313
Amygdala, 20, 21, 23f, 43, 86, 82, 89, 90f, 127, 134–135,
138, 142, 150, 155, 160, 160f, 173, 186–189,
186f, 195, 230–231, 234, 241, 266, 275, 284f,
285, 290, 293, 294f, 295–297
anger and aggression, 180–181
anticipatory anxiety, 291–292, 293f
bipolar disorder, 285–286
chronic stress, 292
emotional memories, 292
fear recognition and management, 291
features, 290
Klüver–Bucy syndrome, 291
life-threatening visual information, 291
long-term potentiation (LTP), 292
pleasure, 153–154
protein synthesis inhibitors, 292
sensory information, 291, 292f
temporal lobes, 290
unconscious/preconscious, 291
Amyloid-β precursor protein (APP), 318, 319f, 322,
323f, 325
Cabernet Sauvignon, 326b
Amyloid plaques, 321–322, 323f, 324–325
A-β-42 amino acid chain, 318
A-β oligomers, 319
amyloid-β/A-β, 318
amyloid-β precursor protein (APP), 318, 319f
diagnosis of, 319
florbetapir F18 (Amyvid), 319–320, 320f
florbetapir PET scan, 320
gene expression, 319b
genetic abnormality, 318
with marmoset monkeys, long-term study, 319, 320f
pharmacologic inhibition, 318
β-Amyloid protein, 201, 318
clinical trials, 322
Amyloid-related imaging abnormalities (ARIAs), 323
Amyvid (florbetapir F18), 319–320, 320f
Androgen insensitivity syndrome (AIS), 210–211, 212f
diagnosis, 212b
Anger and aggression, 17, 39
amygdala, 180–181
attention deficit hyperactivity disorder (ADHD), 184b
defensive attack, medial hypothalamus, 177, 178f
diagnosis, 177
features, 177, 178t
frontal cortex, 179–180, 179f–180f
head trauma, 179b
intermittent explosive disorder, 181b
lateral regions, 177, 178f

lithium, 185b
medial regions, 177, 178f
predatory attack, lateral hypothalamus, 177, 178f
prefrontal cortex (PFC), 17
psychopath, 185–188, 186f–187f
psychosurgery, 180b
Research Domain Criteria, 179
serotonin, 183–185, 185f
temporal lobe epilepsy, 187b
testosterone, 181–183, 182f–183f
types, 177
vasopressin, 183, 184f
violence and age, 180b
Anhedonia, 114, 156, 159, 274, 278, 281
pleasure, 156b
Animal domestication, 2
Animal studies, nonhuman, 89, 97, 110, 118, 134b, 139,
143, 161, 214, 296, 321–322, 324
gene activation markers, 11
knockout mice, silenced genes, 11
optogenetics, 11, 12f
transgenic mice, 11
viral-mediated gene transfer, 11
Anisomycin inhibitor, 238, 239, 239f, 241
Anorexia nervosa, 86b
ANS. *See* Autonomic nervous system (ANS)
Antagonists, 47, 51, 53–54, 58, 100, 124, 134b, 139, 151,
159, 169, 228, 240
Anterior cingulate cortex (ACC), 135, 137f, 265,
266f, 285
Anterograde amnesia, 242, 243f
Anti-amyloid-β monoclonal antibodies, 321
Anticholinergic agents, 48
Anticipatory anxiety, 291–292, 293f
Antidepressants, 47b, 82, 100b, 108, 114, 120, 128, 139,
142, 145–146, 146f, 176, 199b, 203, 218–220,
220b, 275, 277, 278–282, 280f–282f, 291
and anxiety, 296b
psychotherapy, 297, 297f
treatment, 279
Antidiuretic hormone, 183
Antiepileptic drugs, 38b, 56b
Antihistamines, 27, 47, 59, 174, 199
Anti-inflammatory antidepressants, 114b
Anti-inflammatory diet, 116b
Antipsychotic (AP) medication, 43–44, 48b, 59,
175, 224b, 314, 322b
schizophrenia, 305, 305f
Anti-tau medications, 321
Anxiety, 5, 18, 24, 45f, 47f, 48, 55, 56b, 57b, 58, 70,
75, 87, 89–90, 90f, 139, 171, 173, 186, 204b,
218–219, 231, 239, 275, 303
acute stress, 289–290, 289f–290f
alcoholism and, 295b
augmenting psychotherapy, 297–298, 298f
Diagnostic and Statistical Manual (DSM) system,
288, 289t
emotional circuits dysfunction, 39, 39f
GABAergic activity, 43
harmones, 90
heart rates, men, 25b
inhibitory potentials, 35b
monoamines, 49b
neuronal circuitry. *See* Neuronal circuits
neurotransmitters and cell biology, 295–296, 296b
norepinephrine (NE), 46b
obsessive–compulsive disorder (OCD), 298–300,
298f–299f, 300b

Anxiety (Continued)
  optogenetics, 11
  prefrontal cortex (PFC), 17
Apathetic syndromes, 18
  prefrontal lobotomy, 22b
Aplysia's gill-withdrawal reflex
  habituation, 4–5
  sensitization, 4
  slugging and resting state, 4, 5f
  synaptic terminals, 5, 6f
Apoptosis, 75b, 92, 98, 101f, 305
APP (amyloid-β precursor protein), 318, 319f, 322,
      323f, 325
  Cabernet Sauvignon, 326b
Appetite, 59, 199, 218, 275
  cross-sectional analysis, 165, 166f
  dietary treatment interventions, obesity, 164
  eating disorders. See Eating disorders
  energy homeostasis, 164
  genetic predisposition, 164
  homeostatic mechanisms. See Homeostatic
      mechanisms, appetite
  longevity, 174b
  metabolic adaptation, 165
  Minnesota Starvation Experiment, 165
  nutrition and mental health, 175b
  preintervention weight, 164, 165f
  psychiatric medications, 174–175, 174t, 175f
  resting metabolic rate (RMR), 165, 166f
  "set point," 165
  smoking, 170b
  stress, 169b
  thrifty gene, 164–165
  total energy expenditure, 165
ARIAs (amyloid-related imaging abnormalities), 323
Ascending arousal systems, 198–199
Aspartate, 42
Asperger's disorder, 232
Astrocyte cells, 15, 26–27, 37–38, 37f, 106, 111–113, 112f
  epilepsy, 38b
Atomoxetine, 46
ATP (adenosine triphosphate), 29, 56, 57f, 60f
Attention, 2, 18, 22b, 35b, 39, 43b, 47, 69, 79, 102, 119, 129,
      135, 139, 150, 156, 161, 181, 191–192, 215, 225,
      233, 237, 276, 276f, 291–292, 296b, 306
  boredom, 266b
  continuous performance tests (CPTs), 262, 263f
  delayed reward, 265
  dopamine (DA), 266, 267f
  drug addiction, 267
  impulse control, 265
  nucleus accumbens (NAc), 266
  SAT scores, 265
  selective attention, 261, 261f
  self-restraint, 265
  social and academic performance, 265
  stimulant medications, 266
  stopwatches and psychological tests, 261
  working memory. See Working memory
Attention deficit hyperactivity disorder (ADHD), 26, 43b,
      69–70, 161, 175, 204b, 254, 265, 266f
  anger and aggression, 184b
  brain size, 267–268
  in children, 262b
  genetics, 267
  gray matter thickness, 268, 269f
  inhibitory potentials, 35b
  intelligence, 253b

minimal brain dysfunction, 268b
  neglect syndrome, 268b
  prefrontal cortex (PFC), 17
  stimulants, long-term effects, 269–271, 270f–271f
  timing and cerebellum, 269, 270f
Atypical depression, 274
Auditory cortex, 309–310, 310f
Auditory hallucinations
  abnormalities identification, 310
  auditory cortex, 309
  DTI imaging, 310
  ear to cortex pathways, 309, 310f
  functional magnetic resonance imaging (fMRI) scans,
      310, 311f
  language expression deficits, 309
  positive symptoms, 310b
  temporal lobe abnormalities, 309
Autism spectrum, 5, 7, 70
  brain enlargement, 233, 233f–234f
  characteristics, 232
  conditions, 232
  eye aversion, 232–233, 232f
  mirror neurons, 233–235, 234f
  treatment, 235
Autistic Diagnostic Interview, 234f, 235
Autistic-type behaviors, 7
Autoimmune disease, 59b, 115–117, 117f
Autonomic nervous system (ANS), 48, 79, 89, 118, 118f,
      166, 169, 295
  cardiac autonomic activity, 25b
  divisions of, 23, 25f
  parasympathetic division, 23–25
  peripheral noradrenergic neurons, 45
  postganglionic sympathetic neurons, 24
  preganglionic neurons, 24
  sympathetic division, 23–24
  vagus nerve stimulation, 26b
Autoreceptors, 57b, 58
Axon hillock, action potentials, 32–33, 35f,
      36, 53, 125
Axoplasmic transport, 32

B
Basal ganglia, 43, 129
  cortico–striatal–thalamic–cortical circuit, 299
  disorders, 298
  function, 298
  functional imaging studies, 299
  nucleus accumbens (NAc), 299
  structures, 298, 298f
Basal metabolic rate, 165
BBB. See Blood–brain barrier (BBB)
BDNF. See Brain-derived neurotrophic factor (BDNF)
Behavior, parental. See Parental behavior
Beijing Genomics Institute (BGI), 249
Benzedrine/dexedrine, weight loss, 270–271
Benzodiazepines, 54, 56b, 128b, 205, 288, 300
  memory, 238b
  receptor distribution, 295, 295b
BGI (Beijing Genomics Institute), 249
Bifrontal atrophy, 258
Bioelectricity, 125–126, 126f
Biofeedback, 265, 266f
Bipolar depression, 274
Bipolar disorder, 8, 18, 29b, 67, 67f, 70, 117b, 188, 253,
      253f, 274
  amygdala, 285–286

creativity, 257
feature, 285
global activation, 284f, 285
gray matter volume, 285, 285f
intelligence, 252
lithium, 285
monozygotic (identical) twins, 3
and schizophrenia, 284–285
sleep, 204–205
unipolar depression, 284
Blood–brain barrier (BBB), 44f, 51b, 62b, 82, 111, 113, 116, 168, 201, 324
antihistamines, 27
aspartate, 42
astrocyte, 37
endocrine system, 26
high-frequency ultrasound/transcranial magnetic stimulation, 26b
implants, 26b
intranasal delivery, 26b
lipid-soluble substances, 26
P-glycoprotein, 27
tight junctions, 26, 27f
Trojan horse, 26b
Brain banks, 8–9, 308
Brain-derived neurotrophic factor (BDNF), 84, 100, 127, 161, 213, 213f, 220, 285–286, 296, 325
deep brain stimulation (BDS), 282–283, 283f
DNA scarring, 280, 281f–282f
growth factor proteins, 212
ketamine, 281–282
neurogenesis, 279, 280f
psychiatric treatment, 278–279, 279f
utopia, 286b
volume loss, 278, 279f
Brain function, 9, 180
articulate speech, 7–8
Broca's aphasia, 8
facial recognition, 7
localization, 7, 7f
male brain characterization, 8, 8f
Brain reserve
cognitive impairment *vs.* amyloidosis, 324, 324f
neural substrate, 325
Nun Study, 324
Brain shrinking, 117, 278, 306, 314, 317f
Brilliant Madness, 252–253
Brodmann's areas, 16–17, 19f–20f, 305, 309

C
Cabernet Sauvignon, 326b
CAD106 vaccine, 322
Calm down, 35b, 295
Caloric restriction (CR), 174b, 325
Cannabinoid (CB₁) receptor, 51, 170–171
Cardiac autonomic activity, 25b
Cataplexy, 199, 199b
Catecholamine-O-methyltransferase (COMT), 137, 138f
Catecholamines, 47b, 59, 137, 231, 265b
dopamine (DA), 43–44, 43b, 45f, 263
epinephrine, 46
inverse correlation, 264
microdialysis probes, 263
norepinephrine (NE), 44–46, 45f, 46b, 263–264
synthesis, 43, 44f
training phase, 263
vagus nerve stimulation (VNS), 264

CCK (cholecystokinin), 167, 167f, 172
Cell culture, 316b
Central nervous system (CNS), 2, 4, 9, 26–27, 43, 46, 48, 49b, 51, 58, 59b, 85f, 87, 88f, 92–93, 99, 100b, 106, 110–111, 113–114, 116–118, 128, 132, 135, 136t, 140, 143, 160, 166, 171, 174b, 175, 205, 237, 269, 295, 322
aging-related disorders, 316
glial cells, 37–38
hormones, 81–82, 83f–84f
hypothalamus, 23
imaging, noninvasive analysis, 9, 10t
pneumoencephalography, 9
Cerebellum, 26, 137f, 161, 268–269, 278, 295, 314
Cerebral amyloidosis, 319
Cerebral cortex, 11, 26, 29, 30f, 79, 83f, 84, 88f, 94, 134, 144b, 169, 198, 299
γ-aminobutyric acid neurons, 16
amygdala, 21, 23f
Brodmann's areas, 16–17, 19f
cortical neurons, 16
egg fertilization, 15, 16f
gray matter, 16, 18f
hippocampus, 19, 21, 21f
hypothalamus, 22–23, 24f
layers of, 16, 17f
mental illness treatment, 15
mental retardation, 15b
neuroblasts, 15
neurogenesis, 15
prefrontal cortex (PFC), 17–19, 20f
prefrontal lobotomy, 22b
pyramidal neurons, 16
white matter, 16, 18f
Cerebral metabolic activity, 245
Cerebral spinal fluid (CSF), 183–184, 185f, 201, 320b
CG sites (cytosine–guanine sites), 226, 228f
Chemical imbalance, 41b, 122, 274
Chemical imbalance theories, 67
Chemoreceptors, 23
Childhood disintegrative disorder, 232
Children, 15, 37, 68–70, 74, 97, 101, 105, 108, 161, 164, 175, 186, 195b, 207–208, 208f, 222, 224, 233, 235, 249, 250f, 251–252, 254, 261–262, 265, 267–270, 269f–270f, 296b, 305, 305f, 311–312, 312f, 316
congenital adrenal hyperplasia, 210
dyslexia, 255–256, 255f–256f
mental retardation (MR), 255–256, 255f–256f
Chlorpromazine (Thorazine), 302
Cholecystokinin (CCK), 167, 167f, 172
Cholesterol, 79, 86, 87f, 209, 209f
Cholinergic neuronal degeneration, 324
Cholinergic receptors, 59
Chromatin remodeling, 72f, 73
Chronic hallucinations, 302
Chronic mental illness, 303, 304f
Chronic pain, 133, 134b, 144b, 145, 155
gray matter loss, 143, 143f
morphine, 144, 145f
neuropathic pain, 142
nociceptive pain, 142
pain memory, 142–143
safer treatments, 144
terminal illness, 143
Cingulate gyrus, 17, 19, 20f, 22b, 186, 186f, 244–245, 278, 283, 284f, 293, 299
Circadian dysfunction, 203–204

Circuits, 38–39, 38f–39f, 122, 138, 154, 231, 280, 299, 310. *See also* Neuronal circuits
Classic neurotransmitters, 41, 50f, 80
  acetylcholine (ACh), 47–48, 48b
  amino acids, 42–43, 42b, 43f, 48
  monoamines, 43–47, 43b, 44f–47f, 46b–47b
CNS. *See* Central nervous system (CNS)
Cocaine, 58, 109b, 127, 139, 151, 151f, 153–156, 153f, 157f, 158, 158t, 159, 162, 187, 218, 267, 269, 271
Cognition, 26, 43b, 51, 58–59, 156, 187, 191, 195b, 217, 220, 253, 261, 321, 324
  cholinergic system, 48b
  definition, 237
Cognitive ability, in children, 249, 250f
Cognitive-behavioral therapy, 275
Cognitive deficits, intelligence, 254–256, 254f–256f, 274
Cognitive dysfunction, 306
Cognitive tests, 48b, 253–254
Colocalization, 48b
Concentration gradient, 125
Congenital adrenal hyperplasia, 210
Congenital insensitivity
  pain tolerance spectrum, 137–138, 138f
  spectrum of, 137
Consciousness, 54, 126, 130, 191, 192f, 195, 196f, 199
Consolidation, memory, 202, 203f, 238, 238b, 242, 245, 290
Continuous performance tests (CPTs), 262, 263f
Controlled trial, 13–14, 104b, 145, 265, 271, 283, 295
Copy number variation (CNV), 68–69, 69f
Coronal magnetic resonance imaging, 304, 304f
Cortical atrophy
  brain volume loss, 317
  energy metabolism, 318
  examination and coronal slices, 317, 317f
  hair loss, 317
  positron emission tomography (PET), 318, 318f
  sequential magnetic resonance imaging (MRI) scans, 318, 318f
Cortical dysplasia-focal epilepsy, 7
Cortical neurons, 16, 42, 104f, 127, 202, 245, 250, 317
Cortical sensory information, 243
Corticosteroids, 2, 86, 87f, 200
Cortico–striatal–thalamic–cortical circuit, 299
Corticotropin-releasing factor (CRF), 95, 159
Corticotropin-releasing hormone (CRH), 84f, 86, 87b, 88f, 90, 90f, 169, 225, 226f, 276–277, 277b, 295
CPTs (continuous performance tests), 262, 263f
CR (caloric restriction), 174b, 325
Creativity, intelligence, 249, 254
  creative moments, 256
  frontal lobes loosening, 258–259, 259f
  literature review, 256
  and mental illness, 257–258, 257f–258f
  self-criticism, 256
CREB (cyclic adenosine monophosphate responsive element–binding protein), 11, 60f, 81f, 159, 246
CRH (corticotropin-releasing hormone), 84f, 86, 87b, 88f, 90, 90f, 169, 225, 226f, 276–277, 277b, 295
Criminal justice system, 242b
Crystalline intelligence, 250
CSF 5-hydroxyindoleacetic acid (5-HIAA), 183–184, 185f
Cue neurons, 262, 264f
Cushing's disease, 87, 89, 89b, 277b
Cyclic adenosine monophosphate responsive element-binding (CREB) protein, 11, 60f, 81f, 159, 246
Cyclic guanosine monophosphate (cGMP), 49

D-Cycloserine, 54, 239
Cytokines,108–109, 110f, 111, 117–118, 142, 144
  interferon (IFN), 113
  interleukin (IL), 113
  mental illness, 114. *See also* Mental illness
  neural plasticity, 113–114
  role of, 113
  tumor necrosis factor (TNF), 113
  white blood cells, 113, 113f
Cytosine–guanine (CG) sites, 226, 228f

D
Deacetylase enzymes, 239
Declarative memory, 89, 202, 237
  hippocampus, 242–243, 243f
  neocortex, 244, 244f
  system consolidation, 244–245, 245f
Deep brain stimulation (DBS), 125, 129, 155, 278, 299
  brain-derived neurotrophic factor (BDNF), 282–283, 283f
Default mode network, 276, 276f
Defensive attack, anger and aggression, 177, 178f
Delayed-response task, 262–263, 263f–264f
Delay neurons, 262, 264f
Delusions, 303, 306, 309
Dementia, 111, 185, 191, 200–201, 217, 258–259, 302. *See also* Alzheimer's disease (AD)
  causes, 316
  gray matter, 16
Dementia praecox. *See* Schizophrenia
Dendritic spines, 29, 32f, 158, 159f, 212–213, 239–240, 267, 306, 307f
  abnormalities, 254
  arborization, 32b
  morphology, 30
  pathology, 254, 254f
  plasticity, 30
  postsynaptic dendrite, 32
Depolarization, action potentials, 32–33, 36, 34f–35f
Depression, 5, 7, 18, 21, 43, 51, 54, 58, 64, 70, 82, 84, 89b, 100b, 114–115, 116b, 119–120, 124–125, 127, 129, 135, 139, 143–144, 148, 156, 156b, 159, 171, 183, 194, 203, 205, 208, 219, 219f, 257, 257f, 288, 302, 320
  bipolar disorder, 284–286, 284f–285f
  brain biopsy, 274
  brain-derived neurotrophic factor (BDNF), 278–283, 279f–283f, 280b, 286b
  cognitive tasks, 275
  Diagnostic and Statistical Manual of Mental Disorders (DSM) criteria, 274, 288
  dysfunction regions, 274, 275f
  emotional circuits dysfunction, 39, 39f
  emotional responses, 275
  frontal cortex, 275–276, 276f
  functional magnetic resonance imaging (fMRI), 275
  gray matter, 16
  Hippocrates (melancholia), 274
  hormones, 90
  hypothalamic–pituitary–adrenal (HPA) axis, 276–278, 277b, 277f
  meta-analysis, 275
  monoamine hypothesis, 274
  monoamines, 49b
  norepinephrine (NE), 46b
  optogenetics, 11
  overactive amygdala, 275

and pain, 145–146, 145f
positron emission tomography (PET), 275
prefrontal cortex (PFC), 17
during pregnancy, 220
reward dysfunction, 278
serotonin, 47b
serotonin transporter, 283–284, 283f
types, 274
underactive PFC, 275
Depression laboratory test, 277b
Descending pain-modulating circuits, 138, 139f
Developmental disorder, 159–160, 160f, 254
Dexamethasone suppression test, 277b
Diabetes, blood glucose level reduction, calculus
    equations, 29b
Diagnostic and Statistical Manual (DSM) system, 5, 41,
    119, 177, 185, 298
    acoustic probe, 288
    anxious misery spectrum, 288, 289f
    characteristics, 288
    depression, 274
    disorders, 288
    posttraumatic stress disorder (PTSD), 288
    RDoC initiative, 288
Dietary restriction, 325
Diffusion tensor imaging (DTI), 9, 126, 252,
    309–310, 311f
    white matter tracts assessment, 38
    white matter visualization, 38, 39f
5α-Dihydrotestosterone, 209
Disconnected, social attachment
    autism spectrum, 232–235, 232f–234f
    schizophrenic spectrum disorders, 231–232
    social skills impairment, 232
Disinhibited syndromes, 18
Disorganized syndromes, 18
Dissociation, 281–282
Dizygotic (fraternal) twins, 2–3, 4t
DLPFC (dorsolateral prefrontal cortex), 84, 141, 143,
    244, 296, 307f
DNA, 2–3, 11–13, 15, 29, 55, 60f, 64–66,65b–66b, 67–70,
    68f–69f, 71f, 73, 75b, 76, 80, 93–94, 95f, 209b,
    224–225, 228f, 229, 239, 249, 281f, 311–312,
    319, 324
    demethylation, 226
    methylation, 72, 72f, 280, 313, 313b
    microarrays, 12, 12f–13f
    technology, faulty eyewitness identification, 242b
L-DOPA, 43, 44f
Dopamine (DA), 36, 36f, 42b, 44f, 46–48, 57b, 58, 67, 83,
    96–97, 97f, 150–156, 152f–153f, 155f, 159,
    161–162, 167, 169b, 171, 187, 187f, 189, 218,
    224, 224b, 231, 243b, 264, 269, 278
    addictions, 156–157, 157f
    attention, 266, 267f
    -blocking antipsychotic agents, 48
    catecholamines, 263
    hypothesis, 313–314
    mesolimbocortical DA system, 43
    methylphenidate (MPH), 151, 151f
    nigrostriatal/mesostriatal system, 43
    nucleus accumbens, 43b
    pair bonding, 227
    pathways, 43, 45f
    pleasure, 154
    prolactin synthesis and release, 44
    transporter density, 267
    tuberoinfundibular DA system, 44

Dopamine D2/D3 receptor, 271, 271f
Dopamine D4 receptor, 218
Dopaminergic mechanisms, 218
Dorsolateral prefrontal cortex (DLPFC), 84, 141, 143,
    244, 296, 307f
Dream enactment, 201b
Dreaming, 195, 196f, 258
Drug addiction, 267
Drug-seeking behavior, 151
DSM system. *See* Diagnostic and Statistical Manual
    (DSM) system
DTI. *See* Diffusion tensor imaging (DTI)
DTI (diffusion tensor imaging), 9, 126, 252, 309–310, 311f
    white matter tracts assessment, 38
    white matter visualization, 38, 39f
Dysfunctional circuits, 39, 39f
Dyslexia, 254
    in children, 255, 255f
    learning disorder, 255
    phonics-based reading intervention, 255–256, 256f

E
Eating disorders, 86b, 164, 298
    obesity, 171–173, 172t, 173f
    purging, 173
ECT (electroconvulsive therapy), 100, 124, 127, 129, 241,
    275, 276f, 277–278, 280, 282f
    forgetting, 246, 247f
EEG patterns (electroencephalographic patterns), 191–194,
    192f–193f, 194b, 198
    with absence seizures, 127, 128f
    excessive electrical activity, 127–128
    insufficient electrical activity, 128
    synaptic activity, 126, 127f
Electrical brain
    bioelectricity, 125–126, 126f
    chemical imbalance, 122
    electroencephalogram (EEG). *See*
        Electroencephalographic (EEG) patterns
    history of, 122–125, 123f–124f
    stimulation, 128–130, 130f
    withdrawal seizures, 128b
Electrical signaling
    action potential, 33, 35f, 36
    electrochemical signaling, 36–37, 36f
    postsynaptic potentials, 32–33, 34f
    process of, 32
Electrical stimulation, 11, 105, 122–125, 123f–124f, 129,
    130f, 133, 138, 155, 177, 224
Electrochemical communication, 41, 53, 79
Electrochemical signaling, 36–37, 36f
Electroconvulsive therapy (ECT), 100, 124, 127, 129, 241,
    275, 276f, 277–278, 280, 282f
    forgetting, 246, 247f
Electro EEG biofeedback. *See* Neurofeedback
Electroencephalographic (EEG) patterns, 191–194,
    192f–193f, 194b, 198
    with absence seizures, 127, 128f
    excessive electrical activity, 127–128
    insufficient electrical activity, 128
    synaptic activity, 126, 127f
Electrostatic forces, 125
Embryonic stem cells, 12, 95, 97f
Emotional function, 18
    limbic system, 22b
Emotional memories, amygdala, 150, 153–154, 290, 293
Empathy control, 18

Endocannabinoids, 49–51, 142, 154, 170–171
Endocrine system, 26, 118, 118f, 169
Endogenous opioids, 140, 140f, 154, 167
Energy homeostasis, 164, 174
Energy metabolism, 81, 168, 174, 194, 318
Entorhinal cortex, 243–244, 321
Epigenetics, 239
    Agouti gene, 73f–74f, 74–75
    chromatin remodeling, 72f, 73
    DNA methylation, 72, 72f
    environmental events and, 73, 73f
    gene concealing, 70, 72
    mechanisms, 313
    memory, 239
    multifactorial, 75
    telomere, 75b
    transcription factors and RNA polymerase, 70, 71f
Epilepsy, 7, 38b, 43, 124, 126–127, 129, 303
Epinephrine, 43, 46, 57, 79
EPSPs (excitatory postsynaptic potentials), 33, 34f, 36, 53, 60
17β-Estradiol, 209
Excitatory neurons, 36
    action potential, 33, 35f
    glutamate, 42
    monoamines, 43
    postsynaptic potentials, 33, 34f
Excitatory postsynaptic potentials (EPSPs), 33, 34f, 36, 53, 60
Excitatory synaptic density, 308
Excitotoxicity inhibitors, 42b
Exocytosis, 37
Explicit memory, 237, 242, 293
Exposure therapy, 54, 239, 288, 300
Eye aversion, 232–233, 232f

F
Face blindness, 7
Facial recognition, 7
Famine, schizophrenia, 311, 311f
Fast receptors
    acetylcholine (ACh), 53
    amino acid receptors, 53–55, 55f
    γ-aminobutyric acid (GABA), 53
    excitatory postsynaptic potential (EPSP), 53
    glutamate, 53
    glycine, 53
    ion channel, 53, 54f
    types, 53
Fatigue, 59, 89b, 114, 117, 119–120, 253, 322
Faulty eyewitness identification, 242b
Fear, 54, 135, 153, 180, 186–187, 187f, 223, 231, 241, 288, 289f, 292–293, 294f, 296
    acquisition, 297
    extinction, 297, 297f
    memory, 239
    recognition and management, 291
    reduction, 239
Fetal adrenal gland, 210
Fetal alcohol syndrome, 15b
α-Fetoprotein, 209
Fight–flight response control, 24
Finnish Adoption Study, schizophrenia, 311–312, 312f
5-HT neurons (5-hydroxytryptamine neurons), 278
Florbetapir F18 (Amyvid), 319–320, 320f
Fluorescent proteins, 11
Flynn effect, 252b

fMRI. *See* Functional magnetic resonance imaging (fMRI)
Focal disorder, 306
Follicle-stimulating hormone (FSH), 83f–84f, 209, 219
Forgetting, 4, 89, 203, 240–241, 246f
    Alzheimer's disease, 245
    day-to-day clinical practice, 245
    dephosphorylate CREB, 246
    electroconvulsive therapy (ECT), 246, 247f
    forgetting curve, 245
    protein kinases phosphorylate transcription factors, 246
    protein phosphatase 1 (PP1), 246
Fos activity, 225f, 245, 245f
Fos family, 11
Fragile X syndrome, 7
Free-running condition, 196
Frontal cortex, 82, 98, 153, 161, 179–180, 179f–180f, 234f, 235, 245, 251, 252, 262, 266, 278, 279f, 295b, 306–307, 307f, 309, 310f
    addictions, 157–158, 158t
    depression, 275–276, 276f
Frontal lobes loosening, 258–259, 259f
Frontotemporal dementia, 258
FSH (follicle-stimulating hormone), 83f–84f, 209, 219
Functional connectivity imaging technique, 252, 276, 285
Functional magnetic resonance imaging (fMRI), 9, 172, 186, 215, 255, 285, 314
    amygdala, 291, 293, 293f–294f
    auditory hallucinations, 310, 311f
    creativity, intelligence, 256
    depression, 275–276, 276f
    intelligence, 252
    mirror neurons, 234f, 235
    pedophilia, 216

G
GABA. *See* γ-Aminobutyric acid (GABA)
GAD (glutamic acid decarboxylase), 307–308, 308f
Gastric bypass surgery, 144, 167, 172–173, 173f
Gate theory, pain, 133, 136f
Gelatin, 9
Gene activation markers, 11, 245
Gene chips. *See* DNA, microarrays
Gene concealing, 70, 72
Gene expression, 11, 59, 60f, 61, 64, 66, 68, 70, 71f–72f, 72–75, 81, 90, 100, 159, 197, 198f, 211, 218, 224–226, 225f, 239, 246, 280–281, 296, 309, 314
    demethylation, 319b
    memory, 238
    messenger ribonucleic acid (mRNA), 29, 31f
    schizophrenia, 313
    stimulant medication, 270
Gene silencing, 280
Genetics, 3, 7, 11, 164, 247b, 267, 282, 312
    chemical imbalance theories, 67
    copy number variation (CNV), 68–69, 69f
    Human Genome Project. *See* Human Genome Project
    intelligence, 249, 250f
    mental illness heritability, 64, 65t, 66f
    missing heritability, 70
    psychiatric medications, 67
    psychopath, anger and aggression, 188
    schizophrenia, 311
    shared genes, 70
    single genes, linkage studies, 67–68, 67f
    single nucleotide polymorphism (SNP), 68, 68f
    younger gametes, 69–70

Genome-wide association studies, 115, 267, 274, 312, 312f
Genomic effect, 81
Germ theory, 7
Ghrelin, 167, 171–172, 199
Glial cells, 15–16, 99, 106, 112f, 278, 309, 324
  astrocyte, 37–38, 37f
  depression, 280b
  glutamate, 42
  microglia, 37
  oligodendrocyte, 37, 37f
Glial scar, 112–113. *See also* Gliosis
Gliosis, 38, 112, 302
Global activation, bipolar disorder, 284f, 285
Global impairments, addictions, 156, 157f
Glucocorticoid receptors (GRs), 89, 225, 226f, 277, 290
Glucose metabolism, 318, 318f
Glutamate, 38b, 42–43, 42b, 53–54, 55f, 61, 117, 127–128,
    140f, 158, 161, 212, 238, 246, 281, 314
  disorders, 42b
  glial cells, 42
  nitric oxide (NO), 49
Glutamic acid decarboxylase (GAD), 307–308, 308f
Glycine, 36, 42–43, 48, 53–54
P-Glycoprotein, 27
Glymphatic system, 201
Golgi apparatus, neuronal cell, 29, 48
Golgi stain, 9, 9f
Gonadal steroids, 95, 211–212, 220b, 224
Gonadotropin-releasing hormone (GnRH), 84f, 209,
    209b, 219b
Gonads, 209, 209b, 219f, 220
G protein–coupled receptor, types, 55–56, 59
Gray matter, 15–16, 16f, 19, 19f–20f, 29, 30f, 38, 38f, 42,
    94, 98–99, 99f, 111, 112f, 138, 141f, 143, 143f,
    156, 188, 198, 214–216, 252, 268–269, 269f,
    271, 285, 285f, 310, 311f, 313–314, 320
  bipolar disorder, 285, 285f
  intelligence, 251, 251f
  schizophrenia
    during adolescence, 305
    brain imaging techniques, 304
    childhood-onset schizophrenia *vs.* age-matched
      controls, 305
    in children, 305, 305f
    coronal magnetic resonance imaging, 304, 304f
    functional brain imaging, 306–307, 307f
    inhibitory neurons, 307–308, 308f
    Judith Rapoport's laboratory, 305
    process of, 305
    reduced neuropil hypothesis, 305–306, 306f–307f
Growth factor proteins, 59, 99, 105, 111, 127, 137,
    212–213, 213f, 278, 280, 282f, 296, 323–324
Guanosine triphosphate–binding protein, 49, 55
Gut hormones, 166–167, 167f, 172

H
H₁ histamine receptor, 59, 174t, 175
Habituation, pleasure, 155–156, 155f
Hallucinations, 124, 195, 196f, 281, 302–303, 306,
    309–310, 311f
  normal sleep, 195
Head trauma, anger and aggression, 179b
Health care system, 316
Heart rate, 46b, 177, 184, 186–187, 194, 288–289
  men, 25b
Hebb's postulate, 238
Heredity, 2–3, 3f, 4t, 5f, 65

Heroin, 139–140, 157, 159, 269
Heterogeneous pathophysiology, 5, 6f
High-frequency ultrasound/transcranial magnetic
    stimulation, 26b
High vocal center (HVC), 214, 214f, 240, 249, 250f
Hippocampal dentate gyrus, 13
Hippocampus, 19, 21, 21f, 22b, 43, 48, 61, 62f, 82, 84,
    86, 89–90, 92–93, 95, 95b, 96f, 127, 150, 195,
    201–202, 203f, 212f, 225–226, 226f, 239–241,
    244–245, 244f, 266, 277–278, 279f, 291,
    296–297, 297f, 321
  activated HPA axis, 293
  declarative memory, 242–243, 243f
  explicit memory acquisition, 293
  GAD diagnosis, 294
  and memory persistence, 240
  mental illness, 294
  posttraumatic stress disorder (PTSD) score, 293–294,
      294f, 297f
Hippocrates (melancholia), 274
Histamine, 47, 133, 199
  receptors, 59, 174, 174t
Histamine-3 receptor antagonists, 47
Histones acetylation, 239
Home-based sleep monitoring system, 195, 196f
Homeostatic mechanisms, appetite
  adiposity signal, 168
  arcuate nucleus, 168, 169f
  autonomic nervous system (ANS), 166
  downstream effects, 169
  eating pleasure, 167
  endocannabinoids, 170–171
  food intake, 165
  gut hormones, 167, 167f
  lateral hypothalamic (LH) area, 169, 171f
  leptin, 168, 168f
  long-term signals, 167–168
  mechanoreceptors, 166
  neuropeptide Y (NPY), 168–169, 170f
  nutrients, 166
  paraventricular nucleus (PVN), 169, 171f
  proopiomelanocortin (POMC), 168–169
  short-term signals, 166
Homeostatic sleep drive, 200
Hormone replacement therapy (HRT), 217, 217f, 220
Hormones, 2, 23, 26, 41, 46, 48, 48b, 55, 95, 100b, 113–
    114, 118, 127, 166–169, 167f–168f, 172–173,
    173f, 199, 202, 207, 211–212, 214–220, 217f,
    219f, 222, 224, 226f, 231, 240, 241b, 277b,
    281, 289, 289f, 295
  Addison's disease, 89b
  γ-aminobutyric acid (GABA) receptor, 79, 80f
  anger and aggression, 181–183, 182f–184f
  anorexia nervosa, 86b
  autonomic nervous system (ANS), 79
  central nervous system (CNS), 81–82, 83f–84f, 84f
  chemical communication systems, 79, 80f
  cholesterol, 209
  classification, 79, 80t
  Cushing's disease, 89b
  differentiation and activation, 209–210, 211f
  electrochemical connections, 79
  α-fetoprotein, 209
  follicle-stimulating hormone (FSH), 209
  gonadotropin-releasing hormone (GnRH), 209, 209b
  human congenital anomalies, 210–211, 212f
  luteinizing hormone (LH), 209
  male secondary sexual characteristics control, 208–209

Hormones *(Continued)*
  mood disorders, 84b
  neuroendocrine cells, 79
  neurosteroids, 209
  target cells, 80–81, 81f
  testosterone, 209, 209f
  thyroid. *See* Thyroid
  transmitter synthesis/release, 209, 210f
HRT (hormone replacement therapy), 217, 217f, 220
Human congenital anomalies, 210–211, 212f
Human Genome Project
  Caenorhabditis elegans, 65
  gene regulation, 66
  nucleic acids sequence, 65
  protein-coding genes, 65
  RNA world, 65–66, 66b
Human life span, 240, 316b
Human longevity, 316, 316b, 316f
HVC (high vocal center), 214, 214f, 240, 249, 250f
5-Hydroxytryptamine (5-HT) neurons, 46, 48b, 278
Hyperarousal, 204b
Hypercortisolemia, 89, 276–277
Hyperlipidemia, 7
Hyperphosphorylation, tau proteins, 320, 321f
Hyperprolactinemia, 44
Hypertension, 7, 89, 172
Hypoconnectivity, frontoparietal network, 276
Hypocretin, 47, 199
Hypofrontality, 306
Hypoglycemia, 166
Hypomania, 89b, 257, 257f
Hypothalamic–pituitary–adrenal (HPA) axis, 82, 86–90,
    87f–88f, 90f, 95, 114, 119, 119f, 159, 226,
    228f, 275, 275f, 290, 292f, 293, 295
  depression, 276–278, 277b, 277f
  parental behavior, 224
Hypothalamic–pituitary–thyroid (HPT) axis, 82–84,
    82f, 85f, 86t
Hypothalamus, 21, 26, 44, 45f, 47, 79, 81–82, 83f–84f,
    84, 86, 89, 138, 165–168, 169f, 171, 171f, 173,
    177, 179, 178f, 178t, 180f, 180b, 181, 188, 195,
    198–200, 199f, 201, 203, 204b, 209, 215, 218,
    224–225, 230, 277, 291
  chemoreceptors, 23
  control panel, 22
  parasympathetic division, 23–24
  position of, 23, 24f
  sleep–wake cycles, 22–23
  sources of, 23
  steroid hormones and neuropeptides, 23
  sympathetic division, 23–24

I
Immediate memory, 237, 242. *See also* Working memory
Immune function, 89, 200
Immune system, 108, 109b, 111, 113–117, 120f, 126, 200,
    306, 312, 322
Immunity and inflammation
  anti-inflammatory antidepressants, 114b
  anti-inflammatory diet, 116b
  autoimmune disease, 116–117, 117f
  autonomic nervous system (ANS), 118
  components, 108
  cytokines. *See* Cytokines
  electrodes, 111–112, 112f
  endocrine system, 118
  endogenous cortisol, 118

  glial scar, 112–113
  microglia, 111
  protection layers, 111
  rejuvenating capacity, 111
  stress-induced immune dysfunction, 118–120
  substance abuse vaccine, 109b
  syphilis. *See* Syphilis
Immunizations, 322
Impaired communication disorder, 310
Implicit memory, 237, 242
Impulse control, 18, 26, 156, 184, 216, 220, 265–267
Indoleamines, 43, 46, 46f–47f, 47b
Induced pluripotent stem cells, 12–13, 13f
Infantile amnesia, 240–241
Information-processing, sleep
  development, 201–202, 202f
  memory consolidation, 202, 203f
  neurogenesis, 202
  pruning, 97, 202–203, 203f
Inhibitory neurons, 16f, 36f, 54, 56b, 156, 307–308, 308f
  monoamines, 43
  postsynaptic potentials, 33, 34f
Inhibitory postsynaptic potentials (IPSPs), 33, 34f, 36
Insomnia, 47, 89b, 199, 200, 203, 204b, 205, 275
  GABAergic activity, 43
  inhibitory potentials, 35b
Insula cortex, 18–19, 20f
Intellectual abilities, 252
Intelligence, 156, 237
  attention deficit hyperactivity disorder (ADHD), 253b
  bipolar disorder, 252
  brain size, 249–250, 250f
  Brilliant Madness, 252–253
  cognitive deficits, 254–256, 254f–256f
  creativity, 256–259, 257f–259f
  Flynn effect, 252b
  genetics, 249, 250f
  "genius" *vs.* "madness," 252
  "g"/fluid intelligence, 249
  mental illness, 253
  performance enhancement, 253–254
  schizophrenia, 252, 253b
  smartest animal, 250–251, 251f
  smartest humans, 251–252, 251f
  standard deviations, 252, 253f
  tests, 249
  variables, 249
Interferon (IFN), 113
Interleukin (IL), 113, 114
Intermittent explosive disorder, anger and aggression, 181b
Interstitial nuclei of the anterior hypothalamus (INAH),
    215–216, 216f–217f
Intracellular neurofibrillary tangles. *See* Neurofibrillary
    tangles
Intranasal delivery, 26b
In vivo measurement of brain volume, 251
IPSPs (inhibitory postsynaptic potentials), 33, 34f, 36

J
Joubert syndrome, 7
Junk DNA, 65–66, 312

K
Kainate, 54
Ketamine, 54, 139, 281–282
Klüver–Bucy syndrome, 180–181, 291
Knockout mice, silenced genes, 11

L

Labor-intensive three-dimensional analytic tools, 305
Lancet Commission, 325, 325t
Language expression deficits, 309
Latent inhibition, 258, 258f
Learning, definition, 237
Learning disorder, 30, 175, 255
Leptin, 168–172, 168f, 199
LH (luteinizing hormone), 48, 83f–84f, 209
Life expectancy, 316
Limbic lobe, 19, 21, 21f, 22b
Lithium, 13, 82, 100b, 181b, 204, 277–278, 280
    anger and aggression, 185b
    bipolar disorder, 285
Longevity, appetite, 174b
Long-term declarative memories, 242, 244, 244f
Long-term memories, 54, 129, 237–242, 238b, 244, 246
    electroconvulsive therapy (ECT), 246, 247f
Long-term potentiation (LTP), 60–61, 61f–62f, 89, 105,
        292, 296
    memory, 238
Long-term signals, food intake, 167–168
    adiposity signal, 168
    arcuate nucleus, 168, 169f
    leptin, 168, 168f
    proopiomelanocortin (POMC), 168–169
Luteinizing hormone (LH), 48, 83f–84f, 209

M

Magnetic resonance imaging (MRI), 9, 10b, 98–99, 117,
        126, 215–216, 233, 251, 254, 258, 277, 285f,
        293, 299, 323
    attention deficit hyperactivity disorder (ADHD),
        267–268
    cortical atrophy, 318, 318f
    pair bonding, 227
    pedophilia, 216
    schizophrenia, 304–305, 304f, 309, 314
    water movement, 38
Major depression, 18, 21, 70, 278, 284
Maladaptive neuroplasticity, 105, 106f
Mammalian reward system, 149
Mania, 129, 204–205, 285
    GABAergic activity, 43
    inhibitory potentials, 35b
Manic depression, 302
Massachusetts Institute of Technology (MIT), 239
Maturational process, 310
Mean spine density, 306, 307f
Mechanoreceptors, 133, 166
Medial prefrontal cortex (mPFC), 292–293
Medication-resistant depression, 46b
Melanocortin (MC), 167–168, 218
α-Melanocyte-stimulating hormone (α-MSH), 218
Melatonin, 43, 46, 197b, 203–205
Memory, 3, 5, 11, 18, 21, 26, 37–38, 42b, 48, 48b, 54,
        59–61, 89–90, 93, 95, 105, 124, 129, 142–143,
        150, 152–153, 156, 160, 191–192, 195, 202,
        203f, 220, 254, 261–265, 264f, 265b, 267, 282,
        292–297, 300, 306, 308, 312, 317, 319, 320,
        322–324, 326
    alcoholic blackouts, 238b
    amygdala, 292
    consolidation, 238
    D-cycloserine, 239
    declarative memory, 237. *See also* Declarative memory
    definition, 237

    epigenetics, 239
    extinction, 239
    fear reduction, 239
    forgetting. *See* Forgetting
    growth process/metabolic change, 238
    Hebb's postulate, 238
    hippocampus, 21
    immediate memory, 237
    long-term memories, 237–238
    long-term potentiation (LTP), 238
    mnemonist, 247b
    nondeclarative memory, 237
    and pleasure, 243b
    posttraumatic stress disorder (PTSD), 237
    protein synthesis, 238, 239f
    psychotherapy enhancer, 239
    reconsolidation, 241, 242b
    short-term memory, 237
    stress and, 241b
    structural plasticity, 239–241, 240f–241f
    temporal stages of, 237, 238f
    types, 237
Memory consolidation, sleep, 202, 203f
Mental illness, 2, 7–8, 13, 15, 19, 20f, 26, 37, 41b–42b,
        69–70, 74–76, 76f, 82, 108–109, 252–253,
        267, 283, 294, 299, 304f
    and creativity, intelligence, 257–258, 257f–258f
    depression, 114
    heritability, 64, 65t, 66f
    inflammatory response, 116
    schizophrenia, 115–116, 115f
Mental retardation (MR), 9, 15b, 30, 180
    cognitive skills, 254–255
    dendritic pathology, 254, 254f
    deprivation, 254
    dose–response effect, 255, 255f
    environmental impoverishment, 254
Mesolimbic pathway, addictions, 156, 157f
Messenger ribonucleic acid (mRNA), 11–12, 48, 66,
        71f, 308, 313
    brain-derived neurotrophic factor (BDNF), 280, 281f
    genetic instructions, nucleus to cytoplasm, 29, 31f
    ribosome, 29, 31f
Metachromatic leukodystrophy, 309
Methamphetamine, 154, 157, 161, 269–270, 298
N-Methyl-D-aspartate (NMDA), 54, 55f, 61, 62f, 117b,
        212f, 238–240, 281–282
N-Methyl-D-aspartate glutamate receptors, 212
3,4-Methylenedioxymethamphetamine (MDMA), 298
Methylphenidate (MPH), 58, 74, 151, 151f, 161f, 175, 253,
        265, 266b, 269
    placebo controlled trial, 271, 271f
Microarray analysis, 309
Microarray chip, 12, 13f, 309
Microdialysis, pleasure, 151, 151f
Microglia cells, 37, 111
"Minibrains" growth, 13, 13f
Minimal brain dysfunction, 268b
Minimally invasive technique, 22b
Mini-Mental Status Examination, 246
Minnesota Multiphasic Personality Inventory, 257, 258f
Mirror neurons, 233–235, 234f
Mirror-tracing task, 242, 243f
MIT (Massachusetts Institute of Technology), 239
Mitochondria, 29, 33f, 200
Mnemonist, 247b
Modafinil, 47, 174, 199, 253
Monoamine hypothesis, 274

Monoamine oxidases (MAOs), 43
Monoamines, 42b, 43–46, 43b, 44f–47f, 46b–47b, 49b, 50,
     56, 59, 67, 108, 114, 198, 274
  histamine, 47
  orexin/hypocretin (O/H) neurons, 47
Monoclonal antibodies, 117
  A-β oligomers, 323
  A-β PET scan, 322–323, 323f
  aducanumab, 322
  amyloid-related imaging abnormalities (ARIAs), 323
Monozygotic (identical) twins, 2–3, 4t, 5f
  alcoholism, 3
  bipolar disorder, 3
  panic disorder, 3
  schizophrenia, 3, 311
Montreal Procedure, 124
Mood control, 18
Mood disorders, 75b, 84b, 127–128
  bipolar disorder, 204–205
  circadian dysfunction, 203
  depressive symptoms, 219
  estrogen levels alterations, 218, 219f
  hormone replacement, 220
  insomnia, 205
  prevalence of, 218
  seasonal affective disorder (SAD), 203–204
  of sex hormones, 219, 219f
  Veterans Administration (VA) study, 219
mPFC (medial prefrontal cortex), 292–293
MRI. *See* Magnetic resonance imaging (MRI)
mRNA. *See* Messenger ribonucleic acid (mRNA)
α-MSH (α-melanocyte-stimulating hormone), 218
Multicriteria decision analysis, 269
Multiple sclerosis (MS), 37, 100, 116–117, 126, 309
Muscarinic receptor, 24, 59
Muscle tone, 194, 199, 201
Myasthenia gravis, 59b
Myelin, 12, 37, 116, 125–126, 309, 309f
Myelinization process, 37

N
NAc. *See* Nucleus accumbens (NAc)
Narcolepsy, 47, 194, 199–200, 199b, 199f, 253
National Institute of Mental Health (NIMH), 7, 251,
     267, 304
NE. *See* Norepinephrine (NE)
Neglect syndrome, 268b
Neocortex, declarative memory, 244, 244f
Nerve growth factor (NGF), 99–100, 100f, 278, 323–324
  pair bonding, 227, 229f
Nerve growth, sex
  gonadal steroids, 211
  growth factor proteins, 212–213, 213f
  ovariectomized rats, 212, 212f
  transcription factors, 211
Nerve regeneration, 106
Neural plasticity, 113–114, 116
Neuroanatomy, cerebral cortex, 15–23
Neuroblasts, 17f
  cerebral cortex, layers, 15, 16f
  inhibitory interneurons, 15
  neurogenesis, 15
Neurodegenerative disorders, 64, 100, 201b, 302, 316
Neurodevelopmental disruption, 310
Neuroendocrine mechanisms, 231b
Neurofeedback, 265, 266f
Neurofibrillary tangles, 317, 317f, 324

Alzheimer's disease (AD) progression, 320–321, 321f
  microtubules, 320
  tau proteins, 320, 320b, 321f
Neurofibromatosis, 7
Neurogenesis, 15, 89, 98, 106, 114, 240–241, 241b,
     242f, 278
  adult macaque monkeys, 93, 94f
  brain-derived neurotrophic factor (BDNF), 279, 280f
  granule cell layer, 92, 94f
  hippocampus, 21
  information-processing, sleep, 202
  neocortex, 94
  neural stem cells, 92
  postmortem analysis, 94, 95f
  process of, 92, 93f
  rate of, 95, 96f
  stem cells, 95–97, 97f
  subgranular zone (SGZ), 92
Neuronal cell, 50, 92, 97, 307, 317
  axoplasmic transport, 32
  dendrites, 29, 32f. *See also* Dendritic spines
  energy production, 29
  Golgi apparatus, 29
  messenger ribonucleic acid (mRNA), 29, 31f
  mitochondria, 29
  neurotransmitters, 32
  postsynaptic dendrite, 32
  prefrontal cortex (PFC), 29, 30f
  protein synthesis, 29
  synapse, axon terminal end, 32, 33f
Neuronal circuits, 11, 16, 158, 195–200, 197f–199f, 198t,
     197b, 199b, 204, 211–215, 212f–214f
  amygdala, 290–292, 291b, 292f–293f
  hippocampus, 293–294, 294f, 297f
  prefrontal cortex (PFC), 292–293, 293f–294f
  regions of, 290, 291f
Neuronal density, 306, 306f
Neuronal mechanisms, 148, 214, 234
Neuron morphology, 9, 213
Neuropathic pain, 134b, 142, 144–145
Neuropathology, 5, 116, 302
Neuropeptides, 41, 42f, 42b, 48, 49b, 49t, 50f, 79, 140f, 168,
     173, 200, 218, 222, 224, 227–229, 230f, 231
  anger and aggression, 181–183, 182f–184f
  hypothalamus, 23
Neuropeptide Y (NPY), 168–169, 170f
Neuropsychiatric syndromes, 303
Neuropsychological testing, 265, 266f
Neurosteroids, 55, 79–80, 209, 220
Neurotransmitters, 23, 32–33, 33f, 36–37, 53, 54f, 55–56,
     56b–57b, 57f, 59–60, 79, 127, 127f, 155, 172,
     224, 231, 274, 296b
  amines, 41, 42f
  amino acids, 41, 42f
  γ-aminobutyric acid (GABA), 41, 42f, 295
  brain-derived neurotrophic factor, 296
  Ca^{2+} influx, 42
  classic neurotransmitters, 42–48, 42b–43b,
     43f–47f, 46b–48b
  Diagnostic and Statistical Manual of Mental Disorders
     (DSM), 41b
  electrochemical communication, 41b
  neuropeptide, 41, 42f
  neuropeptides, 48, 49b, 49t, 50f
  norepinephrine (NE), 295, 296b
  presynaptic/postsynaptic neuron, 41
  types, 41
  unconventional neurotransmitters, 49–51, 51b

Neurotrophic growth factor (NGF), 99–100, 100f, 227, 229f, 278, 323–324
Neutralizing C fibers, 134b
NGF. *See* Nerve growth factor (NGF)
NIH NeuroBioBank, 8–9
NIMH (National Institute of Mental Health), 7, 267, 304
Nitric oxide (NO), 61
  on behavior and mental disorders, 51b
  glutamate, 49
Nociceptive pain, 133, 142
Nociceptors, 133
Nondeclarative memory, 237
Nongenomic effect, 81
Nonneuronal cells, 94
  astrocyte, 37–38, 37f
  demyelinating disorders, 37
  epilepsy, 38b
  glial cells, 37–38
  microglia, 37
  oligodendrocyte, 37, 37f
Non–rapid eye movement (NREM) sleep, 130, 191
  ascending arousal systems, 198
  brain imaging, 194
  dreaming, 195, 196f
  electroencephalographic (EEG) patterns, 192–194, 193f
  memory consolidation, 202
  muscle tone, 194
  sleepwalking and night terrors, 195b
Noradrenergic neurons, 44–45, 139, 198
Norepinephrine (NE), 24, 41, 42b, 43, 57b, 58, 83, 145, 199, 218, 263, 274
  alertness, 45
  antidepressants and anxiety, 296b
  in anxiety, 46b
  β blocker, 295
  catecholamines, 263–264
  in depression, 46b
  locus coeruleus, 44–45, 46b
  noradrenergic system, 44, 45f
  stress response system, 295
  vagus nerve stimulation (VNS), 46b
Normal sleep
  aging, 195, 196f
  brain imaging, 194
  consciousness as awake, 191
  dreaming, 195, 196f
  electroencephalographic (EEG) patterns, 192–194, 192f–193f, 194b
  long-term shift work, 191
  muscle tone, 194
  neurobehavioral tasks, 191, 192f
  night terrors, 195b
  non–rapid eye movement (non-REM) sleep, 191
  nonsomniacs, 191
  psychiatric community, 191
  rapid eye movement (REM) sleep, 191
  self-reported average duration, 191, 192f
  sleepwalking, 195b
  stages of, 191
NREM sleep. *See* Non–rapid eye movement (NREM) sleep
Nucleus accumbens (NAc), 43, 43b, 45, 150, 150f–151f, 155f, 157f, 159f–160f, 167, 169b, 171, 187, 187f, 189, 218, 224, 274, 326b
  attention, 266
  impulsive behavior, 266
  impulsivity and youth, 266–267, 267f
Nucleus signaling, 59, 60f
Nutrients, 37, 166

O
Obesity, 11, 51, 73f, 74, 89b, 116b, 167, 169, 325
  dietary treatment interventions, 164
  drug treatments, 172, 172t
  gastric bypass surgery, 172–173, 173f
  leptin-deficient humans and rodents, 171
  pulmonary hypertension/valvular disease, 172
  sleep, 199b
  vagus nerve stimulation (VNS), 173
Obsessive–compulsive disorder (OCD), 18, 227, 288, 300b
  basal ganglia, 298–299, 298f
  classification, 298
  heart rates, men, 25b
  OC spectrum disorders, 298
  psychosurgery, 299–300, 299f
  symptoms of, 298
  von Economo's encephalitis, 298
OCD. *See* Obsessive–compulsive disorder (OCD)
OFC (orbitofrontal cortex), 143, 148, 149f, 155, 158, 167, 187, 224, 266, 299
Oligodendrocyte cells, 37, 37f, 106, 111, 309, 309f
Opioids, 109b, 143–144, 148, 152, 167, 171, 204b, 267, 278, 281
  acupuncture, 140–142
  descending pain-modulating circuits, 138, 139f
  endogenous opioids, 140, 140f
  opium, 139
  periaqueductal gray, 138
  placebo, 140, 141f
  pleasure, 154–155
  receptors, 139
  rostral ventral medulla (RVM), 139
  stress-induced analgesia, 142
Optogenetics, 11, 12f
Orbitofrontal cortex (OFC), 143, 148, 149f, 155, 158, 167, 187, 224, 266, 299
Orexin/hypocretin (O/H) neurons, 47, 199–200, 199f, 205
Orexin neurons, 199–200, 199f, 205
Orexin receptor antagonists, 47
Oxytocin, 222–223
  amino acids, 230, 230f
  cuddle hormone levels, 231, 231f
  in hypothalamus, 229–230
  lay press, 231

P
Pain, 49b, 51, 56b, 109, 129, 154b, 155, 172, 185, 218, 241, 278, 324
  acute, 133–137, 134f–137f, 136t
  chronic, 142–144, 143f, 145f
  congenital insensitivity, 137–138, 138f
  depression and antidepressants, 145–146, 145f
  descending pathways and opioids, 138–142, 139f–141f
  GABAergic activity, 43
  neutralizing C fibers, 134b
  postoperative pain, 144b
  prefrontal cortex (PFC), 144b
  schizophrenia, 138
  transcranial magnetic stimulation (TMS), 144b
Pair bonding
  caudate nucleus (CN), 227, 229f
  dopamine (DA), 227
  human male–female affiliation, 231
  monogamy, 226
  nerve growth factor (NGF), 227, 229f
  neuroendocrine systems, 231
  oxytocin, 229–231, 230f–231f

Pair bonding *(Continued)*
 romantic love, 227
 sexual reproduction, 226
 vasopressin, 227–229, 230f
 ventral tegmental area (VTA), 227, 229f
Panic disorder, monozygotic (identical) twins, 3
Paradoxical effect, 175
Parasympathetic division, 23–24
Paraventricular nucleus (PVN), 169, 170, 171, 171f, 222
Parental behavior
 adrenocorticotropic hormone, 224
 corticosterone response, 224
 DNA effect, 225–226, 228f
 dopamine, 224, 224b
 growth and survival, 222
 hormones, 222, 223f
 hypothalamic–pituitary–adrenal (HPA) axis, 224
 hypothalamic region, 224, 225f
 lick and groom behavior, 225, 226f
 maternal behavior, 223
 nulliparous rats, 222, 223f
 offspring's behavior, 224
 preoptic area (POA), 223
 trading places, 225, 227f
Parkinson's disease (PD), 58, 96, 123, 125, 129, 155,
  201b, 298, 316
 benzedrine/dexedrine, weight loss, 270–271
 deep brain stimulation (DBS), 125, 129, 155, 283, 283f
 L-DOPA, 43, 44f
 dopamine (DA) loss, 43
 methamphetamine abuse, 270
Partner Bonding Scale, 229
Parvalbumin neurons, 307–308
Passionate Love Scale, 227, 229f
Peripheral autonomic nervous system (ANS). *See also*
  Autonomic nervous system (ANS)
 acetylcholine (ACh), 48
Personality tests, 2
PFC. *See* Prefrontal cortex (PFC)
Phenylketonuria (PKU), 7
Phonics-based reading intervention, 255–256, 256f
Phosphodiesterase-5 inhibitors, 218
PKU (phenylketonuria), 7
Plasticity and adult development, 3, 42b
 adult neuroplasticity. *See* Adult neuroplasticity
 apoptosis, 92, 98
 cell expansion, 92, 97, 98f
 connection refinement, 92, 97–98
 critical periods, 100–101, 101f–103f
 dendritic spines, 30
 neurogenesis, 92. *See also* Neurogenesis
 neurotrophic growth factor (NGF), 99–100, 100f–101f
 neurotrophins, 100b
 noninvasive magnetic resonance imaging (MRI)
  technology, 98–99, 99f
 personality, 102b
 stroke, 104b
Pleasure, 133, 167, 169b, 187, 187f, 218, 231, 326b
 abuse and pleasant feelings, 152, 152f
 addiction. *See* Addiction
 amygdala, 153–154
 anatomy of, 150, 150f
 anhedonia, 156b
 dopamine, 154
 drug-Seeking behavior, 151
 electrode placement, rat's skull, 149, 149f
 goal-directed behavior, 148, 149f
 habituation, 155–156, 155f

happiness, 148
mammalian reward system, 149
marital conflict, 148b
mesolimbic dopamine (DA) system, 150
methylphenidate (MPH), 151, 151f
microdialysis, 151, 151f
opioids, 154–155
positron emission tomography, 153, 153f
rewarding activities, 154
self-stimulation, 150
voluntary and unconscious behavior, 148
Pneumoencephalography, 9, 10t
Pneumonia, 7
 causes, 274
POMC (proopiomelanocortin), 140b, 168–169, 170b
Positron emission tomography (PET), 9, 10t, 84, 137,
  137f, 141, 153, 153f, 180, 194, 318, 318f,
  319f
 cortical atrophy, 318, 318f
 depression, 275, 276f
 pleasure, 153, 153f
Postganglionic norepinephrine receptors, 24
Postganglionic sympathetic neurons, 24
Postmortem analysis, depressed patients, 94, 95f, 215, 216,
  217f, 278
Poststroke rehabilitation, 264
Postsynaptic dendrite, 32, 61
Postsynaptic neuron, 51, 79, 140f, 161, 238
Postsynaptic potentials, electrical signaling
 depolarization, 33
 excitatory neuron, 33, 34f
 hyperpolarization, 33
 inhibitory neuron, 33, 34f
 postsynaptic synapses (spines), 32–33
Posttraumatic stress disorder (PTSD), 46b, 90, 277, 280,
  290, 293, 294f, 298
 amygdala, 293, 294f
 Diagnostic and Statistical Manual (DSM) system, 288
 hippocampus, 293–294, 294f, 297f
 memory, 237
PP1 (protein phosphatase 1), 246
Predatory attack, anger and aggression, 177, 178f
Prefrontal cortex (PFC), 43b, 84, 97, 129, 144b, 148, 150,
  155, 156, 158, 161, 173, 179, 179b, 180b, 186,
  188, 218, 264, 265b, 267–269, 275, 280b, 285,
  286, 292, 306, 307, 314
 anxiety, 292–293, 293f–294f
 apathetic syndromes, 18
 disinhibited syndromes, 18
 disorganized syndromes, 18
 dysfunction in, 17
 emotional and social functions, 18
 frontal lobe damage, 17–18
 insula cortex, 18–19, 20f
 intelligence, 251, 251f
 myelinization process, 37
 neuronal cell, 29, 30f
 prefrontal lobotomy, 22b
 psychopath, anger and aggression, 186, 186f
 regions of, 17, 20f
 Wisconsin Card Sort test, 307, 307f
 working memory, 262, 263f–264f
Prefrontal limbic governing system, 280
Prefrontal lobotomy, 22b, 181
Preganglionic neurons, 24
Pregnancy, 209, 214–215, 220, 223
Prenatal complications, schizophrenia, 311
Preoptic area (POA), 215, 218, 223

Procedural memory. *See* Nondeclarative memory
Proopiomelanocortin (POMC), 140b, 168–169, 170b
Propeptide precursor, 48, 87
Propeptide proopiomelanocortin, 218, 218f
Prosopagnosia, 7
Protein-coding genes, 65, 66, 68
Protein-coding regions, 11
Protein, fluorescent, 11
Protein phosphatase 1 (PP1), 246
Protein synthesis, 29, 32, 80, 211, 238, 239f, 281, 292
    inhibitors, 238, 239f, 241, 292
Pruning, information-processing, sleep, 97, 202–203, 203f
Psychiatric diagnosis, 7
Psychiatric disorders, 7–9, 21, 25b, 39f, 49b, 64, 65t, 67,
        80, 108, 114, 198
    cognitive decline, 217, 217f
    mood disorders, 218–220, 219f
    pregnancy and depression, 220
    sexual dysfunction, 217–218, 218f
    traumatic brain injury (TBI), 220
Psychiatric Genomic Consortium, 312
Psychoanalytic theory, 302
Psychopath, anger and aggression
    factors, 185
    genetics, 188
    prefrontal cortex and amygdala, 186, 186f
    resting heart rate, 186–188, 187f
    symptoms, 185
    violence pleasure, 185, 187–188, 187f
Psychosis, 5, 89b, 117b, 185b, 253b, 303, 305, 305f, 314
    creativity, 257
Psychostimulants, addictions, 58, 161, 161f
Psychosurgery, 22b
    anger and aggression, 180b
    anterior cingulotomy, 299, 299f
    complications, 299
    cortico–subcortical circuit, 299
    deep brain stimulation (DBS), 299
    supplementary motor area (SMA), 300
    transcranial magnetic stimulation (TMS), 300
    treatment-resistant patients, 299
Psychotherapy, 129, 188, 241
    antidepressant, 297, 297f
    enhancer, 239
    fear extinction, 297
    medications, 297
    3,4-methylenedioxymethamphetamine (MDMA), 298
    phase III trials, 298
    selective serotonin reuptake inhibitors (SSRIs) treatment
        and fear learning, 297
Psychotic depression, 274
Purging, eating disorders, 173
Pyramidal nerve cells, 9, 9f
Pyramidal neurons, 16, 29, 126, 158, 161, 161f, 233,
        307–308

R
Randomized controlled clinical trial, 14, 265
Rapid eye movement (REM) sleep, 130, 191
    aging, 195
    ascending arousal systems, 198
    brain imaging, 194
    consciousness, 130
    dream enactment, 201b
    dreaming, 195, 196f
    electroencephalographic (EEG) patterns, 192–194,
        192f–193f

    memory consolidation, 202
    muscle tone, 194
    sleepwalking and night terrors, 195b
RDoC (Research Domain Criteria), 7, 179, 288
Reconsolidation, 241, 242b
Reduced neuropil hypothesis, 305–306, 306f–307f
Reduction/discontinuation group, 314
Reelin, 313
Refrigerator mother/double-bind. *See* Schizophrenia
Relapse, addictions,159
REM sleep. *See* Rapid eye movement (REM) sleep
Reparative, 200–201
Research Domain Criteria (RDoC), 7, 179, 288
Reserpine, 50–51
Resting heart rate, anger and aggression, 25, 46, 186–188,
        187f
Resting metabolic rate (RMR), 86, 165, 166f, 175
Resting-state functional magnetic resonance imaging,
        276, 276f
Restorative sleep
    energy conservation, 200
    glymphatic system, 201
    homeostatic sleep drive, 200
    immune function, 200
    reparative, 200–201
Reticular activating system, 198
Rett syndrome, 7
Reward dysfunction, 278
Rhythmic motor abnormalities, 269
RMR (resting metabolic rate), 86, 165, 166f, 175
Romantic love, pair bonding, 227

S
SAD (seasonal affective disorder), 203–204
Salivary cortisol levels, acute stress, 289
Salutatory conduction, 126
Schizophrenia, 2–5, 16, 18, 25b, 69, 75b, 114–116,
        138b, 253b
    antipsychotics, 314
    auditory hallucinations, 309–310, 310b, 310f–311f
    and bipolar disorder, 284–285
    brain shrinking, 314
    chlorpromazine (Thorazine), 302
    chronic hallucinations, 302
    chronic mental illness, 303, 304f
    clinical course of, 302, 303f
    conditions, 302–303
    creativity, 257
    delusions, 303
    diagnostic criteria, 302
    disconnected, social attachment, 231–232
    dopamine (DA) blockers, 224, 224b
    dopamine (DA) hypothesis, 313–314
    famine, schizophrenia, 311, 311f
    Finnish Adoption Study, 311–312, 312f
    gene expression, 313
    genetic profile, 2, 3f
    genetics, 311
    genome-wide association studies, 312, 312f
    gliosis, 302
    gray matter, 16. *See also* Gray matter
    hallucinations, 303
    heart rates, men, 25b
    history, 302
    immune system, 312
    impaired communication disorder, 310
    intelligence, 252, 253b

Schizophrenia *(Continued)*
  junk DNA, 312
  maturational process, 310
  monozygotic (identical) twins, 3
  myelination-related genes, 12
  myelinization, 37
  negative symptoms of, mesocortical system, 43b
  neurodevelopmental disruption, 310
  neuropsychiatric syndromes, 303
  in older fathers, 313b
  optogenetics, 11
  pain, 138
  positive symptoms of, mesolimbic system, 43b
  prefrontal cortex (PFC), 17
  prenatal complications, 311
  Psychiatric Genomic Consortium, 312
  psychoanalytic theory, 302
  reduction/discontinuation group, 314
  single nucleotide polymorphisms, 313b
  white matter, 308–309, 308f–309f
Schwann cell, 37
Sclerotic plaques, 317
SCN (suprachiasmatic nucleus), in sleep, 195–196, 197f
Seasonal affective disorder (SAD), 203–204
Secondary messenger cascade, 56, 57f
α-Secretase, 319, 325
β- and γ-Secretases, 318, 325
  DNA sequence coding, 319b
Seizures, 38, 111, 124, 127, 128b, 180b, 187b, 280b
  glutamate, experimental models, 38b
  vagus nerve stimulation, 26b
Selective serotonin reuptake inhibitors (SSRIs), 145, 181, 185, 288, 297
Self-stimulation, pleasure, 150
Sensory-discriminative domain, 133–134, 136f
Serotonergic neurons, 198, 278
Serotonergic system, 46, 47f
Serotonin, 2, 46, 47b, 53b, 83, 145, 274
  anger and aggression, 183–185, 185f
  depression, 283–284, 283f
  receptors, 56–58
Serotonin (5-hydroxytryptamine), 42b, 46, 46f–47f, 47b
Serum hormone levels, acute stress, 289
Sex, 55, 79, 86, 118, 148b, 156
  age-appropriate members, 215
  antidepressants, 220b
  gonadotropin-releasing hormone agonist, 219b
  homosexual males, 215, 216f
  hormones, 208–211, 209f–212f
  humans, 215
  hypothalamus, 215
  interstitial nuclei of the anterior hypothalamus (INAH), 215, 216f
  nerve growth, 211–213, 212f–213f
  pedophilia, 216
  pregnancy, 214–215
  preoptic area (POA), 215
  psychiatric disorders, 217–220, 217f–219f
  sexual dimorphism. *See* Sexual dimorphism
  sexually dimorphic nucleus of the preoptic area (SDN-POA), 215
  songbirds, 213–214, 214f
  transgender, 215–216, 217f
Sexual dimorphism
  bilateral mastectomies, 208
  categories, 207, 208t
  depression, 208
  environment, 208

  etiology, 207, 208f
  psychosocial and psychosexual development, 208
  sexual reassignment, 207
Sexual dysfunction, 217–218, 218f
Sexually dimorphic nucleus of the preoptic area (SDN-POA), 215
Shared genes, 70
"Shared neural substrate," 19
Short-term memory, 237
Short-term signals, food intake
  eating pleasure, 167
  gut hormones, 167, 167f
  mechanoreceptors, 166
  nutrients, 166
Single nucleotide polymorphism (SNP), 68, 68f, 313b
Single photon emission computerized tomography (SPECT), 9, 10b, 275
Sleep, 47, 126, 130
  ascending arousal systems, 198, 198t
  dream enactment, 201b
  hyperarousal, 204b
  information-processing, 200–203, 202f–203f
  melatonin, 197b
  molecular mechanisms, 197–198, 198f
  mood disorders, 203–205
  narcolepsy, 199–200, 199b, 199f
  normal sleep. *See* Normal sleep
  obesity, 199b
  restorative, 200–201
  sleep rebound, 200
  sleep switch, 198, 199f
  suprachiasmatic nucleus (SCN), 195–196, 197f
  ventrolateral preoptic nucleus (VLPO), 198–199
Sleep switch, 198–200, 199f
Sleep–wake cycles, 22–23, 96, 200
Sleepwalking and night terrors, 195b
Slow receptors
  adrenergic receptors, 58–59
  cholinergic receptors, 59
  dopamine (DA) receptors, 58
  "effector" protein, 56
  G protein–coupled receptor, types, 55
  guanosine triphosphate–binding protein, 55
  histamine receptors, 59
  secondary messenger cascade, 56, 57f
  serotonin receptors, 56–58
Slow wave sleep (SWS), 192, 194b, 202
Smartest animal, 250–251, 251f
Smartest humans, 251–252, 251f
Smoking, appetite, 170b
Social attachment, 183
  disconnected, 231–235, 232f–234f
  pair bonding, 226–231, 229f–231f
  parental behavior, 222–226, 223f, 225f–228f
Social dysfunction, optogenetics, 11, 232
Social functions, 18, 309
Sodium–potassium pump, 125
Somatic memory, 237
Somatosensory cortex105, 106f, 137
  acute pain,133, 134f
Songbirds, 95, 213–214, 214f, 240, 249
SPECT (single photon emission computerized tomography), 9, 10b, 275
Spine formation, 161, 202, 217, 238, 306
Spine morphology, 254, 254f
SSRIs (selective serotonin reuptake inhibitors), 145, 181, 185, 288, 297

Steroid hormones, hypothalamus, 23
  hypothalamus, 23
Stress, 95, 159, 169b, 200, 228f, 231b
  aging, 89–90
  appetite, 169b
  chronic, 89, 277
  Cushing's disease, 89
  and genetics cause deviation, 280, 282f
  glucocorticoid receptors (GRs), 89
  hormonal cascade, 231b
  and memory, 241b
  pathologic consequences, 89
Stress, acute, 118
  amygdala, 290
  characteristics, 289
  endocrine responses, 289–290
  of parachute learning, 289, 289f
  placebo-controlled trials, 290
  posttraumatic stress disorder (PTSD), 290
  in public speaking, 290, 290f
  salivary cortisol levels, 289
  serum hormone levels, 289
Stress, chronic, 86, 89, 241, 292
Stress-induced analgesia, 142
Stress-induced immune dysfunction
  endocrine and autonomic signals, 118
  fatigue, 119–120
  hypothalamic–pituitary–adrenal (HPA) axis, 119, 119f
  Whitehall study, 119, 120f
Stress response system, 295
Structural plasticity, 158f
  neurogenesis, 240–241, 242f
  protein molecules, 239–240
  synaptogenesis, 240, 241f
Substance abuse, 9, 11, 100, 109f, 153, 269
  emotional circuits dysfunction, 39, 39f
  nucleus accumbens, 43b
Substance abuse disorder, 18
Suprachiasmatic nucleus (SCN), 23, 154
  sleep, 195–196, 197f
SWS (slow wave sleep), 192, 194b, 202
Sympathetic division, 23–24, 79
Synapse, axon terminal end, 32, 33f
Synaptic plasticity control, 305
Synaptic remodeling, addictions, 158–159, 159f
Synaptogenesis, 97–98, 202, 240, 241f, 282
Syphilis
  adaptive immunity, 109
  complement system, 108, 110f
  inflammation, 109
  phospholipid bilayer cell membrane wall, 110
  progressive neural loss, 111
  tertiary syphilis, 110
  Treponema pallidum, 108, 109f
System consolidation, 244–245, 245f

T
Tau proteins
  cerebral spinal fluid (CSF), 320b
  hyperphosphorylation, 320, 321f
T-cell activation, 322
Telomere, 75b
Temporal information processing, 269
Temporal lobe abnormalities, 309
Temporal lobe epilepsy, anger and aggression, 187b
Testosterone, anger and aggression, 181–183, 182f–183f
Thyroid, 118, 172t

hypothalamic–pituitary–adrenal (HPA) axis and stress, 86–90, 87f–88f, 90f
hypothalamic–pituitary–thyroid (HPT) axis, 82–84, 82b, 85f, 86t
Thyroid-stimulating hormone (TSH), 80t, 82, 83f–85f
Thyrotropin-releasing hormone (TRH), 80t, 82, 84f–85f, 281
Tight junctions, 26, 27f
Timothy syndrome, 7
Tinnitus, 123, 129, 264
TMS (transcranial magnetic stimulation), 26b, 62b,122, 129, 144b, 276, 282f, 300
Total energy expenditure, 165
Transcranial direct current stimulation (tDCS), 123, 129–130
Transcranial magnetic stimulation (TMS), 276, 300
  long-term potentiation (LTP), 62b
  pain, 144b
Transcription factors, 11, 13, 70, 71f, 72–74, 159, 211, 224, 246, 313
Transgender, 215–216, 217f
Transgenic mice, 11
Transient ischemia, 313
Transient receptor potential vanilloid 1 (TRPV1) receptor, 134b
Transmitter-gated ion channel, 53, 54f, 59
Transorbital frontal lobotomy, 22b
Trauma, 3, 73, 74, 98, 113, 116, 127, 146, 179b, 188, 262, 290, 294, 295, 297f, 302
Traumatic brain injury (TBI), 116, 220
Traumatic memories, 241, 245
Trichostatin A, 226, 227f–228f
Tricyclic and monoamine oxidase inhibitor, 274
Tricyclic antidepressants, 24, 47, 58, 59
Trojan horse method, 26b
Tryptophan, 46, 184t
Tuberous sclerosis, 7
Tumor necrosis factor (TNF), 113, 114b

U
Unconventional neurotransmitters, 51b
  endocannabinoids, 50–51
  gases, 49–50
Unipolar depression, 127, 257, 284–286
Utopia, 286b

V
Vaccine, Alzheimer's disease (AD), 322
Vagus nerve stimulation (VNS), 46b, 129, 276
  catecholamines, 264
  norepinephrine (NE), 46b
  obesity, 173
  seizure activity reduction, 26b
Vasopressin, 227–229, 230f
  anger and aggression, 183, 184f
  DNA segment, 229
  huddling, 228
  infusion of, 228
  male prairie vole and meadow vole, 227, 230f
  marital commitment, 229
  Partner Bonding Scale, 229
  receptors, 11, 229
Ventral tegmental area (VTA), 43, 45f, 150, 150f, 151f, 157f, 227, 229f, 243b, 278
Ventrolateral preoptic nucleus (VLPO), 198–200
Verbal and spatial abilities, in children, 249, 250f
Veterans Administration (VA) study, 219, 290

Violence, prefrontal cortex (PFC), 17
Viral-mediated gene transfer, 11
VLPO (ventrolateral preoptic nucleus), 198–200
VNS. *See* Vagus nerve stimulation (VNS)
Voltage-gated calcium channels, 36, 56b
Voltage-gated sodium channels, 36–37, 56b, 125, 127
von Economo's encephalitis, 298

W

Warrior gene, 188
Water maze, 95b, 238, 239f
Western blots, 278, 279f
Whitehall study, 119, 120f
White matter, schizophrenia, 308f
  attention, 262

composition, 308
DTI technology, 309
intelligence, 251, 251f
magnetic resonance imaging (MRI), 309
myelin, 309, 309f
neural signaling disruption, 309
"Wild" mice, 11
Winter depression, 203–204
Wisconsin Card Sort test, 307, 307f
Withdrawal seizures, 128b
Working memory, 18, 192f, 308
  biofeedback, 265, 266f
  catecholamines, 263–264, 264f
  vs. executive function, 265b
  prefrontal cortex (PFC), 262, 263f–264f